ISSUES IN NURSING

GARLAND REFERENCE LIBRARY
OF SOCIAL SCIENCE
(Vol. 295)

ISSUES IN NURSING
An Annotated Bibliography

Bonnie Bullough
Vern L. Bullough
Jane Garvey
Karen Miller Allen
assisted by
Mary Boldt
Janice Fulton

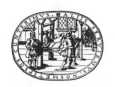

GARLAND PUBLISHING, INC. • NEW YORK & LONDON
1985

Library of Congress Cataloging-in-Publication Data
Main entry under title:

Issues in nursing.

(Garland reference library of social science ;
vol. 295)
Includes index.
1. Nursing—Bibliography. I. Bullough, Bonnie.
II. Series: Garland reference library of social
science ; v. 295. [DNLM: 1. Nursing—abstracts.
ZWY 100 I86]
Z6675.N718 1985 [RT41]   016.61073   84-48758
ISBN 0-8240-8768-2 (alk. paper)

Printed on acid-free, 250-year-life paper
Manufactured in the United States of America

CONTENTS

Preface   xi
Journal Abbreviations   xiii

BIBLIOGRAPHY

Nursing Issues   3

Ethical Issues

   General   8

   Patient's Rights, Informed Consent, and
      Nurse Advocate   41

   Professionalism and Ethics   53

   Birth, Infant, Child Care   58

   Death and Dying   64

   Ethics and Nursing Specialties   72

   Ethics and Mental Illness   76

   Sexuality, Reproduction, Abortion   78

   Aging   82

   Teaching of Ethical Issues   84

   Nursing Research   88

Legal and Regulatory Issues

   General Issues   93

   Malpractice, Liability, Avoiding Liability,
      Standards of Care   103

Nurse Practice Acts, Occupational Licensure, Nurses'
Scope of Function, State Regulation of Nursing   110

Patients' Rights, Informed Consent, Privacy   118

Terminating Life Support, Right to Live, Right to Die,
Handicapped Infants, Genetic Research,
Abortions   122

Labor Law, Nurses' Rights as Employees   126

Prescribing Privileges for Nurses   127

Anti-trust Law, Federal Trade Commission   129

Third Party Reimbursement for Nurses   130

Expert Witness Role   134

Legal Issues Related to Nursing Education   135

Education

Administrative Issues—Perspectives   137

Conflict—Education/Practice   143

Academic Governance   147

Financing   151

Professionalism   160

Credentialing   161

Students   165

Recruitment/Retention   175

Faculty   182

Faculty Practice   192

Graduates   198

Programs

Associate Degree   202

Baccalaureate   204

BSN Completion   214

Contents

Career Mobility 221

Continuing Education 222

Diploma 238

Doctorate 239

Master's 241

Nontraditional 245

Curriculum

Models/Theories 247

Content 257

Nontraditional 268

Teaching Strategies 269

Evaluation 296

Entry into Practice 306

Nursing Research/Nursing Theory 314

Professional Issues

General 334

Collective Bargaining/Unionization 337

Wages/Benefits 346

Job Satisfaction/Dissatisfaction 351

Women/Feminism 354

Power and Politics 363

Image 368

Men in Nursing 375

Racial, Ethnic, or Sexual Minorities in Nursing,
Opportunities/Discrimination 380

Interprofessional Relationships 382

Substance Abuse 386

Physical Fitness   388

International Nursing   388

Organizations   390

Health Care Delivery System

The Delivery of Health Care, Health Policy,
    and Economic Issues   393

Health Care for Members of Racial or Ethnic Minorities
    and Poverty Populations, Transcultural Nursing   402

Health Care for Gay or Lesbian Clients, Homosexuality   411

Standards of Care, Quality Assurance, Peer Review   413

Prospective Payment, Diagnostic Related Groups   416

Consumerism, Self-Help, Self-Care   419

Environmental Issues   421

Supply, Staffing, Manpower, Marketing Nursing
    Services   422

Private Practice, Independent Practice for Nurses   434

Hospital Privileges   436

Nursing Centers   437

Home Health Care   437

Primary Nursing and Team Nursing   438

Competition, Competitive Models, as Nurses
    Alternative to Physicians, HMOs   439

Physician Assistants   443

Physicians   443

Nursing Specialties

Overview   446

Nursing Administration   446

Camp Nursing   447

Cancer Nursing   447

Cardiovascular Nursing   447

Community Health/Public Health Nursing   448

Critical Care, Intensive Care Nursing   449

Emergency Nursing   449

Functional Nursing Roles—Patient Teaching, Clinical
    Teaching, Advocate   450

Geriatrics/Gerontology   451

Maternal/Child Nursing   452

Medical-Surgical Nursing   453

Neurological Nursing   453

Nurse Anesthetist   453

Nurse-Midwifery   454

Orthopedic Nursing   456

Pediatric Nursing   456

Psychiatric, Mental Health Nursing   457

Rehabilitation Nursing   458

Rheumatology Nursing   458

School Nursing   458

Urologic Nursing   459

Specialization—Nurse Practitioners   459

Clinical Issues

Abortion   470

Aging, Geriatrics   471

Alternative Models, Holistic Health Care   473

Biofeedback   474

Compliance   474

Death, Dying, Bereavement, Hospice Care   475

Infants, Children   478

Men   481

Mental Illness   482

Sexuality   483

Social, Psychological Aspects of Care, Stress
    Management, Crisis Intervention   484

Suicide   486

Victims of Rape, Violence, Abuse, Neglect   487

Women's Health, Pregnancy, Childbirth, Menarche,
    Menopause   488

Other Issues   493

Author Index   496

PREFACE

Nursing is in transition from a humble occupation to a profession based on the biological and behavioral sciences as well as a rapidly developing technology. Rapid change creates controversy and nursing issues are being hotly debated. This annotated bibliography attempts to capture some of the flavor of that discussion and to guide readers to both sides of the debates.

Citations are organized around topics which are then clustered to constitute the major issues in nursing. The work is selective rather than comprehensive, with recent and more readily available works being favored over the more difficult to locate and older works. Unpublished papers and dissertations are included only when they fill a gap not covered by published materials. Most citations are American and all are English language. Selected historical works are included as they furnish needed background for an understanding of current issues.

Annotations are brief and suggestive rather than comprehensive. Phrases are often used instead of complete sentences. Materials are cross referenced and an author index is included at the end.

The numbers in parentheses at the end of articles (not books) tell the number of references the author has included. This may furnish a clue as to whether it is a research paper or a more popular article.

JOURNAL ABBREVIATIONS

AANA J
    AANA Journal, American Association of Nurse Anesthetists
AANNT J
    AANNT Journal, American Association of Nephrology Nurses and
    Technicians
ADV NURS SCIENCE
    Advances in Nursing Science
AM J LAW MED
    American Journal of Law and Medicine
AM J NURS
    American Journal of Nursing
AM J PUB HEALTH
    American Journal of Public Health
AM NURSE
    American Nurse
AORN J
    Association of Operating Room Nurses
CAN NURSE
    Canadian Nurse
CANCER NURS
    Cancer Nursing
CARDIOVASC NURS
    Cardiovascular Nursing
CRIT CARE NURSE
    Critical Care Nurse
GERIATR NURS
    Geriatric Nursing
HEART LUNG
    Heart and Lung
INT J NURS STUD
    International Journal of Nursing Studies
INT NURS REV
    International Nursing Review
ISSUES MENT HEALTH NURS
    Issues in Mental Health Nursing
J ADV NURS
    Journal of Advanced Nursing
J ALLIED HEALTH
    Journal of Allied Health
J COMMUNITY HEALTH NURS
    Journal of Community Health Nursing
J CONTIN EDUC NURS
    Journal of Continuing Education in Nursing
J FAMILY PRACTICE
    Journal of Family Practice
J GERONTOL NURS
    Journal of Gerontological Nursing

J MED AND PHIL
  Journal of Medicine and Philosophy
J MED ETHICS
  Journal of Medical Ethics
J NURS ADM
  Journal of Nursing Administrtion
J NURS EDUC
  Journal of Nursing Education
J NURSE MIDWIFE
  Journal of Nurse-Midwifery
J NY STATE NURSES ASSOC
  Journal of The New York State Nurses Association
J PRACT NURS
  Journal of Practical Nursing
J PSYCHOSOC NURS MENT HEALTH SERV
  Journal of Psychosocial Nursing and Mental Health Services
J SCH HEALTH
  Journal of School Health
JEN
  Journal of Emergency Nursing
JOGN NURS
  JOGN Nursing
LAW MED HEALTH CARE
  Law, Medicine and Health Cre
MATERN CHILD NURS J
  Maternal-Child Nursing Journal
MCN
  American Journal of Maternal Child Nursing
MODERN MED
  Modern Medicine
NURS ADM Q
  Nursing Administration Quarterly
NURS CAREERS
  Nursing Careers
NURS CLIN NORTH AM
  Nursing Clinics of North America
NURS DIGEST
  Nursing Digest
NURS ECON
  Nursing Economics
NURS FORUM
  Nursing Forum
NURS HEALTH CARE
  Nursing and Health Care
NURS HOMES
  Nursing Homes
NURS J
  Nursing Journal
NURS LAW AND ETHICS
  Nursing Law and Ethics
NURS LEADERSH
  Nursing Leadership
NURS LIFE
  Nursing Life

NURS MANAGE
  Nursing Management
NURS MIRROR
  Nursing Mirror
NURS OUTLOOK
  Nursing Outlook
NURS RES
  Nursing Research
NURS TIMES
  Nursing Times
NURSE EDUC
  Nurse Educator
NURSE PRACT
  Nurse Practitioner
OCCUP HEALTH NURS
  Occupational Health Nursing
ONCOL NURS FORUM
  Oncology Nursing Forum
ORTHOP NURS
  Orthopaedic Nursing
PED NURS
  Pediatric Nursing
PSYCH NURS
  Psychiatric Nursing
REGAN REP NURS LAW
  Regan Report on Nursing Law
REHABIL NURS
  Rehabilitation Nursing
RES NURS HEALTH
  Research in Nursing and Health
RN
  RN
TODAYS OR NURSE
  Todays OR Nurse
TOP CLIN NURS
  Topics in Clinical Nursing
WEST J NURS RES

Issues in Nursing

NURSING ISSUES

1 Aiken, L., and S.R. Gortner (Eds.). NURSING IN THE 1980's:
   CRISES, OPPORTUNITIES, CHALLENGES. Philadelphia: J.B.
   Lippincott Co., 1982.

   Twenty-seven chapters by a variety of well-known authors
   cover the major current nursing issues. Emphasis is on
   professional issues and the health care delivery system.

2 American Nurses' Association. FACTS ABOUT NURSING 82-83.
   Kansas City, MO.: American Nurses' Association, Pub. No.
   D-73, 1983.

   The 36th edition updates data on registered nurse distribution, nursing education, economic status of registered
   nurses, allied nursing personnel, functions and purposes
   of nursing organizations, and more. New in this edition:
   section on Nurses with Doctorates and a National Help-
   Wanted Advertising Index.

3 _____. ISSUES IN PROFESSIONAL NURSING PRACTICE. Kansas
   City, MO.: American Nurses' Association, Pub. No. NP-68,
   1984.

   1984 monograph series documents nursing's professional
   progress, examines potential role of nursing practice in
   the evolving health care system. Topics include legal
   authority for practice, uniformity versus diversity in
   education, ethical dilemmas in practice, configurations of
   practice arrangements, and the role of nursing theory and
   research in advancing practice. Includes introduction,
   nine monographs, and binder.

4 _____. INVENTORY OF REGISTERED NURSES, 1977-78. Kansas
   City, MO.: American Nurses' Association, Pub. No. D-70,
   1982.

   ANA presents analyses of nurse employment trends, manpower,
   licensure and education data, national, state, and local
   information on professional and personal characteristics of
   registered nurses.

5 _____. NEW DIRECTIONS FOR NURSING IN THE '80s. Kansas
   City, MO.: American Nurses' Association, Pub. No. G-147,
   1980.

   A compilation of thirteen papers presented at the
   1980 ANA Convention that reflect several new and challenging
   directions for nursing in this decade.

6 Bullough, B. and V. Bullough (Eds.). ISSUES IN NURSING.
   New York: Springer Publishing Co., 1966.

   First in a series of four collections on issues done by
   the Bulloughs. Topics covered include education, the role
   of the nurse, the economic problems of the profession, and
   patient centered care.

7 _____. EXPANDING HORIZONS FOR NURSES. New York: Springer
   Publishing Co., 1977.

   Articles on current issues. Topics covered include the
   expanding professional functions of nurses, clinical controversies, legislative issues, nursing education, and the
   women's movement.

   Contains: 790, 795, 888, 923, 1390, 1631, 2018, 2147,
             2152, 2199, 2337, 2491, 2626, 2732, 2768, 2773,
             2789, 2798, 2800, 2802, 2820, 2887, 2892.

8 Bullough, B., V. Bullough and M. C. Soukup. NURSING ISSUES
   AND NURSING STRATEGIES FOR THE EIGHTIES. New York:
   Springer Publishing Co., 1983.

   Papers focused on shortage and turnover among nurses,
   ethical dilemmas, nurse specialists, nursing education,
   and law and politics. Thirty papers, including introductory essays by the editors. The work is the fourth in the
   ISSUES IN NURSING series edited by the Bulloughs since
   1965. Soukup is a new editor for this work. References
   follow each paper.

   Contains: 42, 54, 672, 888, 922, 1060, 1285, 1367,
             1389, 1527, 1781, 1868, 1884, 1889, 2123,
             2239, 2266, 2514, 2559, 2661, 2674.

9 Bullough, V.L. and B. Bullough. HISTORY, TRENDS, AND POLI-
   TICS OF NURSING. East Norwalk, CT.: Appleton-Century-
   Crofts, 1984.

   Provides an overview of how the history, trends and
   politics have affected the field of nursing. Such topics
   as sex discrimination, economics of the profession, nursing
   education, the role of theory in nursing, and the changing
   nursing scene are discussed. These topics are analyzed in
   terms of such issues as the changing nature of hospitals,
   the growing problems in nursing ethics, government intervention in nursing, and the implications of these for political action.

   Contains: 931, 932.

10 Chaska, M. L. THE NURSING PROFESSION: A TIME TO SPEAK.
   New York: McGraw-Hill Book Co., 1983.

Sixty-six papers by a variety of scholars, all of whom
are nurses, provides a comprehensive coverage of the issues
facing the profession. Includes sections on nursing education, research, theory, practice, administration, as well
as the concept of professionalization. Concludes with a
section predicting possible directions for the profession.

Contains: 953, 967, 982, 985, 986, 996, 1098, 1126, 1251,
           1299, 1448, 1491, 1573, 1603.

11 "Commission Earns Points for 'Hearing All Voices, Standing
    Firm on Basics'," AM J NURS (September 1983): 1252,
    1266, 1272, 1274.

    Describes final report--news item. (0)

12 Donnelly, G.F., A. Mengel and D.C. Sutterly. THE NURSING
    SYSTEM: ISSUES, ETHICS AND POLITICS. New York: John
    Wiley and Sons, 1980.

    Analyzes and describes nursing using a systems approach.

13 Duespohl, T.A. (Ed.) NURSING IN TRANSITION. Gaithersburg,
    MD.: Aspen Systems, 1982.

    Covers the major current issues in nursing, including
    practice based research, professionalization, career
    mobility, reality shock, job turnover, quality assurance,
    relationships with physicians, nursing diagnosis, nursing
    accountability and advocacy.

14 Ellis, J.R. and C.L. Hartley. NURSING IN TODAY'S WORLD:
    CHALLENGES, ISSUES AND TRENDS, 2nd Ed. New York: J.B.
    Lippincott, 1984.

    General text covers education, credentialing, health
    care delivery, liability, collective bargaining, organiza-
    tions, and politics.

15 Folta, J. and E. Deck. A SOCIOLOGICAL FRAMEWORK FOR PATIENT
    CARE, 2nd Ed. New York: John Wiley & Sons, 1979.

    This is the second edition of a popular work. It includes
    thirty-seven articles on a variety of topics. Organizing
    framework is the application of sociological insights to the
    solution of nursing problems.

16 Kalisch, P.A. and B.J. Kalisch. THE ADVANCE OF AMERICAN NURS-
    ING. Boston: Little, Brown, 1978.

    An illustrated history of American nursing. Major focus is
    on the twentieth century. Strong points include the cover-
    age of issues related to women, the role of the United States
    Government, and the impact of the political and social cli-
    mate on the history of nursing.

17 Kelly, C. DIMENSIONS OF PROFESSIONAL NURSING, 4th Ed. New
    York: Macmillan Co., 1981.

    Comprehensive overview of issues; now in its fourth edi-
    tion. Strength is in the careful detail furnished about
    nursing organizations. Also includes sections on history,
    law and religion.

18 Lewis, E.P. CHANGING PATTERNS OF NURSING PRACTICE: NEW
    NEEDS, NEW ROLES. New York: The American Journal of
    Nursing Co., 1971.

    A selection of issue oriented articles dating primarily
    from the decade of the 1960's. Selection was from the
    journals published by The American Journal of Nursing
    Company.

19 Lysaught, J.P. ACTION IN AFFIRMATION: TOWARD AN UNAMBI-
    GUOUS PROFESSION OF NURSING. New York: McGraw-Hill, 1980.

    A longitudinal follow up of the recommendation of the
    National Commission for the Study of Nursing Education
    originally made in 1970. Data is presented through 1978.

20 National Commission on Nursing. INITIAL REPORT AND PRIMARY
    RECOMMENDATIONS. Chicago: Hospital Research and Educa-
    tional Trust, 1981.

    A report by thirty commissioners charged to: (1) analyze
    the internal and external forces that influence the environ-
    ment of nurses at work, (2) identify the effects of profes-
    sional issues on nursing practice in health care agencies,
    (3) assess the professional characteristics of nurses in
    relation to the organizational structure of health care
    agencies, (4) explore the motivation and incentives for nurs-
    ing education and nursing practice, (5) analyze the relation
    among education, nursing practice and professional inter-
    action in health care agencies, and (6) plan methods to
    enhance professional status and top management role of the
    nurse.

21 National League for Nursing. PERSPECTIVES IN NURSING--1983-
    1985. New York: National League for Nursing, October,
    1983.

    Papers selected from the 1983 National League for Nursing
    Convention. Included are sections on the history and
    future of the nursing curriculum, competition in health
    care, managing nursing service, models for clinical practice,
    and computers in nursing. References follow each paper.

22 "News: In Final Report, National Commission Reiterates
    Support for BSN and Greater RN Involvement in Policy-
    making," AM J NURS (September 1983): 1252-53, 1272, 1274.

Summarizes major findings of the Institute of Medicine Study of Nursing. The Commission's major findings are summarized in three sets of recommendations: nursing practice, nursing education, and the relationships of the profession to the public. (0)

23 Schnall, D.J. and C.L. Figliola (Eds.). CONTEMPORARY ISSUES IN HEALTH CARE. New York: Praeger Publishers, 1984.

Papers developed from a seminar on contemporary issues. Focus on reforms needed in the health care delivery system in order to contain costs and meet needs of special populations.

See 942.

ETHICAL ISSUES

General

24 Abrams, N. and M.D. Buckner (Eds.). MEDICAL ETHICS: A
    CLINICAL TEXTBOOK AND REFERENCE FOR THE HEALTH CARE PRO-
    FESSIONS. Cambridge, MA.: MIT Press, 1983.

    An anthology of essays from a number of authors. Dis-
    cusses the conceptual foundations of such issues as informed
    consent, paternalism, the definition of death, euthanasia,
    and gives specific issues and situations and alternatives.
    An appendix gives seventy-four cases raising ethical issues,
    a second appendix includes ten professional codes, and a
    third deals with some recent legal decisions.

    Contains: 583

25 Aikens, C.A. STUDIES IN ETHICS FOR NURSES. Philadelphia:
    W.B. Saunders, 1916, 2nd Ed., 1923, 3rd. Ed., 1930, 4th
    Ed., 1937, 5th Ed., 1943.

    Concerned more with nurses in a professional sense than
    the current ethics manuals which concentrate on practice
    issues.

26 Allen, M. "Ethics of Nursing Practice," CAN NURSE 70
    (February 1974): 22-24.

    Twenty-two cases of ethical dilemmas faced by Canadian
    nurses are categorized and analyzed. (0)

27 Allen, P. "Doing What is Right," AORN J 31 (April 1980):
    858, 860, 862, 864, 866.

    A report concerning issues discussed at a conference on
    legal controversies in nursing. Topics include: distinc-
    tion between ethics and law, accountability, reporting
    incompetent physicians, nursing malpractice, and patients'
    rights. (0)

28 American Association of Occupational Health Nurses. "Ameri-
    can Association of Occupational Health Nurses Code of
    Ethics," OCCUP HEALTH NURS 25 (March 1977): 28.

    Gives the Code of Ethics. (0)

29 American Nurses' Association. CODE OF ETHICS FOR NURSING.
    Kansas City, MO.: American Nurses' Association, 1976.

    The 1976 update of the Code.

30 _____. CODE FOR NURSES WITH INTERPRETIVE STATEMENTS.
    Kansas City, MO.: American Nurses' Association, Pub. No.
    G-56, 1976.

    Guidelines adopted by ANA for carrying out nursing respon-
    sibilities consistent with the ethical obligations of the
    profession and quality in nursing care.

31 _____. PERSPECTIVES ON THE CODE FOR NURSES. Kansas
    City, MO.: American Nurses' Association, Pub. No. G-132,
    1978.

    Collection of six papers presented at the 1976 ANA Conven-
    tion at a program sponsored by the Committee on Ethics.
    Provides historical and philosophical perspectives on the
    Code for Nurses, along with considerations from the points
    of view of nursing education, practice, administration, and
    research.

    Contains: 95, 99, 127, 153, 175, 251.

32 _____. ETHICS IN NURSING: REFERENCES AND RESOURCES.
    Kansas City, MO.: American Nurses' Association, 1979.

    An annotated bibliography.

33 _____. ETHICS IN NURSING PRACTICE AND EDUCATION. Kansas
    City, MO.: American Nurses' Association, Pub. No. G-145,
    1980.

    Seven authored papers presented at the 1980 ANA Conven-
    tion in programs sponsored by the Committee on Ethics which
    dealt with ethical decision making and ethics in nursing
    educational curricula.

    Contains: 87, 105, 119, 245, 607, 615.

34 American Nurses' Association, Committee on Ethical Stand-
    ards. "A Code for Nurses," AM J NURS 50 (1950): 196.

    Code and how it was drafted written by the ANA Committee
    on Ethical Standards.

35 American Nurses' Association, Committee on Ethics. GUIDE-
    LINES FOR (NURSES) IMPLEMENTING THE CODE FOR NURSES.
    Kansas City, MO.: American Nurses' Association, 1980.

    An outline of formal and informal disciplinary procedures.

36 _____. ETHICS REFERENCE FOR NURSES. Kansas City, MO.;
   Kansas City, MO.: American Nurses´ Association, 1982.
   A revision of the 1979 bibliography. Contains more than
   600 entries.

37 Annas, G.J. "The Case of Phillip Becker: A Legal Travesty,"
   NURS LAW & ETHICS 1(1) (January 1980): 4, 6.

   Reviews case--issue of right to treatment versus parents´
   rights. (1)

38 Applegate, M.I. "Moral Decisions in Selected Clinical Nursing Practice Situations." Doctoral Dissertation.
   Teachers College, Columbia University, 1981.

   Gives selected clinical practice situations and examines
   moral implictions.

39 Aroskar, M.A. "Anatomy of an Ethical Dilemma: The Theory,"
   AM J NURS 80 (April 1980): 658-60.

   Surveys ethical theories and proposes a procedure for resolving ethical dilemmas. (2)

40 _____."Anatomy of an Ethical Dilemma: The Practice," AM J NURS 80 (April 1980): 661-63.

   Analysis of an ethical dilemma involving the refusal of
   an amputation by an eighty year old woman with gangrene of
   her left foot. (5)

41 _____. "Establishing Limits to Professional Autonomy:
   Whose Responsibility?," NURS LAW & ETHICS 1 (May 1980):
   1-2, 6.

   Argues that professional autonomy in nursing is not an
   end in itself but is a means to enhance personal and professional integrity and improve patient services. (4)

42 _____. "Are Nurses´ Mind Sets Compatible with Ethical
   Practice?," TOP CLIN NURS 4 (April 1982): 22-32.

   Explains four ways that nurses can view the health care
   system and their role in it. Gives the ethical implications
   of these views. (11)

43 _____. "Ethics of Nurse-Patient Relationship." NURSE
   EDUCATOR 5(2) (1980): 18-20. Reprinted in NURSING ISSUES
   AND NURSING STRATEGIES FOR THE EIGHTIES. Edited by B.
   Bullough, V. Bullough and M. C. Soukup. New York: Springer
   Publishing Co., 1983, pp. 95-101.

44 Bandman, E.L. and B. Bandman. BIOETHICS AND HUMAN RIGHTS:
   A READER FOR HEALTH PROFESSIONALS. Boston: Little, Brown
   and Co., 1978.

A multidisciplinary approach to four major topics: (1)
foundations of human rights in health care, (2) the right
to live and boundaries of life, (3) the right to live as
persons and responsibilities for changing behavior, and (4)
right in and to health care.

Contains: 111, 184, 302, 543.

45 Bandman, E. NURSING ETHICS IN THE LIFE SPAN. Norwalk, CT.:
    Appleton-Century-Crofts, 1985.

    Explores the moral problems of everyday nursing practice
    relevant to each developmental stage in a client's life
    span, and the nurse's evaluation and response to such prob-
    lems.

46 Bartsch, J. "Handling Orders That Violate Ethics, Part I,"
    RN 24 (April 1961): 46-49, 76, 78-79; Part II, RN 25
    (February 1962): 58-62, 90-94; Part III, RN 25 (May 1962):
    41-46, 100-105.

    A study of 400 general nurses' responses to three ethical
    dilemmas involving questionable orders. I: A drug order
    by physician; II: an order for a procedure that a nurse be-
    lieves is surgical; III: a nurse refusing to scrub for what
    nurse believes will be a criminal abortion.

47 Beauchamp, T. and L. Walters. CONTEMPORARY ISSUES IN BIO-
    ETHICS. Belmont, CA.: Wadsworth Publishing Co., 1978

    Ethical theory, bioethics, health and disease, patients'
    rights, professional responsibilities, abortion, death,
    euthanasia, the allocation of scarce medical resources,
    human experimentation, behavioral control, genetic inter-
    ventions, and reproductive technologies.

48 Beauchamp, T. and J. Childress. PRINCIPLES OF BIOMEDICAL
    ETHICS. New York: Oxford University Press, 1979.

    A systematic analysis of ethical principles as they apply
    to a broad range of biomedical problems. Present codes of
    ethics and regulations for medicine, nursing and research.

49 Benjamin, M. and J. Curtis. ETHICS IN NURSING. New York:
    Oxford University Press, 1981.

    A textbook by a nurse and a philosopher. Individual cases
    illustrate the application of ethical theory to ethical
    dilemmas in nursing. Topics include moral theory, deception,
    confidentiality, nurse-physician relationships, conscien-
    tious refusal, dilemmas among nurses, institutional policies,
    strikes, and more. Includes ANA and ICN codes and the AHA
    Bill of Rights.

50 Bergman, R. "Evolving Ethical Concepts for Nursing," INT
    NURS REV 23 (July/August 1976): 116-17.

The 1965 ICN Code, its 1973 revision, and what the future code may say.

51   Broadhurst, J.   "Ethics of Nursing," AM J NURS (1917): 792-97.

An outline of topics with commentary for a three year course in ethics. Emphasizes how nursing has changed since all doctors were to be accorded respect and absolute loyalty.

52   Brody, H. ETHICAL DECISIONS IN MEDICINE. Boston: Little, Brown, 1976.

A medical text.

53   Brogan, J.M. ETHICAL PRINCIPLES FOR THE CHARACTER OF A NURSE. Milwaukee: Bruce Publishing Co., 1924.

Included for its historical attitudes. Emphasis then was on moral character, not ethical decision making.

54   Bullough, B. and V.L. Bullough. "Introduction--Dilemmas Inherent in the American Nurses´ Associaion Code of Ethics." Reprinted in NURSING ISSUES AND NURSING STRATE-GIES FOR THE EIGHTIES. Edited by B. Bullough, V. Bullough and M. C. Soukup. New York: Springer Publishing Co., 1983, pp. 89-94.

Gives the American Nurses´ Association Code as of 1976 and looks at dilemmas inherent in attempting to follow the code. (5)

55   Cabiniss, S.H. "Ethics," AM J NURS 3 (1903): 875-79.

"Code of Ethics" does not seem at all to be one of our needs and requirements--nor, in fact, any part of our equip-ment.

56   Cadmus, N.E. "Ethics," AM J NURS 16 (1916): 411-16.

One of the major impediments to developing a good code of ethics is the fact that the training courses of nurses are governed by economic concerns. Concerned with moral charac-ter by nurses.

57   Canadian Nurses Association. BIBLIOGRAPHY: ETHICS. Ottawa: Canadian Nurses Association, 1977.

Includes 291 citation in both French and English.

58   _____. CNA CODE OF ETHICS: AN ETHICAL BASIS FOR NURSES IN CANADA. Prepared by M.S. Roach. Ottawa: Canadian Nurses Association, 1980.

The code of the Canadian Nurses Association with explana-tions and comments.

59 Carper, B.A. "The Ethics of Caring," ADV IN NURS SCIENCE
    1 (April 1979): 11-20.

    Analyzes the concept of caring and models of nurse-
    patient relationships.

60 Carrol, A.M. and R.A. Humphrey. MORAL PROBLEMS IN NURSING:
    CASE STUDIES. Washington, D.C.: University Press of
    America, 1979.

    Includes 214 case studies written by nurses as well as
    chapters on moral theories and decision making and a history
    of the nurse´s professional code.

61 Castles, M.R. "Professional Codes and Personal Values:
    Some Implications of Incongruence." TEACHING AND EVALUAT-
    ING THE AFFECTIVE DOMAIN IN NURSING PROGRAMS. Edited by
    D. Reilly. Thorofare, N.J: Charles B. Slack, 1978, pp. 9-16.
    Reprinted in TODAY´S OR NURSE 2 (May 1980): 11-16,

    Points out the limitations of the code in providing guid-
    ance and explores the possible conflicts between personal
    and professional values.

62 Catholic Hospital Association. ETHICAL ISSUES IN NURSING:
    A PROCEEDINGS. St. Louis: Catholic Hospital Association,
    1976.

    Ten essays on biomedical ethics from a Catholic perspec-
    tive with only tangential reference to nursing.

    Contains: 163, 181, 483.

63 Christman, L. "Moral Dilemmas for Practitioners in a Chang-
    ing Society," J NURS ADM 3 (March/April 1973): 15-17.

    An analysis of the social changes creating problems for
    the health professions and what the responses of nurses
    should be. (1)

64 "Code for Nurses--Ethical Concepts Applied to Nursing,"
    INT NURS REV 20(6) (November/December 1973): 166.

    The 1973 revision of the ICN Code.

65 College of Nurses of Ontario. GUIDELINES FOR ETHICAL BE-
    HAVIOR IN NURSING. Toronto: College of Nurses of Ontario,
    1980.

    A code of ethics that also contains interpretations of
    its statements. Examples of ethical dilemmas are given,
    and an annotated bibliography of twenty-seven items is
    included.

66 Coward, H. and D.E. Larsen (Eds.). ETHICAL ISSUES IN THE
    ALLOCATION OF HEALTH CARE RESOURCES (COMMUNITY SEMINAR
    NO. 2). Alberta, CAN.: The Calgary Institute for Humani-
    ties, University of Calgary, 1982.

    Two topics were discussed during this seminar: the right
    to health care, and justice in the allocation of health
    care resources. The first topic focused on the problems
    of providing long-term health care for the elderly. The
    second topic included problems in choosing priorities in
    the allocation of the health care dollar and considered the
    ethical implications of strikes by health care personnel.

67 Cowart, M.E., R.F. Allen with 6 contributors. CHANGING CON-
    CEPTIONS OF HEALTH CARE: PUBLIC POLICY AND ETHICAL ISSUES
    FOR NURSES. Thorofare, NJ: Slack, Inc., 1981.

    Examines major health policy issues facing the United
    States, ethical and value dilemmas in health care, access-
    ibility and quality of health care services. Also discusses
    justice in child health, nurse and patients' rights, respon-
    sibility of the individual.

68 Cranford, R.E. and A.E. Doudera. "The Emergence of Insti-
    tutional Ethics Committees," LAW MED HEALTH CARE 12
    (February 1984): 13-20.

    History of the institutional ethics committee which began
    to appear in the 1970s and which gives nurses greater respon-
    sibility in decision making. (73)

69 Craven, M.E. "The Work of The Ethics Nursing Committee,"
    INT NURS REV 5 (October 1958): 33-9.

    Report of the development of the ICN Code, surveys con-
    cerning the teaching of ethics, a copy of the 1953 ICN
    Code, and reports of its adoption and distribution.

70 Creighton, H. "ICN's New Code for Nurses," SUPERVISOR
    NURSE 4 (September 1973): 13-15, 18.

    Commentary on the ICN's 1973 revised code which is com-
    pared with the 1968 ANA Code. (4)

71 _____. (Ed.). "Symposium on Current Legal and Pro-
    fessional Issues," NURS CLIN NORTH AM 9 (September 1974):
    391-589 (entire issue).

    Three of the articles deal with ethical issues. They are
    indexed separately.

    Contains: 284, 725, 923, 2152.

72 Crisham, P. "Moral Judgment of Nurses in Hypothetical and
    Nursing Dilemmas." Ph.D. Dissertation. University of
    Minnesota, 1979.

Author used standardized test plus a specially developed one for her dissertation to evaluate moral development in nursing.

73 _____. "Measuring Moral Judgment in Nursing Dilemmas," NURS RES 30(12) (March-April 1981): 104-10.

Author found that level of education and previous involvement with ethical dilemmas were associated with higher levels of principled thinking. (15)

74 Crowder, E. "Manners, Morals, and Nurses: An Historical Overview of Nursing Ethics," TEXAS REPORTS ON BIOLOGY AND MEDICINE 32 (Spring 1974): 173-80.

A history of the development of nursing ethics up to the 1968 revision of the code. (16)

75 Curran, W.J. ETHICS IN MEDICINE: HISTORICAL PERSPECTIVES AND CONTEMPORARY CONCERN. Boston: MIT Press, 1977.

An anthology of readings explores moral and ethical foundations of medical practice and science. The readings are from various disciplines, including philosophy, religion, law, and political science.

76 Curtin, L. "Human Values in Nursing," J NY STATE NURSES ASSOC 8 (December 1977): 33-41. Reprinted in SUPERVISOR NURSE 9 (March 1978): 21-33.

A repetition of what she says elsewhere. (37)

77 _____. "Nursing Ethics: Theories and Pragmatics," NURS FORUM 17 (1978): 4-11.

Institutional and other constraints on ethical nursing practice. (6)

78 _____. "A Proposed Model for Critical Ethical Analysis," NURS FORUM 17 (1978): 12-17.

Proposal for an ethical decision making model. Model explained. (0)

79 _____. "Is There a Right to Health Care?," AM J NURS 80 (March 1980): 462-65.

The nature of rights, including the right to health care. The author argues that although the health care professional has duties to society, the primary focus of concern should remain the individual patient. (12)

80 _____. "Ethical Issues in Nursing Practice and Education." ETHICAL ISSUES IN NURSING AND NURSING EDUCATION. New York: National League for Nursing, 1980, pp. 19-28.

Emphasizes that the freedom of nurses to practice nursing is the key to the significant ethical issues in nursing.

81 Curtin, L. and M.J. Flaherty. NURSING ETHICS: THEORIES AND PRAGMATICS. Bowie, MD.: Robert J. Brady Co., 1982.

The authors review ethical theory in the first half of the book and in the second half they present case studies with analysis and commentary. All but two chapters written by author-editors.

82 Darby, C. and L. Wilton. "Even If the Patient Asks, Nurses Won´t Tell," NURS MIRROR 147 (September 14, 1978): 13-19.

Communication between nurses and cancer patients in a British hospital. Nurses, according to the authors, felt it was not their responsibility to discuss the patient´s diagnosis or prognosis.

83 Davis, A.J. "Ethical Dilemmas and Nursing Practice," LINACRE QUARTERLY 44 (November 1977): 302-11.

Ethical dilemmas faced by hospital nurses; includes commentary on a 1977 survey indicating widespread dissatisfaction among hospital nurses. (9)

84 _____. "Theoretically Realistic." CLINICAL AND SCIENTIFIC SESSIONS, 1979. Kansas City, MO.: American Nurses´ Association, 1979, pp. 3-8.

Description of a moral dilemma and a brief discussion of issues involved.

85 _____. "Ethical Issues in Nursing Practice," WEST J NURS RES 2 (1980): 646-48.

Ethical issues raised by social scientists differ from those raised by biomedical researchers. (2)

86 _____. "Ethical Decision Making: Considerations for Future Activities." ETHICS IN NURSING PRACTICE AND EDUCATION. Kansas City, MO.: American Nurses´ Association, 1980, pp. 23-27.

Author believes that an interdisciplinary approach in the curricula is best combined with ethics rounds in practice contexts.

87 _____. "Ethical Dilemmas in Nursing: A Survey," WEST J NURS RES 3 (1981): 397-407.

Surveyed 205 nurses in order to find out how well nurses understood what a moral dilemma was, the kinds of dilemmas encountered, and their frequency. Results cross tabulated by age, education and position. (4)

88 _____. "Compassion, Suffering, Morality: Ethical
     Dilemmas in Caring," NURS LAW AND ETHICS 2 (May 1981):
     1, 2, 6, 8.

     Examines caring, compassion, quality of life, principles
     of autonomy, sanctity of life, non-maleficence, and bene-
     ficence.

89 _____. "Helping Your Staff Address Ethical Dilemmas,"
     J NURS ADM 12 (February 1982): 9-13.

     Discussion of moral principles and ethical reasoning and
     three methods of ethics rounds. (9)

90 Davis, A.J. and M.A. Aroskar. ETHICAL DILEMMAS AND NURSING
     PRACTICE, 2nd Ed. East Norwalk, CT.: Appleton-Century-
     Crofts, 1983.

     In some thirteen chapters the authors look at many of the
     ethical issues facing nursing today. Included is a chapter
     on values clarification and moral development and guides to
     further reading.

91 Davis, A.J. and J.C. Krueger (Eds.). PATIENTS, NURSES,
     ETHICS. New York: American Journal of Nursing Co., 1980.

     A collection of essays from a 1979 symposium of the Western
     Society of Nurse Researchers. Covers issues related to fed-
     eral regulations, institutional review boards, informed
     consent, and ethics of research with human subjects.

92 Dawson, J.D et al. "Commentary," J MED ETHICS 3 (September
     1977): 119-23.

     Commentary on the ICN Code of Professional Conduct. (5)

93 DECIDING TO FOREGO LIFE-SUSTAINING TREATMENT: PRESIDENT'S
     COMMISSION FOR THE STUDY OF ETHICAL PROBLEMS IN MEDICINE
     AND BIOMEDICAL AND BEHAVIORAL RESEARCH. Washington, D.C.:
     U.S. Government Printing Office, S/N 040-000-00470-0, 1982.

     Covers such topics as who should make the decision, the
     difference between actions and omissions that lead to death,
     seriously ill newborns, moral and legal implications, et al.

94 Densford, K.J. and M.S. Everett. ETHICS FOR MODERN NURSES.
     Philadelphia: W.B. Saunders, 1946.

     Included for its historical value.

95 Dilday, R.C. "The Code for Nurses: An Educational Perspec-
     tive." PERSPECTIVES ON THE CODE FOR NURSES. Kansas City,
     MO.: American Nurses' Association, 1978, pp. 10-17.

     New concern for values in nursing and how this was inte-
     grated into curriculum of one school.

96   Donnelly, G.F., A. Mengel and D.C. Sutterley. THE NURSING
     SYSTEM: ISSUES, ETHICS, AND POLITICS. New York: John
     Wiley, 1980.

     Examines some of the basic dilemmas in nursing practice;
     pays special attention to structure, process, and historical
     evolution and treatment of first and second order change.

97   Doona, M.E. "The Ethical Dimension in ´Ordinary Nursing
     Care´," LINACRE QUARTERLY 44 (November 1977): 320-27.

     Brief history of nursing ethics and consideration of ethi-
     cal problems in patient care. (15)

98   _____ "Ethics: Nursing´s Latest Fad or Its Vitalizing
     Force," FLORIDA NURSE 26 (November 1978): 12-18.

     What constitutes ethics; focuses on everyday aspects of
     ethical practice in nursing.

99   Durand, B. "The Code for Nurses: A Nursing Practice Per-
     spective." PERSPECTIVES ON THE CODE FOR NURSES. Kansas
     City, MO.: American Nurses´ Association, 1978, pp. 18-22.

     The code can be used to improve nursing practice.

100 Edgell, B. ETHICAL PROBLEMS: AN INTRODUCTION TO ETHICS FOR
     HOSPITAL NURSES AND SOCIAL WORKERS. London: Methuen, 1929.

     An early textbook.

101 Edgil, A.E. "Moral Problems in Nursing Practice," JOGN
     NURS 12 (May/June 1983): 210-12.

     Argues that the study of bioethics is essential. (9)

102 "Ethics and Values." Special issue of ADV IN NURS SCIENCE
     (Edited by P. Chinn) 1 (April 1979).

     Contributing authors included elsewhere.

     Contains: 59, 236, 287, 408, 446, 618.

103 "Ethics for Nursing." Special issue of TOP CLIN NURS
     (Edited by S. Ketefian) 4 (April 1982).

     Articles included elsewhere.

     Contains: 43, 110, 193, 373, 591, 594, 650.

104 Fenner, K.M. ETHICS AND LAW IN NURSING: PROFESSIONAL PER-
     SPECTIVES. New York: C. Van Nostrand, 1980.

An introduction and plea for a nurse to study ethical and
legal issues. The last chapter covers problems in bioethics.
Fenner also includes discussion of sexism, racism, and other
forms of discrimination. Suggested readings are annotated.

105 Flaherty, M.J. "Ethical Decision Making in an Interdis-
     ciplinary Setting." ETHICS IN NURSING PRACTICE AND EDUCA-
     TION. Kansas City, MO.: American Nurses' Association,
     1980, pp. 3-10.

     Gives characteristics of professional nurse and scope and
     accountability.

106 _____. "Two Canadian Nursing Codes," WESTMINSTER INSTITUTE
     REVIEW 1 (October 1981): 11.

     Discusses Canadian Nurses Association, Code of Ethics:
     An Ethical Basis for Nursing in Canada and College of Nurses
     of Ontario, Guidelines for Ethical Behaviour in Nursing.

107 Ford, J.G., L.N. Trygstad-Durland and B.C. Nelms. APPLIED
     DECISION MAKING FOR NURSES. St. Louis: C.V. Mosby Co.,
     1978.

     Emphasizes value clarification in decision making.

108 Frey, E.F. "Medicolegal History: A Review of Significant
     Publications and Educational Developments," LAW MED HEALTH
     CARE 10(2) (April 1982): 56-60.

     A short history of medicolegal regulations concentrating
     on period since 1800. Includes forty-four citations. (44)

109 Fromer, M.J. ETHICAL ISSUES IN HEALTH CARE   St. Louis:
     C.V. Mosby Co., 1981.

     Overview of ethical issues, including professional account-
     ability, genetic manipulation, artificial insemination,
     contraception, abortion, behavior control, informed consent,
     organ transplant, death and dying, justice and allocation
     of resources in health care.

110 _____. "Solving Ethical Dilemmas in Nursing Practice,"
     TOP CLIN NURS 4 (April 1982): 15-21.

     Discussion of moral theories, moral principles, and their
     application to a case study. Wants more humanistic material
     in curriculum. (9)

111 Gadow, S. "Nursing and the Humanities: An Approach to
     Humanistic Issues at the Interface of Nursing and the
     Community," CONNECTICUT MED 41(6) (June 1977): 357-61.
     Reprinted in BIOETHICS AND HUMAN RIGHTS. Edited by E.L.
     Bandman and B. Bandman. Boston: Little, Brown, 1978,
     pp. 305-12.

Humanistic issues in nursing as centered around the nurse
and the patient, the nurse and other health professionals,
nurses and nursing, and nurse and the community. (0)

112   _____. "Body and Self: A Dialectic," J MED AND PHIL
5 (September 1980): 172-85.

An application of the philosophy of Merleau-Ponty and
other continental philosophers to the relation of the body
to self in sickness and aging. (7)

113   _____. "Truth: Treatment of Choice, Scarce Resource,
or Patient's Right?," J FAMILY PRACTICE 13(6) (1981):
857-60.

Two approaches are described for addressing ethical problems of truth telling. In neither approach is truth telling
an ethical absolute, but rather a means of attaining the
goal that is assumed for medicine. The first approach is
the view that information is to be disclosed or withheld
according to the anticipated effect upon the patient's well-
being. The second is the view that informed decision making
requires access to all information the patient considers
relevant. (3)

114 Galton, M. "Emergency Resuscitation: Ethics and Legalisms,"
AUSTRALIAN NURS J 10 (September 1980): 44-45.

A brief overview. (0)

115 Ganos, D., R.E. Lipson, G. Warrend and B.J. Weil. DIFFICULT
DECISIONS IN MEDICAL ETHICS. New York: Alan R. Liss,
Inc., 1983.

Utilizes case studies to examine issues in medical ethics.
Contributors from different disciplines provide contrasting
approaches to each topic. Additionally, the editors present
summaries of small group discussions, permitting the reader
to compare his reasoning with that of the participants.
Topics include the obligation to report child abuse, the
right to refuse psychotropic medication, and surrogate
motherhood.

116 Garesche, E.F. ETHICS AND THE ART OF CONDUCT FOR NURSES.
Philadelphia: W.B. Saunder, 1929; 2nd Ed. Rev., 1944.

Included for its historical value to nurses interested
in tracing changing values.

117 Gerds, G. "Making Ideals Tangible," AM J NURS 60 (1960):
672-76.

History of development of ANA Code up to the 1960 revision. Valuable for its historical background. (0)

118 Gladwin, M.E. ETHICS: A TEXTBOOK FOR NURSES. Philadelphia:
     W.B. Saunders Co., 1930; 2nd Ed. 1931; 3rd Ed. 1937.

     Included for comparative historical purposes.

119 Goertzen, I. "A Nursing Administrator's View of Ethics in
     Practice." ETHICS IN NURSING PRACTICE AND EDUCATION.
     Kansas City, MO.: American Nurses' Association, 1980,
     pp. 17-22.

     Responsibility of nursing administrator to provide an
     environment for quality nursing care.

120 Goodall, P.A. ETHICS: THE INNER REALITIES. Philadelphia:
     F.A. Davis, 1942.

     Included for comparative historical purposes.

121 Goodrich, A.W. THE SOCIAL AND ETHICAL SIGNIFICANCE OF NURS-
     ING. New York: Macmillan, 1932; Reprinted, New Haven, CT.:
     Yale School of Nursing, 1973.

     Included for historical comparison.

122 Gorovitz, S., A.L. Jameton, R. Macklin, J.M. O'Connor,
     E.V. Perrin, B.P. St. Clair and S. Sherin. MORAL PROBLEMS
     IN MEDICINE. Englewood Cliffs, NJ: Prentice-Hall, 1976.

     Concentrates on moral problems of physician-patient rela-
     tionship in first part of book; second half includes such
     topics as informed consent and coercion, paternalism, killing
     and letting die, abortion, birth defects, death and dignity,
     right to health care, and allocation of scarce medical re-
     sources.

123 Gounley, M.E. DIGEST OF ETHICS FOR NURSES. Paterson, NJ:
     Anthony Guild Press, 1949.

     Included for historical comparisons.

124 Gruzalski, B. and C. Nelson (Eds.). VALUE CONFLICTS IN
     HEALTH CARE DELIVERY. Cambridge: Ballinger Publishing Co.,
     1983.

     A collection of thirteen essays by different authors empha-
     sizing the need for an interdisciplinary approach to re-
     solve value conflicts. Particular ethical questions are
     discussed in the book along with ways for resolving value
     conflicts.

125 Gulino, C.K. "Existentialist Themes in Nursing Situations."
     Ed.D. Dissertation. Columbia University, Teachers College,
     1979.

     Includes ethics within the existentialist framework.

126 _____. "Entering the Mysterious Dimension of Other:
        An Existential Approach to Nursing Care," NURS OUTLOOK 30
        (June 1982): 352, 357.

        Seminars should be given to nursing students on existen-
        tial themes to help them grapple with humanistic and sub-
        jective problems. (27)

127 Hacker, L.J. "A Nursing Administration Perspective." PER-
        SPECTIVES ON THE CODE FOR NURSES. Kansas City, MO.:
        American Nurses' Association, 1978.

        Obligation of the nurse administrator to disseminate the
        code and make reference to it in standards for accredita-
        tion, in statement of philosophy, objectives, and goals.

128 Hadley, R.D. "ANA Code for Nurses Revised: Greater Focus
        on Nurse, Client," AM NURS 8 (October 1976): 5.

        A new account of the 1976 revision.

129 Harron, F., J. Burnside and T. Beauchamp. HEALTH AND HUMAN
        VALUES: A GUIDE TO MAKING YOUR OWN DECISIONS. New Haven:
        Yale University Press, 1983.

        Covers a complex set of issues arising out of development
        of modern medicine and biomedical research. It is aimed at
        general public and attempts to provide the information
        necessary for participation in debates surrounding the moral
        and public policy questions raised by biomedical develop-
        ments. Annotated bibliography at end of each chapter.

130 _____. BIOMEDICAL-ETHICAL ISSUES: A DIGEST OF LAW AND
        POLICY DEVELOPMENT, SUPPLEMENT TO HEALTH AND HUMAN VALUES.
        New Haven: Yale University Press, 1983.

        A supplement to same authors HEALTH AND HUMAN VALUES sum-
        marizing statutes, court opinion, church policy statements,
        and administrative regulations.

131 _____. HUMAN VALUES IN MEDICINE AND HEALTH CARE:
        AUDIOVISUAL RESOURCES, SUPPLEMENT TO HEALTH AND HUMAN
        RESOURCES. New Haven: Yale University Press, 1983.

        An annotated list of about 400 audiovisual aids, including
        information on purchases and rental costs and distributors.
        Two indices list the materials by topic and format.

132 Hay, H.S. "Concerning Our Ethics," AM J NURS 10 (1910):
        896-902.

        Uses ethics in a different sense than nurses now do.
        Three guiding principles should be "correct evaluation of
        things (the good of humanity and qualities of the heart),
        magnanimity and personal responsibility, and unremitting
        helpfulness."

133 Hayes, E.J., P.J. Hayes and D.E. Kelly. MORAL PRINCIPLES
     OF NURSING. New York: Macmillan, 1964.

     A Catholic text on ethics, includes a discussion of the
     responsibilities of the nurse to the patient, preservation
     of life, and basic principles of ethics.

134 Henderson, V. THE NURSE'S DILEMMA: ETHICAL CONSIDERATIONS
     IN NURSING PRACTICE. Geneva, Switzerland: International
     Council of Nurses, 1977.

     In these first hand accounts, nurses relate the ethical
     dilemmas they have experienced. Intended as a basis for dis-
     cussion among nurses in deciding what is appropriate action
     in the many complex situations they face. Selected readings
     and a bibliography are included.

135 Hillder, M.D. (Ed.). MEDICAL ETHICS AND THE LAW: IMPLICA-
     TIONS FOR PUBLIC POLICY. Cambridge: Ballinger Publishing
     Co., 1981

     A collection of twenty-one papers by twenty-four authors
     stresses economic and public health issues, three chapters
     deal with legal themes and court decision in detail.

136 Hoeffer, B. "The Private Practice Model: An Ethical Per-
     spective," J PSYCHOSOC NURS MENT HEALTH SERV 21 (July 1983):
     31-37.

     Argues that alternatives to private practice model may be
     more congruent with principles of distributive justice. (31)

137 "Hospital Nursing Policy: Guidelines or Mandates," REGAN
     REP NURS LAW 22 (August 1981): 4.

     A brief note emphasizing that a nurse should do anything
     reasonably calculated to save a patient's life, including
     acting contrary to established hospital policy. (0)

138 "How Ethical Are You?, Part I," NURS LIFE 3 (January/February
     1983): 25-33.

     Some 500 nurses were surveyed on a number of ethical
     issues ranging from altering information on medical records,
     pilferage, covering up errors, and response to specific
     situations. Some of the statistics are compared to a 1974
     survey.

139 "How Ethical Are You?, Part II," NURSING LIFE 3 (March/
     April 1983): 46.

     Continuation of reporting of results this time with nur-
     ses' perception of their ethical standards, overdoses of
     narcotics, et al. (0)

140 Deleted.

141 Hull, R.T. "Defining Nursing Ethics Apart from Medical
     Ethics," KANSAS NURSE 55 (September 1980): 5, 8, 20-24.

     Arguments for distinctiveness of nurse ethics. (0)

142 _____. "Ethics: Models of Nurse/Patient/Physician Rela-
     tions," NURSE 55 (October 1980): 19-24.

     In the second article of series, Hull discusses three
     views of humanity and related ethics, as well as three models
     of patient/physician relationships. (15)

143 _____. "Codes or No Codes?," KANSAS NURSE 55 (November
     1980): 8, 18-19, 21.

     Limitation of ANA Code as a moral guide. (20)

144 _____. "The Function of Professional Code of Ethics,"
     WESTMINSTER INSTITUTE REVIEW 1 (October 1981): 12-13.

     Argues language of code should reflect intent and audience;
     it should be descriptive rather than prescriptive, setting
     norms rather than standards. Criticizes the two Canadian
     codes adopted in 1980 in terms of these concepts. (5)

145 _____. "Responsibility and Accountability Analyzed,"
     NURS OUTLOOK 29 (December 1981): 707, 712.

     Courts increasingly are holding nurses as in some ways
     responsible for patients´ losses. Argues that responsibility
     and professionalization go together and nurses need to recog-
     nize this. Proposes schema for doing so. (19)

146 Hynes, K.M. "An Ethical Decision System." PATIENTS, NURSES,
     ETHICS. Edited by A.J. Davis and J.C. Krueger. New York:
     American Journal of Nursing, 1980, pp. 9-21.

     A procedure for resolving ethical dilemmas.

147 Jametown, A. "The Nurse: When Roles and Rules Conflict,"
     HASTINGS CENTER REPORT 7(4) (August 1977) 22-23.

     Argues that standard medical ethics do not answer the
     needs of nurses since there are a number of issues unique
     to nursing or modified by the nursing viewpoint.

148 _____. NURSING PRACTICE: THE ETHICAL ISSUES. Engle-
     wood Cliffs, NJ: Prentice-Hall, Inc., 1984.

     Considers topics such as the concept of professionalism
     in nursing and the obligations of nurses to doctors,
     patients and fellow nurses.

149 Kaserman, I. "A Nursing Committee and the Code for Nurses,"
     AMER J NURS 77 (May 1977): 875-76.

     The setting up of an ethics committee in Tennesee to en-
     force provisions of ANA Code. (0)

150 Keane, N.P. with D.L. Breo. THE SURROGATE MOTHER. New
     York: Everest House, 1981.

     Noel Keane is the "legal father" of the surrogate mother
     phenomenon and this book gives the developments of the con-
     cept from 1976 to 1981. Last quarter of text enumerates
     legal and ethical questions surrounding the phenomenon.

151 Kelley, D.N. "Ethics in a Profession, I," SUPERVISOR NURSE
     9 (May 1978): 7.

     An editorial. (2)

152 _____. "Ethics in a Profession, II," SUPERVISOR NURSE
     9 (June 1978): 7.

     A second editorial. She had done earlier editorials in
     1973 and 1974 in the same journal arguing for the need for
     nurses to become more informed about ethical issues. (0)

153 Ketefian, S. "The Code for Nurses: A Research Perspective."
     PERSPECTIVES ON THE CODE FOR NURSES. Kansas City, MO:
     American Nurses' Association, 1978, pp. 27-34.

     Emphasizes professional obligation to develop the pro-
     fession's body of knowledge.

154 _____. "Moral Reasoning and Moral Behavior Among Selected
     Groups of Practicing Nurses," NURS RES 30(3) (May/June
     1981): 171--76.

     Similar to previous citation, based upon questionnaire
     of seventy-nine practicing nurses. (23)

155 Kluge, E.W. "Nursing: Vocation or Profession?," CAN NURSE
     78 (February 1982): 34-36.

     Discusses the CNA Code of Ethics. The author argues that
     the code has fundamental unclarities and contradictions. (0)

156 Kushner, K.P., H.E. Mayhew, L.A. Rodgers and R.L. Herman.
     CRITICAL ISSUES IN FAMILY PRACTICE: CASES AND COMMENTARY.
     New York: Springer Publishing Co., 1982.

     Describes common ethical, professional, and emotional
     situations faced by practicing physician, followed by criti-
     cal commentaries discussing the problems and alternatives
     for dealing with them. Topics include death and dying,
     medical decision making, and legal and ethical issues in
     practice. Aimed primarily at physicians.

157   Lanara, V.A.   "Philosophy of Nursing and Current Nursing
      Problems," INT NURS REV 23 (March-April 1976): 48-54.

      Nursing philosophy and the dehumanizing forces. (38)

158   Landfield, J.S. and E.P. Seskin.   "The Economic Value of
      Life: Linking Theory to Practice," AM J PUBLIC HEALTH
      72(6) (June 1982): 555-66.

      Human capital estimates of the economic value of life
      have been routinely used in the past to perform cost-
      benefit analyses of health programs.   Recently, however,
      serious questions have been raised concerning the concep-
      tual basis for valuing human life by applying these esti-
      mates.   After reviewing the major approaches to valuing
      risks to life, the paper concludes that estimates based
      on the human capital approach reformulated to add the
      willingness-to-pay criterion is a good standard to use for
      cost-benefit analyses of the risk to life. (58)

159   Levenstein, A. "The Role of Values," SUPERVISOR NURSE 10
      (June 1978): 64-5, 68.

      How roles, responsibilities and value system influence
      perception and decisions. (0)

160   Levine, M.   "Nursing Ethics and the Ethical Nurse," AM J
      NURS (May 1977): 845-49.

      The imposition of one person's values over another's--
      a moral injustice. (6)

161   "Life, Liberty and the Right to Health Care," AM   NURSE 8
      (September 1, 1976): 4.

      Editorial on ANA's Commission on Human Rights.

162   Limbert, P.M.   "Developing a Code of Ethics for the Nursing
      Profession," AM J NURS 32 (December 1932): 1257-63.

      Looks at ANA 1926 Code and makes suggestions.

163   Lumpp, F.   "Ethical Decision Making."   ETHICAL ISSUES IN
      NURSING: PROCEEDINGS.   St. Louis: Catholic Hospital
      Association, 1976, pp. 31-4.

      Brief discussion of ethical decision making from a manage-
      ment point of view.

164   _____.   "Is Health Care a Right?."   NURSING ETHICS:
      THEORIES AND PRAGMATICS.   Edited by L. Curtin and M.J.
      Flaherty.   Bowie, MD.: Robert J. Brady, 1982, pp. 25-34.

      Explores principles of justice as they are involved in
      distribution of health care and right to adequate nursing.

165 _____. "The Role of the Nurse in the Bioethical Decison-
    Making Process," NURS CLIN NORTH AM (March 1979): 13-21.

    Presents two cases and applies an ethical-responsibility
    model. (9)

166 Mahon, K. and S.J. Everson. "Moral Outrage--Nurses´ Rights
    or Responsibility: Ethics Rounds for Nurses," J CONTIN
    EDUC NURS 10 (May-June 1979): 4-7.

    A description of ethics rounds at one Boston hospital. (6)

167 Mahoney, J. BIOETHICS AND BELIEF. Westminster, MD.:
    Christian Classics, 1984.

    A Jesuit view of such issues as fertility control, death
    and dying, medical research and experimentation, and on the
    beginning of life. The author agrees that, in the dialogue
    between religious belief and medicine, both sides have some-
    thing to offer and something to learn. Aimed at student
    level.cc

168 Mappes, E.J.K. "Ethical Dilemmas for Nurses: Physician´s
    Order Versus Patient´s Rights." BIOMEDICAL ETHICS. Edited
    by T.A. Mappes and J.S. Zembaty. New York: McGraw-Hill,
    1981, pp. 95-102.

    Dilemmas that nurses face when a physician´s orders might
    (1) harm the patient, and (2) violate the patient´s rights
    to autonomy.

169 Mappes, T.A. and J.S. Zembaty (Eds.) BIOMEDICAL ETHICS.
    New York: McGraw-Hill, 1981.

    Chapters dealing with nursing issues are cited independ-
    ently. Most issues are not particularly oriented toward
    nurses.

170 Martin, R.M. "Ethical Issues in Present-Day Health Care."
    ETHICAL ISSUES IN NURSING AND NURSING EDUCATION. New
    York: National League for Nursing, 1980, pp. 1-17.

    A proposed method for decison making is discussed.

171 Matejski, M.P. "Ethical Issues in the Health Care System,"
    J ALLIED HEALTH 11 (May 1982): 131-39.

    Emphasizes need for interprofessional cooperation in
    discussion of ethical issues. (10)

172 McAllister, J. ETHICS, WITH A SPECIAL APPLICATION TO THE
    NURSING PROFESSION. Philadelphia: W.B. Saunders Co.,
    1947.

    An early text included for its historical value.

173   McConnell, T.C. MORAL ISSUES IN HEALTH CARE; AN INTRO-
      DUCTION TO MEDICAL ETHICS. Monterey, CA.: Wadsworth
      Health Sciences Division, 1982.

      After a chapter on ethical theory, the author looks at
      patient relationships, informed consent, experimentation,
      euthanasia, abortion, justice, allocation of scarce re-
      sources giving pros and cons for each. Includes the Inter-
      national Code of Nursing Ethics but not the American Nursing
      Code of Ethics.

174   McCormick, R.A. "Ethics Committees: Promise or Peril?,"
      LAW MED HEALTH CARE 12(4) (September 1984): 150-55.

      Examines concept, role and problems related to hospital
      ethics committees that are charged with decisions to con-
      tinue or discontinue treatment to terminally ill persons
      and handicapped infants. (28)

175   McCullought, L. "The Code for Nurses: A Philosophical
      Perspective." PERSPECTIVES ON THE CODE FOR NURSES.
      Kansas City, MO.: American Nurses´ Association, 1978,
      pp. 35-43.

      Holds that the basic supposition of the code is the need
      to respect client rights and treat them in a way that benefits
      them.

176   McFadden, C.J. MEDICAL ETHICS. Philadelphia: F.A. Davis,
      1946; 2nd Ed., 1949; 3rd Ed., 1953; 4th Ed., 1956.

      Primarily aimed at physicians. Included for historical
      background.

177   McIsaac, I. "Ethics in Nursing," AM J NURS 1 (1901): 483-4.

      A pioneering article and indicates how much early nursing
      ethics emphasized importance of character and bringing other
      nurses into line. Did emphasize importance of respect for
      patients regardless of social standing.

178   McKinlay, J.B. (Ed.). LAW AND ETHICS IN HEALTH CARE. Cam-
      bridge: MIT Press, 1982.

      Thirteen articles which appeared in the Millbank Memorial
      Fund Quarterly in the 1970´s and 1980´s. Book has four
      sections: philosophical reflection on relationships of law
      and medicine; antitrust and professional licensure,
      medical malpractice, and ethical quandries arising in health
      care. Only indirectly does it deal with nursing.

179   McShea, M.M.   "Clinical Judgment: An Ethical Issue," J
      PSYCH NURS 16 (March 1978): 52-55.

      Values are inseparable from making clinical judgement and
      urges more research into this area. (12)

180 McVey, W.E. "Nursing Ethics," AM J NURS 14 (September 1914):
     1057-61.

     Physician author utilized some of the principles of the
     AMA to develop a nursing ethic and then draws up suggestions
     on nurse patient relationship.

181 Middleton, C. "Ethical Decision Making." ETHICAL ISSUES IN
     NURSING: PROCEEDINGS. St. Louis: Catholic Hospital
     Association, 1976, pp. 35-45.

     Lists six factors important to a Christian conscience
     and urges hospitals to adopt Christian ethics.

182 Mooney, M.M. "The Ethical Component of Nursing Theory,"
     IMAGE 12 (February 1980): 7-9.

     Analysis of ethical components of four nursing theories.
     (21)

183 Murphy, C. "Levels of Moral Reasoning in a Selected Group
     of Nursing Practitioners." Ed.D. Dissertation. Teachersc
     College, Columbia University, 1976.

     A study of the effects of working environment and position
     of authority on the moral reasoning of nurses.

184 Murphy, C.P. "The Moral Situation in Nursing." BIOETHICS
     AND HUMAN RIGHTS. Edited by E.L. Bandman and B. Bandman.
     Boston: Little, Brown, 1978, pp. 313-20.

     Examines in particular factors that inhibit autonomous
     decision making in nurses and suggests ways to improve
     moral situation.

185 _____. "Models of the Nurse-Patient Relationship."
     ETHICAL PROBLEMS IN THE NURSE-PATIENT RELATIONSHIP.
     Edited by C.P. Murphy and H. Hunter. Boston: Allyn and
     Bacon, 1983, pp. 8-24.

     Three models of nurse patient relationship and their
     ethical implictions.

186 _____. "The Changing Role of Nurses in Making Ethical
     Decisions," LAW MED HEALTH CARE 12(4) (September 1984):
     173-75.

     Reviews two studies of attitudes of nurses spanning last
     decade. Notes a swing away from complete reliance on phy-
     sicians for ethical decision making. Nurse now more con-
     sumer or nurse oriented. (23)

187 Murphy, C.P. and H. Hunter (Eds.). ETHICAL PROBLEMS IN THE
     NURSE-PATIENT RELATIONSHIP. Boston: Allyn and Bacon, 1983.

Contributions by some seventeen authors (most listed
separately in this bibliography). Appendices include ANA
Code, AHA Patient´s Bill of Rights, et al.

Contains: 186, 196, 197, 178, 297, 307, 324, 330, 338,
            376, 526, 545, 652.

188   Murphy, M.A. and J. Murphy. "Making Ethical Decision--
      Systematically," NURSING 76 (May 1976): 13-14.

      Presents a procedure for making ethical decision. (0)

189   Muyskens, J.L. "Collective Responsibility and the Nursing
      Profession." BIOMEDICAL ETHICS. Edited by T.A. Mappes
      and J.S. Zembaty. New York: McGraw-Hill, 1981, pp. 102-8.

      The appeal to collective responsibility can exonerate an
      individual as well as providing a powerful weapon in up-
      grading nursing as a profession and the delivery of health
      care.

190   _____. MORAL PROBLEMS IN NURSING: A PHILOSOPHICAL INVESTI-
      GATION.   Totawa, NJ: Rowman and Littlefield, 1983.

      Defends patient advocate model of nurse in a variety of
      ethical decisions. Case studies provided.

191   National Association for Practical Nurse Education and Ser-
      vice. "Code of Ethics for the Licensed Practical Vocational
      Nurse," J PRACT NURS 21 (June 1971): 33.

      Prints the code of ethics. (0)

192   National League for Nursing. ETHICAL ISSUES IN NURSING AND
      NURSING EDUCATION. New York: National League for Nursing,
      1980.

      Most of the essays are indexed separately.

      Contains: 80, 170, 596, 616.

193   Nelson, M.J. "Authenticity: Fabric of Ethical Nursing Prac-
      tice," TOP CLIN NURS 4 (April 1982): 1-6.

      Authenticity is explained in existential terms and related
      to nursing practice. (9)

194   Nichols, A.W. "Ethics of the Distribution of Health Care,"
      J FAMILY PRACTICE 12(3) (1981): 533-38.
      While the concept of a "right to health care" has been
      evolving in the United States, this should be distinguished
      from "the right to health," guaranteed in the constitutions
      of many socialist countries. In an effort to promote "quality
      of life" for their citizens, governments can, and do, pro-
      vide health care, but this does not always lead to health.
      Distribution of health care discussed.

195 "Nursing Ethics: The Admirable Professional Standards of
     Nurses: A Survey Report," NURSING 74 (September 1974):
     34-44.

     Responses of 11,000 nurses to questions concerning per-
     sonal moral standards, doctor-nurse relationships, sexual
     involvements, et al. Included for historical data base. (0)

196 O'Brien, L. "Allocation of a Scarce Resource: The Bone
     Marrow Case." ETHICAL PROBLEMS IN THE NURSE-PATIENT
     RELATIONSHIP. Edited by C.P. Murphy and H. Hunter.
     Boston: Allyn and Bacon, 1983, pp. 217-32.

     Analysis of a bone marrow transplant case in an ethical
     setting.

197 O'Neil, P.A. "Placebo Administration: An Ethical Issue."
     ETHICAL PROBLEMS IN THE NURSE-PATIENT RELATIONSHIP.
     Edited by C.P. Murphy and H. Hunter. Boston: Allyn and
     Bacon, 1983, pp. 192-214.

     Argues that the use of placebo is in and of itself incom-
     patible with the patient advocacy model of nursing.

198 Osler, W. "Nurse and Patient." AEQUANIMITAS: WITH OTHER
     ADDRESSES TO MEDICAL STUDENTS, NURSES AND PRACTITIONERS
     OF MEDICINE, 2nd Ed. Philadelphia: P. Blakiston's Son
     and Co., 1906, pp. 156-66.

     Osler, the most famous physician of his day, gave this
     talk in 1897. Among other things he comments on confiden-
     tiality, the danger of not resisting the temptation to know
     more about the things you see and hear. He also discusses
     whether nurses should marry. Included in the selections
     are other addresses of Osler with some pertinence to nursing
     ethics, including his discussion of "Doctor and Nurse," pp.
     13-20.

199 Ostheimer, N.C. and J.M. Ostheimer. LIFE OR DEATH--WHOM
     CONTROLS? New York: Springer Publishing Co., 1976.

     Includes some twenty-three articles on such general topics
     as eugenics, abortion, compulsory sterilization, and euth-
     anasia. None of the contributors write from a nursing per-
     spective.

200 Parsons, E. NURSING PROBLEMS AND OBLIGATIONS. Boston:
     Witcomb and Barrows, 1916, 3rd Ed., 1920.
     Includes what could be regarded as ethical issues at that
     time. Included for historical reasons.

201 Parsons, S. "Ethics as Applied to Nursing," AM J NURS 16
     (May 1916): 693-96.

A good benchmark on changing attitudes. Emphasizes character defects that disqualify a person from nursing; urges
application of Golden Rule. (0)

202 Pavalon, E.I. HUMAN RIGHTS AND HEALTH CARE LAW. New York:
     American Journal of Nursing Co., 1980.

     Includes many ethical issues such as informed consent,
     right to refuse treatment, rights of mentally ill, abor-
     tion, sterilization, artificial insemination, prolonging
     life, et al.

203 Payton, R.J. "Pluralistic Ethical Decision Making." CLINI-
     CAL AND SCIENTIFIC SESSIONS, 1979. Kansas City, MO.:
     American Nurses' Association, 1979, pp. 9-16.

     Ethical decision making is presented as a system that
     takes into consideration the ends and means of the action
     presented.

204 Pence. T. ETHICS IN NURSING: AN ANNOTATED BIBLIOGRAPHY. New
     York: National League for Nursing, November, 1983.

     A discussion on a broad range of ethical dilemmas in
     nursing, including abortion, confidentiality and privacy,
     distributive justice and public policy, doctor/nurse/patient
     relationships, human experimentation, informed consent, life
     support systems, and the right to die. (600)

205 Perry, C.M. "Nursing Ethics and Etiquette," AM J NURS 6
     (1906): 448-52, 513-14, 613-16, 861-63.

     Ethics are discussed in terms of virtues: obedience,
     truthfulness, trustworthiness, punctuality, et al.
     Important for historical perspective. (0)

206 "Perspectives: Resolving an Ethical Dilemma," NURSING 80
     (May 1980): 39-43.

     Discussion with hospital staff and a philosopher of an
     ethical problem concerning a fourteen year old boy with
     leukemia whose parents want to take him into Mexico for
     laetrile treatments. (6)

207 Porter, K. "Patient Rights, Nursing Responsibilities,"
     HOSPITALS 47 (June 16, 19973): 102-4, 134. Reprinted in
     NURS DIGEST 1 (October 1973): 4-8.

     American Hospital Association's Patient Bill of Rights
     and commentary on it from an annual meeting of the American
     Society for Hospital Nursing Service Administrators. (0)

208 Poulin, M.A. "Peer Review: Accountability and Legal Impli-
     cations," OCCUP HEALTH NURS 25 (December 1977): 14-17.

Ethical and legal implications of quality assurance accountability and peer review. (6)

209 Prato, S.A. "Ethical Decisions in Daily Practice," SUPER-
VISOR NURSE (July 1981): 18-20.

Argues that the really important decisions in terms of
daily practice have to be made before an answer is required.
Nurse has to be clear in his/her own mind and should involve
patient in plan of care. (5)

210 "Professional Code," NURS TIMES 72 (cSeptember 30, 1976):
1504-5.

The RCN Code of Professional Conduct, and a policy statement what the RCN stands for. (0)

211 Purtilo, R.B. and C.K. Cassell. ETHICAL DIMENSIONS IN THE
HEALTH PROFESSIONS. Philadelphia: W.B. Saunders Co., 1981.

Offers a four step procedure to assist in ethical decision
making. Emphasizes that in spite of the hierarchical organization of health care the patient is supreme. Includes
case studies and dilemmas.

212 Pyne, R.H. PROFESSIONAL DISCIPLINE IN NURSING: THEORY AND
PRACTICE. Oxford: Blackwell Scientific Publications, 1981.

Account of the disciplinary process in England from its
foundation, evolution to current procedures and practice.
Includes a discussion of eleven actual cases plus twenty-two
others in the appendix.

213 Quaife, F.M., and L.E. Gretter. "Ethics of Nursing," AM J
NURS 4 (1904): 520-22.

This is really an exhortation on the character of a nurse.
It raises an interesting ethical problem on its own since
the actual author was L. E. Gretter but Quaife copied it and
submitted it as her own. See AM J NURS 4 (1904): 637. (0)

214 "Questions You Can't Ignore," RN 43 (January 1980): 66-67.

Results of a questionnaire. See R. Sandroff. (0)

215 Rabb, J.D. "Implications of Moral and Ethical Issues for
Nurses," NURS FORUM 15 (February 1976): 168-79.

Nurses confront ethical dilemmas more often than most other
professionals and yet formal discussion of ethics is not
given much attention in nursing schools. (4)

216 Rehr H. (Ed.) ETHICAL DILEMMAS IN HEALTH CARE: A PROFESSIONAL
SEARCH FOR SOLUTIONS. New York: Prodist, 1978.

General work.

34   Ethical Issues

217 Reich, W. (Ed.). ENCYCLOPEDIA OF BIOETHICS. New York:
     Macmillan, 1978.

     A general encyclopedia for all the health professions.
     Article on nursing cited separately in this bibliography.

218 Reilly, D. "Moral/Value Decisions in Nursing Practice,"
     J NY STATE NURSES ASSOC 10 (December 1979): 40-45.

     Calls for humanities in nursing practice, especially values.

219 Reilly, D.E. "Evaluation: Theory and Strategies." TEACHING
     AND EVALUATING THE AFFECTIVE DOMAIN. Edited by D.E.
     Reilly. Thorofare, NJ: Charles B. Slack, 1978, pp. 31-48.

     Examines barriers to evaluating values and explains how
     affective domain can be evaluated.

220 "Revision Proposed in Code for Professional Nurses," AM J
     NURS 60 (January 1960): 77-81

     Proposed revisions to 1958 Code and their rationale. (0)

221 Roach, M.S. "The Act of Caring as Expressed in a Code of
     Ethics," CAN NURSE 78 (June 1982): 30-32.

     Part of a series, a reply to an article by Kluge. (7)

222 Robb, I.H. NURSING ETHICS: FOR HOSPITAL AND PRIVATE USE.
     Cleveland: E.C. Koeckert, 1900; reprinted 1911, 1916,
     1920, 1928.

     A text by one of the early nursing "leaders."

223 Romanell, P. "Ethics, Moral Conflicts, and Choice," AM J
     NURS 77 (May 1977): 850-55.

     Various types of moral conflict examined. (13)

224 Rosen, E. and C. Darocy. "Ethical Issues in Nursing: Your
     Responses to JPN's Fourth Annual Survey," J PRAC NURS 31
     (10) (November-December 1981): 29-33, 36-40.

     Ethical issues involving abortion, birth control, homo-
     sexuality, and the right to die and responses of LPNs. (0)

225 "Royal College of Nursing (RCN) Code of Professional Conduct:
     A Discussion Document," J MEDICAL ETHICS 3 (September
     1977): 115-23.

     The Code and commentators on it. (5)

226 Rule, J.B. "The Professional Ethic in Nursing," J ADV NURS
     3 (January 1978): 3-8.

     Ethical codes are discussed along with ethical concepts. (15)

227 Russell, F. "The Development of a Professional Code of
     Ethics Among Nurses." Master's Thesis. Columbia Univer-
     sity, 1955.

     From Nightingale Pledge in 1898 to the 1926, 1940,
     and 1950 formulations of professional code.

228 Schorr, T.M. "Magna Carta for Nurses Everywhere," AM J NURS
     73 (August 1973): 1329.

     An editorial on the adoption of the ICN's new code of
     ethics. (0)

229 _____. "Speaking of Ethical Behavior," AM J NURS 80
     (March 1980): 421.

     An editorial arguing for the morality of nursing strikes.
     (0)

230 Schrock, R.A. "A Question of Honesty in Nursing Practice,"
     J ADV NURS 5 (1980): 135-48.

     A survey of eighty-three undergraduate nursing and forty-
     eight post basic students' perceptions of moral issues in
     nursing.

231 Scott, R. THE BODY AS PROPERTY. New York: Viking Press,
     1981.

     Raises and responds to three central questions: (1) is
     the use of human tissues for transplantation, therapy and
     other medical and scientific purposes desirable and in
     community interest, (2) is there currently an adequate
     supply of human tissue available, and (3) what acceptable
     steps might be taken to increase the supply.

232 Shelly, J.A. DILEMMA: A NURSE'S GUIDE FOR MAKING ETHICAL
     DECISIONS. Downers Grove, IL.: Intervarsity Press, 1980.

     This is a "Christian" perspective to ethical issues which
     the author feels modifies the value clarification approach.
     Included besides the usual ethical issues is a section on
     evangelism on the job.

233 Shelp, E.E. and C. Ternes. "Moral Integrity for Nurses,"
     NURS LAW & ETHICS 1 (November 1980): 1-2, 6, 8.

     Nurses need to identify role situations that tax their
     integrity in order to develop moral autonomy and moral
     responsibility.

234 Shelp, E.E. (Ed.). BENEFICENCE AND HEALTH CARE. Hingham,
     MA.: D. Reidel Publishing Co., 1982.

A collection of essays exploring the relationship between humanitarian principles and medicine, including Protestant, Catholic, and Jewish ethical views and their relationship of beneficence to health care issues.

235   Siantz, M.L. d Leon (Ed.). "Symposium on Bioethical Issues in Nursing," NURS CLIN NORTH AM 14 (March 1979).

Includes several articles on ethical issues that are cited in this bibliography.

Contains: 165, 235, 341, 355, 507, 513, 582, 603.

236   Sigman, P. "Ethical Choice in Nursing," ADV IN NURS SCIENCE 1 (April 1979): 37-52.

Ethical choice is defined along with ethical systems and it is argued there is a need for teaching them in the nursing curriculum. (76)

237   Silva, M.C. "Science, Ethics and Nursing," AM J NURS 74 (November 1974): 2004-7.

Genetic experimentation and its impact on nursing, test-tube babies, machine-human symbiosis et al., and the need for new developments in ethical codes.

238   _____. "The American Nurses´ Association´s Position Statement on Nursing and Social Policy: Philosophical and Ethical Dimensions," J ADV NURS 8(2) (1983): 147-51.

Includes a discussion of nursing in an ethical setting. (12)

239   _____. "Ethics, Scarce Resources and the Nurse Executive," NURS ECON 2(1) (January/February 1984): 11-18.

To assist nurse executive to equitably distribute scarce nursing resources, several ethical principles inherent in four theoretical perspectives on distributive justice are addressed. These theoretical perspectives offer the nurse executive guidelines for allocating scarce nursing resources, including poetential effects on clients´ care and safety. (10)

240   Simmons, P.D. BIRTH AND DEATH: BIOETHICAL DECISION-MAKING. Philadelphia: Westminster Press, 1983.

This book is one in a series on Biblical perspectives on current issues. It relies upon Biblical authority in discussing such issues as abortion, euthanasia, "biotechnical parenting," and genetics. It lacks a bibliography but has twelve pages of notes.

241   Smith, S. "Three Models of the Nurse-Patient Relationship." NURSING, IMAGES, AND IDEALS. Edited by S.F. Spicker and S. Gadow. New York: Springer, 1980, pp. 176-88.

Offers three models with catch titles: "surrogate
mother," "nurse technician," and "contracted clinician,"
and examines the ethical implictions.

242 Smith, S.J. and A.J. Davis. "Ethical Dilemmas: Conflicts
Among Rights, Duties, and Obligations," AM J NURS 80
(August 1980): 1463-66.

Ethical theories, rights and obligations are defined and
a plea made for ethical dialogue within nursing. (8)

243 Smurl, J.F. "Ethical Decision Making for Everyday Nursing
Problems," NURS LIFE 3 (May/June 1983): 48-52.

Things to consider when making ethical decisons with
case examples.

244 Spicker, O. and D. Gadow. NURSING IMAGES AND IDEALS. New
York: Springer Publishing Co., 1980.

A collection of essays on contemporary conception of nursing and the role of the nurse. Several are cited independently in this collection.

Contains: 226, 241, 2227, 2228, 2260.

245 Stafford, M.J. "Reflections and Questions from a Nurse in
Practice." ETHICS IN NURSING PRACTICE AND EDUCATION.
Kansas City, MO.: American Nurses' Association, 1980,
pp. 11-16.

Presents two cases of dehumanized care for commentary.

246 Stanley, A.T. "Nursing." ENCYCLOPEDIA OF BIOETHICS, Vol.
3. Edited by W.T. Reich. New York: Macmillan and Co.
and the Free Press, 1978, pp. 1138-46.

History of ethics in nursing education, development of
nursing codes, professional values and responsibility, relationships of nurses to other health professionals, and
ethical issues in current nursing practice.

247 Staunton, M. "New Dimensions of Professional Responsibility,"
INT NURS REV 26 (May/June 1979): 84-85.

New technologies and new development in sciences raise
new challenges to nurses. (0)

248 Steele, S.M. and V.M. Harmon. VALUES CLARIFICATION IN NURS-
ING. New York: Appleton-Century-Crofts, 1979.

Discusses values clarification, professional codes, moral
theories, et al. Presents forty-six cases for analysis,
including those dealing with such difficult problems as
quality of life and scarce resources.

249 Sternberg, M.J. "The Search for a Conceptual Framework as
     a Philosophical Basis for Nursing Ethics: An Examination
     of Code, Contract, Context, and Covenant," MILITARY MEDI-
     CINE 44 (1979): 9-22.

     Four concepts identified and analyzed that might serve as
     a philosophic foundation for nursing ethics: code, contact,
     context (the arena in which ethical conflict occurs), and
     convenants (a formalized agreement between persons to do or
     not to do something specific).

250 Sward, K.M. "A Code for Nurses: A Guide for Ethical Nurs-
     Practice," J NY STATE NURSES ASSOC 6 (December 1975): 25-
     32.

     Compares ANA Code of 1968 with ICN Code and discusses
     strategies to move nursing further along the road of ethical
     accountability. (15)

251 _____. "The Code for Nurses: An Historical Perspec-
     tive." PERSPECTIVES ON THE CODE FOR NURSES. Kansas City,
     MO.: American Nurses´ Association, 1978, pp. 1-9.

     Gives a history of the development of the code.

252 Tate, B.L. THE NURSE´S DILEMMA: ETHICAL CONSIDERATION IN
     NURSING PRACTICE. Geneva: International Council of Nurses
     and New York: American Journal of Nursing Co., 1977.

     Presents some fifty-three actual case studies from around
     the world illustrating ethical problems.

253 Taub, S. "Human Life Symposium: A Synopsis and Critique,"
     LAW MED HEALTH CARE 10(3) (June 1982): 129-34.

     A summary of a Human Life Symposium held in Houston,
     March 11-13, 1982 under the sponsorship of the American
     Society of Law and Medicine and the Texas Institute for the
     Interprofessional Study of Health Law. (4)

254 Thompson, J.B. and H.O. Thompson. "The Ethics of Being a
     Female Patient and a Female Care Provider in a Male-
     Dominated Health Illness System," ISSUES HEALTH CARE
     WOMEN 2 (May/August 1980): 25-54.
     Survey of ethical issues dealing with women as receivers
     and givers of health care. (12)

255 _____. ETHICS IN NURSING. New York: Macmillan, 1981.

     An ethics text about moral dilemmas in nursing from gene-
     tic issues to reproductive ones to distributive justice and
     patients´ rights. Chapter notes include much bibliography
     and there is an annotated bibliography. (100+)

256 Uustal, D.B. "The Use of Values Clarification in Nursing
     Practice," J CONTIN EDUC NURS 8(3) (May/June 1977): 8-13.

     Gives a seven step process for values clarification. (12)

257 _____. "Search for Values," IMAGE 9 (February 1977):
     15-17.

     An introduction to values clarification.

258 _____. "Values Clarification in Nursing: Application
     to Practice," AM J NURS 78 (December 1978): 2058-63.

     A description of values clarification and explanation of
     how it helps the nurse, aids patient teaching, et al. (7)

259 Veatch, R.M. CASE STUDIES IN MEDICAL ETHICS. Cambridge,
     MA.: Harvard University Press, 1977.

     Issues of confidentiality, truthtelling, abortion, steriliz-
     ation, contraception, genetics, allocation of scarce re-
     sources, research, psychiatry, consent, right to refuse,
     and death and dying discussed with 112 cases used to illus-
     trate principles.

260 _____. A THEORY OF MEDICAL ETHICS. New York: Basic
     Books, 1981.

     A general framework for medical ethics focused on the
     social contracts between professionals and patients.

261 Warner, S.l. "Code of Ethics: Professional and Legal
     Implications," RADIOLOGIC TECHNOLOGY 52(5) (March/April
     1981): 485-94.

     Primarily concerned with American Society of Radiologic
     Technologists 1980 Code of Ethics but there is a brief dis-
     cussion of the nature and function of codes. (22)

262 Waugh, D. "Moral Development: Theory and Process." TEACH-
     ING AND EVALUATING THE EFFECTIVE DOMAIN IN NURSING PRO-
     GRAMS. Edited by D. Reilly. Thorofare, NJ: Charles B.
     Slack, 1978, pp. 17-30.

     Describes moral development in terms of Kohlberg's con-
     cepts.

263 Way, H. A six part series in NURSING TIMES in 1960, "Ethics
     for Nurses," April 1, April 8, April 15, April 22,
     April 29, and May 6 issues.

     In general it emphasizes that the physician is never con-
     tradicted; medical code requires we save life at all costs,
     and nurses have to obey. Included for historical reasons.

264 Weber, L.J. "Should Physicians and Nurses Give Moral Advice?,'
     HOSPITAL PROGRESS 57 (January 1976): 68-69, 80.

     Moral advice is permissible but there are dangers that it
     is really medical advice. Avoiding giving advice, however,
     encourages the "tolerance ethic." (0)

265 Wells, H. "ICN Nursing Code: An Agreement on Ethical Con-
     cepts," AORN J 20 (July 1974): 25-26, 28.

     Comment on 1973 ICN Code. (2)

266 Wells, R. "Practical Nursing: Who, What, and When to Tell,"
     NURS MIRROR 148 (April 19, 1979): 22-23.

     Claims that nurses (in England) have been excluded from
     ethical decision making because of misperceptions about
     them. (4)

267 "What Are Your Ethical Standards?," NURSING 74 (March 1974):
     29-33.

     This is a questionnaire designed to determine attitudes.
     Results were reported in later issue. (0)

268 Williams, F.C. and C.A. Williams. "Ethical Issues in Health
     Care Policy." CURRENT PERSPECTIVES IN NURSING: SOCIAL
     ISSUES AND TRENDS. Edited by M. Miller and B.C. Flynn.
     St. Louis: C.V. Mosby, 1977, pp. 3-13.

     Ethical issues in the past have centered around personal
     dilemmas; authors argue for group-level decision making and
     moral principles.

269 Winkler, L. and K.A. Fennell. "Values and Nursing Ethics:
     A Bibliography," J PSYCH NURS 19 (April 1981): 19-20.

     Includes sixty-eight entries, most of which are also in-
     cluded here. (68)

270 Winslow, G.R. TRIAGE AND JUSTICE: THE ETHICS OF RATIONING
     LIFE-SAVING MEDICAL RESOURCES. Berkeley, CA.: University
     of California Press, 1982.

     Triage, the rationing of life-saving medical resources,
     is practiced not only in the battlefield, but in the ordinary
     distribution of scarce medical technologies as well. Apply-
     ing John Rawls´ theory of social justice, the author pro-
     poses alternative approaches to the ethical issues facing
     the health care planner. Two hypothetical triage cases
     are discussed. Contrasting utilitarian and egalitarian
     approaches to the allocation of scarce resources.

271   Zuzich, A. " Some Frameworks for Ethical Development."
      TEACHING AND EVALUATING THE AFFECTIVE DOMAIN IN NURSING
      PROGRAMS. Edited by D.E. Reilly. Thorofare, NJ.: Charles
      B. Slack, 1978, pp. 1-8.

      Traditional ethical concepts, situation ethics, et al.
      are described.

Patient's Rights, Informed Consent, and Nurse Advocate

272   Abrahams, N. "A Contrary View of the Nurse as Patient
      Advocate," NURS. FORUM 17 (1978): 258-67.

      Differing views of the meaning of the role of the patient
      advocate are explored. Author argues that nurses are not
      best suited for this role because of the conflicting obli-
      gations and the risks the role may involve. (0)

273   "An End to Benevolent Conspiracy: Nurses and Patients'
      Rights," HASTINGS CENTER REPORT 11(5) (October 1981): 3-4.

      A report on a survey concerning nurse-physician relation-
      ships and patients' rights. (0)

274   Annas, G.J. "Rights of the Terminally Ill Patient," J NURS
      ADM 4 (March/April 1974): 40-44.

      Patient's right to know, confidentiality, privacy, con-
      sent to treatment, are discussed from an ethical and legal
      point of view. (33)

275   _____. "The Patient's Rights Advocate--Can Nurses
      Effectively Fill the Role?," SUPERVISOR NURSE 5 (July
      1974); 20-23, 25.

      Presents a model patient's bill of rights. (3)

276   _____. "Patient Rights: An Agenda for the '80s,"
      NURS LAW AND ETHICS 2 (April 1981): 3.

      Includes five points: no routine procedures, open access
      to medical records, twenty-four-hour-a-day visitor rights,
      full experience disclosure, effective patient advocate.

277   Annas, G.J. and J. Healey. "The Patient's Rights Advocate,"
      J NURS ADM 4 (May/June 1974): 25-31.

      The concept of a patient's rights advocate system are
      outlined. (17)

278   Aroskar, M. "A Nursing Perspective on the Right to Reject
      Treatment." ETHICAL PROBLEMS IN THE NURSE-PATIENT RELA-
      TIONSHIP. Edited by C.P. Murphy and H. Hunter. Boston:
      Allyn and Bacon, 1983, pp. 139-48.

Rejects the "extreme" view of self-determination that re-
duces the role of health care providers to instruments of
the patient's will, but similarly rejects paternalism as
incompatible with respect for individuals.

279 Bejsovec, J.L. "More on the Tuma Case," NURS OUTLOOK
     (January 1978): 8-9.

     Six letters to the editor concerning the Tuma case. (0)

280 Bell, N.K. "Whose Autonomy Is At Stake?," AM J NURS 6
     (June 1981): 1170-73.

     A discussion of the Tuma case where the Idaho Board of
     Nursing suspended a nurse for "interfering in a physician-
     patient relationship." Author argues Board acted wrong-
     fully and agrees with court decision reinstating Tuma. (6)

281 Besch, L.B. "Informed Consent: A Patient's Right," NURS
     OUTLOOK 27 (January 1979): 32-35.

     The history of informed consent, problems involved, the
     difficulty in obtaining it, and the nurse's role. (24)

282 Bihldorff, J.P. "Personalized Care Assures Patient's Rights,"
     DIMENSIONS IN HEALTH SERVICES 52 (July 1975): 36-39.

     The American Hospital Association's Patient's Bill of
     Rights is seen as an attempt to deal with the growing
     depersonalization of hospital services. Solutions such as
     patient care committees and patient advocate are also ex-
     plored. (5)

283 Boyd, K.M. (Ed.). THE ETHICS OF RESOURCE ALLOCATION IN HEALTH
     CARE. Edinburgh: Ediburgh University Press, 1979.

     Ethical aspects of resource allocation in health care
     discussed.

284 Carnegie, M.E. "The Patient's Bill of Rights and the Nurse,"
     NURS CLIN NORTH AM 9 (September 1974): 557-62.

     Includes the American Hospital Association's Patient's
     Bill of Rights and a history of nursing's involvement in
     patient's rights. (15)

285 Chapman, C.M. "The Rights and Responsibilities of Nurses
     and Patients," J ADV NURS 5 (1980): 127-34.

     Nurse-patient relationships are analyzed in terms of a
     social change model. (16)

286 Cote, A.A. "The Patient's Representative: Whose Side Is
     She On?," NURSING 11 (January 1981): 74-78.

The patient's bill of rights, informed consent, the rights to refuse treatment and confidentiality of medical records are subjects for discussion. Author argues that the patient representative is not working against the nurse but merely specializing in a job that previously has been a part of nursing's role. (0)

287 Curtin, L. "The Nurse As Advocate: A Philosophical Foundation for Nursing," ADV IN NURS SCIENCE 1 (April 1979): 1-10.

Philosophically nursing should be defined as a moral art which includes advocacy for patients. Discussion of what such a definition would mean.

288 Davis, A.J. "To Tell or Not," AM J NURS 81 (January 1981): 156-57.

How much should a nurse tell a patient when the family and physician do not want him to be told he is dying. (0)

289 _____. "Whom Can You Tell?," AM J NURS 81 (November 1981): 2078.

Discusses whether it is correct to tell the family but not the patient that the patient has cancer. (2)

290 Dickman, R.L. "The Ethics of Informed Consnet," NURSE PRACT 5 (May/June 1980): 25, 26, 32.

Discussion of informed consent with implications for nurse practitioners. (7)

291 Dodge, J.S. "How Much Should the Patient Be Told--and By Whom?," HOSPITALS 37 (December 16, 1963): 66-67, 70, 74, 76, 79, 125.

A survey of eighty-two physicians, ninety-three patients, and one hundred thirty-six nurses in two hospitals. Included for historical importance. (11)

292 Donohue, M.P. "The Nurse: A Patient Advocate?," NURS FORUM 17 (1978): 143-51.

The historic roots of patient advocacy can be found in nursing's past. Outlines what is needed to more fully develop the role. (9)

293 Fay, P. "In Support of Patient Advocacy as a Nursing Role," NURS OUTLOOK 26 (April 1978): 252-53.

Patient advocacy should be part of nursing role and included in nursing curricula. (6)

294 Ferguson, V. "The Tuma Case: Other Options," NURS OUTLOOK
     26 (March 1978): 142-43.

     A letter to the editor concerning the Tuma case. Other
     letters are included. (0)

295 _____. "Informed Consent: Given the Facts," NURS
     MIRROR 153 (July 1, 1981): 35-36.

     Discussion of Tuma case. (0)

296 Fromer, M.J. "Paternalism in Health Care," NURS OUTLOOK
     29 (May 1981): 284-90.

     Definition and justification of paternalism which has
     been encouraged by nursing education and socialization. (12)

297 Gadow, S. "Existential Advocacy: Philosophical Foundations
     of Nursing." NURSING: IMAGES AND IDEALS. Edited by S.F.
     Spicker and S. Gadow. New York: Springer Publishing Co.,
     1980, pp. 79-101. Reprinted in ETHICAL PROBLEMS IN THE
     NURSE-PATIENT RELATIONSHIP. Edited by C.P. Murphy and
     H. Hunter. Boston: Allyn and Bacon, 1983, p. 4058.

     Argues that "existential advocacy" reject both paternalism
     and consumerism. Instead the true self determination of
     the patient is the aim.

298 Gargaro, W.J. "Informed Consent: The Nurse's Right to
     Inform," CANCER NURS 1 (June 1978): 249-50.

     Why nurses should be concerned about informed consent
     even though they generally have not been held responsible
     for it in courts (up to 1978).

299 _____. "Informed Consent: A Specific Case," CANCER
     NURS 1(4) (August 1978): 329-30.

     Discusses the Tuma case, then on appeal. (0)

300 _____. "Legislating Patients' Rights," CANCER NURS 3
     (October 1980): 401-2.

     Discusses the American Hospital Association's Bill of
     Rights and legislative statutes incorporating patients'
     rights. Emphasizes the value of the document is that it
     makes rights less readily forgotten, not more enforceable.
     (0)

301 _____. "Tuma Revisited," CANCER NURS 5 (April 1982):
     131-32.

     The implications of Supreme Court decision. (0)

302 Gikuuri, J.P. "The Role of the Patient Representative."
     BIOETHICS AND HUMAN RIGHTS. Edited by E.L. Bandman and
     B. Bandman. Boston: Little Brown, 1978, pp. 281-84.

     The patient representative among other things is to pro-
     tect patient rights.

303 Greenlaw, J. "Hospital Policies: Enforcement Equals Endorse-
     ment," NURS LAW AND ETHICS 1 (March 1980): 5-6.

     Many hospital policies are harmful to patients; nurses
     must unite in their efforts to change such institutional
     policies.

304 _____. "Responding to Patient´s Requests for Informa-
     tion," NURS LAW AND ETHICS 1 (April 1980): 6, 8.

     The Tuma case. (1)

305 _____. "Should Hospitals be Responsible for Informed
     Consent?," LAW MED HEALTH CARE 11(4) (September 1983):
     173-76, 187.

     In light of the Magana decision, hospitals bear a greater
     responsibility in getting informed consent. Nurses become
     crucial in enforcing that proper disclosures are given. (28)

306 Halberstam, M.J. "The Patient´s Chart is None of the Patient´s
     Business," MODERN MED 44 (November 1, 1976): 85-86, 88.

     A conservative rection to reforms. Patients should not
     see their charts, the team approach is naive, et al.

307 Healey, J.M. "Patient Rights and Nursing." ETHICAL PROB-
     LEMS IN THE NURSE-PATIENT RELATIONSHIP. Edited by C.P.
     Murphy and H. Hunter. Boston: Allyn and Bacon, 1983,
     pp. 113-21.

     Brief history of patient´s rights movement, a model bill,
     and suggestions for teaching about it.

308 Holder, A.R. and J.W. Lewis. "Informed Consent and the
     Nurse," LAW MED HEALTH CARE 2 (February 1981): 1-2, 8.

     Says courts have determined that the patient´s right to
     be informed is the personal responsibility of the physician,
     not the hospital.

309 Huttmann, B. THE PATIENT´S ADVOCATE. New York: Penguin
     Books, 1981.

     A handbook of patients´ rights for the intelligent lay person.

310   Imbus, S.H. and B.E. Zawacki. "Autonomy for Burned Patients
      When Survival is Unprecedented," NEW ENG J MED 297 (1977):
      308-11.

      While patients are competent during first hours of hospi-
      talization, some treatment choices are available. Way to
      give the patient options. (19)

311   Jenny, J. "Patient Advocacy: Another Role for Nursing?,"
      INT NURS REV 26 (September/October 1979): 176-81.

      Overview of models of patient advocacy and of changes
      needed for this to become part of nurse´s role. (20)

312   "Karen´s Consent Problem," RN 41 (April 1978): 95, 97-98, 100.

      Response of readers to the dilemmas of obtaining consent
      signatures from an uninformed patient. (0)

313   Kastenbaum, B.K. and R.E. Spector. "What Should a Nurse
      Tell a Cancer Patient?," AM J NURS 78 (April 1978): 640-41.

      Discusses the Massachusetts Cancer Nurses´ Group Statement
      of Beliefs Related to Giving Cancer Patients Information. (3)

314   Kelley, K. and E. McClelland. "Signed Consent: Protection
      or Constraint?," NURS OUTLOOK 27 (January 1979): 40-42.

      Authors believe that signed consent was a constraint to
      research. Recommendations offered. (4)

315   Kohnke, M.F. "The Nurse As Advocate," AM J NURS 80 (November
      1980): 2038-40.

      Nurse advocacy is limited to two areas: informing the
      patients and supporting whatever decision they make. (1)

316   _____. "Discussion of ´Consultant/Advocate´ for Medi-
      cally Ill Hospitalized Patient," NURS FORUM 20(2) (1981):
      123-28.

      A commentary on an article by Barbara Smith. (0)

317   _____. ADVOCACY: RISK AND REALITY. St. Louis: C.V.
      Mosby, 1982.

      Wants to limit the role of advocate to merely informing and
      supporting the client; out and out patient advocacy is des-
      cribed as consumerism; author is opposed to values clarification.

318   Kosik, S.H. "patient Advocacy or Fighting the System," AM
      J NURS 72 (April 1972): 694, 698.

      Kosik´s concept and practice of advocacy. (3)

319 Kostro-Marolda, K. "Dilemmas in Practice: Keeping the
     Secret," AM J NURS 84(1) (January 1984): 25-26 with
     comment by A. Davis.

     Student's reaction to last minute operation of a dying
     woman when she knew the operation was useless and in fact
     which residents handled rather than surgeons. Question of
     how much patient and family should know. (0)

320 Krueger, J.C. "Safeguarding the Rights of Human Subjects."
     PATIENTS, NURSES, ETHICS. Edited by A.J. Davis and J.C.
     Krueger. New York: American Journal of Nursing Co., 1980,
     pp. 35-47.

     Surveys issue and offers guidelines.

321 Lebacqz, K. and R. Levine. "Respect for Persons and Informed
     Consent to Participate in Research," CLIN RES 25(3)
     (April 1977): 101-7.

     Essay arguing that the consent requirement is based on
     the ethical principle of respect for persons. Cautions
     against overprotection.

322 Lewis, E.P. "The Patient's Rights," NURS OUTLOOK 21 (February
     1977): 93.

     An editorial on the Bill of Rights of the AHA. (0)

323 _____. "The Right to Inform," NURS OUTLOOK 25 (September
     1977): 561.

     An editorial on the Tuma case. (0)

324 MacIntyre, A. "To Whom is the Nurse Responsible?." ETHICAL
     PROBLEMS IN THE NURSE-PATIENT RELATIONSHIP. Edited by
     C.P. Murphy and H. Hunter. Boston: Allyn and Bacon,
     1983, pp. 79-83.

     Proposes nurse as advocate or translator of patient's
     needs to physician or physician's understanding to patient.
     This would change relationship between physician and nurse,
     demand more humanities in education.

325 Mancini, M. "Nursing, Minors, and the Law," AM J NURS 78
     (Janurary 1978): 124, 126.

     Legal issues which appear in the treatment of minors. (0)

326 Manson, J.N. "The Right of the Patient to Refuse Treat-
     ment," AANA J 51 (June 1983): 302-3.

     Summary of cases concerning refusal of treatment. (0)

327 Marchewka, A.E. "Dilemmas in Practice: When Is Paternalism
     Justifiable?," AM J NURS 83 (July 1983): 1072.

Nurses often claim to decide what is best for patients;
sometimes it is justified and sometimes not. Gives rules
for making decision. (4)

328 May, K.A. "The Nurse as Researcher: Impediment to Informed
     Consent?," NURS OUTLOOK 27 (January 1979): 36-39.

     Another view of the dual role of nurse and researcher
     and its implication on obtaining informed consent. (13)

329 _____. "Informed Consent and Role Conflict." PATIENTS,
     NURSES, ETHICS. Edited by A.J. Davis and J.C. Krueger.
     New York: American Journal of Nursing Co., 1980, pp. 109-15.

     Problems and perceptions of experimental subjects when
     giving consent to nurses who are filling a dual role.

330 McCrann, D.D. "Ethical Issues of Behavior Modification."
     ETHICAL PROBLEMS IN THE NURSE-PATIENT RELATIONSHIP.
     Edited by C.P. Murphy and H. Hunter. Boston: Allyn and
     Bacon, 1983, pp. 187-92.

     Valium is used to obtain a third pelvic examination that
     patient had refused.

331 Miller, B.K., T.J. Mansen and H. Lee. "Patient Advocacy:
     Do Nurses Have the Power to Act as Patient Advocate?,"
     NURS LEADERSH 6 (June 1983): 56-60.

     Until nurses demand autonomy to act as patient care advo-
     cates they will remain primarily care givers. (18)

332 National League for Nursing. NURSING'S ROLE IN PATIENTS'
     RIGHTS. New York: National League for Nursing, 1977.

     The NLN position on patient's rights goes beyond the AHA
     Patient's Bill of Rights.

333 _____. CONSUMERISM AND HEALTH CARE. New York: National
     League for Nursing, 1978.

     Includes six essays and an appendix. Included in the appen-
     dix are the NLN statement of Nursing's Role In Patients'
     Rights, "Guidelines for a Patient's Bill of Rights".

334 Nations, W.C. "Nurse-Lawyer is Patient-Advocate," AM J
     NURS 73 (June 1973): 1039-41.

     A nurse-lawyer develops the role of patient advocate. (1)

335 Neubauer, D.W. "Should the Patient Know the Truth?,"
     ARIZONA MED 22 (March 1965): 215-20.

Included for historical reason. Article is a reprint of
a speech given to Arizona State Nursing Association and
includes a survey of religious views and truthtelling.
Author concludes that nurses should tell the truth but retain hope. (0)

336 Oberst, M.T. "Research Ethics, Part 2: The Concept of Risk
     in Clinical Studies," CANCER NURS 2 (December 1979): 481-82.

     Should informed consent be required for no risk studies. (6)

337 _____. "Rsearch Ethics, Part 3: Risks Associated
     with Researcher Access to Clinical Records," CANCER NURS
     3 (February 1980): 57-58.

     The problems of privacy and confidentiality are discussed
     and policy recommendations are made. (9)

338 Orgel, G.S. "They Have No Right to Know: The Nurse and the
     Terminally Ill Patient." ETHICAL PROBLEMS IN THE NURSE-
     PATIENT RELATIONSHIP. Edited by C.P. Murphy and H. Hunter.
     Boston: Allyn and Boston, 1983, pp. 123-36.

     Claims that nurses must have equal authority in decision
     making to make ethical decision making meaningful.

339 Pankratz, L. and D. Pankratz. "Nursing Autonomy and Patient's
     Rights: Development of a Nursing Attitude Scale," J HEALTH
     AND SOCIAL BEHAVIOR 15 (September 1974): 211-16.

     An additudinal survey of 702 nurses toward professional
     autonomy, advocacy, patients' rights, et al. (22)

340 Pappert, M.S. "The Issue of Confidentiality: A Perspective
     from the Nursing Profession," BULL NY ACADEMY MED 54
     (September 1978): 758-63.

     Commentary on Federal Privacy Act of 1974 and those pro-
     visions which apply to medical records in the private sector.
     (10)

341 Payton, R.J. "Information Control and Autonomy: Does the
     Nurse Have a Role?," NURS CLIN NORTH AM 14 (1979): 23-33.

     Looks at truthtelling, paternalism and autonomy and
     nurse's role in promoting patient autonomy. (9)

342 Peplau, H.E. et al. "Feedback: On the Right to Inform,"
     NURS OUTLOOK 25 (December 1977): 738-43.

     Letters concerning the Tuma case. (0)

343 President's Commission for the Study of Ethical Problems in
     Medicine and Biomedical and Behavioral Research. MAKING
     HEALTH CARE DECISIONS, THE ETHICAL AND LEGAL IMPLICATIONS
     OF INFORMED CONSENT IN THE PATIENT-PRACTITIONER RELATION-
     SHIP, VOL. ONE: REPORT. Washington, D.C.: U.S. Govern-
     ment Printing Office, 1982.

     A history of informed consent in the law and medical
     practice, ethical and legal obligations of health care pro-
     fessionals, communications techniques, and principles for mak-
     ing health care decisions for patients who are incapacitated.

344 Price, R. "Consumerism in Health--Are We Accountable and
     If So How?," AUSTRALIAN NURSES J 10 (April 1981): 50-52.

     The patient's rights movement is active in Australia.
     Interesting for comparison purposes. (13)

345 Quinn, N. and A.R. Somers. "The Patient's Bill of Rights:
     A Significant Aspect of the Consumer Revolution," NURS
     OUTLOOK 22 (April 1974): 240-44.

     A commentary on the American Hospital Association's
     Patient's Bill of Rights and predictions on how nurses will
     respond to the patient's rights movement. Included for
     comparative purposes. (11)

346 Robb, S., M. Peterson and J.W. Nagy. "Advocacy for the
     Aged," AM J NURS 79 (October 1979): 1736-38.

     The personalized account of how three individuals acted
     as patient advocates and were able to compel changes and
     reform. (19)

347 Robb, S.S. "Beware the 'Informed' Consent," Editorial,
     NURS RES 32(3) (May/June 1983): 132.

     Informed consent is failing in its mission of service to
     the elderly in long term care facilities and dulling the
     efforts of researchers responsible for studying the popula-
     tion. (2)

348 Rozovsky, L.E. "A Canadian Patient's Bill of Rights,"
     DIMENSIONS IN HEALTH SERVICE 51 (December 1974): 8-10.

     American Hospital Association's Patient's Bill of Rights
     is examined in light of Canadian law. (6)

349 Sandroff, R. "How the 'Patient Bill of Rights' Makes Honesty
     Easier," RN 41 (August 1978): 42-47.

     An RN survey of 431 nurses about the patients' rights
     movement. (1)

350 Silva, M.C. "Ethics, Informed Consent, and the OR Nurse,"
     TODAY'S OR NURSE 4 (March 1982): 21-22, 24, 62-63.

General summary of issues.

351   Sklar, C. "The Patient's Choice vs. the Nurse's Judgment,"
      CAN NURSE 74 (April 1978): 11-12.

      Discusses a case where nurse overrode a patient's choice
      of pain medication. (0)

352   _____. "Unwarranted Disclosure," CAN NURSE 74 (May
      1978): 6-8.

      Legal liabilities (Canadian) of breach of confidentiality
      and defamation. (5)

353   Smith, B.J. "Consultant/Advocate for the Medically Ill
      Hospitalized Patient," NURS FORUM 20 (1981): 115-22.

      Records an unsuccessful attempt of a psychiatric liaison
      nurse to see that the rights of the patient were observed. (7)

354   Smith, C.S. "Outrageous or Outraged: A Nurse Advocate
      Story," NURS OUTLOOK 28 (October 1980): 624-25.

      A nurse, who became an outspoken patient advocate, found
      almost no support for her advocacy and was entually forced
      to resign in order to avoid being fired. (7)

355   Stanley, A.T. "Is It Ethical to Give Hope to a Dying Per-
      son?," NURS CLIN NORTH AM 14 (1979): 69-80.

      Discusses the Tuma case. (16)

356   Storch, J.L. "Consumer Rights and Health Care," NURS ADM Q
      4 (Winter 1980): 107-15.

      The consumer rights movement and its implication on health
      policy, i.e. patient's rights. (37)

357   Trandel-Korenchuck, K.M. and D.M. Trandel-Korenchuck. "The
      Ethical Implications of Informed Consent,"" NURS ADM Q
      5 (Summer 1981): 101-5.

      Discusses implication and application of informed consent
      for nurses. (5)

358   Tuma, J.L. "Professional Misconduct," NURS OUTLOOK 25
      (September 1977): 546.

      Tuma speaks for herself in a letter to the editor describ-
      ing the incident that brought charges of unprofessional
      conduct when she responded to a cancer patient's request
      for information about alternative treatment. (0)

359   Walsh, M. "Nursing's Responsibility for Patient's Rights."
      CONSUMERISM AND HEALTH CARE. New York: National League
      for Nursing, 1978, pp. 19-27.

Brief account of NLN involvement with patients' rights in early periods, overview of the ANA Patient's Bill of Rights, et al., and the nurse's importance in patients' rights.

360 Walshe-Brennan, K.S. "The Nurse and Confidentiality," NURS MIRROR 146 (April 20, 1978): 32.

Author editorializes that security and confidentiality of psychiatric notes are imperiled by growing layers of administration and new technologies. (9)

361 Watson, A.B. "Informed Consent of Special Subjects," NURS RES 31 (January/February 1982): 43-47.

Historical development of informed consent is briefly examined and its application to nursing research explored. (32)

362 Wilkes, E. "Quality of Life: Effects of the Knowledge of Diagnosis in Terminal Illness," NURS TIMES 73 (September 1977): 1506-7.

Study of 500 dying cancer patients found that patients who knew their condition had a high correlation with better quality care. (4)

363 Yarling, R.R. "Ethical Analysis of a Nursing Problem: The Scope of Nursing Practice in Disclosing the Truth to Terminal Patients. An Inquiry Directed to the National Joint Practice Commission of the AMA and the ANA, Part I," SUPERVISOR NURSE 9 (May 1978): 40-41, 45.

Case studies raising question of scope of nursing practice. Nurse should respond honestly. (14)

364 _____. "Ethical Analysis of a Nursing Problem: The Scope of Nursing Practice in Disclosing the Truth to Terminal Patients. An Inquiry Directed to the National Joint Practice Commission of the AMA and the ANA, Part II," SUPERVISOR NURSE 9 (June 1978): 28-34.

Case studies raising question of scope of nursing practice. Nurse should respond honestly. (33)

365 Youngner, S.J., C. Coulton, B.W. Juknialis and D.L. Jackson. "Patients' Attitudes Toward Hospital Ethics Committees," LAW MED HEALTH CARE 12 (February 1984): 21-25.

First attempt to survey patients' awareness of existence of such committees. Most thought they were useful and seventy-four percent thought that nurses should serve on ethics committees. The group ranked second highest (next to physicians--97%), and above clergy (58%). (20)

See 817, 818, 826, 829, 833, 839, 845, 846, 851, 853, 856, 857 858, 861.

Professionalism and Ethics

366   American Nurses' Association. ACCOUNTABILITY OF THE NURSE.
      Kansas City, MO.: American Nurses' Association, Pub. No.
      NP-43, 1973.

      Four papers presented at the 1972 ANA Convention focus on
      the legal and ethical aspects of the nurse's accountability
      for independent action.

367   Bissell, L., and R.W. Jones. "The Alcoholic Nurse," NURS
      OUTLOOK (February 1981): 96-101.

      Help early in development of alcoholism is important yet
      nurses as a group have not taken care of their own members
      as rapidly as members of male dominated health professions.
      Guidelines on what to do. (17)

368   Blake, B.L.K. "Quality Assurance: An Ethical Responsi
      bility," SUPERVISOR NURSE 12 (February 1981): 32, 37-8.

      A call for nursing to control its own exercises and prac-
      tices, the driving forces behind it, and the forces that
      are restraining the effort of nurses to gain control or
      monitoring the quality of its practice. (16)

369   Connelly, C.E., R.M. Dahlen, L.K. Evans, and N.A. Wieker.
      "To Strike or Not to Strike: A Debate on the Ethics of
      Strikes by Nurses," SUPERVISOR NURSE 10 (January 1979):
      52, 55-59.

      Moral theories are used to examine the "moral" permis-
      sibility of strikes by nurses. (26)

370   Creighton, H. "Liability of a Nurse Floated to Another
      Unit," NURS MANAGE 13 (March 1982): 54-55.

      A hospital and a nurse were held liable for floating a
      nurse to a unit where she was not qualified and where the
      death of a patient resulted. (12)

371   _____. "Refusing to Participate in Abortions," NURS
      MANAGE 13 (April 1982): 27-8.

      Summarizes state and federal regulations allowing hospi-
      tals and nurses to refuse to participate in abortions. (14)

372   Curtin, L.L. "Questioning Drug Orders," SUPERVISOR NURSE
      11 (February 1980): 7.

      An editorial on patients' right to know what they are
      receiving and on the nurse's responsibility in giving medi-
      cation. (0)

373   _____. "Autonomy, Accountability and Nursing Prac-
      tice," TOP CLIN NURS 4 (April 1982): 7-14.

Author argues that neither patients nor nurses are served
by absolute professional autonomy. The difficulties in
obtaining parity in health care endeavor are examined. (30)

374 Cushing, M. "Expanding the Meaning of Accountability,"
     AM J NURS 83(3) (August 1983): 1202-4.

     Skilled hospital personnel have a duty to exercise reason-
     able care in administering services to a patient and have a
     duty to perform acts within their authority to protect the
     health and life of a patient. (4)

375 Daniel, I.Q. "Impaired Professionals: Responsibilities and
     Roles," NURS ECON 2(3) (May/June 1984): 190-93.

     Society has become increasingly aware of the problem of
     impaired professionals, and nursing leaders share this aware-
     ness. When clients are at risk because professional nurses
     practice while impaired, nursing's ethical standards oblige
     colleagues to act. (9)

376 Davis, A.J. "Authority-Autonomy, Ethical Decision Making,
     and Collective Bargaining in Hospital." ETHICAL PROBEMS
     IN THE NURSE-PATIENT RELATIONSHIP. Edited by C.P. Murphy
     and H. Hunter. Boston: Allyn and Bacon, 1983, pp. 63-76.

     Argues that collective bargaining is compatible with
     nurse's primary obligation to the patient.

377 Dock, S. "The Relation of the Nurse to the Doctor and the
     Doctor to the Nurse," AM J NURS 17 (February 1917): 394-96.

     Times have changed. Obedience was the first law corner-
     stone of good nursing and no one can become a reliable nurse
     until they can obey without question.

378 Ensor, B.E., R.C. Dilday, B.M. Harakal, M. Heins, and R.A.
     Bowman. "What the SNAs are Doing...in Maryland, in
     Georgia, in Ohio," AM J NURS 82 (April 1982): 581-94.

     Actions taken by three state nursing associations to help
     their alcoholic colleagues. (5)

379 Erde, E.L. "Notions of Teams and Team Talk in Health Care:
     Implications for Responsibilities," LAW MED HEALTH CARE 9
     (October 1981): 26-28.

     Includes a discussion of whistle blowing among team mem-
     bers.

380 Feliu, A.G. "The Legal Side: Thinking of Blowing the
     Whistle?," AM J NURS 83(11) (November 1983): 1541-42.

Ability to avoid harsh repercussions in whistle blowing
depends upon position in organization, substance of your
complaint, source of the problem, and the rigidity of the
organization. Advice on what to do if there are repercussions. (0)

381 Flaherty, M.J. "Guilt by Association?" NURS MANAGE 12
     (November 1981): 32-33.

     Discusses the case of a nurse who was fired from her job
     because her husband had sold marijuana grown in their home.
     (0)

382 Fulton, K. "Drug Abuse Among Nurses: What Nursing Manage-
     ment Can Do," SUPERVISOR NURSE (January 1981): 18-20.

     Drug abuse is a preventable phenomenon. Nurse adminis-
     trators must examine their own organizations to see where
     exactly they are supporting the phenomenon and then move to
     deal with it. (0)

383 "Going Beyond the Hospital," RN 42 (March 1979): 29.

     A report of the failure of health care professionals in
     New York to report medical misconduct. The result was a
     statute that required physicians to report MD's misconduct.
     For more information see the article listed under Linda
     Stanley. (0)

384 Grand, N.K. "Nightingaleism, Employeeism, and Professional
     Collectivism," NURS FORUM 10(3) (1971): 289-99.

     Though most nurses welcome higher salaries, they reject
     collective bargaining. Conflict is due to different tradi-
     tions. Nurses will be better able to accept bargaining if
     quality of nursing care is included as an issue. (7)

385 Greenlaw, J. "Reporting Incompetent Colleagues," NURS LAW
     AND ETHICS, Part I (February 1980): 4; Part II (May
     1980): 5.

     A nurse has a duty to report incompetent colleagues in
     order to protect patients. Part I is general; Part II
     discusses case of Malone v. Longo. (3)

386 _____. "On Concealing Mistakes," NURS LAW AND ETHICS
     1 (October 1980: 5-6.

     Commentary on the Pisel case.

387 _____. "Enforcing Professional Standards," NURS LAW AND
     ETHICS 1 (December 1980): 3, 7.

Nurses have responsibility to police themselves in order to best serve the public. A strong sense of moral duty is the strongest reason to compel adherence to professional standards.

388   Horsley, J.E.   "When You Can Safely Refuse an Assignment,"
      RN 43 (February 1980): 93-94, 96.

A number of legal cases underscore the point that a nurse must do as instructed and arbitrary refusal to accept duty assignments is never authorized. Nevertheless, when a nurse has a valid personal or professional reason to refuse she can. (0)

389   Hull, R.T.   "Blowing the Whistle While You Work," KANSAS
      NURSE 55 (December 1980): 7, 15, 18-20.

Discussion of issues involved in whistle blowing and of the stand advocated in ANA Code of Ethics. (15)

390   Jaffe, S.   "Help for the Helper: First-hand Views of Recov-
      ery," AM J NURS 82 (April 1982): 578-79.

Discussion with ten recovering alcoholic nurses and six alcoholic nurse patients provide a profile of the parti- cular problems the alcoholic nurse encounters. (2)

391   Jefferson, L.V., and B.E. Ensor.   "Help for the Helper:
      Confronting a Chemically-impaired Colleague," AM J NURS
      82 (April 1982): 574-77.

Under obligation to report.   The wrong thing is to do nothing. (7)

392   Katz, B.F.   "Reporting and Review of Patient Care: The
      Nurse's Responsibility," LAW, MED HEALTH CARE 11(2)
      (April 1983): 76-79.

Responsibility of nurses to bring substandard medical practice to attention of authorities discussed.   Case law related to this obligation reviewed. (22)

393   McClure, M.L.   "The Long Road to Accountability," NURS
      OUTLOOK 26 (January 1978): 47-50.

Three major barriers to nurses taking responsibility: misguided egalitarianism, professional passivity, and lack of meaningful peer review. (6)

394   Murphy, P.   "Deciding to Blow the Whistle," AM J NURS 81
      (September 1981): 1691-92.

Deals with frustration in attempting to blow the whistle on actions of a colleague. (2)

395   Newton, M. and D. Newton.   "Guidelines for Handling Drug
      Errors," NURSING 77 (September 1977): 62-68.

      A study reports that 29 percent of all nurses fail to
      report any type of medication error. This is a commentary
      upon the report. (0)

396   "Nurse Refused to Assist in Abortion: Demoted!," REGAN REP
      NURS LAW 22 (November 1981): 4.

      News report. (0)

397   "Nursing Supervision: Reporting Errant MD´s," REGAN REP
      NURS LAW 21 (November 1980): 1.

      Argues that a nurse cannot be sued, or at least success-
      fully sued by an aggrieved MD if exercising duty to report
      the clinical deficiencies through professional channels. (0)

398   Regan, W.A. "You Don´t Have To Tolerate Substandard Hos-
      pital Practices," RN 44 (January 1981): 99-100, 102.

      Explains how to use the JCAH (Joint Commission on the
      Accreditation of Hospitals) to correct substandard prac-
      tices as well as the legal protection afforded to those who
      use it. (0)

399   Roth, M.D. and L.J. Levin. "Dilemma of Tarasoff: Must Phy-
      sicians Protect the Public or Their Patients?" LAW MED
      HEALTH CARE 11 (June 1983): 104-10, 131.

      This is a legal view of an ethical issue: should the
      professional inform a third party that a patient might be
      dangerous. This raises a conflict between protecting
      patient and protecting public. (47)

400   Sandroff, R. "Protect the MD...Or the Patient?: Nursing´s
      Unequivocal Answer," RN 44 (February 1981): 28-33.

      Some 12, 500 nurses respond to a hypothetical situation
      similar to the Jolene Tuma case, unnecessary surgery and
      hospitalization. (7)

401   Sexton, R. "JCAH Review: Your Most Strategic Moment to
      Speak Out," RN 42 (August 1979): 73-74, 76.

      How the Joint Commission on Accreditation of Hospitals
      works and how it can be used to improve hospital care when
      going through channels does not seem to work. (0)

402   Stanley, L. "Dangerous Doctors: What To Do When the MD
      is Wrong?," RN 42 (March 1979): 23-30.

      What a nurse should do about physicians´ errors. (0)

403 "Unprofessional Nursing Conduct: Legal Definitions," REGAN
     REP NURS LAW 22 (August 1981): 2.

     Brief comment on the case of a nurse whose license was
     suspended because she was convicted of making a false state-
     ment in order to obtain supplemental security income bene-
     fits. (0)

404 "Where Does Loyalty End?," AM J NURS 10 (1910): 230-31.

     This is an editorial on how much loyalty nurses owe to
     physicians. Included for historical information on the
     longevity of the issue.

405 Witt, P. "Dilemmas In Practice: Notes of a Whistleblower,"
     AM J NURS 83(12) (December 1983): 1649-51.

     Personal experiences in a 150 bed private psychiatric
     hospital in which the nurse felt patients were abused.
     Finally agreed to help a patient, was given sick leave, and
     then not recalled, was unemployed and blackballed. Sued
     hospital and administrator and won but took three years. (0)

     See 672, 692, 694, 708, 723, 736.

Birth, Infant, Child Care

406 Bakke, K. "Ethical Dilemmas: Institutionalizing a Sev-
     erely Disabled Child," PED NURS 7 (November/December
     1981): 27-29.

     Analysis of an ethical dilemma involving the institu-
     tionalizing of a nine year old child with hydrocephalus
     and other complications. The ethical theory of William
     Frankena is employed. (3)

407 Capron, A.M. "The New Reproductive Possibilities: Seeking
     a Moral Basis for Concerned Action in a Pluralistic
     Society," LAW, MED HEALTH CARE 12(5) (October 1984): 192-98.

     A variety of new processes involving transfer of ovum
     and/or sperm raise new ethical, legal, and policy issues.
     Books and articles for further reading presented. (32)

408 Chinn, P.L. "Issues in Lowering Infant Mortality, A Call
     for Ethical Action," ADV NURS SCIENCE 1 (April 1979): 63-
     78.

     Ethical issues in the care of neonates.(38)

409 Cushing, M. "Whose Best Interest? Parents vs. Child
     Rights," AM J NURS 82 (February 1982): 313-14.

     Discussion of Green and Becker cases. (0)

410 _____. "Do Not Feed...," AM J NURS 83(4) (April 1983):
         602-4.

     The question of withholding treatment from severely defe-
     ctive newborns, or even allowing them to starve to death is
     examined. Conclusion is that until many of the issues are
     resolved, courts will continue to be petitioned for instruc-
     tions on a case by case basis. (9)

411 Davis, A.J. "When Parents Disagree on Treatment," AM J
         NURS 80 (November 1980): 2080-82.

     A mentally retarded comatose child with renal disease and
     possible brain damage and parents disagree over whether to
     continue treatment. (0)

412 _____. "A Newborn's Right to Life vs. Death," AM J
         NURS 81 (May 1981): 1035.

     Staff has to give information on what infant's life might
     be like with life support and what his death might be like
     without it. (2)

413 Doudera, A.E. "Section 504, Handicapped Newborns, and
         Ethics Committees: An Alternative to the Hotline," LAW,
         MED HEALTH CARE 11(5) (October 1983): 200-2, 236.

     A hospital based ethics committee is proposed as an alter-
     native to the hotline approach of calling the federal gov-
     ernment regarding the rights of severely handicapped infants.
     (35)

414 Drake, D.C. "One Must Die So The Other Might Live," NURS
         FORUM 16 (1977): 228-49.

     Siamese twins who share one and a half hearts and the
     moral deliberation which led up to the surgery. (0)

415 Ellis, T.S. "Letting Defective Babies Die: Who Decides?,"
         AM J LAW MED 7 (Winter 1982): 393-423.

     Explores the decision to withhold treatment from a defec-
     tive newborn. Concludes that legislature should set consis-
     tent guidelines. (113)

416 Garrow, D. "The Severely Handicapped Newborn: A Loving
         Thing To Do," NURS MIRROR 152 (April 30, 1981): 27-28.

     English physician argues parents should be allowed full
     decision making authority regarding treatment or nontreat-
     ment of defective newborns. Babies should not be killed,
     however, instead allowed to die. (0)

417 Grodin, M.A., S.F. Schwartz and I.D. Todres. "Moral Dilemmas
     and Problematic Decision Making in Neonatal Intensive
     Care." THE RIGHTS OF CHILDREN: LEGAL AND PSYCHOLOGICAL
     PERSPECTIVES. Edited by J.S. Henning. Springfield, IL.:
     Charles C. Thomas, 1982.

     Focuses on the dilemmas in dealing with neonates with
     special problems.

418 Gustafson, J.M. "Mongolism, Parental Desires, and the
     Right to Life," PERSPECTIVES IN BIOLOGY AND MEDICINE 16
     (Spring 1973): 529-57.

     Included for historical reasons. Emphasizes nurse´s duty
     to follow orders. (0)

419 Harris, C.E. "Some Ethical and Legal Considerations in
     Neonatal Intensive Care," NURS CLIN NORTH AM 8(3) (September
     1973): 521-31.

     Legal and moral issues in neonate nursing. Author holds
     that it is wrong to operate on a Down´s Syndrome child with
     a bowel obstruction and that parents should not be required
     to make a decision which produces a life vs. death outcome
     for infant. Included for historical reasons. (6)

420 Heymann, P.B. and S. Holtz. "The Severely Defective Newborn:
     The Dilemma and the Decision Process." DECISION MAKING
     AND THE DEFECTIVE NEWBORN. Edited by C.A. Swinyard.
     Springfield: Charles C. Thomas, 1978.

     Discusses three factors to be considered in defining
     reasonable treatment for Myelomeningocele or, as more com-
     monly called, spina bifida cystica. Factors: (1) the inter-
     ests of the infant, (2) the costs to the society both in
     resources and in threats to valued beliefs, and (3) the
     emotional and financial costs to the family of the after
     care of the infant.

421 Horan, D.J. "Infanticide: When Doctor´s Orders Read ´Mur-
     der´," RN 45 (January 1982): 72-76, 78, 81-85.

     Discussion of Danville and other "Baby Doe" type cases
     where orders are written not to feed. (20)

422 Jonsen, A. and M. Garland (Eds.). ETHICS OF NEWBORN INTEN-
     SIVE CARE. San Francisco: Health Policy Program, School
     of Medicine, University of California, 1976.

     The authors seek to raise and explore principal ethical
     and policy issues facing parents, families, physicians,
     nurses, and others who must participate in life-or-death
     decisions in this complex subject.

423 Kleinberger, H. "Children with Meningomyelocele: Some Ethi-
     cal Problems of Care," MED AND LAW 1(4) (1982): 355-58.

Raises and discusses special ethical problems associated with Meningomyelocele.

424   Lorber, J. and R.B. Zachary. "Spina Bifida: To Treat or Not to Treat?," NURS MIRROR 147 (September 14, 1978): 13.

Two pediatricians present opposing views on criteria for selective treatment. (0)

425   Moser, D. et al. "Resolving an Ethical Dilemma: A Child with Leukemia," NURSING 80 (May 1980): 39-43.

Looked at ethical dilemmas from a nursing perspective. As professional practitioners, accountable both to patients and employer. How do you act when ethical behavior toward one seems to conflict with your obligation toward the other? (6)

426   Munzig, N.C. "Dealing with an Ethical Dilemma: A Case in Application," NEPHROL NURSE 3 (January-February 1981): 18-20.

Dialysis of a newborn with a rare fatal disease. (0)

427   Paris, J.J. "Terminating Treatment for Newborns: A Theological Perspective," LAW, MED HEALTH CARE 10(3) (June 1982): 120-24, 144.

A discussion of recent cases from a Catholic point of view by a Jesuit. (23)

428   Paris, J.J. and A.B. Fletcher. "Infant Doe Regulations and the Absolute Requirement to Use Nourishment and Fluid for the Dying Infant," LAW, MED HEALTH CARE 11(5) (October 1983): 210-13.

Authors are a professor of ethics and a professor of child health. Both raise questions about the Infant Doe case arguing that there is no ethical duty to artificially feed hopelessly ill children. (34)

429   Patterson, P. "Fetal Therapy: Issues We Face," AORN 35 (March 1982): 663-68.

New in utero therapeutic interventions often raise new ethical issues. (10)

430   Pothier, P. "Research Involving Children, Fetuses, and the Mentally Retarded." PATIENTS, NURSES, ETHICS. Edited by A.J. Davis and J.C. Krueger. New York: American Journal of Nursing Co., 1980, pp. 149-62.

All three groups share a dependent status and this raises special research problems on consent. Discussion of issues governing such research.

431   Rea, K.   "Suffer Little Children, NURS TIMES 77 (November 25,
        1981): 2044.

        Legal liability of English nurses who comply with orders
        to withhold food from newborns. (0)

432   Rebone, J.W.   "Minimal Quality of Life: Why Parents, Courts
        Chose Infant Doe´s Death," HOSPITAL PROGRESS 63 (June
        1982): 10-14.

        A favorable discussion of the parents of Baby Doe and
        their decision.

433   Roberts, C.S.   "Ethical Issues in the Treatment of Neonates
        with Severe Anomalies," NURS FORUM 18 (1979): 352-65.

        Argues that unless the nurse believes that parents have
        the right to make decisions, the nurse should withdraw.
        Nurse should support parental decision making. (16)

434   Robertson, J.A. "Dilemma in Danville: Defective Newborns,
        To Treat or Not To Treat," HASTINGS CENTER REP 11(5)
        (October 1981): 5-8.

        Discusses Danville case of newborn Siamese twins who were
        taken to nursery to starve. Someone (nurses?) alerted
        authorities and criminal charges were filed against the phy-
        sician and parents. (24)

435   Rothenberg, L.S.   "The Empty Search for an Imprimatur, or
        Delphic Oracles Are in Short Supply," LAW, MED HEALTH CARE
        10(3) (June 1982): 115-17.

        An editorial on implications of decision making involving
        seriously ill newborns. (5)

436   Schowalter, J.E., J.B. Fernholt and N.M. Mann. "The Adoles-
        cent Patient´s Decision to Die," PEDIATRICS 51 (January
        1973): 97-103.

        A sixteen year old girl refused dialysis. Recounts staff
        reaction. (40)

437   Shufer, S. "Dilemmas in Practice: What´s Best for Willie?,"
        AM J NURS 82 (March 1982): 470-72.

        Deciding to take legal action against parents to do what
        an agency believes is the child´s best interest is a diffi-
        cult moral dilemma. Shufer presents her own reaction to
        just such a case. (0)

438   Stinson, R. and P. Stinson. THE LONG DYING OF BABY ANDREW.
        Boston: Atlantic Press, 1983.

A personal account of a parent's struggle to make decisions for and about the life of their newborn son, born four months premature. The child lived for six months and the book deals with their moral struggles but also with the hostile unresponsive health care providers. The need for health care providers to give support becomes all important.

439   Strong, C.   "Defective Infants and Their Impact on Families: Ethical and Legal Considerations," LAW MED HEALTH CARE 11(4) (September 1983): 168-72, 181.

Potential harm to a family is clearly a relevant consideration in decisions to provide aggressive treatment to a defective newborn. (39)

440   The Committee on The Legal and Ethical Aspects of Health Care for Children.   "Comments and Recommendations on the 'Infant Doe' Proposed Regulations," LAW MED HEALTH CARE 11(5) (October 1983). 203-9, 213.

The proposed regulations for reporting discrimination against handicapped infants are discussed by the committee. The committee expresses concerns about the efficacy of this approach. (23)

441   Weir, R.F.   SELECTIVE NONTREATMENT OF HANDICAPPED NEWBORNS: MORAL DILEMMAS IN NEONATAL MEDICINE.   New York: Oxford University Press, 1984.

Aimed primarily at a physician audience but in sections dealing with pediatrician's opinion, different views are presented on how severely disabled newborns should be treated. Argues that the field is rapidly changing and neither the government rules nor this book will be the final word on the subject and argues we need to find new ways to deal with an increasingly complex problem.

442   Zachary, R.   "The Severely Handicapped Newborn: To 'Let Live' or 'Cause to Die'," NURS MIRROR 152 (April 30, 1981): 26-27.

Deals with newborns afflicted with spina bidfida. Surgeon author indicates that administration of large doses of sedatives and "feeding on demand" is to accomplish the death of the baby. Holds that senior nurses should not be allowed to involve themselves or staff in such infanticide. (0)

See: 828, 840, 841, 842, 843, 847, 848, 852, 855, 856, 859, 862, 1969.

Death and Dying

443   Annas, G.J. "Nurses and the Death Penalty," NURS LAW AND
      ETHICS 1 (May 1980): 3.

      Discusses whether nurses should participate in execution
      by lethal injection. Argues that they legally could, but
      that nurses should lead the fight to abolish the death
      penalty once and for all. (4)

444   Aroskar, M.A. "Institutional Ethics Committees and Nursing
      Administration," NURS ECON 2(2) (March/April 1984): 130-36.

      Institutional ethics committees are a relatively new phe-
      nomenon in health care institutions. Nursing administration
      is in a crucial position to advocate for development and
      evaluation of these committees as one institutional response
      to complex ethical issues and questions in patient care and
      policymaking. (12)

445   Backer, B.A., N. Hannon and N.A. Russell. DEATH AND DYING:
      INDIVIDUALS AND INSTITUTIONS. New York: John Wiley & Sons,
      1982.

      A textbook providing an integration of multidisciplinary
      theories and concepts on death, dying, and bereavement with
      an orientation toward care.

446   Bandman, E.L. and B. Bandman. "The Nurse's Role in Protect-
      ing the Patient's Right to Live or Die," ADV NURS SCIENCE
      1 (April 1979): 21-35.

      A survey of different kinds of rights and their applica-
      tion to ethical dilemmas involving the nurse-patient relation-
      ship.

447   Beauchamp, T.L. and S. Perlin (Eds.). ETHICAL ISSUES IN
      DEATH AND DYING. Englewood Cliffs, NJ: Prentice-Hall,
      1978.

      Aimed primarily at a medical audience with no identified
      nurse contributors. Divided into five sections which are
      further divided. Contributors include classical writers as
      Leo Tolstoy and Albert Camus, but mostly current writers.
      Section 1, Definition and Determination of Death, is broken
      down to issues in medicine and issues in the law; Section 2
      deals with suicide; Section 3 with rights of dying patient;
      Section 4 with euthanasia and natural death. There is a
      bibliography of other books on the topic at the end of each
      section and a comprehensive bibliography at the end.

448   Berg, D.L. and C. Isler. "The Right to Die Dilemma: Where
      Do You Fit In?," RN 40 (August 1977): 48-55.

Discussion of the role of the nurse and others in the decision whether to use respiratory support systems on dying
patients and brain-damaged patients. A number of nurses are
interviewed. (0)

449 Bernstein, A.H. "Incompetent's Right to Die: Who Decides?,"
     HOSPITALS (September 1, 1979): 39.

The author presents the dilemma of life-prolonging treatment in the case of the incompetent patient. A number of
case examples are provided. (0)

450 Castledine, G. "The Game of Life (and Death)," NURS MIRROR
     150 (April 24, 1980): 12.

Author argues that legalization of voluntary mercy killing
opens up dangerous abuses, such as the possibility of an
elderly person being persuaded by hard-hearted relatives to
end his/her life. (0)

451 Cawley, M.A. "Euthanasia: Should It Be a Choice?," AM J
     NURS 77 (May 1977): 859-61.

Author presents a case analysis of a dying woman refusing
treatment. Article favors passive euthanasia. (4)

452 Chee, M. "A Child's Right to Die," MCN 7 (March-April 1982):
     81, 84, 88.

A nurse's reaction to the decision of the parents of a
four year old with a progressive neuro-muscular disorder
and pneumonia to decline the use of a respirator.

453 Christensen, R.A. "When Each Extra Day Counts," AM J NURS
     77 (May 1977): 853.

The author argues that the resuscitation of a woman with
terminal leukemia is justified when her children request
it. (13)

454 Collins, V.J. "The Right to Die: Limits of Medical Respon-
     sibility in Prolonging Life," AANA J 41 (February 1973):
     27-36.

Emphasizes that it is the physician's responsibility to
determine when death occurs and whether life is to be pro-
longed. The physician "must remain aloof" from economic,
social, family, emotional, legal, and religious issues and
pursue his art. (Historically important since it appeared
in a nursing journal, and reports physicians' views in
1973.) (12)

455 Cushing, M. "Treatment Beyond Death," AM J NURS 81 (August
     1981): 1527-28.

Discusses Uniform Determination of Death Act and legal
definitions of death. (8)

456   Davis, P.S.   "Medico-Legal Considerations and the Quality
      of Life: Defining Death," TOP CLIN NURS 3 (October 1981):
      79-85.

      Nursing implications of definition of death and quality
      of life. (22)

457   Doudera, A.E. and J.D. Peters.   LEGAL AND ETHICAL ASPECTS
      OF TREATING CRITICALLY AND TERMINALLY ILL PATIENTS.   Ann
      Arbor, MI.:   AUPHA Press, 1982.

      Legal and ethical issues addressed as they relate to a
      variety of critically ill patients.   Landmark cases (Sacke-
      wicz, Brother Fox, Quinlan, etc.) discussed.   Issues
      addressed by thirty-one experts from law, medicine, nursing,
      hospital administration, and public health.

458   Ethics Committee of the American Academy of Neurology.
      "Uniform Definition of Death Act," CONNECTICUT MEDICINE
      46 (May 1982): 259-60.

      Academy endorsed the AMA uniform definition of death. (11)

459   Fletcher, J.   "Ethics and Euthanasia," AM J NURS 73 (April
      1973): 670-75.

      The originator of the term "situational ethics" argues for
      moral permissibility of suicide and mercy killing for reasons
      of compassion. (0)   Note: Excerpts from a chapter in Robert
      H. Williams book ETHICS AND EUTHANASIA.

460   Fromer, M.J.   "The Suicidal Client: Philosophical Basis for
      Nursing Intervention," NURS LAW AND ETHICS 2 (January
      1981): 1-3, 6, 8.

      Author believes that nursing's commitment to client auton-
      omy may mean that nurses should not interfere with autonomous
      suicides. (10)

461   Gadow, S.   "Caring for the Dying: Advocacy or Paternalism?,"
      DEATH EDUCATION 3 (1980): 387-98.

      Instead of traditional paternalism, existentialism advocacy
      is presented as a view toward dying.   Distinction between
      naturalistic, religious, and existential views are described.
      (3)

462   Gargaro, W.J.   "Criminal Prosecution for the Discontinuance
      of Life Support-Part I," CANCER NURS 6 (April 1983): 145-
      46; Part II, CANCER NURS 6 (June 1983): 227-28.

Author is counsel for chief of surgery who is charged with murdering Clarence Herber by discontinuing IVs and hydration. Summary of case and argumentation that action was allowing patient to die with dignity.

463 Gendrop, S.C. "The Order: No Code," LINACRE QUARTERLY 44 (November 1977): 312-19.

Order not to resuscitate, caring for no code patients, and survey responses from thirty-five nurses in a Boston hospital to "no code." (15)

464 Golub, S. and M. Reznikoff. "Attitudes Towards Death: A Comparison of Nursing Students and Graduate Nurses," NURS RES 20(6) (1971): 503-6.

Differences in student and graduate nurse opinions on death were studied. Graduates reported more concern for moral and ethical consideration for the dying (as opposed to prolonging life at all costs), more favorable attitudes towards autopsies, and more focus on the psychological factors associated with death. (22)

465 Greenlaw, J. "Orders Not to Resuscitate: Dilemma for Acute Care as Well as Long Term Care Facilities," LAW MED HEALTH CARE 10(1) (February 1982): 29-31, 45.

DNR (do not resuscitate) orders create legal and ethical dilemmas for nurses, particularly if they are unwritten. DNR orders can be legal if they are in accordance with appropriate guidelines and procedures. (14)

466 Greenstein, L.R. "Bioethics: Occupational Therapy Attitudes Toward the Prolongation of Life," AM J OCCUPATIONAL THERAPY 31 (February 1977): 77-80.

Examines the attitudes of occupational therapists. (24)

467 Gunther, J. DEATH BE NOT PROUD: A MEMOIR. New York: Harper, 1949.

A personal memoir on the death of a child from a fatal disease. Coping mechanisms which proved helpful are mentioned.

468 Harbin, R.E. "Death, Euthanasia and Parental Consent," PED NURS 2 (July-August 1976): 26-28.

Brief overview of issues involved in treatment of defective newborns. Emphasizes quality of life as an issue. (9)

469 Horan, D.J. and D. Mall. DEATH, DYING AND EUTHANASIA. Washington, D.C.: University Publications of America, Inc., 1977.

Thirty-five articles focused on issues related to death, the right to live, and the right to die.

470 Horsley, J.E. "Pulling the Plug Isn't Easy--Explaining It Is Even Harder," RN 43 (December 1980): 69-70, 72, 74.

Nurse's responsibility when pulling the plug discussed by means of a fictional composite case.(0)

471 _____. "When Pulling the Plug Spells Murder," RN 44 (October 1981): 71-72, 74, 76.

Living wills, assisting suicide, allowing to die, withholding treatment, and legal liability of nurses in light of recent cases. (7)

472 Huttman, B.R. "No Code?, Slow Code?, Show Code?," AM J NURS 82(1) (January 1982): 133-36.

Case studies and dilemmas facing nurses. Emphasizes the need for better public education. (0)

473 _____. "The Bitter End," AM J NURS 84(11) (November 1984): 1366-67.

Case discussed; nurse insisted that patient be resuscitated. (0)

474 Johnson, P. "Just What Is Life?," NURSING 76 (June 1976): 28-29.

Discusses favorably a case of passive euthanasia. (0)

475 _____. "The Gray Areas--Who Decides?," AM J NURS 77 (1977): 856-58.

Describes three cases of passive euthanasia.(0)

476 Kasley, V. "As Life Ebbs," AM J NURS 38 (November 1938): 1191-98.

On the physical and psychological comfort of dying patients. An almost pioneering discussion of truthtelling for nurses.

477 Keane, M. "Implication of Euthanasia--A Nursing Perspective," J NY STATE NURSES ASSOC 8(1) (March 1977): 15-18.

A general overview. (3)

478 Kraus, A.S. "Patients Who Want To Die," CANADIAN FAMILY PHYSICIAN 23 (November 1977): 1353-55, 1357-58.

Survey of attitudes of Ontario physicians, nurses, nursing students, and advanced medical students about their attitudes of dying patients and patients who want to die.

479 Kubler-Ross, E. ON DEATH AND DYING. New York: Macmillan,
     1970, many editions.

     The standard classic about death and dying which forced a
     rethinking of the whole topic. The book has twelve chapters
     and a bibliography.

480 _____. "Dying with Dignity," CAN NURSE 67(October
     1971): 31-35.

     Summarizes her stages of dying. (0)

481 Lamerton, R. "The Care of the Dying: A Specialty," NURS
     TIMES 74 (1978): 436.

     Problem is that nurses do not stand up for rights of
     patients, thus the euthanasia "lobby stokes its sinister
     fire." (2)

482 Marcinek, M.A. "The Right to Die: In Support of Passive
     Euthanasia," NURS FORUM 20(2) (1981): 129-37.

     Many of the lives that technology allows us to perpetuate
     are "without quality or without any of the characteristics
     of human life" as this is generally defined. (17)

483 McCarthy, D.G. "Euthanasia: Meaning and Challenge." ETHICAL
     ISSUES IN NURSING: PROCEEDINGS. St. Louis: Catholic Hospi-
     tal Association, 1976, pp. 55-64.

     Catholic perspective.

484 Olson, J. "To Treat or To Allow To Die: An Ethical Dilemma
     in Gerontological Nursing," J GERONTOL NURS 7 (March 1981):
     141-44, 147.

     The case of a ninety-four year old man who is a cardiac
     case is used as an example. (8)

485 "Optimum Care For Hopelessly Ill Patients: A Report of the
     Critical Care Committee of the Massachusetts General Hos-
     pital," SUPERVISOR NURSE 10 (August 1979): 21-22, 25.

     Presents a patient care classification system. (16)

486 Paris, J.J. "Comfort Measures Only for 'DNR' Orders." CON-
     NECTICUT MEDICINE 46 (April 1982): 195-99.

     Improved technology of resuscitation creates problems for
     terminal patients. Discussion. (11)

487 Patey, E.H. "To Care--Or To Kill?," NURS MIRROR 141
     (October 2, 1975): 40-41.

     Included because it comments on the Church of England's
     Study on Euthanasia entitled "On Dying Well." (0)

488   Popoff, D. et al.   "What Are Your Feelings About Death and
      Dying?, Part I," NURSING 75 (August 1975): 15-24; Part II
      (September 1975): 55-62; Part III (October 1975): 39-50.

      Survey of returns from 15,430 nurses about attitudes and
      issues concerning death and dying; also includes information
      on abortion, rights of fetus, passive euthanasia, et al. (0)

489   Rabkin, M.T., G. Gillerman and N.R. Rice.   "Orders Not to
      Resuscitate," SUPERVISOR NURSE 10 (August 1979): 26, 29-30.

      Hospitals urged to consider and implement policies whereby
      orders not to resuscitate may be considered and implemented.
      (0)

490   Ramsey, P. (Ed.).   ETHICS AT THE EDGES OF LIFE: MEDICAL AND
      LEGAL INTERACTION.   New Haven: Yale University Press, 1978.

      Ethical dilemmas related to dying, euthanasia, abortion,
      and newborn problems are discussed.   Text based on Bampton
      lectures which focus on theological questions.

491   "Right to Die," CONNECTICUT MEDICINE 46 (April 1982): 201-5.

      Reviews Quinlan, Belchertown State, Dennerstein and
      Perlmutter cases. (0)

492   Robbins, D.   "Rethinking Ethics for the Incompetent
      Patient," JEN 7 (September-October 1981): 223-24.

      Recent legal decision concerning heroic and other measures
      for incompetents.

493   Russell, O.R.   FREEDOM TO DIE: MORAL AND LEGAL ASPECTS OF
      EUTHANASIA.   New York: Human Sciences Press, 1975.

      An argument for the right of each individual to choose
      whether to live or die, urging legislation to prevent both
      needless suffering and clandestine action.   The author be-
      lieves that there is a time when it should be legally per-
      missable for a physician to end hopeless suffering or pro-
      vide means whereby a patient may do so, but only in accor-
      dance with safeguarding laws which are spelled out.
      Includes a summary of past attitudes on euthanasia.   Among
      appendices is an example of living wills and sample bills.

494   Russell, R.   "Death Without Dignity: This Atrocity Forced
      Me From Nursing," RN 44 (June 1981): 87.

      Describes the case of a terminal cancer patient who wanted
      to be off a respirator but was placed in restraints instead.
      (0)

495   Sandroff, R.   "Is It Right?...To Turn Off Life Support...To
      Keep A Body Alive for Its Organs?...To Give Illegal Nar-
      cotics to the Dying?," RN 43 (December 1980): 24-27, 106,
      108, 110.

      A survey of 12,500 nurses on the above questions. (0)

496   Shepard, M.W.   "This I Believe...About Questioning the
      Right to Die," NURS OUTLOOK 16 (October 1968): 22-25.

      Argues for mercy killing because of compassion and because
      evolution erodes any religious duty to preserve life.   There
      is a reply by Armiger listed in this bibliography. (16)

497   Smith, L.   "Is Useless Treatment Ever Ethical?," NURS LIFE
      3 (May-June 1983): 54-55.

      Gives readers response on whether or not to honor a request
      by a family that a dying patient receive vitamin therapy. (0)

498   Spevlin, G.   "Should a 'No Code' Be A Death Sentence?," RN
      44 (November 1981): 94.

      Calls for a "no code" committee which would approve "no
      code" designation and argues that no physician should
      decide on his/her own on "no code." (0)

499   Storlie, F.J. and others.   "Caring for A Patient Who Wants
      To Die: Should You Let Her?," NURSING 80 (February
      1980): 50-53.

      This is a panel discussion about a patient who wants to
      die. (10)

500   Wallace, S.E. and A. Eser.   SUICIDE AND EUTHANASIA.   Knox-
      ville, TN.: University of Tennessee Press, 1981.

      Papers by philosopher and sociologists on the rights of
      persons to commit suicide or be allowed voluntary euthan-
      asia.

501   Walton, D.N.   ETHICS OF WITHDRAWAL OF LIFE SUPPORT SYSTEMS:
      CASE STUDIES ON DECISION MAKING IN INTENSIVE CARE.   West-
      port, CT.: Greenwood Press, 1983.

      Walton, a physician, distinguishes four groups or kinds
      of decision: declaring the patient dead, when the patient
      wishes heroic measures discontinued, when the family makes
      that decision, and when the physician does.

502   Weber, L.J.   "Ethics and Euthanasia: Another View," AM J
      NURS 73 (July 1973): 1228-31.

      Author replies to Fletcher's article and holds that allow-
      ing patients to die is permissable but rejects direct kill-
      ing. (4)

503 Weir, R.F. (Ed.). ETHICAL ISSUES IN DEATH AND DYING. New
     York: Columbia University Press, 1977.

     Twenty-six articles by authors from life sciences, medi-
     cine, and philosophy focused on truth telling versus protect-
     ing, right to life versus right to die, and the determina-
     tion of death.

504 Whiteworth, R.A. "The Ethics of Suicide Intervention: Seen
     As A Nursing Problem," PSYCH NURS 23 (January-February-
     March 1982): 12-14.

     Holds that society has a moral right to intervene in
     suicide attempts.

505 Will, G.F. "A Trip Toward Death," NEWSWEEK (August 31,
     1981): 72.

     Describes ethical dilemma of giving or withholding treat-
     ment to child with Down's syndrome. (0)

506 Winger, C., F.T. Kapp and R.C. Yeaworth. "Attitudes Toward
     Euthanasia," J MED ETHICS 3 (March 1977): 18-25.

     Examines attitudes toward euthanasia of first year nursing
     students, senior nursing students, registered nurses, first
     year medical students, and college students in general and
     compares them. (17)

     See 844.

Ethics and Nursing Specialties

507 Aroskar, M.A. "Ethical Issues in Community Health Nursing,"
     NURS CLIN NORTH AM 14 (1979): 35-44.

     Ethical dilemmas of community health nurses differ from
     those of other nurses since they have to allocate a scarce
     resource to three needy competency groups: the elderly, the
     deinstitutionalized mentally retarded, and unwed pregnant
     teenagers. Looks at moral problems involved. (5)

508 Ashworth, P. "Ethics in the Intensive Care Therapy Unit,"
     NURS MIRROR 139 (November 14, 1974): 57-61, 63.

     Application of the ICN code to ethical issues in the
     intensive care therapy unit. Issues include prolonging
     life, organ transplant, and attempted suicide. (11)

509 Chavigny, K.H. and A. Helm. "Ethical Dilemmas and the
     Practice of Infection Control," LAW MED HEALTH CARE 10(4)
     (September 1982): 168-71, 174.

     Medical records are significant in different ways to
     diverse groups of individuals. Nurses should document ques-

tionable care but it is best if hospitals have ways of documenting this. Only an up to date record of patient care
protects all concerned. (18)

510   Cohn, S. "The Living Will From the Nurse's Perspective,"
      LAW MED HEALTH CARE 11 (June 1983): 121-24, 136.

      In spite of some legal action, the living will still
      poses basic ethical issues and staff and nurses must be
      able to explain why or why they will not comply. (45)

511   Creighton, H. "Withdrawal from Life Support Systems,"
      SUPERVISOR NURSE 11 (December 1980): 52-54.

      The Dinnerstein, Saikewicz and Brother Fox cases and dis-
      cussion of legal decisions concerning withdrawal of life
      support systems for terminally ill incompetents. (17)

512   Cushing, M. "The Implications of Withdrawing Nutritional
      Devices," AM J NURS 84(2) (February 1984): 191-5.

      Discusses recent California and New Jersey court cases
      and emphasizes the importance of guidelines. (6)

513   Davis, A.J. "Ethics Rounds With Intensive Care Nurses,"
      NURS CLIN NORTH AM 14 (1979): 45-55.

      Issues such as definitions of death, euthanasia, et al.
      of concern to intensive care nurses. (16)

514   _____. "To Make Live or Let Die," AM J NURS 81 (March
      1981): 582.

      Life support systems and patient preferences.(0)

515   Donovan, C.T. "Ethical Issues in Cancer Nursing: II.
      Impediments to Ethical Nursing Practice," ONCOL NURS
      FORUM 7 (Fall 1980): 40-42.

      Recommends the establishment of a nursing ethics committee
      and argues that nurses have to be involved in decision
      making. (2)

516   Drane, J.F. "Ethics and Nurse Anesthetists: Part I," AANA
      J 51 (February 1983): 48-54; Part II, AANA J 51 (April
      1983): 159-66.

      Part I includes a general description of medical ethics
      and what an ethicitist working with health care profes-
      sionals can do. (10) Part II offers guidelines for deci-
      sion making by nurse anesthetists. (15)

517   Elsea, S.J. and P.A. Miya. "Refusal of Blood--An Ethical
      Issue," MCN 6 (November-December 1981): 379-80, 384,
      386-87.

The case of a Jehovah's Witness who refused blood transfusions. (9)

518   Fry, S.T.   "Dilemma in Community Health Ethics," NURS OUT-
      LOOK 31 (May-June 1983): 176-79.

      Author finds a moral tension between the "individualistic"
      emphasis of ANA Code for Nurses and the need for group
      decision and principle of beneficence found in community
      health nursing. (10)

519   Furrow, B.R.   "Diminished Lives and Malpractice: Courts
      Stalled in Transition," LAW MED HEALTH CARE 10(3) (June
      1982): 100-107, 114.

      A summary of some recent cases on "diminished life."
      Two types "wrongful life" suits brought by parents on behalf
      of their child, who in most cases, is born suffering from
      mental or physical defects which could have been detected
      by genetic screening, and "wrongful births" suits, brought
      by parents of a child born as a result of defendant's negli-
      gence. Courts are divided on the first. (78)

520   Gadow, S.   "Ethical Issues in Cancer Nursing: IV. A Model
      for Ethical Decision Making," ONCOL NURS FORUM 7 (Fall
      1980): 44-47.

      Existential advocacy is presented as a philosophy of nurs-
      ing along with its implications. (1)

521   Greenlaw, J.   "Confidentiality--The Psychotherapist's Neme-
      sis," NURS LAW AND ETHICS 1 (November 1980): 5, 8.

      Discussion of Tarasoff and other cases which required
      therapist to warn third parties of threatened harm. (3)

522   Klutas, E.M.   "Confidentiality of Medical Information,"
      OCCUP HEALTH NURS 25 (April 1977): 14-17.

      Dilemmas of occupational health nurses in dealing with
      confidentiality. (6)

523   Lawrence, J.A. and E.H. Farr.   "The 'Nurse Should Consider'
      Critical Care Ethical Issues," J ADV NURS 7 (1982):
      223-29.

      Reports results of a survey given to nurses about a hypo-
      thetical dilemma dealing with the resuscitation of an inten-
      sive care patient. Concludes that differences in opinion
      provide evidence of confusion about ethical issues. (20)

524   Lestz, P.   "A Committee to Decide the Quality of Life,"
      AM J NURS 77 (May 1977): 862-64.

      Uses a fictitious case to illustrate difficulties in
      deciding issues dealing with quality of life. (0)

525 Levine, M.E. "The Ethics of Computer Technology in Health
     Care," NURS FORUM 19 (1980): 193-98.

     Confidentiality of information and depersonalization. (2)

526 Maloney, E.M. "Doctors, Nurses, and Drugs: Notes on the
     Meaning and Ethics of Administration." ETHICAL PROBLEMS
     IN THE NURSE-PATIENT RELATIONSHIP. Edited by C.P. Murphy
     and H. Hunter. Boston: Allyn and Bacon, 1983, pp. 153-64.

     Discussion of drug errors,placebos, and pain management
     and the ethical issues that arise.

527 Mittleman, R., H.S. Goldberg and D.M. Waksman. "Preserving
     Evidence in the Emergency Department," AM J NURS 83(12)
     December 1983): 1652-56.

     Next to saving patient is proper handling of evidence and
     full documentation of what the victim looked like on arrival.
     (3)

528 Penticuff, J.H. "Resolving Ethical Dilemmas in Critical
     Care," DIMENS CRIT CARE NURS 1 (January-February 1982):
     22-27.

     Identifying and resolving ethical dilemmas in critical
     care. (4)

529 Robbins, D.A. LEGAL AND ETHICAL ISSUES IN CANCER CARE IN
     THE UNITED STATES. Springfield, IL.: Charles C. Thomas,
     1983.

     Legal and ethical issues involved in cancer care, cover-
     ing such areas as life support, smoking, hospital licensure
     and accreditation, and palliative care. Patient's rights
     to refuse treatment is discussed, including the Quinlan,
     Saidewicz, Dinnerstein, Spring and Richner cases.

530 Spross, J. "Ethical Issues in Cancer Nursing: III, The
     ANA's Human Rights Guidelines for Nurses in Clinical and
     Other Research," ONCOL NURS FORUM 7 (Fall 1980): 42-44.

     Discusses ANA's human rights guidelines. (4)

531 Steuer, K., K.E. Murphy and M.A. Aroskar. "Dilemmas in
     Practice: The Choice," AM J NURS 82(11) (November 1982):
     1767-70.

     Two personal experiences about no code patients and nurs-
     ing reaction with a comment by Mila Ann Aroskar dealing
     with what a nurse can do. Cases deal with conflict between
     patient and physician with nurse in middle. (0)

532 Thompson, H.O. and J.E. Beebe. "Nurse-Midwifery and Ethics
     ...A Beginning," J NURSE MIDWIFE 21 (Winter 1976): 7-11.

Gives background to ethical issues in abortion, contraception, and sterilization. (20)

533   Thompson, H.S. "Ethics in Private Practice," AM J NURS 6
(1905): 163-66.

Historically important although the prescription essentially advises be loyal to the physician and do not gossip.

534   Whitman, H. "Ethical Issues in Cancer Nursing: I, Defining
the Issues," ONCOL NURS FORUM 7 (Fall 1980): 37-40.

Summary of issues which arise in the care of cancer
patients. (8)

535   Yeaworth, R.C. "The Agonizing Decisions in Mental Retardation," AM J NURS 77 (May 1977): 864-67.

Includes such ethical issues as allocation of resources
and coercion. Author wants nurses to take an informed
stand on such issues. (13)

Ethics and Mental Illness

536   Curtin, L. "Clarity and Freedom: Ethical Issues in Mental
Health," ISSUES MENT HEALTH NURS 2 (1979): 102-8.

Problems involving defining mental health and illness are
discussed as well as the morality of certain behavior control
technologies. (12)

537   Davis, A.J. "The Ethics of Behavior Control," PSYCHIATRIC
NURS 21 (March-April 1980): 12-18.

Behavior control issues and the role of the nurse.

538   Doudera, A.E. and J.P. Swazey. REFUSING TREATMENT IN MENTAL
HEALTH INSTITUTIONS--VALUES IN CONFLICT. Ann Arbor, MI.:
AUPHA Press, 1982.

Professionals from medicine, law, psychiatry, and policy
address the rights of mental health patients to participate
in their own treatment, the right to refuse treatment, the
responsibilities of clinicians to protect patient rights
while ensuring proper treatment and competency, and the role
of law in mental health policy making. Recent federal court
cases involving patient rights to refuse treatment, current
thinking on competency and commitment, and health practitioners' responsibilities and liabilities are reviewed.

539   Kjervik, D.K. "The Psychiatric Nurse's Duty to Warn Potential Victims of Homicidal Psychotherapy Outpatients," LAW
MED HEALTH CARE 9 (December 1981): 11-16, 39.

Argues for duty of nurses to warn potential victims. (78)

540 Lamerton, R. "Vegetables?," NURS TIMES 70 (August 1974):
     1184-85.

     Criticizes term "vegetables" as degrading and as insidi-
     ously affecting nursing attitudes. (5)

541 Norberg, A., B. Norberg and G. Bexell. "Ethical Problems
     in Feeding Patients with Advanced Dementia," BRITISH MED
     J 281 (1980): 847-48.

     The problem posed is when patients deteriorate until spoon
     feeding is no longer safe or possible, and forced feeding
     by intubation or starvation are the alternatives. Brief
     examination of conflicting demands but no final answer given.

542 Parson, L. "Why ECT is an Ethical Issue," NURS TIMES 78
     (March 3, 1982): 352.

     Argues that electroconvulsive treatment is an ethical
     issue and why he refuses to participate in its administra-
     tion. (2)

543 Peplau, H.E. "The Right to Change Behavior: Rights of the
     Mentally Ill." BIOETHICS AND HUMAN RIGHTS. Edited by
     E.L. Bandman and B. Bandman. Boston: Little Brown, 1978,
     pp. 207-212.

     Discusses concept of mental illness and the right to
     treatment or refuse treatment.

544 Schrock, R.A. "The Rights of Mental Patients," NURS TIMES
     76 (May 15, 1980): 884-87.

     Argues that laws never fully protect patients and nurses
     have to become proficient in implementing laws to afford
     greatest protection. (15)

545 Schulkin, J. and R. Neville. "Responsibility, Rehabilita-
     tion, and Drugs: Health Care Dilemmas." ETHICAL PROBLEMS
     IN THE NURSE-PATIENT RELATIONSHIP. Edited by C.P. Murphy
     and H. Hunter. Boston: Allyn and Bacon, 1983, pp. 167-83.

     The use of drugs on mental patients and in drug rehabili-
     tation programs and the ethical issues involved.

546 Siantz, M.L. and L. deLeon. "Human Values in Determining
     the Fate of Persons with Mental Retardation," NURS CLIN
     NORTH AM 14 (1979): 57-67.

     Discussion of mental retardation in general and how value
     judgment affect nursing decisions. Also discussed involun-
     tary sterilization. (33)

547 Simpson, R. "Confidentiality in Psychiatric Nursing," NURS
     TIMES 76 (May 8, 1980): 835-36.

Nurse should be honest in dealing with psychiatric
patients in order to foster trust. (9)

Sexuality, Reproduction, Abortion

548 Allen, D.V. "Factors to Consider in Staffing an Abortion
     Service Facility," J NURS ADM 4 (July-August 1974): 22-27.

     From collected information and their own surveys of nurs-
     ing attitudes toward abortion, the authors make suggestions
     concerning staffing such a service facility. (24)

549 Baron, C.H. "If You Prick Us, Do We Not Bleed?: Of Shylock,
     Fetuses, and the Concept of Person in the Law," LAW MED
     HEALTH CARE 11(2) (April 1983): 52-63, 81.

     Abortion issues, decision and laws reviewed. Concept of
     personhood analyzed. (88)

550 Batchelor, E., Jr. (Ed.). ABORTION: THE MORAL ISSUES. New
     York: The Pilgrim Press, 1982.

     Twenty essays by theologians and ethicists, examining the
     moral, ethical, and social aspects of the debate over abor-
     tion. The essays examine such topics as the voice of women
     in the debate, the rules for the debate, various ecumenical
     views of abortion, and abortion as a socioethic issue.

551 Bayles, M.D. REPRODUCTIVE ETHICS. Englewood Cliffs, NJ:
     Prentice-Hall, 1984.

     Chapters on contraception, genetic choice, abortion,
     childbirth, defective newborns, and other issues. Pro and
     con discussion given; author has preference but indicates
     alternatives.

552 Bell, S. "Is Abortion Morally Justifiable?," NURS FORUM
     20(3) (1981): 288-95.

     The author believes the key issue is whether the unborn
     child is a person and argues that an unborn child fails
     certain criteria for personhood and therefore "an unborn
     child should not be granted all the rights and protections
     due persons." (8)

553 Boyle, J.F. "Statement of the American Medical Association
     to the Subcommittee on Separation of Powers, Judiciary
     Committee, U.S. Senate: Testimony on Human Life and Con-
     ception," CONNECTICUT MEDICINE 46 (June 1982): 343-44.

     Raises problems related to proposed constitutional amend-
     ment declaring that human life begins at conception. (0)

554   Brown, N., D.J. Thompson, R.B. Bulger and E.H. Laws. "How
      Do Nurses Feel About Euthanasia and Abortion?," AM J NURS
      71 (July 1971): 1413-16.

      A survey of 108 nurses. (5)

555   Culliton, B.J. "Genetic Screening: States May Be Writing
      the Wrong Kind of Laws," SCIENCE 191(5) (March 1976):
      926-29.

      A survey of genetic screening programs. In 1976 fourteen
      states had programs for screening newborns for diseases other
      than PKU, and twelve others were interested in broadening
      them. Lists some problem areas which could be screened. (0)

556   Curtin, L.L. and J.A. Petrick. "Reproductive Manipulation:
      Technical Advances, Options and Ethical Ramifications,"
      NURS FORUM 16 (1977): 6-25.

      Discusses ethical issues and moral implications of in
      vitro fertilization, surrogate mothers, and articial wombs.
      (53)

557   Davis, A.J. "Competing Ethical Claims in Abortion," AM J
      NURS 80 (July 1980): 1359.

      Dealing with nurses morally opposed to abortion. (2)

558   Edelwich, J. and A. Brodsky. SEXUAL DILEMMAS FOR THE HELP-
      ING PROFESSIONAL. New York: Brumer/Mazel Publishing, 1982.

      This book is designed to help the professional deal with
      the sexual feelings that can rise in the intimate relation-
      ship between the helping professional and the patient/client.
      The topics covered include seduction, power, opportunity and
      vulnerability, morality, when "referral out" should be a
      solution, relationships among the staff, and legal consid-
      erations.

559   Elder, R.G. "Attitudes of Senior Nursing Students Toward
      the 1973 Supreme Court Decision on Abortion," JOGN NURS
      4 (July/August 1975): 46-54.

      A survey of 264 senior nursing students right after
      Supreme Court decision. Can be used for comparative atti-
      tudes. (8)

560   Fegan, W.A. "Assisting at Abortions: Can You Really Say
      No?," RN 45 (June 1982): 71.

      Reports the case of a nurse who sued the hospital and won
      for demoting her and putting her on half time because of her
      refusal to participate in abortions. (0)

561   Frohock, F.M. ABORTION: A CASE STUDY IN LAW AND MORALS.
      Westport, CT.: Greenwood Press, 1983.

Explains legal, political and experimental aspects of
abortion and discusses possible resolutions of the pro-life
and pro-choice controversy. The book reproduces interviews
to create a simulated dialogue between advocates of each
position. Areas where the two ideologies tend to converge
are identified.

562   Fromer, M.J. "Abortion Ethics," NURS OUTLOOK 30 (April
       1982): 234-40.

       History, legal and moral issue concerning abortion.
       Author favors legal abortions. (9)

563   _____. ETHICAL ISSUES IN SEXUALITY AND REPRODUCTION.
       St. Louis: C.V. Mosby Co., 1983.

       Author, a nurse-philosopher, discusses current issues in
       sexuality and reproduction, including prenatal diagnosis,
       fetal research, genetics, contraception, abortion, and
       homosexuality.

564   Glantz, L.H. "Limiting State Regulation of Reproductive
       Decisions," AM J PUBLIC HEALTH 74(2) (February 1984):
       168-69.

       State challenges to the rights of women for first tri-
       mester abortions established by Roe v Wade in 1973 traced.
       (5)

565   Hendershot, G.E. and J.W. Grim. "Abortion Attitudes Among
       Nurses and Social Workers," AM J PUBLIC HEALTH 64(5)
       (1974): 438-41.

       Examines attitudes towards abortion among samples of
       nurses and social workers. Social workers reported more
       liberal attitudes towards abortion than nurses. (14)

566   Lenow, J.L. "The Fetus as a Patient: Emerging Rights as a
       Person," AM J LAW MED 9 (Spring 1983): 1-29.

       Deals primarily with legal issues, not ethical issues but
       has discussion of legal rights of fetus which has ethical
       implications. Primarily concerned with fetal surgery. (150)

567   Malter, S. "Genetic Counseling: A Responsibility of Health-
       Care Professionals," NURS FORUM 26 (1977): 26-35.

       Ethical implication of reproductive technology. Includes
       a brief historical survey of eugenics.

568   Matheson, H.L.V. "Where Does the Court Stand on Abortion
       and Parental Notification?," AM UNIVERSITY LAW REV 31
       (Winter 1982): 431-70.

       Summary of law cases up to 1982.

569 Moraczewski, A.S. (Ed.). GENETIC MEDICINE AND ENGINEERING:
     ETHICAL AND SOCIAL DIMENSIONS. St. Louis, MO.: The
     Catholic Health Association of the United States and The
     Pope John XXIII Medical-Moral Research and Education Cen-
     ter, 1983.

     These essays examine the current status of genetic research
     and practice and its legal and ethical implications for
     decision makers in Catholic health care facilities. The book
     also delineates decision making guidelines relating to genetic
     diagnosis, counseling, and treatment in Catholic facilities,
     and considers the likely effects of future developments in
     this field.

570 Oberle, J. "Can ´Doctors´ Orders´ Include Voluntary Ster-
     ilization?" RN 45 (January 1982): 34-35.

     Readers responding to the dilemma involving a physician
     decision to sterilize a mentally retarded fourteen year old
     during a Caesarean section and justifying it later to the
     parents as medically necessary. (0)

571 Rowley, P.T. "Genetic Screening: Marvel or Menace?," SCIENCE
     225(4658) (July 13, 1984): 138-46.

     Genetic screening is a systematic search in the population
     for persons of certain genotypes. The usual purpose is to
     detect persons who themselves or whose offspring are at a
     risk for genetic diseases or genetically determined suscepti-
     bilities to environmental agents. Discussion of whether
     genetic screening is a marvel about to free us from the
     scourge of genetic disease or a menace about to invade our
     privacy and determine who may reproduce. (72)

572 Sandroff, R. "Is It Right?," RN 43 (October 1980): 25-30.

     A survey of 12,500 nurses on questions about contraception
     and abortion. (3)

573 Schorr, T.M. "Issues of Conscience," AM J NURS 72 (January
     1972): 61.

     An editorial on the care of abortion patients. (0)

574 Sklar, C. "Teenagers, Birth Control and the Nurse," CAN
     NURSE 74 (November 1978): 14-16.

     Law (Canadian) on consent by minors, birth control coun-
     seling, et al. (13)

575 Strickland, O.L "In Vitro Fertilization: Dilemma or Oppor-
     tunity?," ADV NURS SCIENCE 3 (January 1981): 41-51.

     Pro and con discussion of the implications of in vitro
     fertilization. (27)

576 Tooley, M. ABORTION AND INFANTICIDE. Oxford, ENG.: Claren-
     don Press, 1983.

     Argues in favor of abortion on demand and concludes that
     this argument also might lead to infanticide in some cases.
     Book has interesting case studies and examples, and
     presents the case for abortion on demand after examining
     arguments of anti abortionists and others.

577 Tyrer, L.B. and W.A. Granzig. "The New Morality, Ethics,
     and Nursing," JOGN NURS 9 (September 1973): 54-55.

     The 1972 statement on abortion and sterilization by the
     Nurses Association of the American College of Obstetricians
     and Gynecologists is reprinted. Authors argue that ethical
     principles are only opinions.

Aging

578 Agate, J. "Ethical Issues in Geriatric Care: Family Con-
     flicts in the Management of Old People," NURS MIRROR 133
     (November 1971): 40-41.

     The author maintains that "reasonable independence in
     older people is something to be fostered." Problems with
     death and dying are also discussed.(0)

579 Cogliano, J.F. "Clinical Research in the Nursing Home: One
     Viewpoint," J GERONTOL NURS 5 (November-December 1979):
     39-43.

     Reviews the ethical problems of doing nursing research in
     nursing homes. (20)

580 Cox, C.L. "The Choice," AM J NURS 81(9) (September 1981):
     1627-28.

     The personal feelings of a nurse involved in the decision
     of a ninety-five year old to avoid peritoneal dialysis and
     surgery. (0)

581 Davis, A.J. "Ethical Considerations in Gerontological Nurs-
     ing Research," GERIATR NURS 2 (July-August 1981): 269-72.

     Discusses issues especially relevant to research with the
     elderly. (10)

582 Gadow, S. "Advocacy Nursing and New Meanings of Aging,"
     NURS CLIN NORTH AM 14 (1979): 81-91.

     Philosophical aspects of aging and the application of
     existential advocacy model. (4)

583 _____. "Medicine, Ethics, and the Elderly." MEDICAL
ETHICS: A CLINICAL TEXTBOOK AND REFERENCE FOR THE HEALTH
CARE PROFESSIONS. Edited by N. Abrams and M.D. Buckner.
Cambridge, MA.: MIT Press, 1983, pp. 355-61. Reprinted
in GERONTOLOGIST 20 (1980): 680-85.

Examines what moral principles should be. The primary
guide in caring for elderly. (5)

584 Gunter, L.M., L.H. Heckman, D.H. Moser and M.A. Fasana.
"Issues and Ethics in Geriatric Nursing," J GERONTOL NURS
5 (November-December 1979): 15-20.

Summary of papers given by authors at symposium. (5)

585 Lawton, A.H. "Some Consideration of Bioethics in Geriatrics," J FLORIDA MED ASSOC 69 (April 1982): 310-13.

To achieve a working personal bioethics for the practice
of gerontology and geriatrics, each individual professional
person involved has primarily to be a good, honest, concerned, and loving person himself. The bioethics of society
is totally determined by the ethics of the individuals who
compose that society. Equally, the bioethics of gerontology
and geriatrics results from the ideals of those who care for
the aging and the aged. (2)

586 Lentsche, P.M. "Screening of Older Adults--An Ethical
Issue," J GERONTOL NURS 7 (April 1981): 215-16.

Editorial against health screening since it has the potential of becoming an end in itself, serving the system not
the client. (0)

587 Podnieks, E. "Commentary: Abuse of the Elderly," CAN NURSE
79 (May 1983): 34-35.

Subtle ways in which nursing personnel abuse the elderly
along with suggested preventive measures. (3)

588 Wetle, T. "The Ethical Dimensions of Aging," BUSINESS AND
HEALTH 1(1) (November 1983): 7-9.

A brief overview.

589 Wolanin, M.O. "Research and the Aged." PATIENTS, NURSES,
ETHICS. Edited by A.J. Davis and J.C. Krueger. New York:
American Journal of Nursing Co., 1980, pp. 163-74.

Ethical issues involved in doing research with the elderly.

590 Yarling, R.R. "The Sick Aged, The Nursing Profession, and
The Larger Society," J GERONTOL NURS 3 (March-April 1977):
42-51.

Argues that the care of the sick aged is essentially a
moral question because the aged as a group are powerless
and can only make moral claims upon us. (38)

Teaching of Ethical Issues

591   Berkowitz, M.W.   "The Role of Discussion in Ethics Training," TOP CLIN NURS 4 (April 1982): 33-48.

Argues that most attempts to teach ethics or improve the
ethical thinking of nurses are impractical because they do
not pay sufficient attention to theories of moral development. Kohlberg´s theory of moral development is explained.
(70)

592   Fromer, M.J.   "Teaching Ethics by Case Analysis," NURS OUT-
LOOK 28 (October 1980): 604-9.

Moral principles and theories and their application to a
case study. (8)

593   Fry, S.T.   "Ethical Principles in Nursing Education and
Practice: A Missing Link in the Unification Issue," NURS
HEALTH CARE (September 1982): 363-68.

Argues that the organizational structure of nursing over-
looks the moral commitment of nurses to autonomy, beneficence and justice that are fundamental.

594   Gilbert, C.   "The What and How of Ethics Education," TOP
CLIN NURS 4 (April 1982): 49-56.

What ethics education should be and a methodology for
teaching. (15)

595   Hartigan, E.G.   "Teaching Critical Life Issues in Nursing:
A Philosophical Analysis." Ed.D. Dissertation. Loyola
University of Chicago, 1977.

An analysis of the teaching of critical life issues.

596   House, C.S.   "Ethical Conduct in School Practice." ETHICAL
ISSUES IN NURSING PRACTICE AND EDUCATION. New York:
National League for Nursing, 1980, pp. 53-69.

Recommendations from national reports are applied to nursing education.

597   Jones, E.W.   "Advocacy--A Tool for Radical Nursing Curriculum Planners," J NURS EDUC 21 (January 1982): 40-45.

Questions whether nurses are being trained or educated to
act as proper patient advocates. (7)

598   Kellmer, D.M.   "The Teaching of Ethical Decision-Making in
Schools of Nursing," NURS LEADERSH 5 (June 1982): 20-26.

Author argues that the case study method needs to be sup-
plemented by material in philosophy, classical ethics, and
decision making. (28)

599 Ketefian, S. "Critical Thinking, Educational Preparation,
     and Development of Moral Judgment in Selected Groups of
     Practicing Nursing," NURS RES 30(2) (March-April 1981):
     98-103.

     Some seventy-nine nurses were tested in order to determine
     if there was a relationship between critical thinking, edu-
     cational preparation, and levels of moral reasoning. (27)

600 Krawczyk, R. and E. Kudzma. "Ethics: A Matter of Moral
     Development," NURS OUTLOOK 26 (April 1978): 254-57.

     By presenting ethical dilemmas to nursing students, levels
     of moral development improve. (8)

601 LaForet, E.G. and T.P. O'Malley. "Moral and Philosophic
     Problems of Modern Medicine: A Collegiate Program for Pre-
     Medical and Nursing Students," LINACRE QUARTERLY 42
     (May 1975): 123-27.

     A description of a course on bioethics. (3)

602 Langham, P. "Open Forum: On Teaching Ethics to Nurses,"
     NURS FORUM 16 (1977): 220-27.

     A method for teaching ethics that avoids being absolutistic
     and also subjective. (3)

603 Mahon, K.A. and M.D. Fowler. "Moral Development and Clinical
     Decision-Making," NURS CLIN NORTH AM 14 (March 1979): 3-12.

     Examines Kohlberg's theory and looks at its utility in
     facilitating moral development in clinical education of
     nurses. (13)

604 Mitchell, J.J. "The Use of Case Studies in Bioethics
     Courses," J NURS EDUC 20 (November 1981): 31-36.

     Benefits of case study methods in an undergraduate bio-
     ethics course.

605 Munhall, P. "Moral Reasoning Levels of Nursing Students
     and Faculty in a Baccalaureate Nursing Program," IMAGE 12
     (October 1980): 57-61.

     A survey determining whether or not nursing education in-
     creased the student's level of moral reasoning using
     Kohlberg's theoretical framework. (19)

606 Payton, R.J. A BIOETHICAL PROGRAM OF STUDY FOR BACCALAUREATE
     NURSING STUDENTS. A project in lieu of a dissertation.
     University of Northern Colorado, 1978.

607 _____. "A Bioethical Program for Baccalaureate Nursing
       Students." ETHICS IN NURSING PRACTICE AND EDUCATION.
       Kansas City, MO.: American Nurses´ Association, 1980,
       pp. 53-65.

       Four module approach to integrating bioethics into bacca-
       laureate program.

608 Reilly, D.E. "Teaching Values: Theory and Process." TEACH-
       ING AND EVALUATING THE AFFECTIVE DOMAIN IN NURSING PRO-
       GRAMS. Edited by D.E. Reilly. Thorofare, NJ: Charles B.
       Slack, 1978, pp. 31-48.

       Presents a values clarification strategy.

609 _____. (Ed.). TEACHING AND EVALUATING THE AFFECTIVE
       DOMAIN IN NURSING PROGRAMS. Thorofare, NJ: Charles B.
       Slack, 1978.

       A series of essays about teaching and evaluating attitudes,
       beliefs, and values. Some are cited separately in this bib-
       liography.

       Contains: 61, 219, 262, 271, 608.

610 Ryden, M.B. "An Approach to Ethical Decision Making," NURS
       OUTLOOK 26 (November 1978): 705-6.

       Exploring concrete ethical dilemmas with students by
       example. (0)

611 St. Denis, H.A. "Effects of Moral Education Strategies on
       Nursing Students´ Moral Reasoning and Level of Self Actual-
       izing." Ph.D. Dissertation. Catholic University of
       America, 1980.

       Analysis of consequence of teaching moral precepts to
       nursing students.

612 Schilling, M.J. "Ethics in the Curriculum of Schools of
       Nursing in Texas: A Function of Selected Administrative
       and Institutional Characteristics." Ed.D. Dissertation.
       Texas Tech University, 1979.

       Analysis of curriculum content related to ethics.

613 Schoenrock, N.B. "An Analysis of Moral Reasoning Levels
       and the Implications for Nursing Curriculum." Ph.D. Dis-
       sertation. University of Texas at Austin, 1978.

       Moral reasoning as a curriculum component.

614 Smith, E.D. and R.R. Wieczorek. "How Is the Topic of Pro-
     tection of Human Subjects Taught in Undergraduate and
     Graduate Nursing Research Courses?," NURS RES 27
     (September/October 1978): 328-29.

     Explains the use of a case study approach.(0)

615 Stanley, A.T. "Curriculum Considerations." ETHICS IN
     NURSING PRACTICE AND EDUCATION. Kansas City, MO.:
     American Nurses´ Association, 1980, pp. 39-52.

     A discussion of what ethics education content should
     include and how it should be taught.

616 _____. "Ethics As A Component of the Curriculum."
     ETHICAL ISSUES IN NURSING PRACTICE AND EDUCATION. New
     York: National League for Nursing, 1980, pp. 29-52.
     Reprinted in NURS HEALTH CARE 1 (September 1980): 63-72.

     History and current status of ethics in nursing education,
     how it could be incorporated into the curriculum, and who
     should teach it.

617 Steinfels, M.O. "Ethics, Education and Nursing Practice,"
     HASTINGS CENTER REP 7 (August 1977): 20-21.

     Discusses institutional barriers to ethical practice and
     how ethics should be taught. (0)

618 Sternberg, M.J. "Ethics as a Component of Nursing Educa-
     tion," ADV NURS SCIENCE 1 (April 1979): 53-61.

     Who, what, when, and how of teaching nursing ethics. (18)

619 Stewart, I.M. "Some Fundamental Principles in the Teaching
     of Ethics," AM J NURS 22 (1922): 906-13.

     Emotions should not be eliminated but rather harnessed to
     social ideals. Doing good to others might be harmful to
     patients and without consulting with the patients, nurses
     can violate the most fundamental principles of modern ethics.
     Included for historical reasons. Represents a changing
     concept.

620 Vito, K.O. "Moral Development Considerations in Nursing
     Curricula," J NURS EDUC 22 (March 1983): 108-13.

     Application of moral development theory to nursing curri-
     culum theory and suggestions for future directions. (44)

     See: 1531, 1591, 1595, 1726, 1750.

Nursing Research

621 American Nurses' Association. HUMAN RIGHTS GUIDELINES FOR
     NURSES IN CLINICAL AND OTHER RESEARCH. Kansas City, MO.:
     American Nurses' Association, 1975.

     The ANA position in detail.

622 Armiger, B. "Ethics of Nursing Research: Profile, Princi-
     ples, Perspectives," NURS RES 26 (1977): 330-36.

     A "classic article" on the development of the nursing
     research ethics. (72)

623 Block, D., T.P. Phillips and S.R. Gortner. "Protection of
     Human Research Subjects." PERPECTIVE IN NURSING: SOCIAL
     ISSUES AND TRENDS. Edited by M. Miller and B.C. Flynn.
     St. Louis: C.V. Mosby, 1977, pp. 14-31.

     Brief account of history, guidelines and issues related
     to the protection of human research subjects.

624 Connant, L.H., M.V. Neal and L. Christman. "Readers Response
     to 'Ethical Inquiry in Nursing Research'," NURS FORUM 6
     (1967): 163-77.

     A response to an article by Downs. (9)

625 Corcoran, S. "Should a Service Setting Be Used as a Learn-
     ing Laboratory?, An Ethical Question," NURS OUTLOOK 25
     (December 1977): 771-76.

     After giving arguments for and against, author argues for
     the affirmative conditional upon certain moral constraints.
     (17)

626 Creighton, H. "Legal Concerns of Nursing Research," NURS
     RES 26 (1977): 337-41.

     Codes, regulations, legal cases, and other issues with
     implications for nursing research. (31)

627 Davis, A., J. Benoliel, A. Meleis, A. Mullins and P. Pothier.
     "Ethical Dilemmas and Nursing Research," COMMUN NURS RES
     11 (September 1978): 27-32.

     Research with dying patient, with children, and cross
     culturally is discussed. (4)

628 Davis, A.J. "Ethical Principles of Research." PATIENTS,
     NURSES, ETHICS. Edited by A.J. Davis and J.C. Krueger.
     New York: American Journal of Nursing Co., 1980, pp. 3-8.

     General introduction to subject.

629 _____. "Ethical Issues in Nursing Research," WEST J
      NURS RES 2 (1980): 760-62.

      Social science research and the concept of risk. (5)

630 _____. "Ethical Issues: A Survey of Institutional
      Review Boards," WEST J NURS RES 2 (1980): 536-38.

      Surveys shows that social scientists are more likely than
      biomedical scientists to view IR Boards as unfair. (2)

631 _____. "Ethical Issues in Nursing Research," WEST J
      NURS RES 3 (1981): 247-48.

      Problems of proxy consent in research with children. (3)

632 _____. "Ethical Issues in Nursing Research," WEST J
      NURS RES 3 (1981): 443-44.

      Fellowship opportunities and publications in nursing
      ethics. (0)

633 _____. "Ethical Issues in Nursing Research," WEST J
      NURS RES 4 (1982): 237-39.

      Issues raised by doing research with the elderly. (9)

634 _____. "Ethical Issues in Nursing Research," WEST J
      NURS RES 4 (1982): 317-19.

      Survey of literature relevant to ethics and nursing
      research. (11)

635 _____. "Ethical Issues in Nursing Research," WEST J
      NURS RES 5(2) (Spring 1983): 186-87.

      Pro and con arguments concerning health professionals
      preparing for war. (1)

636 Downs, F.S. "Ethical Inquiry in Nursing Research," NURS
      FORUM 6 (1967): 12-20.

      An early call for setting conditions for ethical research,
      including informed consent, confidentiality, good experi-
      mental design. (3)

637 _____. "Whose Responsibility?: Whose Rights?," NURS
      RES 28 (May-June 1979): 131.

      An editorial on the need to protect the right of research
      subjects. (0)

638 Dunn, L.J. "The Eichner/Storar Decision: A Year's Perspec-
      tive," LAW MED HEALTH CARE 10(3) (June 1982): 117-19, 141.

Eichner case dealt with Brother Joseph Fox who was in a coma and his guardian Father Philip Kichner. His guardian sought authority to discontinue respirator; Storar case involved issue of whether or not a guardian could refuse to allow blood transfusions to be administered to her incompetent ward. The consolidation of two cases in Court of Appeals has created confusion. (30)

639   Fry, S.T. "Accountability in Research: The Relationship of Scientific and Humanistic Values," ADV NURS SCIENCE 4 (October 1981): 1-13.

Emphasizes human rights guidelines and ANA Code. (22)

640   Gallant, D.M. and R. Force. LEGAL AND ETHICAL ISSUES IN HUMAN RESEARCH AND TREATMENT: PSYCHOPARMACOLOGIC CONSIDERATIONS. NewYork: Spectrum Publications, distributed by Halsted Press, 1978.

Based on a symposium which was focused on the ethical and legal aspects of neuropsychopharmacologic research and treatment of patients. Includes an analysis of the statement of principles on the ethical conduct of research by the American College of Neuropsychopharmacology. Chapters on the law by A.A. Stone and N. Chayet. Ethical issues covered by K.A. Lebacquz and the two editors.

641   Jacobson, S.F. "Ethical Issues in Experimentation With Human Subjects," NURS FORUM 12 (1973): 58-71.

Discusses Milgram experiments and deception in psychological research and poses some solutions. (50)

642   Jones, J.H. BAD BLOOD: THE TUSKEGEE SYPHILIS EXPERIMENT. New York: The Free Press, 1981

A classic study of the Tuskegee experiment where syphilis patients were left untreated to observe the progress of the disease even after penicillin and other drugs were available for treatment.

643   Kratz, C. "The Ethics of Research," NURS MIRROR 145 (July 21, 1977): 17-20.

General commentary on nursing research and ethical implications in America, England, Canada, and New Zealand. (8)

644   McKay, R.C. and J.S. Soule. "Nurses as Investigators: Some Ethical and Legal Issues," CAN NURSE 71 (September 1975): 26-29. Reprinted in NURS DIGEST 5 (Spring 1977): 7-9.

Brief overview of legal and ethical issues in nursing research. (0)

645   Meyer, P.B. DRUG EXPERIMENTS ON PRISONERS: ETHICAL, ECONOMIC OR EXPLOITIVE. Lexington, MA.: D.C. Heath, 1976.

An examination of the general question of medical experimentation on humans and the policy dilemmas it creates.
Problems presented by the practice of experimentation on
prisoners in the U.S. also examined.

646   Mitchell, K. "Protecting Children's Rights During Research,"
      PED NURS (January/February 1984): 9-10.

      A summary of the regulations of Department of Health and
      Human Services (HHS) issued June 6, 1983 dealing with
      nurses' responsibilities in protection of children during
      research. (16)

647   Northrop, C. "Human Research and the Law." READINGS IN
      NURSING RESEARCH. Edited by Pavlovich and Krampitz.
      St. Louis: C.V. Mosby, 1981.

      The ethical conduct of research involving human subjects
      requires a balance of society's interests in protecting the
      rights of the human subjects and in developing knowledge
      that can benefit subjects and society as a whole.

648   Oberst, M.T. "Research Ethics, Part I: Randomized
      Clinical Trials," CAN NURS 2 (October 1979): 385-86.

      Brief discussion of ethical issues involved in randomized
      clinical trials. (3)

649   Royal College of Nursing of the United Kingdom. ETHICS
      RELATED TO RESEARCH IN NURSING. London: Royal College
      of Nursing of the United Kingdom, 1977.

      Included because of its official stance.

650   Scott, D.W. "Ethical Issues in Nursing Research: Access
      to Human Subjects," TOP CLIN NURS 4 (April 1982): 74-83.

      Ethical issues involved in using subjects and institutions
      for research. (8)

651   Southby, J.R. "Legal Considerations for Nurse Researchers,"
      AORN J 33 (June 1981): 1278-80, 1285, 1288, 1290.

      Brief overview of ethical guidelines and regulations. (13)

652   Sweezy. S.R. "The Ethical Issue of Informed Consent in
      Human Experimentation." ETHICAL PROBLEMS IN THE NURSE-
      PATIENT RELATIONSHIP. Edited by C.P. Murphy and H. Hunter.
      Boston: Allyn and Back, 1983, pp. 235-45.

      Analyzes the Willowbrook case where retarded children were
      exposed to a strain of hepatitis virus in order to test a
      vaccine.

653   Tilden, V.P.   "Qualitative Research: A New Frontier for
      Nursing."   PATIENTS, NURSES, AND ETHICS.   Edited by A.J.
      Davis and J.C. Krueger. New York: American Journal of
      Nursing Co.,1980, pp. 73-83.

      Discusses special ethical problems that result from re-
      search based upon participant observation.

LEGAL AND REGULATORY ISSUES

General Issues

654 Annas, G.J. "Making Babies Without Sex: The Law and the Pro-
     fits," AM JPUB HEALTH 74(12) (December 1984): 1415-17.

     Discusses legal issues raised by the development of new
     methods of noncoital human reproduction, including surrogate
     embryo transfers, the use of frozen embryos, artificial insem-
     ination by a donor, and in vitro fertilization. Reviews
     current law in United States, Australia and England. (21)

655 Bullough, B. THE LAW AND THE EXPANDING NURSING ROLE (2nd Ed.).
     New York: Appleton-Century-Crofts, 1980.

     Overview of law as it relates to nursing. History, analysis
     and summary of current state nurse practice acts with an empha-
     sis on the coverage of nurse practitioners and other nursing
     specialties by the practice acts.

656 _____. "Legislative Update," PED NURS 9(4) (July/August
     1983): 301.

     Discusses prospective payment (DRGS), the nurse training act
     and proposed legislation for community nursing centers. (1)

657 _____. "Legislative Update," PED NURS 9(5) (September/
     October 1983): 388-89.

     Reports FTC challenge of nurse midwives loss of insurance,
     medicaid costs, and state nurse practice act issues in South
     Carolina. (1)

658 _____. "Legislative Update," PED NURS 10(1) (January/
     February 1984): 85.

     Discusses problem in South Carolina related to an Attorney
     General's opinion of the nurse practice act. Third party re-
     imbursement statutes reported in twelve states. A new Wash-
     ington, D.C. statute allowing hospital privileges for nurse
     practitioners, nurse midwives and anesthetists briefly noted.
     (1)

659 Cazalas, M.W. (Ed.). NURSING AND THE LAW (3rd Ed.). Gaithers-
     burg, MD.: Aspen Systems Corp., 1979.

     Third edition of reference on the law for nurses, nursing
     supervisors, and administrators.

660 Chayet, N.L. and P.C. Sonnenreich. CERTIFICATE OF NEED: AN
     EXPANDING REGULATORY CONCEPT: A COMPILATION AND ANALYSIS OF
     FEDERAL AND STATE LAWS AND PROCEDURES. Washington, D.C.:
     Medicine in the Public Interest, 1978.

     Defines (CON) Certificate of Need. Discusses the principal
     purpose of CON laws.

661 Creighton, H. CHANGING LEGAL ATTITUDES: THE EFFECT OF THE
     LAW ON NURSING. New York: National League for Nursing, Pub.
     No. 20-1512, 1974.

     Discussion of changing legal trends as they impact on nurs-
     ing trends. (49)

662 _____. (Guest Ed.). "Current Legal and Professional
     Issues," NURS CLIN NORTH AM 9 (September 1974).

     Issue devoted to legal and professional issues. Of histori-
     cal interest. Significant changes in nurse practice acts
     after 1974. Changes in liability are fewer.

663 _____. LAW EVERY NURSE SHOULD KNOW. Philadelphia: W.B.
     Saunders, 1981, 4th Ed.

     Probably most well known basic text in the field. Covers
     principles of law, licensure, contracts, liability, the legal
     status of the nurse, torts, misdemeanors, felonies, witnesses,
     dying declarations, and wills. Comprehensive chapter on Cana-
     dian law.

664 Creighton, H. and D. Litt. "Legal Aspects of Nosocomial Infec-
     tion," NURS CLIN NORTH AM 15(4) (December 1980): 789-802.

     Case law related to nosocomial infections reviewed. Author
     urges better infection control standards to prevent these law-
     suits. (45)

665 Curran, W.J., A.L. McGarry and C.S. Petty (Eds.). MODERN
     LEGAL MEDICINE, PSYCHIATRIC, AND FORENSIC SCIENCE. Phila-
     delphia: F.A. Davis Co., 1980.

     Discusses the more traditional areas of trauma-related death
     and suicide investigations as well as modern medicolegal in-
     vestigations such as automobile and airplane deaths, medical
     care related deaths, deaths related to public health hazards,
     and neoplastic diseases. Discusses the importance of thorough
     investigation, impartial reporting, and scientific truth in
     the formulation of findings and conclusions by medicolegal
     professionals and forensic scientists.

666 Cushing, M. "Wronged Rights in Nursing Homes," AM J NURS
     84(10) (October 1984): 1213, 1216, 1218.

     Discussion of recent developments in the law as it relates
     to the rights of nursing homes patients. (11)

667 _____. NURSING JURISPRUDENCE. Englewood Cliffs, NJ:
    Prentice-Hall (Reston), 1985.

    Overview of the current legal issues with a major emphasis
    on case law. Each chapter first identifies the essential legal
    concepts and then relates them to nursing activities. In-
    cludes content on standards of care, safety, medications,
    nursing judgment, communication and documentation, medical
    treatment decisions, care of the mentally ill, abortion,
    impact of the law on nursing practice and educational law.

668 Eccard, W.L. "A Revolution in White--New Approaches in Treat-
    ing Nurses as Professionals," VANDERBILT LAW REVIEW 30
    (1977): 837-39.

    A review of the development of nursing as a profession;
    a discussion of current trends in nursing; a review of legal
    cases in light of these developments and propositions for
    alternatives, approaches to the questions relating to nursing
    malpractice. (219)

669 Fiesta, J. THE LAW & LIABILITY: A GUIDE TO NURSES. New York:
    John Wiley & Sons, 1983.

    An overview of nursing law with an emphasis on liability.
    Case examples used to illustrate principles. Chapters focus on
    various aspects of the legal process as well as issues of
    informed consent, ethical issues, contracts, and professional
    disciplinary actions.

670 George, J.E. LAW AND EMERGENCY CARE. St. Louis: C.V. Mosby
    Co., 1980.

    Covers general legal principles, the duty to provide emer-
    gency care, consent to treatment, triage, scope of emergency
    nursing practice, good samaritan laws, child abuse, rape, the
    psychiatric emergency.

671 Greenlaw, J. "Delivery Rooms: For Women Only?," LAW MED
    HEALTH CARE 9 (December 1981): 28-29, 40.

    Reviews case Backus v. Baptist Medical Center. Gregory
    Backus, R.N. (a man) requested work in the obstetrical/
    gynecological unit of the hospital, and was denied that right
    because of sex. At time article was written he had been denied
    this right at the district court level. However, he subse-
    quently won an appeal. (7)

672 _____. "Reporting Incompetent Colleagues II: Will I Be
    Sued For Defamation?," NURS LAW AND ETHICS (1980): 5. Re-
    printed in NURSING ISSUES AND NURSING STRATEGIES FOR THE
    EIGHTIES. Edited by B. Bullough, V. Bullough and M.C. Soukup.
    New York: Springer Publishing Co., 1983, pp. 102-104.

    Deals with the case of Malone v. Longo in which there was a
    disagreement between two VA nurses over a medication.

673   Heitler, G. "Mandated Benefits: Their Social, Economic, and
      Legal Implications," LAW MED HEALTH CARE 11(6) (December
      1983): 248-52.

      Notes trend and argues against laws which mandate health
      care services such as treatment for alcoholism or hospice care.
      Discusses licensure laws for new types of providers, including
      nurse midwives and nurse practitioners. Argues these new
      workers, along with new delivery mechanisms may be better
      alternatives than mandated benefits. Finally, argues that
      carriers (such as Blue Cross) should have full discretion in
      the type of insurance they write and the type of practitioners
      they cover. (Author is former Vice President and General
      Counsel for Blue Cross and Blue Shield.) (46)

674   Hemelt, M.D. and M.E. Mackert. "Your Legal Guide to Nursing
      Practice," NURSING 79 (October 1979): 57.

      Reprint of Part one of a four part handbook dealing with
      legal issues and nursing. Part two looks at informed consent,
      splitting medications, employee obligation, and resuscitation.
      (0)

675   _____. DYNAMICS OF LAW IN NURSING AND HEALTH CARE. Reston,
      VA.: Reston Publishing Co., 1982, 2nd Ed.

      Second edition of a basic text. In addition to basic prin-
      ciples of liability, it covers abortion, patients´ rights,
      involuntary commitment, confidentiality, health care ethical
      issues, and medical records. Vignettes illustrate principles.

676   Hershey, N. "When Is a Communication Privileged?," AM J NURS
      70 (January 1970): 112-13.

      Whether or not the nurse patient relationship is privileged.
      (0)

677   Holder, A.R. LEGAL ISSUES IN PEDIATRICS AND ADOLESCENT
      MEDICINE. New York: John Wiley & Sons, 1977.

      Discusses medical legal issues peculiar to children broadly
      defined. Includes in vitro fertilization, amniocentisis,
      genetic counseling, fetal research, deformed newborns, and
      their conflicting rights to die and to live, consents to treat
      minors, minors as research subjects, hyperkinetic children,
      minors´ rights to treatment, and contraception, abortion and
      sterilization for minors. Indexes of cases ordered alpha-
      betically and jurisdictionally.

678   Holgate, P. "Strictly Between Ourselves," OCCUP HEALTH 30
      (April 1978): 156-59.

      Confidentiality of medical records. (4)

679 Johnson, S.H. (Ed.). LONG TERM CARE AND THE LAW. Owing
     Mills, MD.: National Health Publishing, 1983.

     Long term health care systems within today's legal struc-
     ture.

680 Jones, A. "The Narciso-Perez Case: Nurse Hunting in Michi-
     gan," THE NATION (December 3, 1977): 584-88.

     Reviews case of two Filipino nurses, Narciso and Perez, who
     were convicted of poisoning their patients. Author argues
     prejudice a major factor in the investigation and trial.

681 Kander, M.L. and R.P. Russell (Eds.). HEALTH ADMINISTRATION
     LAWS, REGULATIONS AND GUIDELINES. Owing Mills, MD.:
     National Health Publishing, 1984.

     A two volume looseleaf resource covering laws and regulations
     that relate to health care facilities. Includes Medicare/
     Medicaid operating standards, reimbursement, prospective pricing
     related to diagnostic related groups (DRGs), policy manual
     requirements, PSROs, labor law, discrimination, occupational
     standards, and standards for home health services.

682 Kapp, M.B. GERIATRICS AND THE LAW. New York: Springer Pub-
     lishing Co., 1984.

     Examins geriatrics practice care from a legal viewpoint.

683 Kerr, A.H. "Nurses' Notes--That's Where the Goodies Are,"
     NURSING '75 (February 1975): 34.

     Kerr provides suggestions and guidelines for accurate and
     informative nursing notes. She views this in terms of its
     importance from a legal standpoint. (0)

684 Klein, C.A. "Informed Consent," NURSE PRACT 9(5) (May 1984):
     56, 58, 60, 62.

     Brief review of case law related to informed consent. (5)

685 Laben, J.K. and C.P. MacLean. LEGAL ISSUES AND GUIDELINES FOR
     NURSES WHO CARE FOR THE MENTALLY ILL. Thorofare, NJ:
     Slack, Inc., 1984.

     Basic legal concepts for psychiatric mental health nurses.
     Coverage includes malpractice, right to refuse treatment,
     access to records.

686 Lesnik, M.J. and B.E. Anderson. NURSING PRACTICE AND THE LAW,
     2nd Ed. with revisions. Philadelphia: J.B. Lippincott Co.,
     1962.

Most well-known text on nursing law during its era. First
edition titled LEGAL ASPECTS OF NURSING published in 1947.
Second edition came out in 1955 and was revised in 1962.
Valuable historical document.

687   Lynk, W.J. "Regulation and Competition: An Examination of
      'The Consumer Choice Health Plan'," J HEALTH POLITICS, POLICY
      AND LAW 6 (Winter 1982): 625-36.

      Arguments against the plan are presented. (18)

688   Machan, T.R. and M.B. Johnson (Eds.). RIGHTS AND REGULATIONS:
      ETHICAL, POLITICAL, AND ECONOMIC ISSUES. Cambridge, MA.:
      Ballinger Publishing Co., 1983.

      Series of essays on the legality and morality of government
      regulation. The authors--legal scholars, philosophers, and
      political theorists--bring differing perspectives to their
      analysis. They examine the goals and assumptions underlying
      the regulation of areas such as health safety and the environ-
      ment, and evaluate the social and economic consequences of
      regulatory schemes.

689   Mancini, M. "The Law and the Occupational Health Nurse," AM J
      NURS (September 1979): 1628.

      Discusses legal issues concerning the occupational health
      nurse, including federal OSHA standards. (4)

690   Mancini, M.R. and A.T. Gale. EMERGENCY CARE AND THE LAW.
      Gaithersburg, MD.: Aspen Systems Corp., 1981.

      Pinpoints the legal issues that come up most often in emer-
      gency care with coverage of many facets and suggested solutions.
      Discusses the growing risks posed by escalating public use of
      emergency room departments.

691   McCaffrey, D.P. OSHA AND THE POLITICS OF HEALTH REGULATION.
      New York: Plenum Publishing, 1982.

      Analyzes the decision and policy-making processes at the
      Occupational Safety and Health Administration (OSHA). The
      author traces the development of OSHA's chemical regulations
      and its handling of several service issues during its first
      ten years of operation, 1971-1981. He then examines what
      happened in those years from the perspectives of three compet-
      ing theories of what ultimately determines government policy:
      the balance of power among private interest groups, the stable
      capital accumulation of survival of the capitalist system, or
      the organizational properties of the government agencies
      themselves.

692   McKinaly, J.B. (Ed.). LAW AND ETHICS IN HEALTH CARE:
      MILBANK READER 7. Cambridge, MA.: MIT Press, 1982.

Selected papers from the Milbank Memorial Fund Quarterly.
Papers were also published earlier in a series put out by
Prodist. These thirteen papers were considered landmark in
quality. Includes sections on antitrust and professional
licensure, malpractice and ethical issues.

693 Miller, R.D. (Ed.). PROBLEMS IN HOSPITAL LAW, 4th Ed.
     Gaithersburg, MD.: Aspen Systems Corp., 1983.

Fourth edition includes regulations and accreditation,
financing and taxation, health planning, reorganization and
closure, medical staff, dying, death and dead bodies, and
other topics.

694 Murchison, I., T. Nichols and R. Hanson. LEGAL ACCOUNTABILITY
     IN THE NURSING PROCESS, 2nd Ed. St. Louis: C.V. Mosby,
     1982.

The book is based on the premise that the law can be a positive force in planning and implementing health care. The
overall theme is one of integrating and incorporating the law
into the nursing process to support independent nursing action.

695 National Health Publishing in cooperation with National Health
     Lawyers Association, edited from their eighth annual sympo-
     sium. HEALTH LAW UPDATE. Owing Mills, MD.: National Health
     Publishing, 1983.

Review and roundup of key developments and their likely
impact on today's health care system.

696 O'Neil, E.A. "Exclusive Referral Agreements for Home Care,"
     NURS ECON 2(5) (September/October 1984): 326-28, 364-65.

Hospital providers may be subject to charges of abandonment
if patients suffer injury as a result of early discharge. To
reduce risks, the use of affiliation agreements for home care
should be considered. (19)

697 O'Sullivan, A.L. "Privileged Communication," AM J NURS 80
     (May 1980): 947-50.

Privileged communication as a legal notion. Questions
whether nurse-client communication is privileged. (26)

698 Peters, J.D., K.S. Fineberg, D.A. Kroll and V. Collins.
     ANESTHESIOLOGY AND THE LAW. Ann Arbor, MI.: AUPHA Press,
     1982.

Liability as it relates to anesthesiology.

699 Reppucci, N.D., L.A. Weithorn, E.P. Mulvey and J. Monahan (Eds.).
     CHILDREN, MENTAL HEALTH, AND THE LAW. Beverly Hills, CA.:
     Sage Publications, Inc., 1984.

Mental health and legal concerns as they affect children
are examined, including child custody, child maltreatment,
reproductive rights, juvenile justice, and education for the
handicapped.

700 Rhodes, A.M. and R.D. Miller. NURSING AND THE LAW, 4th Ed.
     Rockville, MD.: Aspen Systems Corp., 1984.

     Overview of law as it relates to nursing. Includes lia-
     bility, licensure and other credentialing, authorization for
     treatment, issues related to the dying patient, reproduction,
     and patient confidentiality. Earlier editions of this work
     are by other authors. This edition is more comprehensive.

701 Rocereto, L.R. and C.M. Maleski. THE LEGAL DIMENSIONS OF
     NURSING PRACTICE. New York: Springer Publishing Co., 1982.

     A brief legal guide for professional nurses. Covers standards
     of care, informed consent, liability and record keeping. Legal
     questions are posed and answered by summarizing case law or
     relevant statutes.

702 Roemer, R. and G. McKray. LEGAL ASPECTS OF HEALTH POLICY:
     ISSUES AND TRENDS. Westport, CT.: Greenwood Press, 1980.

     Comprehensive coverage of issues related to public health
     policy. Basic authority for health law reviewed, including
     police powers of states and federal constitutional powers.
     Regulation of health personnel through licensing and federal
     mechanisms reviewed. Legal issues discussed, including access
     to health care, right to treatment, civil rights, abortion,
     family planning, medicaid, cost control, peer review, and
     medical malpractice. Concludes with an essay relating law and
     health policy.

703 Rubenfeld, M.G., Sr. R. Donley, E.G. Falinski, B.R. Herpin,
     P. Horn and S. Walker. "The Nurse Training Act: Yesterday,
     Today, and ...," AM J NURS (June 1981): 1202-4.

     A history of the Federal Nurse Training Act from 1965 to
     1981. (18)

704 Sadoff, R.L. LEGAL ISSUES IN THE CARE OF PSYCHIATRIC PATIENTS.
     New York: Springer Publishing Co., 1982.

     Author is a forensic psychiatrist. Brief work covering the
     legal regulations which apply to mental health practice, in-
     cluding confidentiality, involuntary hospitalization, patients'
     rights, suicide, evaluation of competence, liability, and
     criminal law.

705 Schweitzer, B. "Legislative Update," PED NURS 7(4) (July/
     August 1980): 47, 53.

Update on block grants and nurse training act. Reports un-
favorable Attorney General's opinion on the right of California
nurse practitioners to prescribe. (0)

706 _____. "Legislative Update," PED NURS 8(1) (January/
February 1982): 66.

Funding for federal maternal child health programs reported.
The IOM Study of Nursing and pro-competition proposals discussed. (0)

707 Schweitzer, B. and H.M. Griffith. "The New Federalism and
Health Care," PED NURS 7(6) (November/December 1981): 35-36,
52.

Capitol Hill nurses comment on the emerging health policy
and politics of the Reagan Administration. Emphasis is on competition, cost reduction. Judy Buckalew, Shiela Burke, and
Deborah Turner were interviewed. (0)

708 Sidley, N.T. (Ed.). LAW AND ETHICS. New York: Health Sciences
Press, Inc., 1984.

A survey of law as it relates to health professionals.
Covers issues related to liability in detail. Chapters on
ethics also included.

709 Smith, D.B. LONG TERM CARE IN TRANSITION: THE REGULATION OF
NURSING HOMES. Ann Arbor, MI.: Health Administration Press,
School of Public Health, The University of Michigan, 1981.

As the American population ages, long-term care has moved to
the forefront of changes in regulation within the health care
industry. This case study focuses on the history and experience of regulating long-term care in New York. It analyzes
different strategies of control and their effectiveness,
focusing on professional standards, fiscal controls, criminal
enforcement, and consumer controls.

710 Southwick, A.F. and G.J. Siedell, III. THE LAW OF HOSPITAL
AND HEALTH CARE ADMINISTRATION. Ann Arbor, MI.: Health
Administration Press, University of Michigan, 1978.

Comprehensive work on hospital administrative law. Major
topics covered include an introduction to the legal system;
the hospital as a corporation, professional liability; hospital
liability; and the relationship of the hospital and the physician. Target audience appears to be hospital administrators/
students.

711 Thoford, S.M. and R.D. Miller, Jr. NURSING AND THE LAW.
Gaithersburg, MD.: Aspen Systems Corp., 1984.

Revision of a general text for nurses. Cases used to illustrate principles.

712   Trandel-Korenchuk, D.M. and K.M. Trandel-Korenchuk.   "Current
      Legal Issues Facing Nursing Practice," NURS ADM Q (1980):
      37-55.

      Summarizes and analyzes the state laws related to expanded
      nursing roles, examines prescriptive authority for nurses, and
      discusses issues related to third party reimbursement and mal-
      practice insurance. Table analyzes state nurse practice acts.
      (13)

713   _____. "Informed Consent and Mental Incompetency: Legal
      Forum," NURS ADM Q 8(1) (Fall 1983): 76-78.

      When a patient is not mentally competent a legally recognized
      substitute must be obtained.(3)

714   Trocchio, J. "Nursing Home Deregulation: Regulatory Reform
      Efforts," NURS ECON 2(3) (May/June 1984): 185-89.

      Regulatory reform has been a major policy objective during
      the past two presidential administrations. In the health arena,
      one of the most dramatic reform efforts focused on nursing
      homes. This regulatory reform activity is reviewed. (18)

715   Verville, R.E. "The New Medicare Regulations and the Impact
      They Will Have on Nurse Anesthetists," AANA J 50(6) (December
      1982): 585-88.

      Discusses how Medicare regulations of 1982 will affect nurse
      anesthetists. Summarizes the AANA's position on the new regu-
      lations. (0)

716   "Washington Focus: National Institute for Nursing Could Help
      Fight Their War on Health Costs," NURS & HEALTH CARE 4
      (October 1983): 436-37.

      Arguments supporting the establishment of a National Insti-
      tute of Nursing within the National Institutes of Health are
      presented. (0)

717   Weisstub, D.N. (Ed.). LAW AND PSYCHIATRY. New York: Pergamon
      Press, 1978.

      Addresses issues related to revision of mental health legis-
      lation and redefinitions of patients' rights, the limits of
      professional obligations, and authority. Emphasizes the shift
      from the needs of society to the protection of the rights of
      the individual.

718   Wexler, D.B. MENTAL HEALTH LAW: MAJOR ISSUES. New York:
      Plenum Press, 1981.

      Covers various aspects of mental health law. Good dis-
      cussion of Tarasoff case.

719 Wiley, L. "Liability for Death: Nine Nurses' Legal Ordeals,"
     NURSING 81 1(9) (September 1981): 34-43.

     Reviews several cases in which nurses were charged with
     murder or lost their jobs because of suspicion. Negative pub-
     licity and the naivete of the nurses about their situation
     seems to be common to the cases. (0)

     See 104, 129, 140, 141, 145, 150, 174, 202, 208, 259, 358, 377,
     380, 382, 383, 396, 397, 399, 400, 405, 419, 443, 445, 447,
     450, 510, 527, 538, 574, 626, 640, 647, 651, 993, 997, 1027,
     1071, 1135, 1180, 1182, 1228, 1947, 2107, 2110, 2143.

Malpractice, Liability, Avoiding Liability,
Standards of Care

720 Blumenreich, G.A. and D. Benkob. "Liability of a Surgeon When
     Working With a Nurse Anesthetist," AANA J 52 (June 1984):
     335-36.

     Vicarious liability of surgeon for a nurse anesthetist dis-
     cussed with cases. Surgeon not ordinarily liable. (0)

721 Bowyer, E.A. "The Liability of the Occupational Health
     Nurse," LAW MED HEALTH CARE 11(5) (October 1983): 224-28.

     Occupational health nurses face some risks of liability not
     encountered in ordinary nursing settings. They necessarily
     make independent judgments, they must deal with worker's com-
     pensation laws, and they are occasionally pressured by employers
     to breach confidentiality. (37)

722 Campazzi, B.C. "Nurses, Nursing and Malpractice Litigation:
     1967-1977," NURS ADM Q 5 (Fall 1980): 1 10.

     Appealed cases that were reported in the FEDERAL REGISTER
     during the ten year period from January 1, 1967 to January 1,
     1977 were analyzed to determine how often nurses were involved.
     A total of 390 cases were found. Most cases involving nurses
     occurred in general hospitals. In forty-six cases the nurse
     was the first named defendant, in the others the nurse was
     named in addition to other defendents. Nursing personnel were
     held responsible in seven cases with judgments ranging from
     $400 to $100,000. (26)

723 Chavigny, K. and A. Helm. "Ethical Dilemmas and the Practice
     of Infection Control," LAW MED HEALTH CARE 10 (September
     1982): 168-71, 174.

     Argues that nurse epidemiologists have a duty to act as
     patient advocates. Yet hospital nurses in charge of infection
     control sometimes find themselves in a dilemma; proper control
     of infections includes tracing their source, yet this informa-
     tion could establish liability for the hospital in malpractice
     litigation. (18)

724 Cohn, S.D. "Legal Issues in School Nursing Practice," LAW MED
     HEALTH CARE 12(5) (October 1984): 219-21.

     Statutes covering school nurses summarized and liability
     discussed. (23)

725 Creighton, H. "Malpractice Problem," NURS FORUM 9 (September
     1974): 425-33.

     Review of selected malpractice cases brought against nurses.
     (20)

726 Curran, W.J. "Closed-Claims Data for Malpractice Actions in
     the United States," AM J PUB HEALTH 71(9) (September 1981):
     1066-67.

     Closed-claims data for a three and one-half year period ana-
     lyzed. Dollar amounts awarded increasing but physicians and
     hospitals continue to win most of the verdicts. Physicians
     paid seventy-one percent of the awards, hospitals twenty-five
     percent, and other health professionals (including nurses and
     dentists) four percent of the awards. (5)

727 Cushing, M. "A Judgment on Standards," AM J NURS (April 1981):
     797-98.

     Reviews a case, Pisel v. Stamford Hospital et al., involving
     a woman on a psychiatric unit who had wedged her head between
     the bed rail and the mattress, asphyxiated, and sustained per-
     manent damage. Written standards of care an important factor
     in the case. (1)

728 _____. "Legal Side: A Matter of Judgment," AM J NURS 82(6)
     (June 1982): 990-92.

     Case deals with a nurse who urged the family of a patient to
     take her to another hospital twenty miles away as quickly as
     possible, and failed to notify the physician on emergency call.
     Nurse lost her license for failure to stabilize patient's con-
     dition and failure to call physician even though facilities at
     hospital were inadequate (probably) to deal with situation. (5)

729 _____. "Legal Side: When Medical Standards Apply to Nurse
     Practitioners," AM J NURS 82(8) (August 1982): 1274, 1276.

     Two cases of negligence involving nurse practitioners re-
     viewed, one a Kaiser Permanente case involving a patent with a
     myocardial infarction, the second involving a patient with a
     Dalcon shield. In both cases nurse practitioners were held to
     the same standard of care as physicians. (2)

730 _____. "Legal Side: Legal Lessons in Patient Teaching," AM
     J NURS 84(6) (June 1984): 721-22.

Fear of law suits has lead many providers to write out home
care instructions. Nurses should, however, still give good
oral instructions to avoid liability. (5)

731 Fineberg, K.S., D. Peters, J.R. Willson and D.A. Kroll.
     OBSTETRICS/GYNECOLOGY AND THE LAW. Ann Arbor, MI.: AUPHA
     Press, 1984.

     Concepts of liability discussed as they relate to obstetrical
     gynecological practice. Federal and state regulations that
     apply to this practice setting reviewed (including those which
     apply to midwives).

732 Greenlaw, J. "Malpractice Insurance for Nurses: Legal,
     Ethical and Professional Issues," NURS LAW AND ETHICS 2
     (June/July 1981): 7-8.

     Ethical (and legal and professional) resons why nurses
     should carry malpractice insurance.

733 _____. "Failure to Use Siderails: When Is It Negligence,"
     LAW MED HEALTH CARE 10(3) (June 1982): 125-28.

     An examination of legal issues involved in use of siderails.
     Provides some recommendations for use of siderails and other
     restraints. (18)

734 _____. "Documentation of Patient Care: An Often Under-
     estimated Responsibility," LAW MED HEALTH CARE 10(4)
     (September 1982): 172-74.

     Documenting care on the chart is an important nursing respon-
     sibility. Inadequate documentation can lead to the loss of a
     malpractice suit. (18)

735 _____. "Liability for Nursing Negligence in the Operating
     Room," LAW MED HEALTH CARE 10(5) (October 1982): 222-24.

     Discusses captain of the ship doctrine and indicated its
     growing erosion as far as nurses in operating rooms are con-
     cerned. Increasing liability for nursing negligence will
     be appropriately attributed to the party having the right to
     control the nurse's conduct. (10)

736 _____. "Nursing Negligence in the Hospital Emergency
     Department," LAW MED HEALTH CARE 12(3) (June 1984): 118-21,
     132.

     Reviews malpractice litigation against hospital emergency
     room nurses. Triage responsibilities and problems in communi-
     cation with physicians often involved in these cases. Standards
     of care discussed. (31)

737 Hackler, E.T. "Expansion of Health Care Providers Liability:
     An Application of Darling to Long Term Health Care Facili-
     ties," CONNECTICUT LAW REV 9(3) (Spring 1977): 462-81.

     Industry-wide standards are being established for the nursing
     home industry. Author credits the influence of the Darling
     case, HEW standards, and Joint Commission accreditation as
     causal factors in the development of these standards. (139)

738 Hershey, N. "Pitfalls in Liability Insurance," AM J NURS
     (September 1966): 2002.

     Hershey recommends that no matter what type of setting a
     nurse works in he or she must determine what coverage she has
     and obtain a certificate of insurance if covered. Two examples
     of liability cases involving nurses are cited. (0)

739 _____. "Nurses Notes--They Can Play a Critical Role in
     Court," AM J NURS (November 1969): 2403.

     The case of Toth v. Community Hospital is presented and the
     importance of nurses´ notes as they relate to it. (0)

740 _____. "The Influence of Charting Upon Liability Determina-
     tions," J NURS ADM (March/April 1976): 35.

     Discusses the importance of the patient´s chart in malpractice
     and negligence cases. Several case reports are given as ex-
     amples. (0)

741 Hogue, E. NURSING AND LEGAL LIABILITY: CASES AND COMMENTARY.
     Owings Mills, MD.: National Health Publishing, 1984.

     A basic guide for nurses to the problem of legal liability,
     including malpractice. Illustrations from key court decisions
     which relate to the practice of nursing.

742 Holder, A.R. MEDICAL MALPRACTICE LAW. New York: Wiley, 1978
     (2nd Ed.).

     Comprehensive coverage of medical malpractice. Major focus
     on physician liability but fairly good coverage of nursing and
     hospital liability.

743 "Jeanne E. Gugino Sued the Harvard Community Health Plan and
     Two of Its Employees, Dr. Thomas Mahoney and Susan Daggett,
     R.N., A Nurse Practitioner," THE REGAN REPORT ON NURS LAW
     21(3) (August 1980).

     Reviews Gugino v. Harvrd Community Health Plan involving a
     patient who developed problems with a Dalcon shield. The
     nurse practitioner in the case was held responsible for the
     same standard of care as a physician. (1)

744 Kehrer, B.H. and M.D. Intriligator. "Malpractice and Employ-
     ment of Allied Health Personnel," MEDICAL CARE XIII(10)
     (October 1975): 876, 883.

     Cost of malpractice insurance thought to be a deterrent to
     the employment of allied health personnel in physicians
     offices. However, authors point out that malpractice insurance
     costs vary within only a narrow range. (38)

745 Kieffer, M.J. "Legal Brief: 'The Law and Specialty Health
     Practitioner'," AANA J 51 (December 1953): 562-64.

     Notes trend in nurse practice acts to broaden definitions.
     Sees same trend in case law to hold nurse responsible for own
     acts. Cites 1981 Louisiana case Hughes v. St. Paul Fire and
     Marine Insurance Company in which CRNA's negligence led to a
     patient death. Courts found attending physician free of wrong-
     doing.

746 Klein, C.A. "Assault and Battery," NURSE PRACT 9(7) (July
     1984): 47, 50, 52.

     Cases reviewed. Handling patients who do not want to be
     touched can lead to litigation. (11)

747 _____. "False Imprisonment," NURSE PRACT 9(9) (September
     1984): 41, 44.

     Reviews case law on false imprisonment. Holding a patient
     without legal cause is an intentional tort and it may result
     in a significant claim for damage. (4)

748 Law, S. and S. Polan. PAIN AND PROFIT: THE POLITICS OF MAL-
     PRACTICE. New York: Harper & Row Publishers, 1978.

     Argues that the medical malpractice crisis of the 1970's was
     caused by a variety of factors. Reviews case law related to
     malpractice decisions. Examines the role of lawyers and insur-
     ance companies in the escalating malpractice claims. Discusses
     approaches to management of the problem.

749 Lombardi, T. with G.N. Hoffman. MEDICAL MALPRACTICE INSURANCE:
     A LEGISLATOR'S VIEW. Syracuse, NY: Syracuse University
     Press, 1978.

     A New York State Senator's investigation of the medical mal-
     practice issue. Author was most interested in evaluating leg-
     islative solutions to the problem.

750 "M.D. Liability for R.N. Errors: The Ohio Rule," THE REGAN
     REPORT ON NURS LAW 23(1) (June 1982): 4.

     Discusses implications of a case in which patient suffered
     damage from an intubation done by a nurse anesthetist. Surgeon
     held responsible only for his own acts. (0)

751 O'Neil, E.A. "Release of Liability Forms: Will The Courts
     Listen?," NURS ECON 1(1) (July/August 1983): 29-33, 69.

     The use of release of liability forms, designed to protect
     providers from patient claims, is on the increase. This has
     given the courts ample opportunity to distinguish among differ-
     ent forms: exculpatory clauses signed by the patient prior to
     treatment, releases based on settlement of claims, and releases
     signed by patients who wish to terminate medical treatment.
     Legal reasons for the distinctions are discussed for the pur-
     pose of encouraging intelligent use of forms. (7)

752 Perry, S.E. "Managing to Avoid Malpractice," J NURS ADM
     (August 1978): 43.

     Describes preventive management and defensive nursing tech-
     niques to help staff nurses and nurse managers avoid problems
     which may lead to litigation. (19)

753 Regan, W.A. "Law Forum," HOSP PROGRESS (March 1978): 32.

     Regan presents two court cases. The first deals with "fore-
     seeability" as an important determinant of malpractice and the
     second case discusses a hospital held negligent by the court
     for failing to examine a new patient. (0)

754 Roach, W.H., Jr. "Responsible Intervention: A Legal Duty to
     Act," J NURS ADM (July 1980): 18-24.

     Nurses responsibilities to check questionable orders and to
     call physicians to come to care for patients are discussed.
     Illustrative cases which resulted in the nurse or the hospital
     being found liable are presented. (17)

755 Rubenstein, H.S., F.H. Miller, S. Postel and H.B. Evans.
     "Standards of Medical Care Based on Consensus Rather Than
     Evidence: The Case of Routine Bedrail Use for the Elderly,"
     LAW MED HEALTH CARE 11(6) (December 1983): 271-76.

     Questions routine use of bedrails. Data from one hospital
     indicates bedrails can, in fact, be a cause of patient falls.
     However, review of liability cases indicates malpractice
     claims often made when fall occurs and bedrails were not used.
     Suggests larger study be done. (37)

756 Salman, S.L. "Risk Manager Must Interact With Infection Con-
     trol Expert," HOSPITALS (March 16, 1980): 52-53.

     Suggests that the infection control practitioner and the
     risk manager work together on an infection control committee.
     This provides better patient care enabling the hospital to
     deal with or avoid malpractice cases involving nosocomial
     infections. (0)

757 _____. "Committee Is An Important Tool in Risk Manage-
     ment," HOSPITALS (September 16, 1980): 45-50.

     Discusses the issue of "claims management" efforts within
     the risk management program and suggests the formation of a
     medical incident review committee. (0)

758 _____. "The Impact of Comparative Negligence on Mal-
     practice," HOSPITALS (March 16, 1981): 46-49.

     The concept of comparative negligence is discussed along
     with its application to risk management and medical malprac-
     tice. (9)

759 Scanlan, K.M. "The Nurse and Malpractice: Legal Problems in
     the Nursing Profession," WESTERN STATE UNIVERSITY LAW REV
     9(2) (Spring 1982): 227-38.

     The issue of standard of care is crucial in determining
     nurses and/or hospital liability. Recent cases tend to demand
     a higher standard of care and more judgment on the part of
     nurses. (35)

760 Sklar, C.L. "The Legal Significance of Charting," CAN NURSE
     (March 1978): 10.

     The importance of charting from both a medical and legal
     standpoint are discussed. (0)

761 Titus, A.C. "Governmental Responsibility for Victims of
     Atomic Testing: A Chronicle of the Politics of Compensation,"
     J HEALTH POLITICS, POLICY LAW 8(2) (Summer 1983): 277-92.

     Since 1945 the U.S. government has conducted extensive atomic
     testing for purposes of protecting the national security and
     developing industrial uses of nuclear power. Newly available
     information indicates that many citizens were unwittingly
     harmed by exposure to radioactive fallout from this testing.
     This article analyzes the politics of the atomic compensation
     movement, from its beginnings through the 97th Congress. It
     concludes that, barring the enactment of specific legislation,
     atomic victims stand little chance of gaining financial compen-
     sation or moral satisfaction. (53)
     Editors Note: A 1984 decision gave compensation to selected
     Utah residents for fallout related malignancies.

762 "The Darling Case," J AM MED ASSOC 206 (November 11, 1968):
     1665-66.

     Landmark case reviewed. Injured leg negligently treated in
     a small hospital. Standards of care, including those of JCAH,
     the state licensing act, and the hospital standards used in
     case. Nursing care cited because of failure to inform chief
     of staff of problems. (1)

763 "The Darling Case Revisited," J AM MED ASSOC 206 (November 18,
     1968): 1875-76.

     Darling case compared to previous cases. Its landmark
     characteristics pointed out. (5)

764 Trandel-Korenchuk, D. and K. Trandel-Korenchuk. "Borrowed
     Servant and Captain-of-the Ship Doctrines," NURSE PRACT
     (February 1982): 33-34.

     Traces the history of the "borrowed servant" doctrine which
     held that physicians were responsible for the liability of
     nurses even though they were employed by a hospital rather
     than the physician. Courts are now less likely to accept this
     doctrine. (1)

765 Viles, S.M. "Liability for the Negligence of Hospital Nursing
     Personnel," NURS ADM Q (1980): 83-93.

     Reviews history of nursing liability and its assignment to
     the physician or the hospital. Analyzes the concept of negli-
     gence and gives examples. (41)

     See 370, 381, 398, 402, 667, 2332.

Nurse Practice Acts, Occupational Licensure,
Nurses´ Scope of Function, State Regulation
of Nursing

766 American Nurses´ Association. CRITICAL REQUIREMENTS FOR SAFE/
     EFFECTIVE NURSING PRACTICE. Kansas City, MO.: American
     Nurses´ Association, Pub. No. B-41, 1978.

     Performance data based on approximately 11,150 incidents to
     be used in developing tests that examine the validity of the
     State Board Test Pool.

767 _____. THE NURSING PRACTICE ACT: SUGGESTED STATE LEGISLATION.
     Kansas City, MO.: American Nurses´ Association, 1981.

     A model nurse practice act developed by an ad hoc committee
     of the American Nurses´ Association gives rationale for the
     proposed wording for state laws.

768 _____. QUESTIONS AND ANSWERS: SUNSET LAWS AND NURSING.
     Kansas City, MO.: American Nurses´ Association, Pub. No.
     G-155, 1982.

Using a question-and-answer format, this publication discusses
the development of sunset laws, the pros and cons of sunset
evaluation, the implications of the law for state boards of
nursing, and the measures state nurses' associations can take
in preparing for their participation in the evaluation process.
A bibliography is included.

769 _____. STATUTORY DEFINITIONS OF NURSING PRACTICE AND THEIR
CONFORMITY TO CERTAIN ANA PRINCIPLES. Kansas City, MO.:
American Nurses' Association, Pub. No. D-81, 1983.

State-by-state analysis of nursing practice acts, reviewed
for congruity with ANA principles. Includes definitions and
comments as to language omitted, at variance, or added, followed
by analysis of variables within definitions.

770 _____. THE REGULATION OF ADVANCED NURSING PRACTICE AS PRO-
VIDED FOR IN NURSING PRACTICE ACTS AND ADMINISTRATIVE RULES.
Kansas City, MO.: American Nurses' Association, Pub. No.
D-76, 1983.

Report on current methods used by state boards of nursing in
regulating practice of advanced practitioners, including sections on qualifications and regulations government nurse anesthesia practice, nurse midwifery practice, nurse practitioner
practice, clinical nurse specialist practice.

771 _____. STATE LEGISLATIVE REPORT--A QUARTERLY REVIEW OF
LEGISLATIVE ACTIVITIES OF INTEREST TO THE NURSING PROFESSION.
Kansas City, MO.: American Nurses' Association, Pub. No.
D-78, Vol. 1, 1983; Vol. 2, 1984.

Surveys legislative activities affecting nursing practice,
health care financing, public health and safety, with reference to pertinent publications, readings, conferences.

772 _____. LICENSURE TO PRACTICE NURSING. Kansas City, MO.:
American Nurses' Association, Pub. No. B-17, 1984.

Outlines the purpose of licensure and the procedures for
obtaining and renewing a license. Includes directory of all
state boards of nursing.

773 Begun, J.W., E.W. Crowe and R. Feldman. "Occupational Regulation in the States: A Causal Model," J HEALTH POLITICS,
POLICY LAW 6(2) (Summer 1981): 229-54.

An analysis of the state regulation of optometry. The power
of the optometry interest group is analyzed as it impacts on
the regulation of optometrists. (79)

774 Bullough, B. "The Law and the Expanding Nursing Role," AM J
PUB HEALTH 66(3) (March 1976): 249-54.

Outlines the three phases in nursing licensure as conceptualized by the author and surveys recent changes in state
nurse practice acts aimed at coverage of expanded nursing
roles. (68)

775 _____. "Legislative Update: Good News In Missouri,"
    PED NURS 10(2) (March/April 1984): 162.

Reports and comments on favorable decision by the Missouri
Supreme Court in Sermchief v. Gonzales. (1)

776 _____. "Legislative Update: Louisiana Board of Nursing
    Hanging In There," PED NURS 10(3) (May/June 1984): 235-36.

Describes efforts by the Louisiana Medical Society to keep
the Board of Nursing from issuing regulations covering the
advanced practice of nursing. (9)

777 _____. "Legislative Update: Legal Restrictions as a Barrier
    to Nurse Practitioner Role Development," PED NURS 10(6)
    (November/December 1984): 439-42.

Legal actions against nurse practitioners have escalated in
recent years. Most of the challenges have come from medical
societies, medical boards, or attorney generals. Outcomes
have varied. (24)

778 Cohn, S.D. "Revocation of Nurses´ Licenses: How Does It
    Happen?," LAW MED HEALTH CARE 11(1) (February 1983): 22-24.

Grounds for revocation of nurses licenses in the states reviewed. Difficult to operationalize the concept "unprofessional
conduct." Nurses licenses seldom revoked. (41)

779 Cohn, S.D., N. Cuffehy, N. Kraus and S.A. Tom. LEGISLATION
    AND NURSE-MIDWIFERY PRACTICE IN THE USA: REPORT OF A 1983
    SURVEY CONDUCTED BY THE POLITICAL AND ECONOMIC AFFAIRS COM-
    MITTEE OF THE AMERICAN COLLEGE OF NURSE MIDWIVES. Washington,
    D.C.: American College of Nurse Midwives, 1984. Published
    as a special issue of THE JOURNAL OF NURSE-MIDWIFERY 29(2)
    (March/April 1984).

Certified Nurse-Midwives have established a legal basis for
practice in all but two jurisdictions. The variety of laws
and rules that exist in the states are presented in a state-by-
state format. Nurse midwives are most often regulated by boards
of nursing but a variety of other regulatory agencies are noted,
including boards of medicine and public health. The American
College of Nurse-Midwifery favors a separate authority for nurse-
midwives. Introductory article analyzes several parameters,
including reimbursement, prescription writing, and educational
requirements.

780 Donovan, P. "Medical Societies vs. Nurse Practitioners,"
     FAMILY PLANNING PERSPECTIVES 15(4) (July/August 1983):
     166-71.

     In several states legal challenges to nurse practitioners are
     coming from medical boards. The author suggests that these
     challenges are based upon an economic threat. (43)

781 Doyle, E. and J. Meurer. "Practicing Medicine Without a
     License," NURSE PRACT 8(6) (June 1983): 41-42, 44.

     Describes and gives background information about the case
     against two Missouri family planning nurse practitioners. At
     the time the article was written the nurse practitioners had
     lost at the County Circuit Court level. (Eventually the Supreme
     Court ruled in favor of the nurse practitioners.)(6)

782 Ennen, A.G L. "Interpreting Missouri's Nursing Practice Act,"
     ST. LOUIS UNIVERSITY LAW JOURNAL 26 (June 1982): 931-47.

     Overview and analysis of the 1975 Missouri Nurse Practice
     Act, particularly as it relates to nurse practitioners. (102)

783 Grobe, S.J. "Sunset Laws," AM J NURS (July 1981): 1355-59.

     Nurse practice acts and nursing boards in thirty-five states
     face some type of periodic process, with the possibility of
     termination if a public need is no longer being served. Nurses
     are urged to monitor this process in their own states in order
     to preserve nursing licensure. (2)

784 Gross, S.J. OF FOXES AND HEN HOUSES: LICENSING AND THE HEALTH
     PROFESSIONS. Westport, CT.: Greenwood Press, 1984.

     The purposes and attributes of various professions, licensing
     boards, and their interaction with health care professions are
     scrutinized; the history of licensing is outlined; and the
     definition and measurement of competency and the effects of
     licensure on the quality of care is examined. Alternatives to
     licensure: professional disclosure, accountability, regula-
     tion of procedure rather than profession, are explored. Gross
     believes a phased deregulation of the professions can enhance
     both competition and accountability resulting in increased
     quality, reduced cost, and improved public self-protection.

785 Haggerty, V.C. "Doctrine of Delegated Medical Acts," NURSE
     PRACT 8(4) (April 1983): 9, 12.

     Argues against using the concept of delegated medical acts
     to legitimize advanced nursing practice. (6)

786 Hall, V.C. STATUTORY REGULATION OF THE SCOPE OF NURSING PRAC-
     TICE--A CRITICAL SURVEY. Chicago, IL.: The National Joint
     Practice Commission, 1975.

A review of nurse and medical practice acts as they relate
to an expanded scope of function for registered nurses. (66)

787 _____. "The Legal Scope of Nurse Practitioners Under
Nurse Practice and Medical Practice Acts." THE NEW HEALTH
PROFESSIONALS. Edited by A.A. Bliss and E.D. Cohen. German-
town, MD.: Aspen Systems Corp., 1977, pp. 106-39.

Classifies the legal approaches used to accommodate nurse
practitioners as follows: additional acts amendments, total
redefinitions, and a repeal of the prohibition against medical
practice. Favors the additional acts clause. (7)

788 Hansen, H.R. MEDICAL LICENSURE AND CONSUMER PROTECTION: AN
ANALYSIS AND EVALUATION OF STATE MEDICAL LICENSURE. Washington: Group Health Association of America, 1962.

Discusses legal basis of licensing and summarizes individual
state medical licensure laws.

789 Hershey, N. "Professional Practice Acts and Professional
Delusion," J NURS ADM (July/August 1974): 36-39. Reprinted
in EXPANDING HORIZONS FOR NURSES. Edited by B. Bullough
and V. Bullough. New York: Springer Publishing Co., 1977,
pp. 187-95.

Supports institutional licensure and closer ties to medicine in place of individual licensure. (0)

790 _____. "Defining the Scope of Nursing Practice: Actors,
Criteria and Economic Implications," NURS LAW & ETHICS 1(7)
(August/September 1980): 3, 10-12.

Argues that the first criterion for determining scope of
practice should be public interest. It is in the public interest to expand the nursing role. Nursing boards and nursing
organizations sometimes present barriers to this expansion.
Hershey observes that this type of behavior tends to be seen
less often in other professions. (6)

791 Hughes, B.S. "Role Evolution vs. Legislation," NURSE PRAC
8(3) (March 1983): 9-12.

Author argues against statutes for advanced nursing practice.
Uses Florida nurse practice act amendments and subsequent
efforts by physicians to control nurse practitioners to demonstrate argument. (0)

792 Hyde, E. "Territorial Imperatives in Health Care," NURS
OUTLOOK 32(3) (May/June 1984): 136-37.

Legal challenges to nurse midwives from physicians reported.
(2)

793 "Jolene Tuma Wins; Court Rules Practice Did Not Define 'Unpro-
     fessional Conduct'," NURS OUTLOOK (June 1979): 376.

     Reviews Tuma case, announces that the Idaho Supreme Court
     ruled in her favor. (0)

794 Keating, S., V.L. Nevin, C. Pakatar and R. Wang. "New York's
     Game of Power and Politics," NURSE PRACT 9(4) (April 1984):
     11-14.

     Legal problems of nurse practitioners in New York reviewed.
     Attorney for the State Education Department has narrowly inter-
     preted the 1972 Nurse Practice Act as not allowing medical
     diagnosis or treatment. Authors do not, however, favor chang-
     ing the law. (13)

795 Kinkela, G.G. and R.V. Kinkela. "Institutional Licensure:
     Cure All or Chaos," J NURS ADM (May/June 1974): 16-19. Re-
     printed in EXPANDING HORIZONS FOR NURSES. Edited by B.
     Bullough and V. Bullough, New York: Springer Publishing
     Co., 1977, pp. 195-203.

     Discusses the issues of institutional licensure. Institu-
     tional licensure was based on the assumption that it was the
     best solution to observed defects in the system but questions
     whether this is so without drawing conclusions. (28)

796 Kissam, P.C. "Physician's Assistant and Nurse Practitioner
     Laws for Expanded Medical Delegation." THE NEW HEALTH PRO-
     FESSIONALS. Edited by A.A. Bliss and E.D. Cohen. German-
     town, MD.: Aspen Systems Corp., 1977, pp. 116-49.

     Survey of both medical and nurse practice acts. Argues
     most legislation to date is unduly restrictive of nurse prac-
     titioners and physicians' assistants. (38)

797 Kucera, W.R. "A Defining of Terms: Collaboration vs. Super-
     vision," J AANA (December 1980): 547-48.

     Reports and discusses 1980 Maryland decision ruling the
     terms "supervision" and "collaboration" synonymous as they
     relate to the relationship between physicians and nurse anes-
     thetists. (0)

798 Mallison, M.B. "Time To Talk About Licensure," AM J NURS
     84(11) (November 1984): 1353.

     Notes that the National Federation of Licensed Practical
     Nurses voted in 1984 to move to the Associate Degree education
     for Licensed Practical Nurses by 1990. Implications for
     registered nurse licensure discussed. (0)

799 Monheit, A.C. "Occupational Licensure and the Utilization of
     Nursing Labor: An Economic Analysis," ADV HEALTH ECON AND
     HEALTH SERVICES RES 3 (1982): 117-42.

Examines the effects of occupational licensure on the utilization of registered nurses and practical nurses. Distinguishes between mandatory and permissive licensure, and notes
that nearly all states had passed mandatory registered nurse
laws by 1970. (33)

800   Moniz, D.M. and G.R. Tarutis. "Making Law, Not Breaking Law,"
      NURSE PRACT 8(9) (October 1983): 66-68.

      Cautions nurses that they can have their license revoked for
      practice beyond the legally sanctioned scope of function.
      Suggests further legislation, insurance, and mutual support
      among nurses. (0)

801   "News: Nebraska Legislature Says NP Roles Must Be Set By Law,
      Not Regulations," AM J NURS (August 1981): 1446.

      New Nebraska legislation authorized nurse practitioners and
      nurse anesthetists roles and settles a six year dispute between
      the attorney general and nurse practitioners. (0)

802   "News: State Board Regulations for NPs Become Legal Issue in
      Two States," AM J NURS (August 1981): 1432-34.

      Regulation of nursing specialties challenged by state
      medical societies in Kansas and Louisiana.(0)

803   Nichols, A.W. "Physician Extenders, The Law and The Future,"
      J FAMILY PRAC 11(1) (January 1980): 101-8.

      The possibilities of physician extenders evolving to a more
      independent model involving licensure are discussed. This
      would decrease the employing physician's vicarious liability
      but increase the liability for the physician extender. If
      physician extenders seek independence, confrontation with the
      physician community is inevitable and failure is likely. (33)

804   "Nurse Practitioners: Here Today....Gone Tomorrow?," NOVA
      LAW J 6 (Winter 1982): 365-83.

      Legislation covering nurse practitioners in Florida is
      analyzed and compared to that of other states. Author con-
      cerned about future possibility of malpractice litigation. (77)

805   O'Neil, E.A. "A Gavel Falls for Nursing: Sermchief v.
      Gonzales," NURS ECON 2(2) (March/April 1984): 102-4.

      Although nearly forty states have passed statutes that ex-
      pand the realm of permissable nursing activities, there has
      been little litigation in this area. Recently, however, the
      Supreme Court of Missouri handed down an opinion in Sermchief
      v. Gonzales that may be precedent-setting. (3)

806   Roemer, R. "The Nurse Practitioner in Family Planning
      Services: Law and Practice," FAMILY PLANNING/POPULATION
      REPORTER 6(3) (June 1977): 28-34.

Overview of laws and regulations covering nurse practitioners and nurse midwives who deliver family planning services. (37)

807   Rottenberg, S. (Ed.). OCCUPATIONAL LICENSURE AND REGULATIONS. Washington, D.C.: American Enterprise Institute for Public Policy Research, 1980.

Conservative analysis of occupational licensure by variety of authors many of whom favor abolishing licensure.

808   Schweitzer, B. "Legislative Update," PED NURS 7(7) (November/ December 1980): 45

Reports decision of California Board of Nursing to allow nurses to prescribe using protocols; veto of reimbursement in New York; and conflict in Texas over nurse practitioner functions. (0)

809   _____. "Legislative Update," PED NURS 7(5) (September/ October 1981): 66.

Lawsuit by Louisiana State Medical Society against Board of Nursing for adopting nurse practitioner regulations reported. Problems of Colorado nurses with possible limitation on ratio of nurse practitioners to physicians discussed, plus Washington news. (0)

810   "State Board Regulations for NPs Become Legal Issue in Two States," AM J NURS 81(8) (August 1981): 1432-33.

Legal battles over nurse practitioner regulations in Kansas and Louisiana. (0)

811   Thomas, C. "State Report," NURSE PRACT (9) (October 1983): 12.

Reports failure of nurse practitioner legislation in New York; a decision not to seek new nurse practitioner regulations in West Virginia; and Board of Nursing support for nurse practitioners in Louisiana. (0)

812   Thomas, M.J. "New York's Power and Politics," NURSE PRACT 9(11) (November 1984): 61.

A letter written as a rebuttal to the article by Keating et al. "New York's Game of Power and Politics." Author argues that law should be changed to allow advanced nursing practice. (3)

813   Toth, R.S. "New Health Professionals: The Physician Assistant and Advanced Nurse Practitioner in Texas," SOUTH TEXAS LAW J 22 (1982): 132-54.

The history and current role of physician assistants and
nurse practitioners are presented. Texas physician assistant
statute and the nurse practice act revisions covering the advanced nurse practitioner are presented and contrasted. Liability for the two types of "new health professionals" is discussed. Author expresses concern about their level of competence. (274)

814   Trandel-Korenchuck, D. and K. Trandel-Korenchuck. "How State
      Laws Recognize Advanced Nursing Practice," NURS OUTLOOK
      (November 1978): 713-19.

      Overview of coverage of advanced practice in the states.
      Discussion of various mechanisms. (44)

815   Watchorn, C. "Midwifery: A History of Statutory Suppression,"
      GOLDEN GATE UNIVERSITY LAW REV 9(2) (1978-1979): 631-43.

      Traces the legal status of midwives in California. Focus is
      primarily on lay midwives. (55)

816   Wolff, M.A. "Success in Missouri: Court Recognition of Nurses'
      Independent and Collaborative Roles," PED NURS 10(3) (May/
      June 1984): 183-85.

      A discussion of the decision by the Missouri Supreme Court
      in the case of Sermchief v. Gonzales. Ruling overturned lower
      court decision and held that nurses diagnosing and treating
      patients in accordance with standing orders and protocols is
      legal in Missouri. (7)

      See 280, 295, 298, 301, 355, 1280, 2191.

Patients' Rights, Informed Consent, Privacy

817   Annas, G.J. THE RIGHTS OF HOSPITAL PATIENTS. New York:
      Avon, 1975.

      Discusses patients' rights under present law and offers
      suggestions on how patients can protect their rights.

818   _____. INFORMED CONSENT TO HUMAN EXPERIMENTATION: THE
      SUBJECT'S DILEMMA. Cambridge: Ballinger Publishing Co.,
      1977.

      Analyzes the legal system as it attempts to articulate the
      law of informed consent relating to human experimentation on
      various types of subjects. It looks not only at the dilemmas
      faced by the subject, but at the dilemmas facing investigators,
      lawyers and judges as they attempt to implement the require-
      ments of informed consent.

819   _____. "The Emerging Stowaway: Patients' Rights in the
      1980s," LAW MED HEALTH CARE 10(1) (February 1982): 32-35, 46.

Supports increased patients´ rights. Reviews development of patients´ rights movement, analyzes current barriers and suggests strategies for change. (19)

820 Appelbaum, P.S. "Is The Need for Treatment Constitutionally Acceptable as a Basis for Civil Commitment?," LAW MED HEALTH CARE 12(4) (September 1984): 144-49.

Traces history of commitment laws, and notes a recent trend to focus on need for treatment as a criterion for commitment. (67)

821 Apperson, M. (Ed.). PRIVACY AND CONFIDENTIALITY: CAN THEY BE PROTECTED? Boston, MA.: Public Responsibility in Medicine & Research, 1982.

A report from the conference "Privacy and Confidentiality: Can They Be Protected?" held in Boston in 1981. It contains a summary of each presentation and workshop.

822 Baram, M.S. "The Right to Know and the Duty to Disclose Hazard Information," AM J PUB HEALTH 74(4) (April 1984): 385-90.

A discussion of the employees right to know about health hazards and what should be told him, including what an occupational nurse should say.(38)

823 Cohrssen, J.J. and L.E. Kopolow. COURT SCREENING AND PATIENT ADVOCACY: A HANDBOOK OF PRINCIPLES. Washington, D.C.: U.S. Department of Health, Education and Welfare, National Institute of Mental Health, DHEW Pub. (ADM) 79-157, 1979.

Covers commitment process and patient advocacy.

824 Comment, O´Bannon vs. Town Court Nursing Center. "Patients´ Right to Participate in Nursing Home Decertification," AM J LAW & MED 7 (Winter 1982): 469-92.

Analyzes the Supreme Court decision about the right of nursing home patients in the decertification process. Suggests alternate methods of asserting these patients rights. (156)

825 Cushing, M. "Wronged Rights in Nursing Homes," AM J NURS 84(10) (October 1984): 1213, 1216, 1218.

Overview of statutes and regulations which relate to patients in nursing homes. (11)

826 Fried, C. "Rights and Health Care--Beyond Equity and Efficiency," NEW ENG J MED 293 (July 31, 1975): 241-45.

Economic analysis has difficulty accommodating the concept
of rights. Familiar arguments based on resource constraints do
not prove that rights cannot reasonably be recognized. Rights
in medical care are different from rights to medical care, and
must be respected. That such rights may be overriden in
emergencies does not mean that respect for rights is not a
constraint upon the pursuit of equity and efficiency. (13)

827 Furrow, B.R. "Damage Remedies and Institutional Reform: The
     Right to Refuse Treatment," LAW MED HEALTH CARE 10 (September
     1982): 152-57.

     Recent court decisions have given institutionalized mental
     hospital patients the right to refuse treatment. Cases related
     to this right are presented.

828 Gaylin, W. "The Competence of Children: No Longer All or
     None," HASTINGS CENTER REPORT 12 (April 1982): 33-38.

     Defines limits and identifies principles to decide if a
     person is competent enough to make decisions about their health
     care, disregarding legal age. (4)

829 Herr, S.S. RIGHTS AND ADVOCACY FOR RETARDED PEOPLE. Lexington,
     MA.: D.C. Heath and Co., 1983.

     Past and current law to protect retarded persons presented.
     Legal battles to achieve rights described. Continuing needs
     for advocacy discussed.

830 Herr, S.S., D.P.S. Arons and W. Wallace, Jr. LEGAL RIGHTS AND
     MENTAL HEALTH CARE. Lexington, MA.: D.C. Heath and Co.,
     1983.

     Describes the development and current status of issues
     affecting the legal rights of the mentally ill, including the
     right to treatment, the right to refuse treatment, the special
     problems and rights of children, and the manner in which lawyers
     and clinical professionals resolve dilemmas involving the
     mentally ill.

831 Hogue, E. NURSING AND INFORMED CONSENT: CASES AND COMMENTARY.
     Owing Mills, MD.: National Health Publishing, 1983.

     Legalities of informed consent.

832 Kapp, M. "Adult Protective Services: Convincing the Patient
     to Consent," LAW MED HEALTH CARE 11(4) (September 1983):
     163-67, 188.

     Society should try to avoid coercive elements of protective
     services; self determination is best served when a competent
     individual uses the durable power of attorney to dictate who
     will make medical decisions for him or her; goal is not to
     obtain protective services but to ensure quality and appro-
     priateness of services. (44)

833   Kucera, W.R.   "The Strange Case of Informed Consent and the
      Standard of Care," J AANA 46 (June 1978): 291-93.

      State's Supreme Court considered issues concerning informed
      consent for anesthesia procedures and the standard of care
      against which a medical practitioner's conduct will be measured.
      (0)

834   Lidz, C.W., A. Meisel, E. Zerubavel, M. Carter, R.M. Sestak
      and L.H. Roth. INFORMED CONSENT: A STUDY OF DECISION MAKING
      IN PSYCHIATRY. New York: The Guilford Press, 1984.

      Empirical study of decision making among psychiatric patients.
      Though the findings varied somewhat from setting to setting,
      overall the authors found little that approximated the decision
      making patterns prescribed by the doctrine.

835   Marmor, et al.   "Medical Care and Procompetitive Reform,"
      VANDERBILT LAW REV 34 (May 1981): 1010-21 (excerpt).

      An excerpt discussing methods to possibly increase consumer
      sovereignty in medical care and encouraging alternative organi-
      zations for providers. (80)

836   Rosoff, A.J. INFORMED CONSENT. Rockville, MD.: Aspen
      Systems Corp., 1981.

      Provides quick answers to questions regarding the law and
      informed consent as well as providing a starting point for
      more detailed legal research.

837   Rozovsky, F.A. CONSENT TO TREATMENT: A PRACTICAL GUIDE.
      Boston: Little, Brown and Co., 1984.

      Comprehensive coverage of the law related to informed con-
      sent to treatment. Includes general information as well as
      issues related to special patient populations.

838   White, W.D. "Informed Consent: Ambiguity in Theory and
      Practice," J HEALTH POLITICS, POLICY AND LAW 8(1) (Spring
      1983): 99-119.

      Indicates there are problems related to the current law
      related to informed consent. Issues on the law of informed
      consent. Discusses three tests that might be made of whether
      a law is a good law. Concludes that the law of informed con-
      sent does not pass any one of these tests. Sees a need for
      both physician's and patient's protection. (51)

839   Ziegenfuss, J.T., Jr. PATIENTS' RIGHTS AND PROFESSIONAL
      SERVICE. New York: Van Nostrand Co., 1983.

Guidelines for staff conduct as it affects patients' rights.
Patients' rights with respect to such matters as admission,
treatment, confidentiality, freedom of movement, and civil
rights are outlined. The author presents examples of viola-
tions of these rights and discusses preventive measures.

See 168, 305, 308, 326, 343, 357, 521, 1281.

Terminating Life Support, Right to Live, Right to Die,
Handicapped Infants, Genetic Research, Abortions

840 Annas, G.J. "The Baby Doe Regulations: Government Interven-
     tion in Neonatal Rescue Medicine," AM J PUB HEALTH 74(6)
     (June 1984): 618-20.

     Examines Baby Doe regulations. (7)

841 _____. "The Case of Baby Jane Doe: Child Abuse or
     Unlawful Federal Intervention?," AM J PUB HEALTH 74(7)
     (July 1984): 727-29.

     A summary of the issues dealing with the Baby Jane Doe
     born October 11, 1983, suffering from spina bifida, hydro-
     cephaly, and microcephaly and upon which the federal efforts
     to intervene more directly in health care were based. (9)

842 _____. "Ethics Committees in Neonatal Care: Substantive
     Protection or Procedural Diversion?," AM J PUB HEALTH 74(8)
     (August 1984): 843-45.

     Argues that ethics committees will probably be as accurate
     as the current doctor patient model and more accurate if they
     can gather relevant information that might not otherwise be
     considered.

843 Bullough, B. "Legislative Update: Baby Doe Regulations,"
     PED NURS 10(3) (May/June 1984): 235.

     Describes latest version of controversial "Baby Doe Regula-
     tions" prohibiting discrimination against handicapped infants.
     (1)

844 Campos-Outcalt, D. "Brain Death: Medical and Legal Issues,"
     J FAMILY PRACTICE 19(3) (1984): 349-54.

     Irreversible cessation of brain function has become a widely
     accepted criterion of death. Case law, state statutes, and
     medical opinion, backed by clinical studies, all support the
     use of brain death criteria as a means of determining death.
     Current state statutes are in need of some uniformity, as
     twelve different statutory approaches to brain death are cur-
     rently in use. Brain death should not be confused with the
     still unresolved issue of termination of life support to ter-
     minally ill, mentally incompetent patients, or those who are
     comatose yet do not meet brain death criteria.

845 Cohn, S.D. "The Living Will From the Nurse's Perspective,"
     LAW MED HEALTH CARE 11(3) (1983): 121-24, 136.

     Lists those states which then had Right to Die laws.
     Although clinical situations to which a living will applies
     are not very common, they are among those which many people
     fear most. By understanding the concept of a living will a
     nurse will be able to more effectively give sensitive care.
     (45)

846 Creighton, H. "Terminating Life Support: Law for the Nurse
     Supervisor," SUPERVISOR NURSE (January 1977): 66.

     Briefly discusses the Quinlan case and provides explicit
     policies from two hospitals regarding resuscitation. It also
     presents California legislation on a "Right to Die" bill. (19)

847 Feldman, E. and T.H. Murray. "State Legislation and the Handi-
     capped Newborn: A Moral and Political Dilemma," LAW MED
     HEALTH CARE 12(4) (September 1984): 156-63.

     Reviews state laws about handicapped newborns. Finds they
     are characterized by problems in implementation. Relates this
     to new federal regulations and law. (60)

848 Furrow, B.R. "Impaired Children and Tort Remedies: The Emer-
     gence of a Consensus," LAW MED HEALTH CARE 11(4) (September
     1983): 148-54.

     Wrongful life suits involving "impaired" children are losing
     intensity as a debatable issue. Courts are recognizing the
     merits of tort litigation in the wrongful life cases. Tort
     suits are not purely compensatory but provide incentives for
     change. (41)

849 Glantz, L.H. "Limiting State Regulation of Reproductive Deci-
     sions," AM J PUB HEALTH 74(2) (February 1984): 168-69.

     A summary of the issues involved in abortion cases. (5)

850 Hoyt, J.D. and J.M. Davies. "A Response to the Task Force on
     Supportive Care," LAW MED HEALTH CARE 12(3) (June 1984):
     103-5, 134.

     A critique of supportive care plan of the Minnesota task
     force. Argues the guidelines discriminate against elderly
     and disabled persons. (18)

851 Kapp, M.B. "Response to the Living Will Furor: Directives
     for Maximum Care," AM J MED 72 (June 1982): 855-59.

     Discusses decision making concerning the extent of medical
     treatment that should be provided to a terminally ill patient.
     The "right to die" and "death with dignity," ethical and legal
     dilemmas. (23)

852 Milunsky, A. and G. Annas (Eds.). GENETICS AND THE LAW.
     NATIONAL SYMPOSIUM ON GENETICS AND THE LAW. New York:
     Plenum Press, 1980.

     Discusses moral and legal problems generated by the impact
     of genetic research on medical practice and social policy.
     The moral and legal problems that may be generated by the
     research itself rather than by its application are also dis-
     cussed.

853 Robertson, J. "Legal Criteria for Orders Not to Resuscitate:
     A Response of Justice Liacos," MEDICOLEGAL NEWS (February
     1980): 4.

     This is a comment by Robertson in response to an article by
     Justice Liacos, entitled "Dilemmas of Dying" which dealt with
     the Saikewicz decision.(5)

854 Robertson, J.A. THE RIGHTS OF THE CRITICALLY ILL. Cambridge,
     MA.: Ballinger Publishing Co., 1983.

     A work in the series sponsored by the American Civil Liberties
     Union to educate the public regarding their legal rights.
     Issues covered include truth telling and confidentiality,
     treatment and control of medication, suicide, refusing treat-
     ment, stopping treatment for incompetent patients, living wills,
     organ transplants, autopsies, experimentation, resource allo-
     cation, and cost control.

855 Shaw, M.W. and A.E. Doudera (Eds.). DEFINING HUMAN LIFE:
     MEDICAL, LEGAL AND ETHICAL IMPLICATIONS. Ann Arbor, MI.:
     AUPHA Press, 1983.

     Contributors from law, medicine, philosophy, biology, embry-
     ology, and genetics explore the issue of personhood. The
     implications of the definition for law, medicine discussed.
     Issue of the rights of the unborn, the right to choose abortion,
     and the responsibility of the legal and medical professionals
     in defining human life.

856 Taub, S. "Withholding Treatment From Defective Newborns,"
     LAW MED HEALTH CARE 10(1) (February 1982): 4-10.

     The Danville case of Siamese twins joined below the waist
     reviewed. A "do not feed" order was reported to the state.
     Parents and physician were charged with attempted murder,
     although charges were dismissed. Discussion of issues and
     related cases. (49)

857 "The Right to Refuse Treatment: A Model Act," (Compiled by the
     Legal Advisors Committee of Concern for Dying, George J.
     Annas, Chair.) AM J PUB HEALTH 73(8) (August 1983): 918-21.

Patient's right to refuse treatment is often thwarted either because the patient is unable to competently communicate or because providers insist on treatment. To overcome this some states enacted the so called "living will" or "natural death" statutes, but the committee wants to move beyond these models and propose a Model Act that clearly ennunciates an individual's right to refuse treatment and does not limit its exercise to the terminally ill or to heroic measures and provides a mechanism by which individuals can set forth their wishes in advance and designate someone to enforce them. (34)

858   The Task Force on Supportive Care. "The Supportive Care Plan--
      Its Meaning and Application: Recommendations and Guide-
      lines," LAW MED HEALTH CARE 12(3) (June 1984): 97-102.

      A position paper done by a Minnesota task force on suppor-
      tive care for persons who can benefit from no further treat-
      ment efforts. A supportive care decision means care aimed at
      comfort, hygiene, and dignity but not aimed at prolonging life.
      Conditions that fit the definition are discussed and proce-
      dures for protecting the individual's rights are outlined. (3)

859   Waters, J. "Wrongful Life: The Implications of Suits in Wrong-
      ful Life Brought by Children Against Their Parents," DRAKE
      LAW REV 31 (1981/1982): 411-34.

      Discusses the problems raised by a California court's deci-
      sion to allow children born with degenerative genetic diseases
      to sue and recover damages from their mothers for the uniquely
      feminine decision to give birth. (186)

860   Westfall, D. "Beyond Abortion: The Potential Reach of a
      Human Life Amendment," AM J LAW & MED 8(2) (Summer 1982):
      97-135.

      In Roe v. Wade, the Supreme Court held that the constitu-
      tionally protected right to privacy includes a woman's right
      to terminate pregnancy. Following the decision, anti-abortion
      groups turned to Congress to limit or negate that right. As
      a result of their efforts, several "human life" statutes and
      constitutional amendments have been proposed. This article
      focuses on the implications of proposed amendments that seek
      to ban or limit the availability of abortions indirectly by
      broadening the definition of "person" to include newborn indi-
      viduals. The article discusses the potentially serious effects
      such an amendment would have in areas unrelated to abortion.
      (242)

861   Yarling, R.R. "Ethical Analysis of a Nursing Problem: The
      Scope of Nursing Practice in Disclosing the Truth to Terminal
      Patients, An Inquiry Directed to the National Joint Practice
      Commission of the AMA and the ANA, Part I," SUPERVISOR NURSE
      9 (May 1978): 40-41, 45-50. Part II, SUPERVISOR NURSE 9
      (June 1978): 28-34.

A two part article which poses a question for the National
Joint Practice Commission regarding nurses' rights and obligations to answer questions posed by terminal patients. Situation is a complex one, particularly when the nurses and physicians disagree or when the patients, families, nurses, and
physicians disagree about how much information the patient
should have. Legal and ethical issues are involved. Because
the law regarding patients right to information is changing,
the articles are out of date in some details, but basic analysis is still sound. (14); (33)

862 Zaslow, J. "Wrongful Conception, Wrongful Birth, and Wrongful
      Life: The Parameters of Liability," LEGAL ASPECTS OF MEDICAL
      PRACTICE 10 (May 1982): 4, 7.

      Recent court decisions about cases involving children who
      were born to "sterilized" parents, or in which children were
      born defective. (8)

      See 371, 410, 413, 417, 446, 449, 454, 455, 456, 457, 458, 462,
      465, 491, 493, 495, 500, 503, 505, 511, 512, 517, 519.

Labor Law, Nurses' Rights As Employees

863 Annas, G.J., L.H. Glantz and B.F. Katz. THE RIGHTS OF DOCTORS,
      NURSES AND ALLIED HEALTH PROFESSIONALS. New York: Avon
      Books, 1981.

      Basic coverage of the legal rights and responsibilities of
      health professionals. Part of the series sponsored by the
      American Civil Liberties Union. Aimed at a general audience.
      Covers liability, licensure, the living will, the union move-
      ment in the health occupations, informed consent, drugs, human
      experimentation, medical records, privacy, the care of the
      dying, childbirth, abortion, and sterilization.

864 Cooper, C.G. and N.J. Brent. "The Nursing Profession and The
      Right to Separate Representation," CHICAGO-KENT LAW REV
      58(4) (1982): 1053-81.

      Reviews the National Labor Relations Act as it relates to
      nurses. The lack of jurisdiction between 1947 and 1974 over
      most hospital employees means that most policies of the National
      Labor Relations Board are recent. Major legal controversy has
      been over whether registered nurses could constitute a separate
      collective bargaining unit. Relevant case law discussed. Most
      recent decision supports registered nurses as a separate unit.
      (111)

865 Manson, J.N. "Legal Briefs: Statutory Rights Governing Employ-
      ment Relationships in the Health Care Field," AANA J 49(5)
      (October 1981): 529-31.

Notes that it is the Fair Labor Standards Act which establishes the fundamental concept that employees are entitled to
compensation for "working time," that requires equal pay for
equal work by different employees, and that establishes minimum
wages and maximum working hours. Examines how the Fair Labor
Standards Act applies to nurse anesthetists. (0)

866 Moskowitz, S. "Pay Equity and American Nurses: A Legal Analy-
     sis," SAINT LOUIS UNIVERSITY LAW J 23 (1983): 801-55.

Comprehensive overview of the legal issues related to nurses
salaries. Pay equity litigation including Lemons v. The City
and County of Denver and the 1981 decision of the Supreme
Court on County of Washington v. Gunther are reviewed. State
statutes and collective bargaining are discussed. (337)

867 Moskowitz, S. and L.D. Moskowitz. "Protecting Your Job," AM
     J NURS 84(1) (January 1984): 54-58.

What nurses can do if they have no contract and they are
arbitrarily fired. (32)

868 Shepard, I.M. and A.E. Doudera (Eds.). HEALTH CARE LABOR LAW.
     Ann Arbor, MI.: AUPHA Press, 1981.

Law, labor relations, collective bargaining, arbitration,
equal employment opportunity and union organization campaigns
are discussed as they affect the health care industry. Includes unions and management views on unionization.

Prescribing Privileges for Nurses

869 American Nurses' Association. PRESCRIBING PRIVILEGES FOR
     NURSES: A REVIEW OF CURRENT LAW. Kansas City, MO.: American
     Nurses' Association, Pub. No. D-80, 1984.

Surveys regulations presently governing nurses' prescriptive
authority. Includes state-by-state summary, legal authorities
and governing bodies, limitations and restrictions, and requirements for physician supervision.

870 Batey, M.V. and J.M. Holland. "Impact on Structural Autonomy
     Accorded Through State Regulatory Policies on Nurses' Pres-
     cribing Practices," IMAGE: THE JOURNAL OF NURSING SCHOLAR-
     SHIP XV (Summer 1983): 84-90.

Nurse practitioner prescribing practices in five states are
analyzed and found to be similar in spite of variations in the
enabling legislation in the five states. (25)

871 Bigbee, J.L., S. Lundin, J. Corbett and J. Collins. "Prescip-
     tive Authority for Nurse Practitioners: A Comparative Study
     of Professional Attitudes," AM J PUB HEALTH 74(2) (February
     1984): 162-63.

Assessed the attitudes of Wyoming physicians, pharmacists, nurses, and nurse practitioners about granting prescriptive authority to nurse practitioners. Support for the issue was mixed, with physicians expressing the strongest disagreement. All groups supported limitation of authority to a specific drug formulary, collaborative regulation, and mandatory certification and continuing education if prescriptive authority is granted to nurse practitioners. (5)

872   Bigbee, J.L. "Territoriality and Prescriptive Authority for Nurse Practitioners," NURS & HEALTH CARE 5(2) (February 1984): 106-10.

Uses the concept of territoriality to discuss nurse practitioners' current struggle for prescription writing privileges. Argues that nurse practitioners and physicians may be able to amicably share this territory in spite of the surplus of physicians reported by the GMENAC Report. (8)

873   Bullough, B. "Prescribing Authority for Nurses," NURS ECON 1 (September/October 1983): 122-25.

Laws in fourteen states authorize nurses to prescribe drugs. The privilege is limited to nurses in advanced specialty practice and there are limitations on the drugs that can be prescribed. Suggestions are offered for nurses who are planning to seek legislation. (22)

874   _____. "Legislative Update," PED NURS 9(6) (November/ December 1983): 462-64.

Column describes the current status of prescribing privileges for nurses. Sixteen states give some authority but the limitations vary. (22)

875   Christensen, D.B. "Legal Recognition of Prescriptive Authority for Pharmacists," U.S. PHARMACIST (March 1982): H-13- H-15.

Reviews state laws which allow pharmacists to prescribe. Pharmacists position often similar to nurses position regarding prescribing. (10)

876   Cowen, D.L. "Pharmacy and Freedom," PHARMACY IN HISTORY 26(2) (1984): 70-82.

A history of pharmacy laws and regulations. Furnishes background to an understanding of current pharmacy laws. (81)

877   Moniz, D.M. and G.R. Tarutis. "Making Law, Not Breaking Law," NURSE PRAC 8 (October 1983): 66, 68.

The legal status of nurses prescribing using standing orders
was questioned by the Washington Board of Nursing at licensure
revocation proceedings. Washington law neither allows nor
prohibits this practice. The case was dismissed but the authors
warn that prescribing using protocols involves legal risks to
nurses. (O)

878   "News: Utah Nurse Practitioners Conducting Pilot Project in
      Prescription Writing," AM J NURS 81(8) (August 1981): 1424,
      1448.

      News item. (O)

Anti-trust Law, Federal Trade Commission

879   Barnes, E.G. "Federal Trade Commission-American Medical Asso-
      ciate Case and Other Related Activities," FOOD, DRUG AND
      COSMETIC LAW J 37 (April 1982): 237-43.

      Barnes was the administrative judge for the FTC trial against
      the AMA. His article presents the FTC's action against the AMA
      as well as other health related activities. (32)

880   Bernstein, A.H. "Staff Privileges and Anti-trust Laws,"
      HOSPITALS (September 1, 1982): 76-78.

      Discusses cases of health care institutions charged with
      antitrust violations for denial of hospital privileges. (13)
      Bernstein, a hospital attorney in Oakland, California, writes
      a regular feature article for HOSPITALS dealing with legal
      issues in health care.

881   Foster, H.S. "Exclusive Arrangements Between Hospitals and
      Physicians: Antitrust's Next Frontier in Health?," SAINT
      LOUIS UNIVERSITY LAW J 26 (1982): 535-59.

      To date only a few antitrust challenges of the exclusive
      arrangments between hospitals and staff physicians have
      occurred. However, more are expected in the future. (111)

882   Havighurst, C. "Antitrust Enforcement in the Medical Services
      Industry: What Does It All Mean?," MILBANK MEMORIAL FUND Q
      58 (Winter 1980): 89-124.

      Describes and attempts to explain recent movements to enforce
      the antitrust laws in the health care sector of the economy.
      (45)

883   Thompson, M.J. ANTITRUST AND THE HEALTH CARE PROVIDER.
      Rockland, MD.: Aspen Systems Corp., 1979.

      This text explores a variety of facets of antitrust law that
      have proved to be of concern to health care providers.

Third Party Reimbursement for Nurses

884   American Nurses' Association. REIMBURSEMENT FOR NURSING
      SERVICES: A POSITION STATEMENT OF THE COMMISSION ON ECONOMIC
      AND GENERAL WELFARE. Kansas City, MO.: American Nurses'
      Association, Pub. No. EC-139, 1977.

      Proposes an informational and conceptual framework within
      which ANA can formulate strategies for the attainment of reim-
      bursement objectives.

885   _____. THIRD-PARTY REIMBURSEMENT LEGISLATION FOR SERVICES
      OF NURSES: A REPORT OF CHANGES IN STATE HEALTH INSURANCE
      LAWS. Kansas City, MO.: American Nurses' Association, Pub.
      No. D-77, 1983.

      Overview and analysis of current legislation, with review
      of legislation introducted into state legislatures in 1983.
      Summarizes each law and bill, with statutory references.

886   _____. OBTAINING THIRD-PARTY REIMBURSEMENT: A NURSE'S GUIDE
      TO METHODS AND STRATEGIES. Kansas City, MO.: American
      Nurses' Association, Pub. No. NS-29, 1984.

      Preparatory guidelines for the nursing professional working
      toward legislative and nonlegislative policies for third-party
      payment. Includes overview of systems, professional nursing's
      involvement, and detailed discussion of strategies for obtain-
      ing direct payment to nurses by health insurers.

887   Baker, N. "Entrepreneurial Practice for Nurses: A Response
      to Hershey," LAW MED HEALTH CARE 11(6) (December 1983): 257-
      69, 283.

      Points out the weakness in some of Hershey's arguments against
      nurses. Points out that although nursing and medical care
      overlap, expanded nursing care given by nurse practitioners
      is different from medical care. (16)

888   _____. "Reimbursement for Nursing Services: Issues and
      Trends," NURS LAW & ETHICS 1 (April 1980): 1, 2, 4. Reprinted
      in NURSING ISSUES AND NURSING STRATEGIES FOR THE EIGHTIES.
      Edited by B. Bullough, V. Bullough, and M.C. Soukup. New
      York: Springer Publishing Co., 1983, pp. 305-311.

      Stresses the need for the consumer to become acquainted with
      different aspects of the health care system. Nurses have a
      responsibility to do more of this since they are both in the
      position to do so and the victims of failing to do so. (13)

889   Brown, B.S. "Editorial: Devilish Options," PED NURS 8(1)
      (January/February 1982); 7.

      Dilemmas related to the reported future oversupply of phy-
      sicians and third party reimbursement for nurse practitioners
      discussed. (10)

890 Bullough, B.   "Legislative Update," PED NURS 8(6) (November/
     December 1982): 431-32.

     Federal and state laws covering reimbursement for nurse
     practitioners reviewed. (15)

891 Campbell, J.M.   "Practice Management: Reimbursement Basics,"
     PED NURS 8(6) (November/December 1982): 424.

     Discusses methods of processing claims for third party reim-
     bursement for nurses, and notes that techniques for reimburse-
     ment are complex and that reimbursable procedure eligibility
     changes often.(3)

892 Cohn, S.D.   "Survey of Legislation on Third Party Reimburse-
     ment for Nurses," LAW MED HEALTH CARE 11(6) (December 1983):
     260-63, 286.

     Reviews federal CHAMPUS and Medicaid laws which reimburse
     nurse midwives. In addition, laws have been passed in fifteen
     states which either mandate coverage or benefits to certain
     nurses. Most commonly covered are nurse midwives, five states
     mention nurse practitioners, two include nurse anesthetists,
     one psychiatric/mental health nurse, and in three states regis-
     tered nurses are covered. Author concludes that there is a
     growing trend to directly reimburse nurses. (35)

893 "Fact Sheet--House Bill 1456: An Act Providing Reimbursement
     for Services of Certain Health Care Providers," MASSACHUSETTS
     NURSE 49(4) (April 1980): 1, 6.

     Discusses the effect that legislation allowing third party
     reimbursement for nurses in Massachusetts would have on health
     care. Notes that consumers' health care needs can be met more
     adequately when they have the freedom to choose between quali-
     fied providers. (0)

894 Goldwater, M.   "From a Legislator: Views on Third-Party Reim-
     bursement for Nurses," AM J NURS 82 (3) (March 1982): 411-14.

     Examines the history of third party payments and summarizes
     Maryland's recent legislation providing for third party reim-
     bursement for certain nurses. Written by the legislator who
     introduced the landmark bill to the Maryland legislature. (3)

895 Griffith, H.M.   "Strategies for Direct Third-party Reimburse-
     ment for Nurses," AM J NURS 82(3) (March 1982): 408-11.

     Summarizes the legislative history of how Maryland became
     the first state to mandate third party reimbursement for nurse
     practitioners and nurse midwives without direct physician
     supervision. (11)

896 Hackley, B.K.   "Independent Reimbursement from Third-party
     Payers to Nurse-Midwives," J NURSE-MIDWIF 26(3) (May/June
     1981): 15-23.

Discusses the implications of differing payment mechanisms,
analyzes precedents in nurse—midwifery reimbursement and
current legislative proposals before Congress, and outlines
suggested strategies to precipitate change. Without independent reimbursement, which is a cornerstone of independent
practice, the freedom of nurse—midwives to engage in their
chosen profession is seriously jeopardized. (40)

897 Hershey, N. "Entrepreneurial Practice for Nurses: An Assess-
     ment of the Issues," LAW MED HEALTH CARE 11(6) (December
     1983): 253-56, 285.

     Argues against mandated "free choice" laws for third party
     reimbursement which would allow nurse practitioners to bill
     independently of physicians. Argues that research about the
     quality of care given by nurse practitioners would not apply
     with mandated third party reimbursement because that research
     was done when nurse practitioners were employed in organized
     health care settings under physician supervision. Is less
     negative about nurse midwives and nurse anesthetists. (25)

898 Jennings, C.P. "Nursing's Case for Third Party Reimbursement,"
     AM J NURS 79(1) (January 1979): 110-14.

     Observes that funding methods and reimbursement practices
     can alter health care patterns. Present reimbursement schemes
     favor costly hospitalization and physician care. Emphasizes
     that nurses need to convince legislators that they are of sub-
     stantial economic consequence and essential providers of care.
     (11)

899 LaBar, C. THIRD-PARTY REIMBURSEMENT FOR SERVICES OF NURSES.
     Kansas City, MO.: American Nurses' Association, Pub. No.
     D-72G, 1983.

     Reviews progress in achieving changes in the health care
     financing and delivery systems that enable third-party reim-
     bursement for nurses' services. (34)

900 "Landmark Maryland Nurse-Midwife Reimbursement Bill Passed,"
     J NURSE MIDWIF 23 (Fall 1978): 19.

     Provides a brief summary of a Maryland law affecting nurse
     midwives. (0)

901 McCarty, P. "Nurses Eligible for Direct Payment in 13 States,"
     AM NURSE 15(6) (June 1983): 1, 19.

     Reports that thirteen states (Montana, Alaska, Maryland, New
     Jersey, New Mexico, New York, Pennsylvania, Utah, Washington,
     Mississippi, Oregon, California, and West Virginia) now include
     provisions for direct payment to nurses, or to certain cate-
     gories of nursing in statutes governing health insurance. (0)

902 "New Jersey Nurse Entrepreneurs Now Eligible for Third Party
     Reimbursement," AM J NURS 84(3) (March 1984): 377.

     Reports that New Jersey nurses in private practice will begin
     receiving third party reimbursement in April, 1984. The new
     law extends Blue Shield reimbursement to all "eligible services
     by a registered professional nurse, within the scope of the
     nurse´s practice." (0)

903 "News: Hospitals Must Cost Out Nursing Care Under Landmark
     Maine Law," AM J NURS (September 1983): 1251, 1262.

     Describes a 1983 Maine hospital prospective reimbursement
     law which will require hospitals to separate out the nursing
     costs. This is the first such law in the nation. (0)

904 "Nurse-Midwife Payments Oked with Medicare-Medicaid Bill,"
     AM J NURS (March 1981): 448, 466.

     Medicaid payments to nurse midwives were authorized in 1981
     amendments to the social security law.

905 Peterson, M.L. "The Institute of Medicine Report: A Manpower
     Policy for Primary Health Care," ANNALS OF INTERNAL MED
     92(6) (June 1980): 843-51.

     Provides comments on accreditation for nurse practitioner
     education programs, information about state licensing laws for
     nurse practitioners, and recommendations for reimbursement
     for primary care. (13)

906 Pulcini, J. "Perspectives on Level of Reimbursement for
     Nursing Services," NURS ECON 2(2) (March/April 1984): 118-23.

     Observes that nurses have a particular disadvantage in the
     health care market because they are potential competitors of
     physicians. Encourages nurses to continue to work towards
     direct reimbursement, and provides an historical and political
     perspective of reimbursement for primary health care. (24)

907 Schweitzer, B. "Legislative Update," PED NURS 7(2) (March/
     April 1981): 58.

     Reimbursement options for nurses under CHAMPUS and for nurse
     midwives reported. Other federal legislative activities also
     covered. (0)

908 Tripp, S. and C. Proctor. "3rd Party Reimbursement for Nurses:
     A Piece of the Pie," MASSACHUSETTS NURSE 49(1) (January
     1980): 6-7.

     Explores the present system of health care costs and forms
     of reimbursements and presents information on third party
     reimbursement. Proposes possible options available to nurses.
     (0)

909   "Wash. Law Requires Blue Cross, Shield to Pay RNs Directly for
      Own Services," AM J NURS (September 1981): 1557, 1566.

      Third party reimbursement for nurses who perform reimburs-
      able services. Bill passed in 1975, was vetoed by governor
      when Blue Cross/Blue Shield argued they would pay nurses with-
      out legislation. Resubmitted it to the legislature and signed
      into law this time. (0)

910   Weston, J.L. "Distribution of Nurse Practitioners and Physi-
      cian Assistants: Implications of Legal Constraints and Reim-
      bursement," PUBLIC HEALTH REPORTS 95(3) (May/June 1980):
      253-58.

      Observes that the distribution of nurse practitioners and
      physician assistants is not adequate in medically underserved
      areas. Discusses the effect of state reimbursement policies
      and legal constraints on the distribution of NPs and PAs.
      Provides information about specific state regulations regarding
      prescription of drugs and direct reimbursement. (5)

911   Wriston, S. "Nurse Practitioner Reimbursement," J HEALTH
      POLITICS, POLICY AND LAW 6(3) (Fall 1981): 444-62.

      Addresses problems related to nurse practitioner reimburse-
      ment and the Rural Health Clinic Services Act of 1977. It is
      considered important that the Act recognizes the nurse prac-
      titioner as a reimbursable provider of traditional medical
      service, but it is still necessary to clarify nurse practi-
      tioner reimbursement policies. Discusses controversy surround-
      ing third party payer practices and medical society opposition
      to such payment to nurse practitioners. (141)

      See 2108, 2117.

Expert Witness Role

912   Northrop, C. and A. Mech. "The Nurse as Expert Witness,"
      NURS LAW & ETHICS 2(3) (March 1981): 1, 2, 6, 8.

      Describes the role of the expert witness. Cites cases which
      used nurses who served as expert witnesses. (8)

913   Perry, S. "If You´re Called As An Expert Witness," AM J NURS
      (March 1977): 458.

      Provides general information to help the increasing number
      of nurses who are being called as witnesses and expert wit-
      nesses in legal proceedings dealing with malpractice. (0)

Legal Issues Related to Nursing Education

914   Bullough, B.   "The Entry Into Practice Resolution," PED
      NURS 5(5) (September/October 1979): 25-28.

      Historical background and current discussion of the resolu-
      tions. (12)

915   "CE Now Required for Relicensure in 16 States," AM J NURS
      82(11) (November 1982): 1668, 1675.

      Overview of mandatory continuing education laws. (0)

916   Creighton, H.   "Physical Handicaps: Law for the Nurse Super-
      visor," SUPERVISOR NURSE (March 1980): 44.

      Deals with the issue of whether physical disabilities must
      be disregarded when employing nurses or admitting them to
      schools of nursing. Three cases are presented. (12)

917   Dodge, G.H.   "Legislators Look Askance at Mandatory CE,"
      AORN J 31(6) (May 1980): 1080, 1082, 1083, 1086-87, 1090-91.

      Negative view of mandatory continuing education laws. Slow-
      ing of trend to pass such laws reported. (2)

918   Podratz, R.O.   "A Student Sues," AM J NURS (September 1980):
      1604.

      A nurse educator presents her own experience with a law suit
      filed against the school by a student failing a course. (0)

919   Pollock, C., G. Poteet and W. Whilan.   "Students' Rights,"
      AM J NURS (April 1976): 600.

      Discusses legislation and judicial decisions which emphasize
      students' rights to privacy and due process with schools
      carrying the burden of proof in disciplinary action. (20)

920   Pollock, C., et al.   "Faculties Have Rights Too," AM J NURS
      (April 1977): 636.

      Presents many court decisions involving faculties and students
      with the recent trend being decisions upholding faculty rights
      as well as students. (16)

921   Rudy, C.A.   "Update: Mandatory Continuing Education," PED
      NURS 7(1) (January/February 1981): 37-38.

      Overview of mandatory continuation laws; states which accept
      NAPNAP and other continuing education programs listed. (4)

922   Stuart, C.T.   "Mandatory Continuing Education for Relicensure
      in Nursing: Issue of the Eighties?" NURSING ISSUES AND
      NURSING STRATEGIES FOR THE EIGHTIES.   Edited by B. Bullough,
      V. Bullough, M.C. Soukup.   New York: Springer Publishing
      Co., 1983, pp. 312-25.

      Discusses the pros and cons of mandatory continuing educa-
      tion, and the need to insure nursing competence. (11)

923   Whitaker, J.G.   "The Issue of Mandatory Continuing Education,"
      NURS CL NORTH AM 9 (September 1974): 475-83.   Reprinted in
      EXPANDING HORIZONS FOR NURSES.   Edited by B. Bullough and
      V. Bullough.   New York: Springer Publishing Co., 1977,
      pp. 178-86.

      Raises questions about mandatory continuing education for
      renewal of license and indicates the cautions that need to be
      exercised. (10)

      See 1422.

EDUCATION

Administrative Issues - Perspectives

924 American Academy of Nursing. STRUCTURE TO OUTCOME: MAKING IT
     WORK. Kansas City, MO.: American Nurses' Association, Pub.
     No. G-158, 1983.

     Collection of five major papers presented at the American
     Academy of Nursing's first annual Nursing Faculty Practice
     Symposium; presentations focus on values and structures of
     organizations, offer definitions of practice, and address from
     a variety of perspectives the pertinent issues and concerns
     confronting nursing faculty.

925 Aydelotte, M.K. "The Future Health Delivery System and the
     Utilization of Nurses Prepared in Formal Educational Pro-
     grams." THE NURSING PROFESSION: VIEWS THROUGH THE MIST.
     Edited by N.L. Chaska. New York: McGraw-Hill Book Co.,
     1978, pp. 349-58.

     The present and future needs for nurses within the health
     care delivery system requires clarification of the knowledge
     and competencies of various educational preparations. A match
     between educational preparation and needs for nursing prac-
     tice will help to maximize utilization.

926 Barkauskas, V.H. "Public Health Nursing Practice--An Educator's
     View," NURS OUTLOOK (July/August 1982): 384-89.

     A discussion of issues related to public health nursing
     includes students, faculty, curriculum planning and content,
     roles and functions of master's program graduates, faculty-
     agency relationships, and clinical research. Changing student
     composition, diminishing faculty specialists, and the uncertain
     future are explored. (19)

927 Brown, B.J. "Reviewing the Past and Current Status of Nursing's
     Role in Influencing Governmental Policy for Research and
     Training in Nursing." CURRENT ISSUES IN NURSING. Edited
     by J.C. McCloskey and H.K. Grace. Scranton, PA. Blackwell
     Scientific Publications, 1981, pp. 497-503.

     Nurses need to unite as a political force to influence leg-
     islation to improve education, research and patient care. (2)

928 Brown, B.J. and P.L. Chinn (Eds.). NURSING EDUCATION: PRACTICAL
     METHODS AND MODELS. Rockville, MD.: Aspen Publications, 1982.

A collection of articles which address some of the current
problems facing nursing education. Specific sections explore
curricular aspects, administrative aspects, the schism between
education and nursing service and continuing education.

929 Brown, E.L. NURSING FOR THE FUTURE. Philadelphia: W.F. Fell
     Co., 1948.

     In a study of the nursing and health needs of society, the
     investigators found inadequate nursing service in most hospi-
     tals. Poor educational programs were blamed for these defi-
     ciencies. It was recommended that educational programs for
     nurses be conducted in colleges and universities and that
     these programs be nationally classified and accredited. Prac-
     tical nursing programs should also be encouraged.

930 Brown Report. (See Brown, E. L. NURSING FOR THE FUTURE.)

931 Bullough, V.L. and B. Bullough. "Sex Discrimination and
     Nursing Education," HISTORY, TRENDS AND POLITICS OF NURSING.
     Edited by V. Bullough and B. Bullough. Norwalk, CT.:
     Appleton-Century-Crofts, 1984, pp. 25-32.

     A discussion of the development of educational programs in
     nursing and the influence the sex of its membership on its
     quest for acceptance in universities and colleges.

932 Bullough, V.L. and B. Bullough. "Nursing Education." HISTORY,
     TRENDS AND POLITICS OF NURSING. Edited by V. Bullough and
     B. Bullough. Norwalk, CT.: Appleton-Century-Crofts, 1984,
     pp. 51-68.

     Reviews the historical development of nursing education as
     it impacts on current issues and problems. Particular focus
     is directed toward entry into practice resolutions, career
     ladder options, and doctoral preparation for nurses.

933 Chaska, N.L. "Not Crystal Clear." THE NURSING PROFESSION:
     VIEWS THROUGH THE MIST. Edited by N.L. Chaska. New York:
     McGraw-Hill Book Co., 1978, pp. 407-27.

     A review of the status of critical areas of nursing as they
     relate to future planning in professionalism, education, re-
     search, theory and practice. (3)

934 Christman, L. "Alternatives in the Role Expression of Nurses
     That May Affect the Future of the Nursing Profession." THE
     NURSING PROFESSION: VIEWS THROUGH THE MIST. Edited by
     N.L. Chaska. New York: McGraw-Hill Book Co., 1978, pp.
     359-65.

     Changes are forecast for the educational preparation for
     nurses. Economic necessities will in all likelihood eliminate
     all but the health science university programs. Nurse prac-
     titioners will manage primary care centers and entry into
     nursing practice will be at the graduate level. (0)

935 Committee for the Study of Nursing Education. NURSING AND
     NURSING EDUCATION IN THE UNITED STATES. Edited by J.
     Goldmark. New York: Macmillan Co., 1923.

     The Goldmark Report, as this study is referred to, identi-
     fied poor educational practices in existing schools of nurs-
     ing in the United States. The problems were largely due to
     training schools being conducted in hospitals rather than edu-
     cational institutions. This system led to overproduction of
     nurses who were inadequately selected and imperfectly educated.

936 Committee on the Grading of Nursing Schools. Final Report.
     NURSING SCHOOLS TODAY AND TOMORROW. New York: n.p., 1934.

     A committee was organized to address the problems of over-
     production and undereducation which were identified in the
     Goldmark Report. It was organized to provide grading of nurs-
     ing schools with the goal of raising professional standards.
     The committee found nearly all the schools were owned and con-
     trolled by hospitals. Programs were used to meet service needs
     rather than the educational needs of students. It was recom-
     mended that schools of nursing be conducted under the aegis of
     colleges and universities.

937 Conway-Rutowski, B. "Future Trends in Post-Basic Education,"
     J NURS EDUC 21(6) (June 1982): 5-10.

     Technology will allow for the maximizing of faculty effective-
     ness. Fewer traditional aged students will be enrolled and
     adult learners will increase proportionately. Economic aid
     will decrease and management will become more centralized.
     Programs will focus more on learning than teaching and part-
     time students will have flexible scheduling. (13)

938 Fasano, N.F. and M.J. White. "Future Scenario: Commencement
     Address to the Class of 2010," J NURS EDUC 21(3) (March
     1982): 20-25.

     The extension of current trends and situations to a futuris-
     tic perspective envisions changes in nursing, health care and
     society. The author expects eradication of disease, a highly
     technological and depersonalized society and increased longe-
     vity. (8)

939 Goldmark Report. (See 936: NURSING AND NURSING EDUCATION IN
     THE UNITED STATES.)

940 Hartley, C.L., N.B. Hechenberger, J.A. Bryson and J.A. McCluskey.
     "Educators Strive for Unity," NURS HEALTH CARE 5(2) (February
     1984): 76-83.

     A report of interviews of chairpersons and vice chairpersons
     of the NLN Councils of Associate Degree, Baccalaureate and
     Higher Degree, Diploma and Practical Nurse Programs focuses on
     common concerns and issues in the area of nursing education. (0)

941   Huber, M.L.   "Associate Degree Nursing: Implications for the
      1980s and Beyond," J NURS ED 21(6) (June 1982): 24-33.

      Through knowledge of issues, interpretation of trends and
      consideration of alternatives, community college leaders may
      plan for the future of associate degree nursing programs. A
      focus on the originally intended practice role, leaving com-
      munity health and leadership preparation to baccalaureate pro-
      grams, and preparing for increased student enrollments are
      some of the factors which must be considered in future planning.
      (8)

942   Jacox, A.   "Significant Questions," NURS OUTLOOK 31(1)
      (January/February 1983): 28-33.

      The study of nursing being conducted by the Institute of
      Medicine seeks to determine the need to continue financial
      support to nursing education and determine the reasons nurses
      leave the profession or fail to practice in medically under-
      served areas. The use of "old" data; data collected for other
      purposes, and underrepresentation of the professional group in
      the study committee affects the credibility of the study find-
      ings. (16)

943   Leininger, M.   "Futurology of Nursing: Goals and Challenges
      for Tomorrow." THE NURSING PROFESSION: VIEWS THROUGH THE
      MIST. Edited by N.L. Chaska. New York: McGraw-Hill Book
      Co., 1978, pp. 379-96.

      Leininger predicts areas of anticipated change which have
      implications for the future of nursing and recommends actions
      which will serve to shape the future of nursing practice. (17)

944   Masson, V.   "International Collaboration in Nursing Education:
      The People to People Approach," J NURS EDUC 19(5) (May 1980):
      48-54.

      Describes the nursing programs of Project Hope, their struc-
      ture, operation and philosophy. Reviews the structure of
      nursing education programs in the developing nations. Twenty-
      five programs currently operate at eleven sites in seven coun-
      tries. (5)

945   Mauger, B.L. and K. Higgins.   "Developing and Implementing
      Collaborative Nursing Education Research in the South,"
      NURS RES 29(3) (May/June 1980): 189-92.

      A project funded by the Department of Health, Education and
      Welfare provided for the development of a regional research
      project in the southern states. The focus of the project was
      to identify educational research issues. Clinical performance
      evaluation, graduate follow-up, and curriculum were the major
      areas of interest. Nineteen research groups developed studies
      on issues in nursing education. (0)

946 Mauksch, I.G. "An Analysis of Some Critical Contemporary
     Issues in Nursing," J CONTIN EDUC NURS 14 (1983): 4-8.

     In the past, the nursing profession has underplayed compe-
     tence differences between registered nurses and aides. In the
     future, the nursing profession should prevent sub-professionals
     from carrying out nursing tasks of a professional nature.
     Nurses' increasing competence with technical gadgetry has been
     associated with increased autonomy, accountability, and asser-
     tiveness, and that technology has increased physicians' depend-
     ence on the judgment of nursing specialists. (0)

947 McNeil, J. "An Administrator's View of Staff Educational
     Needs," NURS OUTLOOK 26(10) (October 1978): 641-45.

     Nurse administrators are in these positions without advanced
     formal education. Well prepared master's graduates do not
     have experience and cannot find the positions Efforts must
     be made to provide formal education which is meaningful to the
     administrator role and grant degrees to current administrators
     in public health.

     Staff nurses in public health need physical assessment skills
     and specialty preparation as nurse practitioners to enhance the
     community health background. (6)

948 Morris, A.L., D.A. Hastings and K.R. Crispell. "The Role of
     the Nursing School in the Academic Health Center: Report of
     a Study," J NURS EDUC 22(4) (April 1983): 152-60.

     A major study surveyed top administrative officials in aca-
     demic health centers regarding the structural components and
     hierarchal relationships present. Highlights of this study
     are reported focusing on areas of particular interest to nurs-
     ing students. (0)

949 Nahm, H. E. "History of Nursing-A Century of Change." CURRENT
     ISSUES IN NURSING. Edited by J.C. McCloskey and H.K. Grace.
     Scranton, PA.: Blackwell Scientific Publications, 1981,
     pp. 14-25.

     Traces the development of nursing education programs, pro-
     fessional organizations, licensure and accreditation and con-
     siders the directions for future development of nursing educa-
     tion and research. (27)

950 NLN PERSPECTIVES FOR NURSING AND GOALS OF THE NATIONAL LEAGUE
     FOR NURSING 1979-1981. New York: National League for
     Nursing, 1979.

     A year long effort of a committee of the National League for
     Nursing focused on key issues in health care as they affect
     nursing and a reevaluation of the goals of the organization.

951 NURSING AND NURSING EDUCATION IN THE UNITED STATES. Report of
     the Committee for the Study of Nursing Education. New York:
     Macmillan Co., 1923.

     Report of a cooperative work between the League of Nursing
     Education and a committee appointed by the Rockefeller Founda-
     tion. Findings identified poor educational practice in exist-
     ing schools of nursing in the United States directly attributed
     to their adjunct relationship to hospitals as service institu-
     tions rather than educational institutions. Such conditions
     were responsible for overproduction of nurses, inadequately
     selected and imperfectly educated. (Also known as the Gold-
     mark Report.)

952 Peterson, C.J. "Issues in Allied Health Education." THE
     NURSING PROFESSION: VIEWS THROUGH THE MIST. Edited by N.L.
     Chaska. New York: McGraw-Hill Book Co., 1978, pp. 135-151.

     Major issues in the education of allied health practitioners
     are described as: "health" as the coming perspective, curri-
     culum development, individualized instruction, clinical educa-
     tion, continuing education, educational mobility, and maldis-
     tribution of person power. These issues are explored in depth
     and other issues related to future planning identified. (43)

953 _____. "Overview of Issues in Nursing Education." THE
     NURSING PROFESSION: A TIME TO SPEAK. Edited by N.L. Chaska.
     New York: McGraw-Hill Book Co., 1983, pp. 91-100.

     Considers current problems and future needs in nursing edu-
     cation. (4)

954 Rawnsley, M.M. "The Goldmark Report: Midpoint in Nursing His-
     tory." NURS OUTLOOK 21(6) (June 1973): 380-83.

     Reviews educational issues of past and considers current
     issues in light of the Goldmark Report. Identifies the need
     for nurses to determine policy and settle issues as an inde-
     pendent professional group; excessive clinical hours reminis-
     cent of apprenticeship education, lack of correlation between
     theory and practice; the need to stress prevention of illness
     within nursing curricula; and inferior quality of teachers
     were all issues noted in the Goldmark Report which continue
     unsettled at the present time. (18)

955 Safier, G. "Leaders Among Contemporary U.S. Nurses: An Oral
     History." THE NURSING PROFESSION: VIEWS THROUGH THE MIST.
     Edited by N.L. Chaska. New York: McGraw-Hill Book Co.,
     1978, pp. 81-92.

     Interviews with twelve nursing leaders most over age seventy
     provide insight into nursing's past. Educational structures
     and historical events are described in terms of personal im-
     pact. Current and future professional issues are explored.
     (9)

956   Sovie, M.D. "Nursing: A Future to Shape." THE NURSING
      PROFESSION: VIEWS THROUGH THE MIST. Edited by N.L. Chaska.
      New York: McGraw-Hill Book Co., 1978, pp. 366-378.

      The women's movement, consumerism, health planning and the
      knowledge explosion are current societal forces which are
      moving nursing to plan its future. Within this changing envir-
      onment nursing is progressing toward increased professional
      stature. (33)

957   Stewart, I. THE EDUCATION OF NURSES. New York: Macmillan
      Co., 1948.

      Traces the development of nursing education from primitive
      times to 1933.

958   West, M. and C. Hawkins. NURSING SCHOOLS AT THE MID-CENTURY.
      New York: National Committee for the Improvement of Nursing
      Services, 1950.

      A mid-century survey reported a wide range of practices among
      schools of nursing in the United States. The need for clearer
      definition of educational standards was identified as basic to
      the improvement of nursing service.

      See 998, 1451.

Conflict- Education/Practice

959   Baker, C.M. "Moving Toward Interdependence: Strategies for
      Collaboration," NURSE EDUC 6(5) (September/October 1981):
      27-31.

      A survey of the literature identified the need for maximum
      voluntary collaboration by nurses in practice and education
      since current efforts are not successful. The principal
      obstacle is the tradition of commitment to one or the other.
      The major functions of professional nursing are depicted in a
      model which might be used to foster collaboration. (18)

960   Blanchard, S.L. "The Discontinuity Between School and Prac-
      tice," NURS MANAGE 14 (1983): 41-43.

      Argues that nursing educators and nursing administrators
      should work to reduce the discrepancy new graduate nurses
      experience between ideal situations and actual conditions of
      nursing practice by providing students with more exposure to
      actual clinical situations under the guidance of an instructor.
      (5)

961   Carter, L.B. "Improving Relationships Between Nursing Service
      and Education in the Clinical Agency," J NURS EDUC 18(7)
      (September 1979): 7-12.

Communication, informal socialization and shared interest
between nurse educators, nursing service personnel and students
are discussed which can serve to promote a common goal of improved patient care. (5)

962 Chaska, N.L. "Status Consistency and Nurses´ Perception of
     Conflict Between Nursing Education and Practice." THE
     NURSING PROFESSION: VIEWS THROUGH THE MIST. Edited by N.L.
     Chaska. New York: McGraw-Hill Book Co., 1978, pp. 100-11.

     A study of 303 nurses considered educational preparation,
     status of position and income as factors influencing their per-
     ception of conflict between nursing education and nursing
     practice. (24)

963 Curran, C.L. and C. Metcalf. "Combining Resources," NURS
     MANAGE 14(1) (January 1983): 33-36.

     A new model of collaboration based upon identifying and
     sharing resources is proposed to promote understanding of the
     interdependence of clinicians and academicians. The basic
     components of the organizational model are parallel committees
     in both settings so that faculty participate on nursing ser-
     vice committees and clinicians participate on academic com-
     mittees. (0)

964 Dexter, P.A., and J. Laidig. "Breaking the Education/Service
     Barrier," NURS OUTLOOK 28(3) (March 1980): 179-82.

     A group of associate degree faculty found collaboration with
     nursing service administrators enriched their understanding of
     quality assurance and enabled them to strengthen their own
     knowledge and that of their students. (0)

965 Douglas, D.J. "Nursing Practice and Nursing Education: Realism
     Versus Idealism." THE NURSING PROFESSION: VIEWS THROUGH THE
     MIST. Edited by N.L. Chaska. New York: McGraw-Hill Book
     Co., 1978, pp. 129-34.

     Various types of models are described which may be used to
     create curricula with practical and theoretical utility. Such
     models may help to close the gap between education and ser-
     vice. (0)

966 Eschbach, D. "Role Exchange: An Exciting Experiment," NURS
     OUTLOOK 31(3) (May/June 1983): 164-67.

     Discusses the program REEP (Role Exchange/Education Practice)
     which was developed and implemented at Saddleback College in
     1980. For an eight week period a nurse educator is assigned
     to carry out the job of a nurse in a hospital, while a prac-

ticing nurse is assigned to carry out the job of the nurse
educator. The purpose is to update the clinical skills of
faculty, provide opportunities for practicing nurses to learn
about nursing education, and to bridge the gap between service and educator. (21)

967 Ezell, A. S. "Future Social Planning for Nursing Education
     and Nursing Practice Organizations." THE NURSING PROFESSION:
     A TIME TO SPEAK. Edited by N.L. Chaska. New York: McGraw-
     Hill Book Co., 1983, pp. 764-77.
     Goal disparity between nursing practice and nursing education
is growing. Discomfort with this gap should lead both to
choose between two organizational choices: long-range social
planning which will adapt nursing to the environment and hence
gain external consistency; or organizational future-responsive
social learning which will strive for internal consistency at
the expense of environmental conflicts. (17)

968 Fishel, A.H. and G.A. Johnson. "The Three-way Conference--
     Nursing Student, Nursing Supervisor and Nursing Educator,"
     J NURS EDUC 20(6) (June 1981): 18-23.

     Conflicts between expectations of nursing education and nurs-
ing service causes stress in student nurses. Utilization of
three way conferences between the student and these two factions
allowed for direct confrontation of conflicts and assisted
students in integrating theory and practice. (7)

969 Fortune, M. and C.S. Torres. "Service-Education Collaboration
     in a Community Health Agency," NURS HEALTH CARE 4(8) (October
     1983): 448-49.

     Recounts collaborative efforts of faculty from five schools
of nursing to resolve problems related to processing of information in a community health agency. Their goal was to satisfy
the educational needs of nursing students by streamlining,
clarifying and unifying agency policies. (0)

970 Grace, H.K. "Unification, Reunification, Reconciliation or
     Collaboration--Bridging the Education/Service Gap." CURRENT
     ISSUES IN NURSING. Edited by J. McCloskey and H.K. Grace.
     Scranton, PA.: Blackwell Scientific Publications, 1981,
     pp. 626-43.

     Uses conceptual models to depict changes in the education-
service role in nursing education from the first programs in
the United States to present. It is necessary in bridging the
gap between education and service to recall the history behind
the separation and prevent the recreation of the same problems.
(9)

971 Jarratt, V.R. "'The Time Has Come,' The Walrus Said, 'To Talk
     of Many Things'." NURS HEALTH CARE 4(9) (November 1983):
     498-503.

Nursing service and nursing education continue to assume
adversary roles. The roots of conflict are traced. Specific
solutions are proposed to resolve conflict and serve to unite
these two groups. (0)

972 Johnson, J. "The Education/Service Split: Who Loses?," NURS
     OUTLOOK 28(7) (July 1980): 412-15.

     The gap between service and education is of recent origins.
     Separation of "our" problems and "your" problems becomes less
     evident in joint appointment models. Nursing service is
     demanding more of the educational institutions in exchange
     for use of clinical resources. Whether faculty choose to be
     proactive or reactive in resolving service problems, the time
     is near when such demands will be mandated. (22)

973 Mezey, M.D., J.E. Lynaugh and J.E. Cherry. "The Teaching Nurs-
       ing Home Program," NURS OUTLOOK 32(3) (May/June 1984):
       146-50.

     Describes the characteristics of eleven teaching nursing home
     programs co-sponsored by the Robert Wood Johnson Foundation and
     the American Academy of Nursing. These programs seek to bridge
     the gap between education and practice through sharing and
     involvement in a joint venture. (4)

974 Nayer, D.D. "Unification: Bringing Nursing Service and Nurs-
       ing Education Together," AM J NURS 80(6) (June 1980): 1110-14.

     Recounts the historical background from which faculty prac-
     tice emerged, variations in models currently utilized and the
     recent resolution of the American Academy of Nursing endorsing
     unification or reconciliation of service and education. (0)

975 Riddell, D. and K. Hubalik. "Bridging the Gap: Responsibility
       of Education or Service?" CURRENT ISSUES IN NURSING. Edited
       by J.C. McCloskey and H.K. Grace. Scranton, PA.: Blackwell
       Scientific Publications, 1981, pp. 621-26.

     Argues educators are principally to blame for promulgating
     conflict between educators and administrators. However, both
     need to work to bridge the gap and unify nursing. (10)

976 Schmalenberg, C.E. and M. Kramer. "Dreams and Reality: Where
       Do They Meet?" J NURS ADM 6 (June 1976): 35-43.

     Explores the two subcultures of the nursing world and des-
     cribes the phenomenon of reality shock as found in a nationwide
     sample of graduate nurses. Discussions focus on the impli-
     cations of reality shock for nursing and for society, and
     suggestions for remediations are presented. (8)

977 Wagner, D.L. "Nursing Administrators´ Assessment of Nursing
       Education," NURS OUTLOOK 28(9) (September 1980): 557-61.

An examination of dissatisfactions between nursing service
and nursing education with recommendations for resolution of
conflict. (7)

978 Walker, D. and J.T. Bailey. "'Pay-offs' and 'Trade-offs':
     Reflections of a Nursing Administrator and a Nursing Educator
     on a Collaborative Study in the Practice of Nursing," J NURS
     EDUC 19(6) (June 1980): 54-57.

A discussion between representatives from nursing service
and nursing education who participated in a jointly funded
research project points out the need for continued collaborative studies which should help bridge the gap and conflict
between education and administration. (10)

979 Werner, J. "Joint Endeavors: The Way To Bring Service and
     Education Together," NURS OUTLOOK 28(9) (September 1980):
     546-50.

A discussion of the rift between the goals of nursing education and the service areas. A shared vision is necessary
which commits both factions to nursing care, accountability
and reconciliation. Power, strength, and success as a profession require unification. (7)

980 White, C., R. Knollmueller and S. Yaksich. "Preparation for
     Community Health Nursing: Issues and Problems." NURS OUTLOOK
     28(10) (October 1980): 617-23.

Findings of a national survey of nursing programs and community health nursing agencies are highlighted which document
current patterns of collaboration in providing for the education of community health nurses in baccalaureate nursing
programs. A widening gulf between education and practice is
identified. Suggestions are offered which could serve to
strengthen this relationship. (0)

See 969, 1302, 1345, 1443, 1671.

Academic Governance

981 Baj, P.A. "The Role of the Academic Nursing Administrator in
     Baccalaureate Programs for the Registered Nurse," NURS
     LEADERSH 6(1) (March 1983): 16-21.

Argues that the dean of a baccalaureate nursing program for
RNs needs an understanding of organizational theory in order
to provide the climate and programs which will foster professional growth. (26)

982 Baker, C.M. "Faculty Unionism: Issues and Impact." THE NURS-
     ING PROFESSION: A TIME TO SPEAK. Edited by N.L. Chaska.
     New York: McGraw-Hill Book Co., 1983, pp. 778-91

Collective bargaining in nursing education is becoming
increasingly common. The impact of unionism on academic
governance, employm,ent conditions, and quality of education
are discussed. (19)

983 Bridgewater, S.C. "Organizational Autonomy for Nursing Educa-
     tion," J NURS EDUC 18(1) (January 1978): 4-8.

When nursing programs are contained within medical or other
institutional schools they become subordinate. Lack of contact in equal fashion with other professional programs, lack
of decision-making and lack of control curtail professional
autonomy. It is therefore recommended that no collegiate
nursing program remain in a subordinate relationship with
another educational unit. (30)

984 Conway, M.E. and O. Andruskiw. ADMINISTRATIVE THEORY AND
     PRACTICE: ISSUES IN HIGHER EDUCATION IN NURSING. Norwlk,
     CT.: Appleton-Century-Crofts, 1983.

Addresses timely issues facing deans and administrators in
schools of nursing in light of changing times and diminishing
resources. Describes a socio-humanistic model for decision
making.

985 Ezell, A.S. "Anarchy and Revolution Within Educational Organi-
     zations of Nursing." THE NURSING PROFESSION: A TIME TO
     SPEAK. Edited by N.L. Chaska. New York: McGraw-Hill Book
     Co., 1983, pp. 70-90.

Organizational behaviors and patterns of interaction in
schools of nursing are discussed with particular attention to
anarchy and machiavellian types. (45)

986 Fagin, C.M. and D.O. McGivern. "Building a Network of Support
     in Order to Strengthen the Position of the Dean." THE NURS-
     ING PROFESSION: A TIME TO SPEAK. Edited by N.L. Chaska.
     New York: McGraw-Hill Book Co., 1983, pp. 749-63.

The longevity of deans in schools of nursing is decreasing.
The development of support networks is critical to the success
of the dean's role. These networks are described in terms of
level, function, and strategies. (6)

987 Finneran, M.D. "Trends in the Evaluation of Nursing Deans,"
     NURS OUTLOOK 31(3) (May/June 1983): 172-75.

A survey of deans reported that sixty percent were being
formally evaluated. The purposes of administrative evaluation
was to assess the deans' overall performance. Productivity,
effectiveness, performance in role, leadership, and management
skills were the most frequently cited criteria for evaluation.
(8)

988 Griffith, J.W. "Organizational Patterns of Baccalaureate
     Nursing Programs," J NURS EDUC 19(5) (May 1980): 55-60.

     Compares and analyzes the organizational patterns of five
     baccalaureate nursing programs. The programs were found to
     differ substantially in goals and faculty advancement. The
     network of relations and decision making processes was
     similar in the institutions studied. (11)

989 Hall, B.A., R. deTornyay and B. Mitsunaga. "Deans in Nursing:
     How Do They See Their Future?," J NURS EDUC 22(7) (September
     1983): 274-77.

     A comparison of deans in 1970 and in 1980 revealed that fewer
     expect to stay in the position until retirement. Age and the
     number of years in the current deanship were found to be major
     predictors of whether a dean aspires to top level university
     positions. (3)

990 Hawken, P.L. "Growing Our Own: A Way to Prepare Deans,"
     NURS OUTLOOK 28(3) (March 1980): 170-72.

     On the job experience from the dean's perspective is a use-
     ful method of preparing for the realities of the dean's role.
     (0)

991 Higgs, Z.R. "Expectations and Perceptions of the Curricular
     Leadership Role of Administrators of Nursing Education
     Units," NURS RES 27(1) (January/February 1978): 57-63.

     A survey of deans and faculty regarding the curricular leader-
     ship role of the dean identified agreement as to the dean's
     role in curricular design and evaluation. There was no agree-
     ment, however, within either group as to how the dean should
     function in curriculum implementation. (21)

992 Hollshwander, C.H. "Models in Administration and the Dean's
     Exercise of Power and Leadership," J NURS EDUC 22(7)
     (September 1983): 289-91.

     A review of organizational models is presented. The human
     resources model was judged most appropriate for nursing educa-
     tion. This model utilizes power to enhance the sphere of
     influence which includes the personal life and achievement of
     each member of the group. (6)

993 Limandri, B.J. "Academic Procedural Due Process for Students
     In The Health Professions," J NURS EDUC 20(2) (February
     1981): 9-18.

     Describes and discusses cases of due process which deal with
     establishing the institutional right and grounds for due pro-
     cess in education and health education. (19)

150   Education

994 Martin, E.J. "Selection of Nursing Deans," NURS OUTLOOK 31(3)
     (May/June 1983): 168-72.

     A survey of sixty-three deans reveals some interesting new
     trends. Advantages and disadvantages of internally and exter-
     nally selected candidates are discussed. Over seventy-five
     percent of the deans appoint associate/assistant deans and
     tend to choose internal candidates. (4)

995 Miller, Sr. P. "Student Grade Appeals: Procedure and
     Process," J NURS EDUC 21(6) (June 1982): 34-38.
     When a faculty member and student dispute a grade, an appeals
     procedure may assist in resolving the differences of opinion.
     Such a procedure allows the student the right of due process,
     maintains the academic freedom of faculty, and facilitates a
     just decision. (11)

996 Murphy, J.F. "The Academic Deanship in Nursing: Challenge or
     Capitulation." THE NURSING PROFESSION: A TIME TO SPEAK.
     Edited by N.L. Chaska. New York: McGraw-Hill Book Co.,
     1983, pp. 739-48.

     The role of the dean requires technical, human, and concep-
     tual skills. The needs for these skills vary within specific
     schools, however, current pressures require conceptual skills
     to a greater extent than technical skills. The focus of human
     skills have moved from intra to inter group concerns. (5)

997 "NC's PHNs Fight to Save a University's Public Health Nursing
     Department," AM J NURS 83(12) (December 1983): 1711.

     Public health nurses in the State of North Carolina success-
     fully fought a plan at the University of North Carolina to
     replace the Department of Public Health Nursing by an inter-
     disciplinary nursing curriculum. University officials per-
     ceived the legislative infringement in violation of academic
     freedom. (0)

998 Partridge, R. "The Decanal Role: A Dilemma of Academic Leader-
     ship," J NURS EDUC 22(2) (February 1983): 59-61.

     The role of the dean varies within institutions and with
     personal preferences. Many wish to align their identity with
     faculty expressing temporary administrative service. Distinc-
     tions exist between leadership and management within the dean's
     role and many alternatives are evidenced. (13)

999 Redman, B.K. and Z.A. Barley. "On the Governance System of
     University Schools of Nursing," J NURS EDUC 17(7) (September
     1978): 27-31.

School of nursing governance must be viewed in the larger
context of the entire school. Conceptualization of this framework is necessary in dealing with issues that confront sub-
units of the larger system. As external pressures and accountability in use of resources face universities, schools of
nursing should move to maximize their governance in efficient
ways. (1)

1000   Spink, L.M. "Due Process in Academic Dismissals," J NURS EDUC
       22(7) (September 1983): 305-6.

       Educational institutions should provide due procedures in
       instances of academic dismissals. Several cases are reported.
       Although there is the doctrine of judicial non-interference in
       academia, procedures for evaluation should be fair and reason-
       able. Guidelines are proposed. (5)

1001   "Turmoil at Wright State University Follows Word on New BSN
       Program," AM J NURS 80(3) (March 1980): 385, 390.

       The Board of Trustees of Wright State University issued a
       directive that a second nursing program for registered nurses
       be planned outside the administration of the School of Nursing.
       This announcement was followed by the resignation of the dean
       and associate dean. Twenty of the thirty faculty gave notice
       of their intent to leave at the conclusion of their present
       contracts. The dean saw this action as an attempt to place
       the School of Nursing under the control of the School of
       Medicine. (0)

       See 1398.

Financing

1002   "ANA Tells Congress Shut-off of Funds May Signal Disaster,"
       AM J NURS 81(5) (May 1981): 907, 945-46.

       Further cuts in funds to nursing education proposed by the
       Reagan administration threaten the continuation of programs
       already underway. Despite federal assistance, nursing short-
       ages still exist particularly in the areas of clinical nurse
       specialists, nurse educators, nurse researchers, and nursing
       service administration.(0)

1003   "Appropriations is Next Step for Federal Nursing Funds," AM J
       NURS 81(10) (October 1981): 1773-74.

       The Budget Reconciliation Bill appropriated $63 million for
       federally backed nursing programs. Nurses must urge their
       local representatives in Congress to back this funding for the
       nursing components as it is feared further cuts may be in-
       flicted. (0)

1004   Boehret, A.C. and A. LaRowe. "Class Size and Cost in ADN Pro-
       grams." NURS OUTLOOK 26(6) (June 1978): 389-91.

Small numbers of students within a given class are not cost effective. Class admissions between forty-nine and sixty students maximize use of faculty and resources. (4)

1005   Brown, B.J., W.F. Lasher and C.L. Embrey. "A Costing Method-
       ology for Schools of Nursing," NURS OUTLOOK 27(9) (September
       1979): 584-89.

A systematic approach to cost analysis for a school of nursing is presented as a method of understanding current financial structure and projecting future needs. (0)

1006   Brown, E. "The Cost of Nursing Education." CURRENT ISSUES IN
       NURSING. Edited by J.C. McCloskey and H.K. Grace. Scranton,
       PA.: Blackwell Scientific Publications, 1981, pp. 531-38.

Over the years many studies have been conducted to measure
the cost of educating a nursing student in diploma, associate
degree, and baccalaureate programs. Costs varied greatly and
the studies were found to be incomplete and inconsistent. (17)

1007   "Carter Asks Congress to Cut 25 Percent of Nursing Budget,"
       AM J NURS 80(6) (June 1980): 1064,1066.

Carter has proposed drastic cuts to health and social programs. Congress was asked to reduce appropriations for capi-
tation funds and nursing research. (0)

1008   "Carter's Budget Signals Fight on Nursing Funds," AM J NURS
       80(3) (March 1980): 375, 398, 400.

Patricia Harris, Secretary of Health, Education and Welfare
stated that President Carter intends to dismantle nursing education support efforts, pending approval of Congress. She
identified a distributional problem with trained nurses who
are not practicing and feels educational support encourages
this. (0)

1009   "Congress Balks at Cuts; Restores some NTA Funds," AM J NURS
       79(4) (April 1979): 569, 584.

The Carter administration proposed cutting funds to nursing
education by $84 million. The House Appropriations Committee
and the House of Representatives reduced the cutback to $22.3
million. Congress is currently debating the issue. (0)

1010   "Congress Expected to 'Continue' Nursing Funds," AM J NURS
       80(8) (August 1980): 1387, 1392.

Congress is expected to continue federal aid to nursing education. Bills to combine the Nurse Training Act with other
health professions education were not approved. A compromise
between a bill of Senator Kennedy and one of Senator Schweiker
was forwarded to the Senate for vote. (0)

1011 "Congress Okays Funds for Nursing Education Through June,"
      AM J NURS 81(2) (February 1981): 278.

      A continuing resolution passed by the 96th Congress assured
      funding of federally supported programs through June. (0)

1012 Creason, N. "Effects of Government Funding on Instructional
      Components in Nursing Education." CURRENT ISSUES IN NURSING.
      Edited by J.C. McCloskey and H.K. Grace. Scranton, PA.:
      Blackwell Scientific Publications, 1981, pp. 489-97.

      Federal funding for nursing education is decreasing. A re-
      examination of program offerings in respect to mission and
      goals of the school is necessary in light of decreased external
      funding. Through planning, educational administrators may
      become actors rather than reactors in political decisions. (18)

1013 Derby, V.L. "Financing Nursing Education," NURSE EDUC 5(2)
      (March/April 1980): 21-25.

      Costs for education are rising at alarming rates while at
      the same time financial support is decreasing. Funding is
      explored in the areas of tuition and federal, state and private
      contributions. Recommendations for the most effective use of
      resources as suggested by the Carnegie Commission are pre-
      sented. The PLANTRAN II computer model is presented which
      will help analyze the financial status of a school and facili-
      tate planning. (23)

1014 Detherage, K.S. and M. Thobaben. "Nursing Fellowship Oppor-
      tunities for Advanced Studies," NURS OUTLOOK 30(2) (February
      1982): 115-21.

      Lists current fellowships available to nurses for post
      master's research, practice and educational pursuits. Iden-
      tifies purpose, eligibility requirements, conditions of award
      and period of support for each fellowship. (3)

1015 "DHHS Allocates $9.9 Million to Capitation," AM J NURS 81(10)
      (October 1981): 1741, 1758.

      Capitation money was awarded to 405 baccalaureate programs,
      555 associate degree programs and 148 diploma programs.
      Traineeship awards for 1981-82 total $12.8 million. (0)

1016 "Dramatic Increase in Faculty Pay Cited in Recent AACN Survey,"
      AM J NURS 79(7) (July 1979): 1181, 1200.

      A survey of 6,297 full-time faculty positions in 189 schools
      revealed dramatic increases in salaries of doctorally prepared
      faculty since previously reported data five years ago. Com-
      parison figures are provided. (0)

1017 "Expiring Congress OKs $48.9 Million for Nurse Training," AM
      J NURS 83(2) (February 1983): 195, 304.

Although not entirely satisfactory, federal appropriations
for nurse training was considerably more than the $12.5 million
suggested by the Reagan administration. (0)

1018   "Faculty Salaries Rise 5-6% in BSN and Grad Programs: AACN
       Voices Concern Over Low Doctoral Differential," AM J NURS
       83(8) (August 1983): 1132.

       A comparison of salaries of doctorally and non doctorally
       prepared faculty showed little differentiation. Variations
       were noted in geographic regions, type of institutions and
       type of degree programs offered. (0)

1019   Farrell, M. and J. Eckert. "Zero-based Budgeting in Nursing
       Education," NURS OUTLOOK 27(12) (December 1979): 792-95.

       By requiring justification of anticipated costs, nursing
       education can make decisions relative to program changes with
       better awareness of cost-benefit outcomes. Such an effort is
       described in which four alternative proposals were reviewed
       and ranked and a course of action selected. (4)

1020   "Federal Nursing Programs Face 6 Percent Across-the-Board Cut,"
       AM J NURS 82(2) (February 1982): 211, 240.

       Continued decreases in federal appropriations to nursing
       programs are anticipated. (0)

1021   "Funding Cuts Will Worsen Shortage, ANA Tells Senate," AM J
       NURS 81(6) (June 1981): 1090, 1106.

       Dr. Verla Collins testified before the Senate Labor and Human
       Resources Committee that nursing education and nursing services
       will be critically affected by lack of federal funds. (0)

1022   "Funds for Nursing Slashed in Proposed Reagan Budget," AM J
       NURS 81(5) (May 1981): 907, 937, 945.

       Decreases in federal funds for nursing are proposed and not
       expected to influence currently enrolled students. Proposed
       block grants would consolidate fifteen individual health pro-
       gram appropriations to states for discretionary distribution.
       Continued HHS budget slashing still leaves substantial
       increases for fiscal 1982. (0)

1023   Ginzberg, E. "The Economics of Health Care and the Future of
       Nursing," NURS EDUC 6(3) (May/June 1981): 29-32.

       The impact of a strained economy on the health care system
       requires action by nursing leaders. Increases in baccalaureate
       prepared nurses, changes in nurse practice acts, and profes-
       sional recognition are necessary to offset the economic impact
       on education, reimbursement and utilization. (0)

1024   "Hearings on Aid to Education Begin: ANA Cites Shortage," AM J
        NURS 81(4) (April 1981): 651, 692, 694.

        Constance Holleran of ANA spoke at a congressional hearing
        regarding continued federal funding for nursing education.
        She suggested that Congress stimulate studies which may remedy
        problems related to retention and job satisfaction. (0)

1025   "Heaviest Yet Budget Cutbacks Loom in Federal Nursing Funds,"
        AM J NURS 82(4) (April 1982): 517, 524.

        President Reagan's proposed budget cuts drastically reduce
        appropriations to nursing education. (0)

1026   "HEW Budget Would Slash Nursing Funds," AM J NURS 78(3) (March
        1978): 345, 350, 371.

        Proposed budget cuts in the Carter administration threaten
        to decrease enrollments in schools of nursing. A severe blow
        to nursing students receiving federal loans, scholarships and
        traineeships would be felt. Proposed budget distribution is
        described. (0)

1027   "High Court Action Frees Salary Data in Sex-Bias Suit," AM J
        NURS 81(12) (December 1981): 2117, 2220.

        The U.S. Supreme Court's refusal to consider an appeal of
        the University of Pittsburgh in a salary discrimination based
        on sex allows the Equal Employment Opportunity Commission
        access to salary scales of male and female employees in the
        schools of nursing, pharmacy, social work and other health-
        related professions. The University has been charged with
        paying women faculty with equal or similar qualifications less
        than their male colleagues. (0)

1028   "House Bill Boosts Budget for Nursing by $41 Million Over
        Senate's Version," AM J NURS 81(8) (August 1981): 1421, 1445.

        The current federal budget for nursing education is roughly
        $100 million. Lengthy debates in the House ended with the
        acceptance of the "Dingell package" which allotted larger
        amounts for nursing education than did the Senate earlier
        this year. (0)

1029   "House Rejects Recission of Health Professions Education
        Funding," AM J NURS 80(7) (July 1980: 1244, 1272.

        The House of Representatives rejected President Carter's
        request to slash appropriated funds for health professions
        education. Rep. Waxman's bill designating $103 million for
        federal support to nursing education was approved by the House
        of Representatives. Two health manpower bills submitted by
        Senators Kennedy and Schweiker have as yet not been approved.
        A continuing resolution is expected. (0)

1030 "IOM Study Sees Need for Funds in Graduate, Specialty Areas,"
      AM J NURS 83(3) (March 1983): 343, 344, 454.

      The study by the Institute of Medicine Committee on Nursing
      and Nursing Education concluded that federal support to nursing
      education should focus on graduate study. Key points of the
      study are described. (0)

1031 "Institute of Medicine Will Report on Nursing Education," AM
      J NURS 81(1) (January 1981): 9, 165.

      A plan developed by the Committee of the Institute of Medi-
      cine will seek answers to questions regarding national nursing
      shortages and educational needs. (0)

1032 "Landslide of Support Saves MSU College of Nursing," AM J NURS
      81(6) (June 1981): 1087, 1095, 1096, 1100.

      Financial difficulties forced a decision to close Michigan
      State University College of Nursing. This decision was re-
      versed when some 7,000 nurses protested the closure. (0)

1033 Lash, A.A. "Federal Financing and Its Effect on Higher Nurs-
      ing Education." CURRENT ISSUES IN NURSING. Edited by J.C.
      McCloskey and H.K. Grace. Scranton, PA.: Blackwell Scienti-
      fic Publications, 1981, pp. 474-89.

      Concern for an adequate supply of nurses to meet the nation's
      health needs has been evident in federal appropriations of
      funds since World War I. These funds have served to improve
      the quantity of nurses by providing capitation grants, school
      start-up programs, financial distress grants, student assist-
      ance programs, and utilization of educational talent programs.
      The quality has been improved through professional trainee-
      ships, accreditation requirements for federal funding, research
      funds, specialty programs, and teaching improvement projects.
      The time has come for scholarly documentation of the effects
      of federal financing on nursing and nursing education. (20)

1034 Lazinski, H. "The Effects of Clinical Teaching on the Budgets
      of Schools of Nursing," J NURS EDUC 18(1) (January 1979):
      21-24.

      Examines ways in which clinical teaching can be more cost
      effective and less time consuming. Increase in student-faculty
      ratios, grouping assignments or assigning the morning of clini-
      cal laboratory and eliminating anecdotal notes in favor of
      student diaries are suggested. (3)

1035 Leininger, M.M. "Creativity and Challenges for Nurse
      Researchers in This Economic Recession," NURSE EDUC 8(1)
      (Spring 1983): 13-14.

      Economic realities require innovative approaches to securing
      monies for research. Suggestions are given to help nurse re-
      searchers economize and maximize resources. (0)

1036   Moore, J.B. "The Unhealthy Financial Aid Situation for Health
       Science Careers," J NURS EDUC 22(7) (September 1983): 291-95.

       A review of previous and present financial aid sources for
       nursing students demonstrated reduced resources. The Coleman
       Report is reviewed with specific attention to high school stu-
       dents´ plans for financing nursing education.(8)

1037   "Nurse Credentialors Say No To Coalition, Yes to More
       ´Dialog´," AM J NURS 82(7) (July 1982): 1023, 1054, 1056-57.

       A task force to study implementation of a credentialing center
       for nursing has completed their work. Nursing organizations
       are willing to continue discussion but as yet not ready to
       pledge their money. Problems inherent in such a center are
       explored. (0)

1038   "Nurse Lobbyists Face Double Battle," AM J NURS 79(2) (February
       1979): 204.

       President Carter´s recent veto of the Nurse Training Act is
       considered just one segment of a larger issue which involves
       continued federal funding of health and social welfare pro-
       grams. (0)

1039   "Nurses Spark Drive to Save NTA," AM J NURS 79(2) (February
       1979): 203-4.

       Efforts to mobilize nurses across the nation to protest
       President Carter´s veto of the Nurse Training amendments are
       decribed. Serious and long-term negative effects on future
       health care services are feared. (0)

1040   "Nurse Training Act Extension Is Likely," AM J NURS 78(5)
       (May 1978): 765, 778.

       Chances for funding of the Nurse Practice Act look good this
       year. Although there are some indications that the nurse
       employment market is saturated, overall anyone seeking employ-
       ment in nursing is absorbed. (0)

1041   "Nurse Training Act Extension Sought," AM J NURS 78(3) (March
       1978): 345.

       Although the Carter administration seeks to discontinue
       federal funding to nursing programs, a consensus bill has been
       introduced to the House and Senate which seeks a two year ex-
       tension of the current program. (0)

1042   "Nurse Training Act is Reported Out of House Health Sub
       Committee," AM J NURS 78(6) (June 1978): 974.

The Nurse Training Act bill for two year renewal favorably
reported out of the House Interstate and Foreign Commerce Committee subcommittee on health and the environment. A section
was added to provide for nurse anesthetists and a study of
nursing manpower needs. (O)

1043   "Nurse Training Act Passes U. S. House Almost Unanimously,"
        AM J NURS 78(11)(November 1978): 1823, 1826.

        Both houses passed a $208 million Nurse Training Act. Stu-
        dent loans will be forgiven if a nurse practices in an under-
        served area. An extensive study of the nation's nursing needs
        was called for in the new law. (O)

1044   "Nurse Training Funds Integrated With Others in Schweiker
        Bill," AM J NURS 80(3) (March 1980): 375, 396.

        Senator Richard Schweiker (R., PA.) introduced a bill that
        would combine the Nurse Training Act into a larger "Health
        Professions Education Assistance and Nursing Training Act of
        1980." Capitation grants to medical and nursing students would
        end and although the level of federal fundings would be about
        the same, allocations would differ. Senator Edward Kennedy
        (D. MA.) and Representative Henry Waxman (D. CA.) are expected
        to introduce similar bills. (O)

1045   "Nursing Education Fares Well as 95th Congress Winds Up," AM
        J NURS 78(12) (December 1978): 2001, 2020-22, 2033.

        The Nurse Training Act passed a $208 million budget in both
        houses on the last day of the 95th Congress. It is speculated
        that President Carter will veto the Nurse Training Act. (O)

1046   "Nursing Education Support Meager in Reagan Budget," AM J NURS
        83(4) (April 1983): 497, 628.

        A review of President Reagan's proposed budget reveals con-
        tinued reductions in allocation of funds for nursing.(O)

1047   "Nursing Funds Stay With Health in New DHHS," AM J NURS 79(12)
        (December 1979): 2076.

        The newly created Department of Health and Human Services
        replaces the Department of Health, Education and Welfare.
        Nursing student loans and scholarship programs will not be
        transferred to the new education department but remain with
        HSS, Division of Manpower Training. (O)

1048   "Nursing Schools Face Crackdown on Student Loan Delinquencies,"
        AM J NURS 82(11) (November 1982): 1663, 1685.

        Plans are underway to enforce loan repayment by nursing stu-
        dents. Guidelines for schools of nursing will be ready in
        December which will restrict further student loans to schools
        of nursing who do not reduce their delinquency rates. (O)

1049 "Nursing Students Join in Massive Lobbying Effort," AM J NURS
      82(4) (April 1982): 517, 543, 676.

      Nursing students lobbied in Washington, D.C. as federal cuts
      to nursing education threatened continuation of studies. (0)

1050 "President Carter Signs NTA," AM J NURS 79(11) (November
      1979): 1899.

      Nurse Training Amendments were signed by President Carter
      granting $103 million to nursing education programs. Congress
      will begin a total overhaul of health manpower support programs
      in 1980. (0)

1051 Rinke, L.T. "It Could Happen Again," NURS OUTLOOK 28(7)
      (July 1980): 449-51.

      A group of graduate students, undergraduate students and
      faculty describe how they were able to positively influence
      legislators to rescind federal cuts to nursing education and
      research. (0)

1052 Deleted.

1053 "RWJ Project Links Nursing Home Care to Nursing Schools," AM J
      NURS 81(9) (September 1981): 1557, 1587.

      The Robert Wood Johnson Foundation has funded a $5 million
      Teaching Nursing Home Program which will seek to affiliate
      nursing homes and nursing schools. This is intended to ulti-
      mately upgrade long-term care. Grants of up to $500,000 each
      will be awarded to ten university nursing schools with graduate
      nursing programs. (0)

1054 "Skidmore's Students Fight Move to Close Their Program," AM J
      NURS 82(4) (April 1982): 518, 667, 668, 670, 675.

      A fifty percent drop in applications over a five year period
      with accompanying fiscal losses were given as reasons for clos-
      ing a sixty year old baccalaureate nursing program. Faculty,
      students and parents challenged these findings. (0)

1055 "Statewide Budget Cuts Threaten UCLA Nursing Programs," AM J
      NURS 82(4) (April 1982): 518, 662, 664, 666-67.

      A state level deficit led the Chancellor at UCLA to propose
      drastic cuts in financial support to the nursing programs which
      would eliminate the undergraduate program, reduce graduate
      school enrollment in nursing by fifty percent and eliminate
      twenty faculty lines. Nurses protested which led to a revised
      plan. (0)

1056 "Student Loan Crackdown Hits Nursing Programs," AM J NURS
      82(10) (October 1982): 1478, 1492-93.

Schools with high loan default rates will be barred from receiving further loans from the National Direct Student Loan Program. Any educational institution that failed to collect twenty-five percent or more of the NDSL Loans will be disqualified. The Black colleges are affected the most. A list is provided of baccalaureate and associate degree nursing programs affected. (0)

1057   Swanson, E.A. and S.S. Sweeney. "Private Support: A Vital Role in the Future of Nursing." CURRENT ISSUES IN NURSING. Edited by J.C. McCloskey and H.K. Grace. Scranton, PA.: Blackwell Scientific Publications, 1981, pp. 539-50.

Declining enrollments, continued or increased inflation, and public concern for the costs of education are producing financial crises in public and private institutions. Schools of nursing must explore various sources of funding and develop skills in fund raising to meet the financial needs of their programs. (29)

1058   "$21 Million Added to Reagan Budget for Nursing Support," AM J NURS 81(7) (July 1981): 1251-52, 1256.

Although $21 million has been added to the nursing budget proposed by President Reagan, federal support could drop to less than half its current level in fiscal, 1982. Nursing shortage problems are under study by the Institute of Medicine, however, problems of low pay and lack of autonomy cannot be resolved through federal funds. Federal support to other health programs is threatened with cuts. (0)

1059   "Veto of NTA Points Profession to Edge of Crisis," AM J NURS 79(4) (April 1979): 569-70, 581.

Individual programs report on the effects of loss of institutional support and student assistance which accompanies the president's veto of the Nurse Practice Act. Available statistics indicate an impending crisis for nursing education and nursing practice if funding is withheld. (0)

See 984, 1654.

Professionalism

1060   Bullough, B. and V. Bullough. "Educational Issues: Background Paper." NURSING ISSUES AND NURSING STRATEGIES FOR THE EIGHTIES. Edited by B. Bullough, V. Bullough, and M.C. Soukup. New York: Springer Publishing Co., 1983, pp. 179-89.

Discusses the historical development and social factors that influenced the development of nursing education. Current educational issues evolve from the development of multiple nurse education programs. The entry into practice resolution has become the basis for heated arguments from dissenting groups. (13)

1061 Christensen, G.J. "Professional Interaction in Academic Health
      Centers," J NURS EDUC 17(8) (October 1978): 11-19.

      A study of five university health centers found the attitudes
      and behaviors of students, faculty and administrators in den-
      tistry, medicine, nursing, and basic science relative to shared
      learning, facilities and rights differed among professions,
      among various statuses of persons within the professions, and
      among the administrative structures. (7)

1062 Christman, L. "Accountability and Autonomy Are More Than
      Rhetoric," NURS EDUC 3(4) (July/August 1978): 3-6.

      In order for nursing to become accountable and autonomous,
      the entry into practice issue must be resolved; educational
      programs must be reduced in number and improved in quality;
      faculty must be engaged in practice; decentralization of auth-
      ority must be stressed and individual autonomy must be pro-
      moted. Nurses must understand the need for continued life
      long learning. (0)

1063 Cotanch, P.H. "Self-Actualization and Professional Socializa-
      tion of Nursing Students in the Clinical Laboratory Exper-
      ience," J NURS EDUC 20(8) (October 1981): 4-14.

      A survey of nursing students at two southeastern universities
      was conducted to determine if self-actualization was associated
      with the process of professional socialization. A positive
      correlation was found. (23)

Credentialing

1064 "ANA Task Force Sees Support for Nursing Credentialing Center,"
      AM J NURS 81(8) (August 1981): 1424.

      Of 147 nursing, health, and educational organizations only
      nine did not endorse the concept of a credentialing center for
      nursing. Seventy nursing and health related organizations have
      contributed $50,615 to underwrite the work of the Task Force
      on Credentialing until a grant can be secured. (0)

1065 "ANA Will Move to Set Up Nursing Credentialing Center, Says
      Board," AM J NURS 82(5) (May 1982): 745, 760.

      The American Nurses' Association is looking to establish a
      separate incorporated national credentialing center for nurs-
      ing. The center will be involved in licensures, registration,
      certification and accreditation. Professional support was
      sought and assured. (0)

1066 "A New Licensing Exam for Nurses," AM J NURS 80(4) (April
      1980): 723-25.

An interview with the executive director and chairperson of
the National Council of State Boards of Nursing, Inc. provides
insight into the new test plan for registered nurse licensure.
(0)

1067   American Nurses´ Association. THE STUDY OF CREDENTIALING IN
       NURSING: A NEW APPROACH, VOL. I, THE REPORT OF THE COMMITTEE.
       Kansas City, MO.: American Nurses´ Association, Pub. No.
       G-136, 1979.

       Reports a twenty-four month study conducted for ANA consider-
       ing credentialing definitions, a model for credentialing in
       nursing, principles and positions on credentialing, use of
       designated nursing credential forms, and the establishment of
       a national nursing credentialing center.

1068   _____. THE STUDY OF CREDENTIALING IN NURSING: A NEW APPROACH,
       VOL. II, STAFF WORKING PAPERS. Kansas City, MO.: American
       Nurses´ Association, Pub. No. G-138, 1979.

       Developed by the staff of the Committee for the Study of
       Credentialing in Nursing and by commissioned consultants.

1069   "California Board Votes to Develop Licensing Exam," AM J NURS
       81(5) (May 1981): 909.

       The California Board of Registered Nurses voted to develop a
       separate California RN licensing examination to be used in
       place of the State Board Test Pool Examination. California´s
       BRN question the "job-relatedness" of the SBTPE. Continued
       nursing shortages in the state and problems of foreign-trained
       and minority-group nurses in passing the current examination
       prompted this action. (0)

1070   "California´s Board Postpones Its Plan for Test Production,"
       AM J NURS 81(8) (August 1981): g 1422.

       Plans to develop a California licensing exam in place of
       the State Board Test Pool Examination have been discontinued
       for the present. California nurses protested the plan which
       was an attempt to remove the adverse impact on foreign-born
       and minority groups. (0)

1071   Chambers, C.M. "Confidentiality and Disclosure in Accredita-
       tion: A Precis of the Legal Issues and Risks," NURS HEALTH
       CARE 4(8) (October 1983): 445-47.

       An examination of the legality of confidentiality in accredi-
       tation of schools of nursing and the legal issues and risks
       involved in the disclosure of such information. (10)

1072   "Credentialing in Nursing: A New Approach," AM J NURS 79(4)
       (April 1979): 674-83.

A report of the Committee for the Study of Credentialing in
Nursing reveals progress to date on the development of a credentialing center, its purpose and proposed jurisdiction. (O)

1073   Dunbley, P.H.   "The ANA Certification Program," NURS CLIN
       NORTH AM 9 (September 1974): 485-95.

       In 1973 ANA initiated its voluntary certification program.
       Article important for history of certification. (6)

1074   McQuaid, E.A. and M.T. Kane.   "How Do Graduates of Different
       Types of Programs Perform on State Boards?," AM J NURS 79(2)
       (February 1979): 305-8.

       A comparison of State Board Examination scores of diploma,
       associate degree and baccalaureate graduates revealed that
       diploma graduates had the highest mean on four of the five
       tests. Differences in range among programs was not as wide as
       differences within programs. (16)

1075   "NLN Recommends Significant Changes in Program Accreditation,"
       AM J NURS 82(3) (March 1982): 390.

       Summarizes a three year NLN accreditation study which calls
       for the development of more uniform and precise accreditation
       policies, practices and procedures. In addition, broader par-
       ticipation by eductional programs at many stages of the accredi-
       tation process were recommended. (O)

1076   "New York Exam Decision Prompts Investigation by Other Boards,"
       AM J NURS 79(10) (October 1979): 1680.

       A report of investigative actions by various states prompted
       by New York State's decision to reject the July RN licensing
       results. In those states where investigations have already
       been conducted, there were no indications that test results
       differed from those of other exams. (O)

1077   "92% Pass NCLEX," AM J NURS 82(11) (November 1982): 1664.

       First-time writers of the new state licensure examination
       were more successful than their predecessors taking the old
       examination. (O)

1078   "Nurses Go To Court Over N.Y. Decision to Void RN Exam," AM J
       NURS 79(11) (November 1979): 1900, 1930.

       Petitions by nurses in New York State have been presented to
       State Supreme Court demanding that the New York State Education
       Department show cause why the July licensing examination was
       invalidated. A request was made for a reversal of the decision
       and licensure of candidates who passed. Investigations of
       alleged cheating are in progress. (O)

1079   "RN July Licensing Exam Invalidated in New York," AM J NURS
       79(10) (October 1979): 1671, 1680, 1684.

       The Commissioner of Education of the State of New York re-
       ported that 12,000 nurses who took licensing exams in July 1979
       will have to retake the exam in February, 1980 because of
       alleged charges that the test booklets were being sold prior
       to the test date. An investigation by the State Police Depart-
       ment Bureau of Criminal Investigation has been requested.
       This action means that none of the 100,000 applicants who took
       the July exam in other states can be licensed in New York. (0)

1080   Schmidt, M.S. "Why a Separate Organization for State Boards?,"
       AM J NURS 80(4) (April 1980): 725-26.

       Traces the development of State Board licensing bodies for
       nurses over the past eighty years and focuses on the new
       National Council of State Boards of Nursing, Inc. which re-
       cently replaced the American Nurses´ Association, Council of
       State Boards of Nursing. (8)

1081   "State Boards Pick CTB/McGraw-Hill to Produce Exam," AM J NURS
       81(8) (August 1981): 1421-1422, 1438.

       The California Testing Bureau/McGraw-Hill was chosen over
       other contractors as the new national testing service for the
       State Board Test Pool Examination. Criterion referenced scor-
       ing is being explored for some parts of the tests. A machine
       scored booklet will be used which will eliminate separate score
       sheets and improve security. Diagnostic profiles of students
       who fail will be provided without additional charge. (0)

1082   "Task Force on Credentialing Asks for "Commitment from Nursing
       Groups´," AM J NURS 80(12) (December 1980): 2125, 2146, 2152.

       Nursing resource groups are being asked for written state-
       ments of commitment and financial contributions to support
       the ANA Task Force on Credentialing. NLN´s position is dis-
       cussed.(0)

1083   "Washington Dean Heads Task Force on Credentialing," AM J NURS
       79(10) (October 1979): 1671, 1700.

       A task force to direct activities of the Study of Creden-
       tialing in Nursing will convene groups to study the recommended
       principles and positions of a national nursing credentialing
       center. They will be responsible for educating nurses and the
       public about the study and conducting a cost analysis. (0).

Students

1084   Allen, M.E.M. "The Problem of Communication in a Summer Work-
       shop for Foreign Nurses," J NURS EDUC 19(1) (January 1980):
       8-12

       Describes interactional problems experienced by foreign
       nurses during an eight week workshop in psychiatric nursing.
       Verbal and written communications are described in patient,
       student and teacher interactions which prove frustrating to
       the foreign student. (8)

1085   Anderson, A. "One Step at a Time," J NURS EDUC 20(4) (April
       1981): 22-27.

       A nursing instructor describes her experience in planning
       clinical learning for a handicapped student. Resistance of
       faculty and clinical agencies to accepting handicapped stu-
       dents and federal legislation building academic practices is
       described. (1)

1086   Aquino, N.S., P.J. Trent and J.E. Deutch. "Factors Related to
       Foreign Nurse Graduates Test-Taking Performance," NURS RES
       28(2) (March/April 1979): 111-14.

       A study of test format, English proficiency and anxiety
       among foreign nurses as factors influencing performance on
       State Board Examinations found only one of the factors, English
       proficiency, to be influential. (14)

1087   Auster, D. "Sex Differences in Attitudes Toward Nursing Edu-
       cation," J NURS EDUC 18(6) (June 1979): 19-28.

       A survey of differences in attitudes toward nursing education
       based on sex, revealed sex role socialization, cultural values
       and sex typing of occupations are deterrents to men entering
       nursing. (23)

1088   Awtrey, J. "From Somebody to Nobody," NURS OUTLOOK 27(11)
       (November 1979): 718-20.

       Recounts the discomfort in assuming a student role after
       having been a faculty member in the same institution. (0)

1089   Baker, A. and G. Cook. "Stress, Adaptation, and the Black
       Individual: Implications for Nursing Education," J NURS EDUC
       6 (June 1983): 237-42.

       Reports a study identifying methods used by Black individuals
       to handle stress. Identifies the need for curricular content
       addressing cultural diversity in stress and adaptation within

programs that prepare health care providers and particularly
nurses. Argues that nursing interventions in assisting
patients to deal with stress must be done with an awareness
of cultural uniqueness. (25)

1090   Balogh, E. et al. "RN Students Analyze Their Experiences,"
       NURS OUTLOOK 28(2) (February 1980): 112-15.

       Twelve RN students reflect on the frustrations and turmoil
       experienced during a baccalaureate completion program. The
       process of transition from comfort in the subordinate posi-
       tion to eventual comfort in the leadership role occurred in
       the final semester of the senior year. (4)

1091   Barnes, S.Y. "Problems Foreign Nurses Encounter in Passing
       Psychiatric Nursing on U. S. Exams for Licensure," J NURS
       EDUC 19(1) (January 1980): 19-26.

       Problems encountered by foreign nurses in a course designed
       to prepare them for state board examinations in psychiatric
       nursing are identified. Cultural differences led to very poor
       nurse-patient interactions. They experienced difficulty in
       dealing honestly with patients and setting limits. (13)

1092   Benda, E. "When the Postpartum Nursing Student is Male--A
       Challenge to Maternity Instructors," J NURS EDUC 20(4)
       (April 1981): 5-8.

       A nursing instructor provides suggestions to be used as a
       guide and resource for nurse educators planning postpartum
       clinical experiences for male nursing students. Identifying
       anxiety producing situations and selection of teaching strate-
       gies which will promote initial comfort are recommended. (5)

1093   Blainey, C.G. "Anxiety in the Undergrduate Medical-Surgical
       Clinical Student," J NURS EDUC 19(8) (October 1980): 33-36.

       A faculty member describes her experiences in identifying
       and intervening in anxiety situations experienced by student
       nurses. It is important for teachers to recognize and deal
       with anxiety as it interferes with learning. (5)

1094   Bronner, M. "Bridges or Barriers to Success: The Nature of
       the Student Experiences in Nursing," J NURS EDUC 21(7)
       (September 1982): 38-41.

       A survey of foreign students who studied in American graduate
       programs in nursing found that students from nations whose
       first language was not English, namely the Orient, Asia, South
       America and Africa, experienced isolation, homesickness, lone-
       liness, and culture shock. Strategies should be developed to
       meet the needs of these students via social and support struc-
       tures. (3)

1095   Carmack, B.J. "Resolving an Incident of Academic Dishonesty:
       Plagiarism," NURS EDUC 8(1) (Spring 1983): 9-12.

       A nurse educator reports her experience of plagiarism with
       student nurses. The processes of confrontation, conflict, and
       conflict resolution are described and guidelines for faculty
       who encounter similar problems proposed. (1)

1096   Choi, S.C., S.B. Boxerman and L. Steinburg. "Nurses´ Prefer-
       ence of Terminal Digits in Data Reading," J NURS EDUC 17(9)
       (November 1978): 38-41.

       Analysis of data reported by 120 student nurses on 7300 high
       school students demonstrated a tendency to round off blood
       pressure and weight data. Zero is the preferred digit. (0)

1097   Claerbaut, D. "Expansion Trends in Health Care and The Role
       of Minority Students: A Challenge for Nursing Eduction,"
       J NURS EDUC 17(4) (April 1978): 42-47.

       A study of Black students in a midwestern college conference
       found that nursing majors differed in attitudes from the Black
       students in general. Powerlessness and normlessness were not
       perceived as problems in nursing majors, however, disorienta-
       tion and loneliness were problematic to sixty percent of the
       sample studied. (10)

1098   Dalme, F.C. "Nursing Students and the Development of Profes-
       sional Identity." THE NURSING PROFESSION: A TIME TO SPEAK.
       Edited by N.L. Chaska. New York: McGraw-Hill Book Co.,
       1983, pp. 134-45.

       A study of 250 baccalaureate nursing students examined stu-
       dents' perception of the influence of peers, faculty, and
       staff nurses on the development of professional identity.
       Peers were a significant influence in both first and second
       year students, however, second year students were also
       influenced by faculty and staff nurses. (21)

1099   Durrant, L. "The Student of Nursing Needs--The Consumer of
       Education," J NURS EDUC 17(6) (June 1978): 15-19.

       A discussion of allegiance by faculty to student or patient
       needs concludes that students as consumers of education should
       receive priority. In attending to student needs faculty are
       ultimately preparing them to attend to patient needs as gradu-
       ate nurses and thus effecting a long term contribution to the
       quality of patient care. (10)

1100   Ferrell, B. "Attitudes Toward Learning Styles and Self-
       Direction of ADN Students," J NURS EDUC 17(2) (February
       1978): 19-22.

       An associate degree program designed for licensed practical
       nurses was begun at the Southern Illinois Collegiate Common
       Market. A study was undertaken in order to determine which

learning styles were preferred and the preference for dependent
versus self-directed learning. The least preferred learning
style was simulation whereas peer learning received the highest
composite score. Students tended to prefer self-directed
learning experiences. (0)

1101 Finley, B. and S. Mynatt. "Faculty Intervention Into Suicidal
      Crisis," NURSE EDUC 6(2) (March/April 1981): 12-16.

      Adolescents, girls and students are high suicide risks.
      Nurse faculty need to be aware of crisis in students. Two
      faculty recount an experience of successful crisis intervention
      with a nursing student. (22)

1102 Fishbein, E.G. "Female Gender as a Variable in the Educational
      Process: A Review," J NURS EDUC 21(5) (May 1982): 43-48.

      Although females demonstrate intellectual and achievement
      advantages over boys during childhood, males surpass females
      at the adult performance level. Social influences appear to
      cause this phenomenon. (14)

1103 Fishel, A.H. "Graduation/Termination," AM J NURS 81(6) (June
      1981): 1156-58.

      Graduation is similar to other developmental rites of passage
      and is accompanied by a grieving process. Denial, anger and
      depression precede acceptance. Anxiety and coping are dis-
      cussed and guidelines provided to assist new graduates ter-
      minate their student role. (0)

1104 Foote, R.H. "Double Standards?," AM J NURS 80(9) (September
      1980): 1610.

      A male student and subsequent registered nurse recounts his
      experiences with sex discrimination in nursing. He found the
      greatest problems with female nurses and not with patients or
      allied health personnel. (0)

1105 Grassi-Russo, N. and P.B. Morris. "Hopes and Fears: The Atti-
      tudes of Freshman Nursing Students," J NURS EDUC 20(6) (June
      1981): 9-17.

      A study was done to identify hopes and fears of 102 freshmen
      nursing students in a diploma school in an attempt to promote
      awareness of attitudes and provide early support. Fear of
      failure in school was most frequently identified (46.3%). (19)

1106 Kahn, A.M. "Modifications in Nursing Student Attitudes as
      Measured by the EPPS: A Significant Reversal from the Past,"
      NURS RES 29(1) (January/February 1980): 61-63.

      A change in the nursing profile was observed in an experi-
      mental study matching nursing and non nursing majors of the
      same age groups. Similarity was found between the two groups

on autonomy and deference which differs from previous data
(1964-1970) when nursing students were found to have higher
deference needs and lower autonomy needs than other college
women. (16)

1107   "Kansas Attorney General Limits Use of Nursing Students at UK
        Hospital," AM J NURS 82(3) (March 1982): 378-79.

        The Attorney General of Kansas moved to halt the University
        of Kansas Medical Center from employing senior nursing students
        to work without faculty supervision. (0)

1108   Kayser-Jones, J., H. Abu-Saad and E.G. Nichols. "Canadian and
        European Students in the United States," J NURS EDUC 21(7)
        (September 1982): 26-31.

        A survey of European and Canadian students studying nursing
        in the United States revealed factors which contributed to a
        satisfactory adjustment. Friends and relatives in the United
        States, the ability to speak English, helpful classmates, and
        helpful faculty were rated most helpful. (9)

1109   Kayser-Jones, J., H. Abu-Saad and F.N. Akinnaso. "Nigeria:
        The Land, Its People, and Health Care," J NURS EDUC 21(7)
        (September 1982): 32-37.

        Differences in social values and social customs, and finan-
        cial problems were most frequently identified problems of
        Nigerian students in adjusting to the American culture. Com-
        petitiveness, inflexibility, and the rapid pace of the program
        were identified as problems experienced in the American nursing
        programs. The needs of these students include excellent teach-
        ing, leadership, and problem-solving skills as they assume
        multiple, important positions upon returning to their homeland.
        (9)

1110   Leonard, A.M. and I. Rogers. "Role Imagery: A Delicate
        Balance," J NURS EDUC 17(3) (March 1978): 42-46.

        A survey of student nurses and experienced nurses sought to
        determine how professional nurses evaluated various nursing
        functions. Both students and experienced nurses ranked tradi-
        tional activities high. The need for the development of
        communication skills in order to provide emotional support to
        patients was recommended by both groups. (7)

1111   Leone, L.P. "Orienting Nurses from Other Countries to Graduate
        Education in the United States," J NURS EDUC 21(7) (September
        1982): 45-47.

        A planned orientation for foreign students anticipated their
        needs for understanding a wide variety of institutional, health
        care, and cultural systems in the United States. It was felt
        that such orientation eased their adjustment and contributed
        to positive learning experiences. (0)

1112 Lillard, J. "The Socialization Process: A Student's Viewpoint," NURSE EDUC 7(4) (July/August 1982): 11-12.

Faculty need to ratify student behavior and serve as role
models. Students select role models who display enthusiasm
for nursing, convey an interest in students as individuals,
facilitate growth and value student ideas. (4)

1113 Little, M. and S. Brian. "The Challengers, Interactors and
Mainstreamers: Second Step Education and Nursing Roles,"
NURS RES 31(4) (July/August 1982): 239-45.

A longitudinal study of 236 registered nurse students enrolled in baccalaureate completion programs revealed that
students on entry to the programs vary greatly in professional
orientations. Three groups were identified as challengers,
interactors, and mainstreamers based on varying nursing styles,
sociopolitical views and personality characteristics. All
three groups perceived themselves as more professionally com-
mitted and competent when they graduated. (17)

1114 Malarkey, L. "The Older Student-Stress or Success on Campus,"
J NURS EDUC 18(2) (February 1979): 15-19.

A significant increase in the enrollment of women over
twenty-five years of age in a basic nursing program requires
faculty understanding of the unique strengths and needs of
this learner group. High motivation and maturity of judgment
are often accompanied by fears and anxiety. (8)

1115 Mancini, J., C. LaVecchia and R. Clegg. "Graduate Nursing
Students and Stress," J NURS EDUC 22(8) (October 1983):
329-34.

The effects of relaxation, response, imagery and diaphrag-
matic breathing on stress response was measured in thirty
female graduate nursing students. (30)

1116 Mauksch, I.G. "Paradox of Risk Takers," AORN J 25 (1977):
1289, 1292-93, 1296-97, 1300-1, 1304, 1307-8, 1312.

Summarizes personality profile studies of nurses in past in
terms of changes that should be made in order to cultivate
risk taking and accountability. (0)

1117 McKay, S.R. "A Review of Student Stress in Nursing Education
Programs," NURS FORUM 27(4) (1978): 376-93.

A review of the literature reveals that stress has always
accompanied nursing education. Faculty need to reverse this
trend and develop support structures for nursing students. (31)

1118 McMorrow, M.E. "Nursing Faculty Response to Open-Door Policy,"
J NURS EDUC 17(7) (September 1978): 32-34.

The change in student population which occurred as a result
of open admission policies requires faculty to reexamine their
teaching strategies to provide support for unprepared students. (2)

1119   Moore, D.S., S.D. Decker and M.W. Dowd. "Baccalaureate Nursing
       Students' Identification with the Women's Movement," NURS
       RES 27(5) (September/October 1978): 291-95.

       A study of 291 baccalaureate nursing students revealed that
       students identified with the feminist movement increasingly as
       they moved through the program and continued to increase this
       identification following graduation. They regarded the
       "typical" nurse as less professional than themselves. (19)

1120   Morris, P.B. and N. Grssi-Russo. "Motives of Beginning Stu-
       dents for Choosing Nursing Schools," J NURS EDUC 18(5) (May
       1979): 34-40.

       Beginning students perceive differences in motivating factors
       between self and others as depicted in a rank ordering of ten
       factors. An early experience in sharing perceptions, attitudes
       and expectations of fellow nursing students will help students
       recognize that these differences are misconceptions. (12)

1121   Morrison, B.L. "Conflicts and Frustration Influencing Nurses
       from Other Countries," J NURS EDUC 19(1) (January 1980):
       12-19.

       Explores the concept of motivation in foreign nurses as well
       as the sources of conflict these motivations create for the
       nurse and the employing institutions. Mistaken expectations
       of modern well-staffed hospitals; inadequate educational pre-
       paration; unfamiliar equipment; and state board examinations
       combine to cause anxiety in foreign nurses wishing to practice
       in the United States. Institutional problems are created
       by lack of understanding of common English and cultural pre-
       judices of patients. (5)

1122   Ostmoe, P.M., H.L. Van Hoozer, A.L. Scheffel and C.M. Crowell.
       "Learning Style Preferences and Selection of Learning Stra-
       tegies: Consideration and Implications for Nurse Educators,"
       J NURS EDUC 23(1) (January 1984): 27-30.

       Baccalaureate nursing students in this study prefer tradi-
       tional, teacher-directed, well organized teaching strategies
       in which students assume a passive role. Their preference for
       non-traditional and innovative strategies decreased as they
       moved through the program. (11)

1123   Packard, K.L., A.I. Schwebel and J.S. Ganey. "Concerns of
       Final Semester Baccalaureate Nursing Students," NURS RES
       28(5) (September/October 1979): 302-304.

A study of the personal, professional and academic concerns of a group of senior baccalaureate nursing students found personal concerns most prevalent and client-related concerns infrequent. (7)

1124   Parlocha, P. and A. Hiraki. "Strategies for Faculty: Teaching the RN Student in a BSN Program," J NURS EDUC 21(5) (May 1982): 22-25.

RN students are different in their characteristics and learning needs than generic nursing students. They require consistent reinforcement, integration and application of nursing concepts into clinical practice. Faculty must understand their needs and assist students in making cognitive connections. (4)

1125   "RN Students Analyze Their Experiences," NURS OUTLOOK 28(2) (February 1980): 112-15.

RN students moved through stress and frustration within a baccalaureate program. A senior year seminar was influential in reducing the discomfort associated with the leadership identity. (3)

1126   Sargis, N.M. "Upper-Division or Completion Programs for RN's." THE NURSING PROFESSION: A TIME TO SPEAK. Edited by N.L. Chaska. New York: McGraw-Hill Book Co., 1983, pp. 111-20.

The education of registered nurse graduates in baccalaureate nursing degree programs poses yet another issue of diversity in preparation. These problems are explored and solutions offered. (21)

1127   Sime, A.M., S.A. Corcoran and M.A. Libera. "BSN vs. Non-BSN Students and Success in Graduate Study." J NURS EDUC 22(5) (May 1983): 190-94.

A study of entry and progression characteristics of graduate students comparing baccalaureate in nursing degree prepared nurses to non baccalaureate nursing degree students. Considers a number of variables. Sample numbers were small (N=28, N=4). Concluded that there were no differences between the two groups. (8)

1128   Slavinsky, A., D. Diers and J. Dixon. "College Graduates: The Hidden Nursing Population," NURS HEALTH CARE 4 (September 1983): 373-78.

College graduates are entering nursing programs in increasing numbers. A Yale survey reports college graduates represent one in every twenty students enrolled in nursing programs. Eighty-eight percent are enrolled in regular rather than special programs. Special programs are offered at eight sites across the United States, predominantly in private institutions in the Northeastern central quadrant. Two grant the BSN degree

after one year of study; five offer the master´s degree after
two or more years of study; and one offers the doctorate degree
after three years of study. Graduates of these programs are
estimated to represent five percent of currently practicing
nurses. (12)

1129   Smullen, B.B.   "Second-Step Education for RNs: The Quiet
       Revolution," NURS HEALTH CARE 3(7) (September 1982): 369-73.

RNs who return for baccalaureate degrees are frustrated,
anxious and confused. Nurse educators can assist them in
transition to the professional role through understanding the
learner, applying learning to the health care delivery system
and assisting in implementing modest change efforts. (9)

1130   Stacklum, M.M.   "New Student in Psych," AM J NURS 81(4) (April
       1981): 763.

An instructor describes the phases of adjustment experienced
by student nurses engaged in clinical practice in the psychiatric setting. (0)

1131   Stein, R.F.   "The Emerging Graduate," THE NURSING PROFESSION:
       VIEWS THROUGH THE MIST. Edited by N.L. Chaska. New York:
       McGraw-Hill Book Co., 1978, pp. 21-34.

A three year longitudinal study of two classes of nursing
students identifies transformations in attitudes and values
which occur during an educational program as they contribute
to role socialization. The personality traits of students
entering nursing changed during the study period. Characteristics of nurturance and deference to authority were re-
placed by traits of autonomy, exhibitionism and heterosexu-
ality. This made them similar to other college students. (29)

1132   Stoller, E.P.   "Preconceptions of the Nursing Role: A Case
       Study of An Entering Class," J NURS EDUC 17(6)) (June 1978):
       2-14.

Identifies the preconceptions of the nurse role of entering
students and compares findings to a group of graduating seniors
in a diploma program. Differences were noted between the two
groups which can be attributed in part to the schooling process. Further study is recommended. (18)

1133   Strauss, S.S. and E.B. Hutton.   "A Framework for Conceptualiz-
       ing Stress in Clinical Learning," J NURS EDUC 22(9)
       (November 1983): 367-71.

Proposes and describes the Transactional Model to use as a
method of understanding stressful experiences in nursing students. Such understanding will contribute to the identification of coping patterns and the interventions which will facilitate effective adaptation. (11)

1134   Stuebbe, B.   "Student and Faculty Perspectives on the Role of
        a Nursing Instructor," J NURS EDUC 19(7) (September 1980):
        4-9.

        A student examined the theoretical and actual role of a nurs-
        ing instructor as an assignment within a senior management
        career path elective. Within the study, freshman, junior and
        senior students and instructors ranked eighteen characteris-
        tics of teacher, person and nurse. Faculty ranked teacher
        characteristics highest while students ranked nurse character-
        istics highest. (11)

1135   "Supreme Court Rules Against All-Woman Nursing School," AM J
        NURS 82(8) (August 1982): 1187, 1283.

        The Mississippi University for Women was charged with sex
        discrimination for refusing admission to a male nurse. The
        historical stereotyping of nursing as a women´s profession
        entered into the decision at the Supreme Court level which
        ruled in favor of the student. (0)

1136   Tien, J.   "Surviving Graduate Nursing Programs in the United
        States--A Personal Account of an Asian-American Student,"
        J NURS EDUC 21(7) (September 1982): 42-44.

        The personal experiences of a foreign student enrolled in
        master´s and doctoral programs in nursing in the United States
        are reported. Language difficulties, cultural differences,
        and dietary changes caused considerable stress for the author.
        (0)

1137   Tumminia, P.A.   "Teaching Problems and Strategies With Male
        Nursing Students," NURSE EDUC 6(5) (September/October
        1981): 9-11.

        Nurse faculty must recognize and address the unique problems
        of male nursing students and support them in their profes-
        sional role development. Conflict in role stereotype, min-
        ority status in a female dominated group and lack of male
        role models require specific teaching strategies to minimize
        their impact on learning. (18)

1138   Uphold, C.R.   "Using an Individualized Clinical Evaluation
        Strategy to Motivate the RN Student," J NURS EDUC 22(9)
        (November 1983): 397-400.

        The author proposes a different approach to evaluation of
        RN students in baccalaureate completion programs which more
        clearly measures their goal attainment as well as program
        goals. (17)

1139   Waltz, C.F.   "Faculty Influence on Nursing Students´ Pre-
        ferences for Practice," NURS RES 27(2) (March/April 1978):
        89-97.

Seeks to establish a relationship between faculty preferences and the emergence of students preference for nursing
practice at three time intervals. (39)

1140 Watson, J. "Conceptual Systems of Undergraduate Nursing
      Students as Compared with University Students at Large and
      Practicing Nurses," NURS RES 27(3) (May/June 1978): 151-55.

A study of the characteristics of abstractness over con-
creteness in junior level nursing students found them similar
to other college students and more abstract than practicing
nurses. (26)

1141 Williams, M.A., D.W. Bloch and E.M. Blair. "Values and Value
      Changes of Graduate Nursing Students: Their Relationship to
      Faculty Values and to Selected Educational Factors," NURS
      RES 27(3) (May/June 1978): 181-89.

After one year of study the values of students in a graduate
nursing program changed. Increases in values of support,
recognition, and independence were accompanied by decreases
in values of benevolence, conformity and practical mindedness.
The influence of educational factors on these changes was not
clear. (23)

1142 Woolley, A.S. "From RN to BSN: Faculty Perceptions," NURS
      OUTLOOK 26(2) (February 1978): 103-5.

RN students move through stages of compliance, identification and internalization in the route to socialization to a
new nursing identity. Faculty support change which requires
unfreezing, changing and refreezing by support of the RN and
an understanding of the change process they are experiencing.
(11)

See 944, 1094, 1101, 1114, 1117, 1133, 1191, 1208, 1234, 1681.

Recruitment/Retention

1143 Abu-Saad, H. and J. Kayser-Jones. "Applicability of Nursing
      School Programs in Meeting Foreign Students´ Needs and Ex-
      pectations," J NURS EDUC 21(7) (September 1982): 4-10.

A survey of foreign nursing students in the United States
indicated that their expectations were fairly closely met.
Differences in personal and professional socialization were
found and lack of congruence between the school´s and the stu-
dent´s expectations. Suggestions for improving the orientation and education of foreign students are given. (8)

1144 Abu-Saad, H., J. Kayser-Jones and J. Tien. "Asian Nursing
      Students in the United States," J NURS EDUC 21(7) (September
      1982): 11-15.

Different social customs, differences in values and loneliness were identified as factors which caused difficulty
among Asian students in adjusting to the American culture.
Friends and relatives in the United States, helpful classmates and faculty, the ability to speak English well and the
presence of other foreign students were identified as helpful
in adjustment. (12)

1145   Abu-Saad, H. and J. Kayser-Jones. "Middle Eastern Nursing
       Students in the United States," J NURS EDUC 21(7) (September
       1982): 22-25.

Cultural differences experienced by foreign students from
Middle Eastern countries studying in American schools of nursing caused difficulties. Understanding of cultural values and
support of faculty and classmates were found most needed for
satisfactory adjustment. (6)

1146   Abu-Saad, H., J. Kayser-Jones and Y. Gutierrez. "Latin Amer-
       ican Nursing Students in the United States," J NURS EDUC
       21(7) (September 1982): 16-21.

Loneliness was the greatest difficulty identified by Latin
American nursing students in their adjustment in the United
States. Factors helpful in adjustment were identified as:
American friends, financial security, support groups in the
community, knowing the area, and host families. (6)

1147   Alichnie, M.C. and J.T. Bellucci. "Prediction of Freshman
       Students' Success in a Baccalaureate Nursing Programs," NURS
       RES 30(1) (January/February 1981): 49-53.

A sample consisting of two freshman nursing classes at Wilkes
College, Wilkes-Barre, Pennsylvania was used to determine cognitive and noncognitive variables which best predicted GPA and
withdrawal at the conclusion of the freshman year. The Apt-
itude Test for Nursing was found to be the best predictor of
academic achievement. Science GPA had the highest correlation with withdrawal from the nursing program. (19)

1148   Beale, A.V. and A.F. McCutcheon. "On Becoming a Nurse," J
       NURS EDUC 19(4) (April 1980): 28-32.

A survey of admission criteria to schools of nursing in the
State of Virginia found specific high school units and secon-
dary grade point average were considered most important.
However, each institution tended to value certain criteria
more than others and considerable differences were found between institutions. This poses a problem in advising high
school students interested in nursing. (4)

1149   Binger, J.L. "Practical Suggestions for Applying to Doctoral
       Programs," NURSE EDUC 6(7) (December 1981): 34-37.

Nurses interested in a doctoral program should gather information on program requirements, faculty and students currently
enrolled. When requesting letters of recommendation, professional productivity should be stressed. The application
and statement of purpose should communicate critical information regarding the individual's past and future career.
Exploration of funding resources should begin at the time of
interview. (27)

1150 Buckley, J. "Faculty Commitment to Retention and Recruitment
      of Black Students," NURS OUTLOOK 28(1) (January 1980): 46-50.

A survey of 40 integrated and predominantly Black schools
of nursing revealed that Black faculty had the greatest influence on the recruitment and retention of Black students.
Commitment to this goal by faculty and the presence of
flexible and innovative programs had a positive effect on
recruitment, admission and retention. (3)

1151 Claerbaut, D. "New Directions in the Education of Minority
      Nursing Students," J NURS EDUC 19(3) (March 1980): 11-15.

Minorities in the health care delivery setting are frequently
cared for by nurses of the dominant culture. Recommendations
for increasing enrollments of minorities in schools of nursing
include suggestions for recruitment, financial assistance,
academic assistance, role modeling by nurses of minority cul-
tures, curricular focus on the social sciences and research by
and about minorities. (13)

1152 Curran, C.L., M. Habeeb and E. Sobol. "Selecting a Doctoral
      Program for a Career in Nursing," NURSE EDUC 6(1) (January/
      February 1981): 11-15.

The variety of doctoral programs available to nurses today
may be confusing to prospective candidates. Thoughtful consideration of the school, faculty, possibility of acceptance
and completion, nature of the research program, personal
impressions of student experience and the relationship of
graduation and attainment of personal and professional goals
are necessary prior to selection of a program. (20)

1153 Davis, W.E. Jr. "ODWIN Expansion Program: A Study in Sucess,"
      NURS RES 27(4) (July/August 1978): 230-32.

An eight week pre nursing program for high school graduates
with marginal credentials demonstrated a positive influence
on enrollment and successful completion of a nursing program.
(7)

1154 Drice, A.D., V. Hunter and B.S. Williams. "The Influence
      of Academic Support Programs on Retention of Minority Nursing
      Students 1971-1974: A Descriptive Study," J NURS EDUC 17(3)
      (March 1978): 22-35.

An evaluation of the academic support services for minority students at UCLA School of Nursing indicated that these services influenced increases in academic averages. (16)

1155   Dustan, L.C. "Buyer Beware: The RN As Baccalaureate Student," NURSE EDUC 6(3) (May/June 1981): 10-13.

In selecting a college or university, registered nurse students need to examine the quality of faculty, the methods of granting credit for prior learning, the quantity and quality of academic services available, the quality of the general education and science courses offered, and the cost of the program. (3)

1156   Ferguson, C.K. "Reading Skills versus Success in Nursing School," J NURS EDUC 18(3) (March 1979): 6-12.

Deficiencies in reading skills were contributing to failure in the associate degree program at San Antonio College. An analysis of the readability level of the textbooks used led to the use of the Nelson Denny Reading Test for students on admission. Students scoring lower than tenth grade level were advised to take a remedial reading course prior to beginning the nursing curriculum. A twelfth grade level was needed for success in the program. (3)

1157   Fong, M.L. "The Group Interview: A Tool for Nursing Student Selection," J NURS EDUC 17 (7) (September 1978): 35-40.

The use of a group interview for admission screening of applicants was found more accurate than individual interviews in assessing interpersonal skills, group skills, communication skills, and the ability to speak clearly. (6)

1158   Hayes, E.R. "Prediction of Academic Success in a Baccalaureate Nursing Education Program," J NURS EDUC 20(6) (June 1981): 4-8.

A multiple regression equation approach was used to identify valid predictor variables of success in baccalaureate education. Cognitive variables are the most powerful predictors. Through advisement of high risk students, attrition may be reduced and maximum utilization of resources attained. (6)

1159   Holtzclaw, B.J. "Crisis: Changing Student Applicant Pools," NURS HEALTH CARE 4(8) (October 1983): 450-54.

Student applicants are changing. Decreases in college aged population are expected to continue and research has indicated that students of today hold different values and are attracted to different incentives than their predecessors. Early recruitment through positive imagery of nurses in young school

children both male and female, the development of career lad-
der programs, and attractive programs for adult learners
are necessary for the future of nursing education and nursing
practice. (12)

1160   Hutcheson, J.D., Jr., L.M. Garland and L.S. Lowe.
       "Antecedents of Nursing School Attrition: Attitudinal Dimen-
       sions," NURS RES 28 (1) (January/February 1979): 57-62.

       A study of the influences of attitudinal factors on attrition
       in one school of nursing found traditional measures of scho-
       lastic aptitude were not good indicators. Attitudinal meas-
       ures studied were found to have little direct impact. Acad-
       emic performance was found the strongest and most consistent
       indicator of attrition. (17)

1161   Knopke, H.J. "Predicting Student Attrition in a Baccalaureate
       Curriculum," NURS RES 28(4) (July/August 1979): 224-27.

       A model is proposed to predict attrition and retention in
       nursing schools. Achievement, learning style, and psycholog-
       ical variables were examined over a six year period. Signifi-
       cant differences were found in combined variables between
       drop out and continuing students. (18)

1162   McNally, J.M. "The Improvement of Licensure Results of
       Minority BSN Students," J NURS EDUC 18(6) (June 1979): 8-18.

       A project is described which provides for socio-economically
       disadvantaged nursing students to promote success in complet-
       ing a program leading to licensure. Academic remediation,
       cultural enrichment, personal counseling and participation in
       formulation and implementation of the program were utilized.
       Students found the supportive spirit most helpful. (8)

1163   Moore, B.M. and W.L. Pentecost. "CSULB Nursing: Education-
       ally Disadvantaged Students Can Succeed," J NURS EDUC 18(6)
       (June 1979): 50-58.

       Experience in advising academically disadvantaged students
       at California State University at Long Beach began with crisis
       intervention and evolved into planned anticipatory guidance.
       (3)

1164   Niedringhalls, L. and D.L. O'Driscoll. "Staying Within the
       Law--Academic Probation and Dismissal," NURS OUTLOOK 31
       (May/June 1983): 156-59.

       Guidelines to comply with the court's position on the ap-
       plication of academic sanctions are specified. Case histories
       are presented and procedural safeguards to be used by admin-
       istrators before dismissing a student for academic reasons
       are provided.

1165   Norris, C.G. "Characteristics of the Adult Learner and
          Extended Higher Education for Registered Nurses," NURS
          HEALTH CARE 1(2) (September 1980): 87-93.

          A national trend toward increased enrollment of adults in
          higher education programs is apparent. Access to education
          for these individuals has been hampered by lack of financial
          aid and some alienation on the part of university professors.
          Moves are underway to provide quality programs to students in
          areas distant from college and university campuses. (12)

1166   Outtz, J.H. "Predicting the Success on State Board Examin-
          ations for Blacks," J NURS EDUC 18(9) (November 1979):
          35-40.

          A study of predictive variables of the performance of Black
          nurses on State Board Examinations found the college cummul-
          ative GPA was the best predictor of success followed by the
          SAT verbal score. (12)

1167   Paduano, M.A. "A Closer Look at Freshman Attrition in an
          Urban AD Nursing Program and the Questions It Raises," J NY
          STATE NURSES ASSOC 11(2) (June 1980): 14-17.

          Concern for high attrition at Pace University prompted a
          study of one freshmen class. A 36 percent attrition rate
          was found. Contributing to this attrition was diversity in
          educational preparation in previous college coursework. Marked
          differences in academic standards were noted among these
          colleges. Faculty must be aware of student needs for remed-
          iation and restrict AD curriculum to that content and level
          of proficiency commensurate with the philosophy of the AD
          a program (4)

1168   Schoen, D.C. "Predictors of Success for ADN Graduates," NURS
          LEADERSH 6(4) (December 1983):   104-12.

          A study of predictors of clinical competency for a graduat-
          ing class of associate degree nurses two and one-half years
          after graduation found the strongest predictor was the length
          of time taken to complete the ADN program. Final year
          clinical evaluations by ADN program instructors had some
          a predictive validity as did grade point average, however,
          state board scores did not. (9)

1169   Schwirian, P.M. and S.R. Gortner. "How Nursing Schools
          Predict Their Successful Graduates," NURS OUTLOOK 27(5)
          (May 1979): 352-58.

          Assesses the relationship between achievement in school and
          performance after graduation in selected nurse graduates of
          associate degree, diploma and baccalaureate programs. A
          change in the selection process noted greater concern for

academic performance and chronological and emotional maturity
as opposed to submissive, cautious behaviors previously sought.
Students thus selected and apprised of their progress in the
program are more likely to be successful graduates. (3)

1170 Seither, F.F. "Prediction of Achievement in Baccalaureate
      Nursing Education," J NURS EDUC 19(3) (March 1980): 28-36.

      A study of valid predictors of academic success in a bac-
      calaureate nursing program identified grade point average in
      the biological and behavioral sciences and high school per-
      centile rank as most predictive. Few of the variables proved
      predictive of on-the-job performance. (11)

1171 Sime, A.M., S.A. Corcoran, and M.B. Libera. "Predicting
      Success in Graduate Education," J NURS EDUC 22(1) (January
      1983): 7-11.

      A report of indices of predictive validity of selected
      measures for three groups of students admitted to the graduate
      program in nursing at the University of Minnesota. Bac-
      calauareate GPA was found to be modestly predictive of the
      Master's GPA but was not predictive of faculty rating of
      students on characteristics which one might expect to be
      associated with grades. (14)

1172 "Slack Economy Spurs Part-time, RN Enrollments in BSN Prog-
      rams," AM J NURS 82(8) (August 1982): 1190, 1194.

      Full time enrollments in undergraduate and graduate degree
      programs continue to decline while part-time enrollments are
      increasing. Generic baccalaureate enrollments have declined
      while RNs in baccalaureate and master's programs have in-
      creased. (0)

1173 Sobol, E.G. "Self-Actualization and the Baccalaureate
      Nursing Student's Response to Stress," NURS RES 27(4) (July/
      August 1984): 238-44.

      A study of 144 senior nursing students demonstrated that
      the level of self-actualization is a factor in the differen-
      tial perception of evaluative events as stressful. Implica-
      tions for recruitment and selection of baccalaureate nursing
      students are discussed. (59)

1174 Story, B.W. "The I AM Model for Retention of Minority Nursing
      Student," NURSE EDUC 3(6) (November/December 1978): 16-20.

      An affirmative action plan is described which assisted
      minority students in gaining admission, completing degree
      requirements, and obtaining appropriate job placement. (1)

1175 Ventura, W.P. "Non-Nurses in an MSN Program: Comparing
      Liberal Arts and Science Majors," NURSE EDUC 4(5) (Septem-
      ber/October 1979): 28-33.

      A comparison of performance on state board examinations by
      graduates of the master's degree program at Pace University
      demonstrated high achievement levels by students with under-
      graduate degrees in liberal arts education. It was concluded
      that the liberal arts undergraduate major provides a good
      academic base for master's level nursing education. (2)

1176 Vinson, K.S. "Organizational Transformation: Using Organ-
      izational Development (OD) in Nursing Education and Train-
      ing," J NURS EDUC 23(3) (March 1984): 130-32.

      Organizational Development strategies and technologies
      proved effective in reducing staff turnover and stress in a
      military program which prepares practical nurses. (6)

1177 Weinstein, E.L., I. Brown and M.W. Wahlstrom. "Character-
      istics of the Successful Nursing Student," J NURS EDUC 19(3)
      (March 1980): 53-59.

      High attrition rates in Ontario led to a study of demographic
      variables and behavioral antecedents characteristic of suc-
      cessful nursing students. A review of transcripts found the
      number of pure and applied science courses an applicant com-
      pleted was the best predictor of success in a nursing program.
      Average high school English grades and mathematics grades
      were also good predictors. (5)

1178 Weinstein, E.L., L. Brown and M.W. Wahlstrom. "Selection
      Procedures and Attrition," J NURS EDUC 18(4) (April 1979):
      38-46.

      A research study conducted in Ontario sought to reduce
      attrition in schools of nursing through improvement of the
      selection process. Predictive capabilities of a multiple of
      variables were examined, and an index of campus success rate
      determined based on selection procedures. (4)

1179 Wilson, H.S. and J. Levy. "Why RN Students Drop Out," NURS
      OUTLOOK 26(7) (July 1978): 437-41.

      An examination of factors which lead to withdrawal of RN
      students identifies personal adjustment as critical to contin-
      uation. Matching and balancing processes can be facilitated
      by sound personal and career counseling before and during
      nursing program attendance. (8)

Faculty

1180 "After Five Years Sex Discrimination Suit Comes to Court,"
      AM J NURS 79(6) (June 1979): 1040.

Faculty at the University of Washington School of Nursing
charged the University with sex discrimination in pay
scales. (0)

1181 Allbritten, D., M.E. Megal, K.A. Buckley, M.R.C. Scalone
and S. Panwar. "Faculty Peer Review: An Evolving Process,"
J NURS EDUC 22(7) (September 1983): 296-99.

A pilot project of voluntary, collegial peer review of
nursing faculty found it helpful in assisting in the improvement of teaching skills. In order to document the merits
of such a project, measurement of the overall quality of
teaching behaviors before and after implementation of peer
review is necessary. (9)

1182 "Arizona Nursing Board Dismisses Complaint vs.College," AM
J NURS 83(4) (April 1983): 506,634.

A report of the investigative actions and findings of the
State Board of Nursing in a faculty complaint. Excessive
workload,age and sex discriminations were dismissed. (0)

1183 Bach, C.A., L. Bell and T. Fernandez. "Who Teaches Foundations in an Integrated Curriculum?," NURS OUTLOOK 27(2)
(February 1979): 112-15.

The assignment of specialty faculty to a foundations of
nursing practice course caused anxiety in faculty. However,
benefits were derived from the experience and students were
able to identify positive aspects from the faculty mix. (0)

1184 Brannigan, C.N. "Revamping the Peer Review Process," J NURS
EDUC 22(7) (September 1983): 287-89.

A tool for peer evaluation is proposed which is equitable
and easy to use. This instrument broadens the evaluative
input of faculty to include colleagues and contributes to
goal determinations. (5)

1185 Brown, S.T. "Faculty and Student Perceptions of Effective
Clinical Teachers," J NURS EDUC 20(9) (November 1981): 4-15.

A study was conducted to identify student and teachers
perceptions of important characteristics of the clinical
teacher. Lack of congruence was found in some areas. Students
regarded relationships with students as most important whereas
faculty regarded professional competence as most important. (28)

1186 Bueche, M.N. "Academic Tenure: A Reexamination for the
Eighties," NURSE EDUC 8(1) (Spring 1983): 3-7.

Issues surrounding the process of tenuring faculty are discussed and strategies to assist faculty in preparing for
tenure presented. (39)

1187   Busl, L.D. "The Teacher as Manager of the Learning Environ-
       ment," J NURS EDUC 20(5) (May 1981): 42-47.

       In organizing the learning environment, the teacher should
       be aware of the principles of learning and choose and adapt
       teaching to meet the learning style of the student. The role
       of teaching is not merely the transmission of knowledge but
       one of facilitating learning. (9)

1188   Christman, L. "The Practitioner-Teacher," NURS EDUC 4(2)
       (March/April 1979): 8-11.

       Describes four components of the professional role as ser-
       vice, education, consultation and research, and the support
       structure utilized at Rush University to achieve integration.
       The need for similar models is stressed as critical to the
       achievement of full professional status. (1)

1189   Clarkson, J.A. "Confessions of a Nursing Instructor," J
       NURS EDUC 22(7) (September 1983): 295-96.

       A personal recount of the frustrations and rewards of teach-
       ing nursing. (3)

1190   Cohen, B.J. "Strategies for Dealing with Conflict: Faculty
       and the Law," J NURS EDUC 17(5) (May 1978): 16-20.

       Discusses contractual arrangements and their legality, the
       procedure of due process and the powers of collective bargain-
       ing in respect to nurse faculty. (12)

1191   Collins, P.B. "Strategies for Dealing with Conflict: Crisis
       Intervention," J NURS EDUC 17(5) (May 1978): 39-46.

       A model is proposed by which faculty members can restore
       equilibrium in stressful situations. (6)

1192   Coudret, N.A. "Determining Faculty Workload," NURSE EDUC
       6(2) (March/April 1981): 38-41.

       A survey of nurse faculty workload and existing workload
       policies in associate degree and baccalaureate programs re-
       vealed the formula approach was preferred. Contact hours were
       preferred to credit hours as a basis for establishing workload.
       When necessary, a conversion measure should be used to equate
       nursing faculty workload with other faculty workload in the
       institution. (4)

1193   Crawford, M.E., G. Laing, M. Linwood, M. Kyle A. DeBlock.
       "A Formula for Calculating Faculty Workload," J NURS EDUC
       22(7) (September 1983): 285-86.

A formula is presented to calculate faculty workload in its
component parts. Lecture, clinical teaching, research, committee activities, and publishing are weighted for undergraduate teaching faculty as a baseline for determining equitable
load. (2)

1194   Creason, N. "Registration and Voting Participation of Four
       Faculty Groups," NURS RES 27(5) (September/October 1978):
       325-27.

       A study compares registration and voting behavior among
       nurse faculty and other female and male dominant faculties to
       gain understanding of the relationship of voting practices to
       professional prestige and power. (18)

1195   Creighton, H. "Education of Instructors," NURS MANAGE 14
       (1983): 48-49.

       Presents a legal case involving an instructor whose contract
       was not renewed because her master's degree was not in nursing.
       The college was held to be within its rights in doing so. (12)

1196   Curran, C.R. and D.W. Riley. "Faculty Practice Plans: Will
       They Work for Nurses?," NURS ECON 2(5) (September/October
       1984): 319-24.

       Approximately $1 billion will be generated by medical facul-
       ty practice plans in 1984. Nursing faculty practice plans
       could provide financial incentives to practitioners and create
       a system to balance research, teaching, and patient care.(6)

1197   Davenport, N.J. "The Nurse Scientist--Between Two Worlds,"
       NURS OUTLOOK 28(1) (January 1980): 28-31.

       Nurses with doctorate degrees in physiology are few in
       number and experience overload in the faculty role. The
       nature of their research is time consuming and often fails to
       be immediately applicable to nursing practice. They are
       therefore frustrated and misunderstood when requesting release
       time from heavy faculty loads to engage in research. (5)

1198   Dennis, C.M., A. O'Hearn, B.J. Hatcher and A.M. Hilton.
       "Peer Evaluation: A Process of Development," J NURS EDUC
       22(2) (February 1983): 93-95.

       The development of a peer evaluation method is described
       which was created to assist faculty in the evaluation of
       teaching effectiveness. It was found that the successful de-
       velopment of such a method required regular total faculty
       awareness and approval of the developing instrument. (6)

1199   Fleming, J.W. "Tenure Today," AM J NURS 83(2) (February
       1983): 279-80.

Establishing quotas, developing contracts, varying the
tenure and nontenured classifications, making temporary appointments, avoiding tenure commitments, and adopting early
retirements are useful strategies for planning program needs
for faculty. (8)

1200 Flynn, P. "That First Teaching Job," AM J NURS 79(11)
      (November 1979): 1996-97.

      A nurse recounts her first experiences in teaching identify-
      ing successes and problems encountered. (0)

1201 Gaevert, H.S. "Striking Balance Between Content and Method
      in Nursing Education," NURS FORUM 27(3) (1978): 245-57.

      A discussion of Alfred North Whitehead's philosophy of educ-
      ation adapted to the preparation of nurse educators. Students
      need assistance in applying theoretical concepts to the prac-
      tice setting. The nurse educator must be both a "knower"
      and a "doer." (10)

1202 Garrity, M., V. Miller, M. Osborn and M. Vanderlinden.
      "Developing Criteria for Promotion and Tenure," NURS OUTLOOK
      28(3) (March 1980): 187-91.

      One faculty group reports on a long, arduous, and frustrating
      project of gaining faculty consensus regarding criteria for
      appointment, promotion and tenure. (4)

1203 Gay, J.T. "Faculty Release Time Quarter," NURS HEALTH CARE
      5(1) (January 1984): 37-39.

      A mechanism developed at the University of Alabama School
      of Nursing provides a release time quarter (R+Q) in which
      faculty contract for professional development activities
      which will be of personal benefit as well as of benefit to the
      school and the students. The advantages of such a policy are
      discussed as well as the challenges it proposes. (0)

1204 Heller, B.R. "Associate Degree Nursing: Faculty Preparation
      and Commitment," NURS OUTLOOK 30(5) (May 1982): 310-11.

      Educational requirements for nurse faculty in associate
      degree programs are less than that of other disciplines in
      community colleges. Ill prepared faculty do not identify
      differences between diploma, associate degree, and baccalaur-
      eate programs. They have not been prepared to teach and
      their lack of commitment to the technical level of teaching
      serves to perpetuate confusion in graduates and employing
      agencies. (4)

1205 Helmuth, M.R. and T.D. Guberski. "Preparation for Preceptor
      Role," NURS OUTLOOK 28(1) (January 1980): 36-39.

Early nurse practitioner programs utilized physician preceptors. As nurses became experienced in the role, they were
able to assume the preceptor role and after teaching beginning
students on a one-to-one basis, moved to structure the teaching of beginning students by advanced students. Confidence
and skill in the nurse practitioner role are essential to the
role of preceptor. (0)

1206 Holzemer, W.L., V.H. Barkauskas and V.M. Ohlson. "A Program
       Evlauation of Four Workshops Designed to Prepare Nurse
       Faculty in Health Assessment," J NURS EDUC 19(4) (April
       1980): 7-18.

       Provides instruments used in the evaluation of workshops to
       prepare nurse faculty in primary care. Findings indicated
       that the programs were successful in preparing faculty in
       health assessment and all faculty were directly or indirectly
       working with health assessment skills six months following the
       program. (9)

1207 Kelley, L.K. and J.M. Baker. "Women in Nursing and Academic
       Tenure," J NURS EDUC 19(2) (February 1980): 41-48.

       Explores the issue of academic tenure in schools of nursing.
       Nursing faculty must be informed and assertive in seeking
       tenure. (13)

1208 Kielinen, C.E. "Conflict Resolution: Communication--Good,
       Withdrawal--Bad," J NURS EDUC 17(5) (May 1978): 12-15.

       Conflicts exist which cannot be resolved through communica-
       tion. In situations where conflict persists, withdrawal may
       be the right decision. (39)

1209 Kinsey, D.C. "Implementation of Peer Review Within a Bac-
       calaureate Nursing Program," J NURS EDUC 20(5) (May 1981):
       29-33.

       A peer evaluation program at Cedar Crest College was begun
       to acknowledge excellence in teaching; to identify and evaluate
       behaviors that constitute excellence; and, to utilize eval-
       uation to improve teaching effectiveness. A Peer Evaluation
       Tool is provided. Other schools implementing such a process
       should tailor peer evaluation to the character of the depart-
       ment; thoroughly review the effort of others; and, strive
       through peer evaluation to improve the instructional program. (4)

1210 Lacefield, W.E. and R.D. Kingston. "Relationships Between
       Faculty Evaluations and Faculty Development," J NURS EDUC
       22(7) (September 1983): 278-84.

A discussion of remediation methods for improving faculty teaching skills. A diagnostic/prescriptive use of evaluation instruments which measured practical, day-to-day teaching skills by student evaluations had a significantly greater impact than traditional methods. (8)

1211   Leftwich, R.E. "The Nurse as Grievance Officer," J NURS EDUC 22(7) (September 1983): 301-3.

Interpersonal, critical thinking and leadership skills which are taught in baccalaureate and higher degree nursing programs provide nursing faculty with the skills necessary to assume the position of grievance officer. (2)

1212   Lenhart, R.C. "Faculty Burnout--and Some Reasons Why," NURS OUTLOOK 28(7) (July 1980): 424-25.

Decreasing funds and decreasing enrollments are increasing faculty pressure. Recruitment and progression of unqualified candidates contribute to faculty burnout and poor program image. (0)

1213   Lenz, E.R. and C.F. Waltz. "Patterns of Job Search and Mobility Among Nurse Educators," J NURS EDUC 22(7) (September 1983): 267-73.

A survey of 790 faculty in southern schools of nursing is reported which seeks information regarding factors which influence job changes. Salary, geographic location, administrative leadership style and the school's reputation were the most important factors identified in choosing the present position. Job dissatisfaction was not a major reason for leaving the present position. (11)

1214   Luginbill, C. "Nurse-Instructors for Medical Students," AM J NURS 78(5) (May 1978): 868-70.

A nurse instructor describes her experiences in providing clinical instruction to third year medical students in a hospital based teaching program. (0)

1215   Marriner, A. "Factors of Importance in Determination of Faculty Salaries," J NURS EDUC 20(5) (May 1981): 34-41.

A survey was conducted to determine faculty perceptions of equitable wages and factors which should be considered in wage differentials. The majority of the 83 faculty surveyed felt dissatisfied with their pay but satisfied with their jobs. A variety of factors should be considered in determining faculty salaries. (16)

1216   Mauksch, I.G.   "The Socialization of Nurse Faculty," NURSE
       EDUC 7(4) (July/August 1982): 7-10.

       Nurse faculty members occupy a complex role greater than
       that of teacher of nursing. Conflicts common to the role
       include professional-bureaucratic conflict and demands of
       career, jobs and family. A planned process of socialization
       is needed. (7)

1217   McQueen, J.   "In Support of Part-time Faculty," NURS OUTLOOK
       29(2) (February 1981): 102-3.

       Part-time faculty are substantial in numbers and yet are not
       accorded equity within academe. Study of the characteristics,
       value and contributions of this professional group is war-
       ranted. (2)

1218   Nieswiadomy, R.M.   "Nurse Educators' Involvement in Research,"
       J NURS EDUC 23(2) (February 1984): 52-56.

       A report of a study of the research productivity of nurse
       educators showed that doctorally prepared faculty with 16-20
       years in nursing employed in institutions with graduate prog-
       rams were most likely to be engaged in research activities. (0)

1219   "Nursing Faculty Salaries Increase, AACN Survey Finds," AM J
       NURS 82(3) (March 1982): 358,388.

       A survey of faculty salaries in baccalaureate and graduate
       programs revealed an 8 to 10 percent increase over the 1980-81
       level. Salaries in the western states are substantially
       higher and salaries in universities that offer master's or
       doctoral level nursing programs are higher. Salaries are
       comparable to other departments within the university.
       Average salaries by rank and educational preparation are pro-
       vided. (0)

1220   O'Connor, A.   "Sources of Conflict for Faculty Members," J
       NURS EDUC 17(5) (May 1978): 35-38.

       Faculty members encounter conflict situations involving
       students, other faculty and administrative personnel as well
       as internal conflict related to their role. A discussion of
       these various sources of conflict is provided and construc-
       tive actions proposed. (11)

1221   O'Kane, P.K. and Sr. M. Meyer. "Sharing a Faculty Position,"
       NURS OUTLOOK 30(7) (July/August 1982): 411-13.

       Two nurses who negotiated a shared faculty position see
       this as a viable option by which to free time for other pro-
       fessional and personal commitments. Many problems that were
       encountered may be reconciled in future endeavors. (3)

1222 O´Shea, H.S. "Role Orientation and Role Strain of Clinical
      Nurse Faculty in Baccalaureate Programs, NURS RES 31(5)
      (September/October 1982): 306-13.

      Study explored relationship between role orientation and
      role strain of 453 nurse faculty teaching in 41 baccalaureate
      programs. (15)

1223 Ostrand, L. and W. Willis. "Faculty Preparation: An MPH or
      MSN Degree?," NURS OUTLOOK 26(10) (October 1978): 637-40.

      Faculty with a master´s in public health degree were com-
      pared to faculty with a master´s of science in nursing degree.
      A survey of public health graduates found 58 percent felt
      their´s was better than or as good as the nursing degree
      whereas 43.9 percent of the deans and chairpersons who res-
      ponded concurred with the graduates. (0)

1224 Page, S. and J. Loeper. "Peer Review of the Nurse Educator:
      The Process and Development of a Format," J NURS EDUC 17(9)
      (November 1978): 21-29.

      A tool for use in peer review of nurse faculty is provided
      and the method of development described. (7)

1225 Parsons, M.A. and C.R. Collison. "This Process of Change
      in Curriculum Evaluation," J NURS EDUC 19(7) (September
      1980): 36-38.

      Faculty growth was noted as a result of participation in a
      project to create a comprehensive evaluation framework for
      both baccalaureate and master´s programs. The anxieties en-
      countered in this process are described. (7)

1226 Perry, S.E. "A Doctorate--Necessary but Not Sufficient,"
      NURS OUTLOOK 30(2) (February 1982): 95-96.

      Nursing fails to gain faculty status in the university com-
      munity because they do not require the same credentials. The
      doctorate degree preferably in nursing should be the minimum
      academic credential for a faculty position. Beyond this
      scholarship should be demonstrated through research, pub-
      lication, and dissemination of findings. (0)

1227 Phillips, J.R. "Surviving Faculty Abuse," J NURS EDUC 22(7)
      (September 1983): 303-5.

      Abuse occurs in academic settings. Greater understanding
      of how this abuse presently occurs and awareness of strategies
      for surviving it are presented to help faculty deal with such
      situations. (0)

1228 Podratz, R.O. "A Student Sues," AM J NURS 80(9) (September
      1980): 1604-5.

      A faculty member describes her anxieties related to a
      threatened law suit by a student she failed in a clinical
      course. (0)

1229 Porth, C. "Peer Review for Nursing Faculty," J NY STATE
      NURSES ASSOC 9(4) (December 1978): 48-53.

      An orderly and accountable method of peer review is needed
      within the evaluation of nursing faculty. Criteria used to
      assess faculty competence are generally the same from one
      institution to another and include education, clinical exper-
      tise and research. The expectations of the individual
      institution within these areas should be made clear to faculty
      from the time of appointment. (9)

1230 Saylor, A.A. et al. "Guidelines for Faculty Workload," AM
      J NURS (May 1979): 902-4.

      Provides a definitive breakdown of work hours to determine
      faculty workload. (2)

1231 Solomons, H.C., N.S. Jordison and S.R. Powell. "How Faculty
      Members Spend Their Time," NURS OUTLOOK 28(3) (March 1980):
      160-65.

      A survey of nursing faculty in one institution identified
      the distribution of time spent in four major areas: teaching,
      scholarly productivity and research, service, and professional
      growth. Teaching was the major activity for all faculty
      regardless of rank. Professors and associate professors spent
      more time in scholarly productivity and research and less
      time in professional growth activities than the lower ranked
      faculty. Deterrents to research are identified. (25)

1232 Sorcinelli, M.D. and M.L. Logothetis. "Faculty Development
      in Nursing Education: A Teaching Consultation Service," J
      NURS EDUC 21(4) (April 1982): 35-41.

      A teaching-consultation process utilized at Indiana Univer-
      sity Northwest included four major assessment of teaching,
      analysis of data, improvement of efforts and a final review.
      Participation in this process led to increased awareness of
      teaching skills which motivated improvements. Student feed-
      back indicated that the consultation resulted in improved
      teaching abilities. (4)

1233 Sweeney, S.S. and P.M. Ostmoe. "Academic Freedom: A
      Relevant Concept for Collegiate Nursing Education," NURS
      FORUM 19(1) (1980): 4-18.

A review of the history of academic freedom and nursing's
movement to collegiate programs. Issues affecting academic
freedom and future implications are discussed. Nurse faculty
members need to be aware of these issues and implications
in order to plan for an uncertain future. (17)

1234 Tappen, R.M. "Strategies for Dealing with Conflict Using
        Confrontation," J NURS EDUC 17(5) (May 1978): 47-52.

        Defines confrontation and different techniques which are
        appropriate for faculty to use based on the source of conflict.
        This effective method of conflict resolution can be successful
        in gaining increased self-esteem, increased autonomy, oppor-
        tunities for self-actualization, and a greater awareness and
        understanding of other people. (8)

1235 Turnbull, E. "Rewards in Nursing: The Case of Nurse Precep-
        tors," J NURS ADM 13 (January 1983): 10-13.

        The author describes a framework for identifying and de-
        veloping effective reward mechanisms and applies it to a
        specific situation--the nursing preceptorship. (7))

1236 Van Ort, S.R. "Developing a System for Documenting Teaching
        Effectiveness," J NURS EDUC 22(8) (October 1983): 324-28.

        Faculty evaluations are gaining increasing importance in
        academe. Congruence of evaluation to institutional and program
        goals must be considered. Criteria for faculty evaluation and
        sources of input are proposed within a model to measure teach-
        ing effectiveness. (7)

1237 Wood, V. STUDENT ISSUES: A CASE BOOK. London, Canada: The
        University of Western Ontario, 1984.

        A case book aimed at helping potential nurse educators
        develop ways of anticipating and responding to student and
        personal problems. (0)

        See 1018, 2325.

Faculty Practice

1238 Anderson, E. and P. Pierson. "An Exploratory Study of Faculty
        Practice: Views of Those Faculty Engaged in Practice Who
        Teach in an NLN Accredited Baccalaureate Program," WEST
        J NURS RES 5(2) (Spring 1983): 129-40.

        Reviews history of faculty-practice as an issue, identifies
        several models which incorporate faculty practice, and reports
        the results of a survey of practicing faculty's perceptions
        about various factors related to that practice. (23)

1239   Archer, S.E. and R.P. Fleshman. "Faculty Role Modeling,"
       NURS OUTLOOK 29(10) (October 1981): 586-89.

       Role modeling within one graduate program was achieved
       through working with faculty in the community in both needs
       assessment activities and planning for needed programs. These
       graduate students assisted in writing a grant proposal which
       was subsequently funded. The students served as codirectors
       of the funded project and are now role models to other graduate
       students. (6)

1240   Blazeck, A.M., J. Selekman, M. Timpe and Z.R. Wolf.
       "Unification: Nursing Education and Nursing Practice."
       NURS HEALTH CARE 3(1) (January 1982): 18-24.

       Lack of unity between educators and practitioners is both
       real and chronic. Unification models both within and outside
       nursing differ. These differences are described by comparing
       Rush University, the University of Rochester and Case Western
       Reserve University and their approach to unification. Clear
       definition of terms and responsibilities is needed. Eleven
       strategies are proposed to resolve problems. (16)

1241   Chicadoz, G.H., E.G. Bush, K.E. Korthuis, and S.W. Utz.
       "Mobilizing Faculty Toward Integration of Practice into
       Faculty Roles," NURS HEALTH CARE 11(10) (December 1981):
       548-53.

       Describes the transformation of a school of nursing that
       used traditional faculty roles into a joint practice model.
       Lends insight into the structuring and process of change,
       problems and problem resolution within the adoption of a
       unification model. (23)

1242   Christman, L. "On The Scene: Uniting Service and Education
       at Rush-Presbyterian-St. Luke's Medical Center," NURS ADM
       Q 3(3) (Spring 1979): 7-13.

       Argues that the full clinical role of a professional in-
       cludes service, education, consultation, and research. When
       large numbers of people do this the profession becomes di-
       chotomized. Formulas are given for role expression of know-
       ledge, group professional power, and innovative potential. (0)

1243   Christy, T.E. "Clinical Practice as a Function of Nursing
       Education: An Historical Analysis," NURS OUTLOOK 28(8)
       (August 1980): 493-97.

       Current concern for faculty to maintain clinical skills
       by on-going practice prompts a historical account of such
       practice. Prior to World War II nursing service personnel
       provided for the teaching needs of students. Problems with
       this practice led to the separation of service and faculty
       functions. Reinstating the dual role will undoubtedly create
       similar problems as previously encountered. (17)

1244 Collison, C.R. and M.A. Parsons. "Is Practice A Viable Faculty Role?," NURS OUTLOOK 28(11) (November 1980): 677-79.

A variety of options are proposed for faculty to engage in clinical practice. One option might be to acknowledge a faculty member's ultimate responsibility for care rendered by students under their clinical supervision as representing a practice component. Administrative support for faculty practice is critical to a workable arrangement. (10)

1245 Dickens, M.R. "Faculty Practice and Social Support," NURS LEADERSH 6(4) (December 1983): 121-28.

Several methods for faculty practice are available. These include: joint appointment, dual appointment, moonlighting, group practice, private practice, and university operated nursing clinics. Support needs include: informational, emotional, instrumental, and appraisal. A survey of 74 schools in the southeast revealed that approximately one-third of the faculty were practicing mostly during summers, recesses, and weekends. There was little indication of institutional support found in the survey sample. (28)

1246 Fasano, N. "Joint Appointments: Challenge for Nursing," NURS FORUM 20(1) (1981): 72-85.

Supports the need for joint appointment and presents rationale for involving faculty members in clinical practice. Four models are proposed and include: nurse preceptor, nurse administrator, nurse clinician, and faculty practitioner. (16)

1247 Hollshwander, C.H., D. Kinsey and M. Paradowski. "Teacher-Practitioner-Researcher," NURS HEALTH CARE 5(3) (March 1984): 144-49.

A report on the planning, development and implementation of a joint practice program initiated by two Pennsylvania colleges. (21)

1248 Holm, K. "Faculty Practice--Noble Intentions Gone Awry?," NURS OUTLOOK 29(11) (November 1981): 655-57.

The author describes the satisfactions and frustrations which occur when faculty assume dual roles. Pride in clinical expertise and credibility as a practitioner are offset by overwork and inadequate release time. Financial rewards should accompany the heavier workload. (3)

1249 Kuhn, J.K. "An Experience with a Joint Appointment," AM J NURS 82(10) (October 1982): 1570-71.

A nurse faculty member discusses her experiences with joint
appointment. Working one day a week at the hospital where she
had students helped increase professional confidence, student
respect, and staff collegiality. Problems encountered in
joint appointment are identified and strategies for resolution
proposed. (1)

1250 Langford, T.L. "Faculty Could Practice If--And Other Myths,"
      NURS HEALTH CARE 4 (November 1983): 515-17.

      Author argues that many of the reasons faculty members give
      for avoiding clinical practice are myths. Eight myths are
      presented with strategies for rebutting them or changing the
      situation. (0)

1251 MacPhail, J. "Collaboration/Unification Models for Nursing
      Eduction and Nursing Service." THE NURSING PROFESSION: A
      TIME TO SPEAK. Edited by N.L. Chaska. New York: McGraw-
      Hill Book Co., 1983, pp. 637-49.

      The need for faculty practice is defended. The three major
      examples of collaboration/unification models are: Case
      Western Reserve, Rush University, and the University of
      Rochester. Similar approaches are needed to assure quality
      in education and practice. (16)

1252 Mauksch, I.G. "Faculty Practice: A Professional Imperative,"
      NURSE EDUC 5(3) (May/June 1980): 21-24.

      Faculty practice is a vital component of the nursing role
      as nurses assume increasing responsibilities within the health
      care delivery system. Identifies practice in other profes-
      sional roles and considers conditions that led to separation
      of teaching and practice within nursing. Total preoccupation
      with acceptance and respect within academia led nursing to
      neglect the practice role. Practice should be meshed with
      clinical teaching and some of the clinical teaching should
      be delegated to clinical personnel. (5)

1253 McCarthy, P.A. "Will Faculty Practice Make Perfect?," NURS
      OUTLOOK 29(3) (March 1981): 163.

      Demands for faculty to devote time to clinical practice
      places yet another burden on this overworked and underpaid
      professional group. This latest requirement is a rational-
      ization of a quest for perfection which has always been
      present in nursing. (0)

1254 Mills, B.B. and T.A. Free. "Nursing Practice," PED NURS
      10(3) (May/June 1984): 212-14.

      A model of faculty practice with practical suggestions. (4)

1255   Ossler, C.C., M.E. Goodwin, M. Mariani and C.L. Gilliss.
       "Establishment of a Nursing Clinic for Faculty and Student
       Clinical Practice," NURS OUTLOOK 30(7) (July/August 1982):
       402-5.

       Faculty at the Catholic University of America set up a
       nursing clinic in order to provide community health experiences
       to students. They found the clinic of benefit to faculty,
       students, and clients and plans for expansion are underway.
       (0)

1256   "Primary Care Faculty Fellows Say Practice of New Skills Is
       Limited," AM J NURS 79(8) (August 1979): 1368.

       Nurse faculty prepared as primary care nurse practitioners
       perceive difficulties in assuming positions which will utilize
       their skills on return to their respective schools of nursing.
       (0)

1257   "RWJ Fellowships Aim to Promote Faculty Practice," AM J NURS
       82(11) (November 1982): 1676, 1680.

       Nine clinical scholars fellowships are being offered which
       seek to prepare doctorally prepared registered nurses for
       more effective clinical teaching, practice, and research.
       Candidates will participate in clinical care and research at
       the University of California at San Francisco, the University
       of Pennsylvania, or the University of Rochester for a two
       year period and receive stipends equal to their current
       salary. (0)

1258   Sherman, J.E. "Role Modeling for FNP Students," NURS OUTLOOK
       28(1) (January 1980): 40-42.

       Although the joint appointment of practitioner faculty to
       a practice setting has its advantages, it is fraught with
       problems that involve faculty, students, patients, and ad-
       ministrative networks in college, clinic, and medicine. (8)

1259   Smith, G.R. "Compensating Faculty for Their Clinical
       Practice," NURS OUTLOOK 28(11) (November 1980): 673-76.

       Nursing education can benefit from examining faculty
       practice plans used in medical schools. A time plan can be
       used to develop a feasible structure prior to initiation.
       The plan should accommodate various specialty areas in a
       variety of practice settings. (4)

1260   _____. "Faculty Practice Plans: Latent Obstacles to
       Success." CURRENT ISSUES IN NURSING. Edited by J.C.
       McCloskey and H.K. Grace. Scranton, PA.: Blackwell
       Scientific Publications, 1981, pp. 551-57.

The success of a faculty practice plan depends upon the numbers of faculty who subsequently engage in practice. Barriers to practice include mythologies of academic nursing, priorities, commitments, legitimacy, institutional arrangements and financial incentives. Practice must be defined by faculty and be broad enough to fit a variety of practice areas.(10)

1261 Sorenson, G., A. Gassman and M. Walters. "An Experiment in a Working Relationship Between Nursing Education and Nursing Service," J NURS EDUC 23(2) (February 1984): 81-83.

A cooperative nursing service-nursing education project was undertaken between a Veterans Administration Medical Center and a College of Nursing and sought to provide for more involvement of faculty and students in nursing service and more participation of hospital nursing staff in the education of students. Strengths and weaknesses within such an approach are explored. (0)

1262 Spilotro, S. "A Unified Role for Nursing," NURS ADM Q 3(3) (Spring 1979): 21-25.

Describes the successful implementation of a unification model at Rush-Presbyterian-St. Luke's Medical Center. Practitioners/teachers assume responsibilities within university and service settings and participate in the committee activities of both. One hundred and fifty faculty are currently practicing this role within Rush and provide a unified role for nursing which encompasses service, education, research, and consultation. Research is optional for the Rush faculty, however, the other three components are required. (0)

1263 Wahlquist, G.I., K.R. Flynn and P.T. Horvath. "Clinical Practice and the Graduate Nursing Faculty," J NURS EDUC 22(9) (November 1983): 394-96.

Yale University School of Nursing has since its inception legitimized faculty practice. All faculty hold a triple commitment to teaching, practice, and research. Logistics of planning and implementing such a model are discussed. (7)

1264 Wakefield-Fisher, M. "The Issue: Faculty Practice," J NURS EDUC 22(5) (May 1983): 207-10.

Pros and cons of faculty practice are explored in terms of realistic expectations and the benefits to service and education. Role strain and role overload are discussed. Methods to facilitate the implementation of faculty practice are suggested. Research is necessary to determine if this issue is a step forward or backward for the profession of nursing. (29)

See 966, 970, 973, 1188.

Graduates

1265   Alhadeff, G. "Anxiety in a New Graduate," AM J NURS 79(4)
       (April 1979): 687-88.

       A new graduate recounts her anxiety and approaches to
       establishing confidence in her professional role. (0)

1266   Balint, J., K. Menninger and M. Hurt. "Job Opportunities for
       Master's Prepared Nurses," NURS OUTLOOK 31(2) (March/April
       1983): 109-14.

       Most nurses undertaking graduate study major in the clinical
       specialist area. A survey of advertised positions for
       master's prepared nurses over a three year period revealed
       greater opportunities in teaching and administration. The
       number of nurses prepared as clinical specialists far out-
       number the positions available. (14)

1267   "Board Okays Temporary Permits for Foreign Educated Nurses in
       California," AM J NURS 80(7) (July 1980): 1243.

       Nurses licensed in foreign countries will be able to work
       with temporary permits in the State of California. These
       permits previously only available to graduates awaiting State
       Board test scores will be valid until the next exam for per-
       manent licensure. This action was prompted by a 20 percent
       shortage of nurses in the state. (0)

1268   Cantor, M.M., D.M. Schroeder and S.W. Kurth. "The Ex-
       perienced Nurse and the New Graduate: Do Their Learning
       Needs Differ?," NURSE EDUC 6(7) (December 1981): 17-22.

       A study of learning needs of graduates of various nursing
       programs revealed diversity within as well as among programs.
       Inconsistencies were noted in the kinds and amounts of
       clinical experiences afforded students. Adjustments in
       program content are recommended. (10)

1269   Castle, J. "That's Not The Way We Do Things Around Here,"
       AM J NURS 81(7) (July 1981): 1348.

       One person's reality shock. A new ADN graduate reports what
       happened. (0)

1270   Goldstein, J.O. "Comparison of Graduating AD and Bac-
       calaureate Nursing Students' Characteristics," NURS RES
       29(1) (January/February 1980): 46-49.

       Graduating seniors from five associate degree and five bac-
       alaureate programs were tested to determine differences in
       self-actualization as measured by the Personal Orientation
       Inventory. Baccalaureate students scored higher on all scales
       which was considered a positive attribute for leadership
       roles. (27)

1271 Howell, F. "Employers Evaluations of New Graduates," NURS
      OUTLOOK 26(7) (July 1978): 448-51.

      An associate degree nursing graduate conducted a state-wide
      survey of directors of nurses to identify perceptions of
      differences between AD, diploma and baccalaureate graduates
      by employers. The baccalaureate degree nurse was considered
      to function best in large institutions and education was
      important in advancement. In small institutions the diploma
      nurse was judged superior and advancement was determined by
      individual capability not education. Correlation was found
      between the education of the respondent and perceptions of
      superiority based on education. (0)

1272 Kramer, M. REALITY SHOCK: WHY NURSES LEAVE NURSING. St.
      Louis: C.V. Mosby, 1974.

      A report of eight years of study and research into the con-
      flicts experienced by new graduate nurses between their
      schooling and the expectations in the work place. A planned
      anticipatory socialization program is described which proposes
      strategies for smoothing transition from school to work.

1273 McCloskey, J.C. "Nursing Education and Job Effectiveness,"
      NURS RES 32(1) (1983): 53-58.

      The purpose of this study was to determine whether nurses
      from different educational preparation differ in job effec-
      tiveness. Head nurses rated 299 staff nurses on job effec-
      tiveness by comparing them to each other and to ideal, best
      and worst nurses. Years of schooling had a significant but
      small effect on job performance. (7)

1274 Meisenhelder, J.B. "The New Graduate Socialization," J
      CONTIN EDUC NURS 12(3) (1981): 16-22.

      Presents the theoretical basis, content, structure, and
      detailed guidelines for implementing an orientation program
      designed to facilitate conflict resolution and adjustment
      to a practice setting. (4)

1275 Munro, B.H. "Job Satisfaction Among Recent Graduates of
      Schools of Nursing," NURS RES 32(6) (November/December
      1983): 350-55.

      Responsibility defined as the importance and challenge of
      the work was found to be the strongest predictor of job satis-
      faction in 329 employed registered nurse gradutes of diploma,
      associate degree, and baccalaureate programs. Working con-
      ditions was found to be the second most important predictor.
      No significant differences were found based on program. (32)

1276 Murray, L.M. and D.R. Morris. "Professional Autonomy Among
      Senior Nursing Students in Diploma, Associate Degree, and
      Baccalaureate Nursing Programs," NURS RES 31(5) (September/
      October 1982): 311-13.

A questionnaire was administered to nurses at five institutions and to 206 nursing administrators to test dependence vs. independence. Nurses in community hospitals, who
were primarily diploma graduates, came out lowest on three
dimensions of dependence; nursing administrators highest. (7)

1277   "NY Revises Decision, Accepts July Exam Scores," AM J NURS
       79(12) (December 1979): 2067, 2080-81.

       A state police investigation into alleged cheating in New
       York State RN licensing exam revealed no evidence of miscon-
       duct. A decision to reject the test results was reversed. (0)

1278   Raker, L. "Treating Reality Shock," AM J NURS 79(4) (April
       1979): 688.

       A prescription for reality shock is paralleled to the treat-
       ment of physiological shock. (1)

1279   "Role and Competencies of Graduates of Diploma Programs in
       Nursing," NURS OUTLOOK 26(8) (August 1978): 520.

       Utilizes the nursing process to identify competencies of
       diploma program graduates. A revised statement prepared by
       the Council of Diploma Programs in Nursing of the National
       League for Nursing. (0)

1280   Rottkamp, B.C. "Survey of Nurse Attitudes Toward Profes-
       sional Nursing Practice," J NURS EDUC 19(5) (May 1980):
       32-38.

       A survey of graduate nurse students reactions to the New
       York State Nurse Practice Act found agreement in 96.5 percent
       of the sample. Differences were found between students
       majoring in education and those majoring in supervision
       and administration regarding impediments to professional
       nursing practice. (0)

1281   "SBTP Exam Bows Out: NCLEX Readied for July Candidates," AM
       J NURS 82(3) (March 1982): 366.

       A new licensure examination will be known as the NCLEX
       (National Council Licensure Examination) instead of the State
       Board Test Pool Examination (SBTP). The new exam will focus
       on application of knowledge and specific nursing behaviors.
       Questions will be categorized according to five steps: as-
       sessment, analysis, planning, implementing, and evaluating.
       The locus of decision-making in nurse, client and instances
       shared by nurse and client will be tested. (0)

1282   Sasmor, J.L. "Postdoctoral Blues," NURS OUTLOOK 27(11)
       (November 1979): 720-21.

New doctoral graduates experience symptoms of subacute grief
which results from the separation from the group status of
doctoral candidates. Recognizing the existence of the
problem, anticipatory and transition guidance can help reduce
this phenomena. (0)

1283   Schoen, D. "Predictors of Success for ADN Graduates," NURS
        LEADERSH 6(4) (December 1983): 104-12.

        Reports of study findings on fifty-five Associate Degree
        nurse graduates relative to the predictive ability of in-
        structor evaluations, length of time for program completion,
        grade point average and state board examination results on
        clinical competence two years after graduation. Only in-
        structor evaluations and length of time taken to complete
        the program were found predictive of future on the job suc-
        cess. (9)

1284   Snyder, D.J. "New Baccalaureate Graduates' Perceptions
        of Organizational Conflict," NURS RES 31(5) (September/
        October 1982): 300-5.

        Study explores process of professional socialization in
        a sample of newly graduated baccalaureate nurses whose
        first experience as practicing professionals was in a hospital
        organizational system. Professional socialization defined
        in terms of concept of identity.

1285   Soukup, M.C. "Reality Shock Alleviation: Student Experience
        in Preceptored Advanced Clinical Nursing Practicum."
        NURSING ISSUES AND NURSING STRATEGIES FOR THE EIGHTIES.
        Edited by B. Bullough, V. Bullough, and M.C. Soukup.
        New York: Springer Publishing Co., 1983, pp. 266-278.

        Reality shock is lessened by initiating students into the
        reality of nursing. Discusses a course entitled Advanced
        Clinical Nursing designed to do this. (7)

1286   Soules, H.M. "Professional Advancement and Salary Dif-
        ferentials Among Baccalaureate, Diploma, and Associate
        Degree Nurses," NURS FORUM 27(2) (1978): 184-201.

        A comparative study of opportunities for professional
        advancement and salary differentials for graduates of three
        basic nursing programs in sixteen San Francisco hospitals
        revealed that few baccalaureate nurses held head nurse or
        management positions. No salary differential was present
        based on education. Graduates from all three programs are
        filling the same positions, are promoted equally, and receive
        the same salary. (6)

1287   Vacek, P. and T. Ashikaga. "Educational Program Evaluation:
        The University of Vermont Family Nurse Practitioner
        Program," NURS RES 27(1) (January/February 1978): 36-41.

A study of graduates of a family nurse practitioner program
sought to compare the nursing activities performed by this
group with nurses practicing outside the specialty area.
Widespread differences were found. (12)

See 1265, 1278, 1460, 1800.

Programs

Associate Degree

1288 "Boston University Part of Project to Improve African Health
      Care," AM J NURS 79(3) (March 1979): 400.

      Describes the involvement of Boston University School of
      Nursing in developing curricula, continuing education and
      consultation to 10 central and western African nations which
      is a part of a larger effort to improve the delivery of
      health care services. (0)

1289 Fabayo, A.O. "Nursing and the Community College Movement,"
      NURS FORUM 19(2) (1980): 181-92.

      A review of the community college movement, the development
      of associate degree programs in nursing and the dilemmas these
      programs propose in terms of requiring a baccalaureate degree
      for entry into professional nursing practice. (19)

1290 Hilbert, G.K. "Experiences in a Weekend Program," NURS
      OUTLOOK 27(7) (July 1979): 476-78.

      A 32 month weekend associate degree nursing program offers
      an unique opportunity for a nursing education. Although some
      disadvantages have been noted in terms of quality and schedul-
      ing of clinical experiences, one community college has contin-
      ued the program for four years and find the advantages out-
      weigh the disadvantages. (3)

1291 "Kellogg-Funded Project Aims to Add Clinical Skills to ADN
      Curricula," AM J NURS 82(11) (November 1982): 1772.

      Grants totaling $6.5 million have been awarded by Kellogg
      to establish competencies of AD graduates, redesign curricula
      accordingly and prepare AD faculty at the master's degree
      level. Participating programs and regional groups are spread
      across the United States. (0)

1292 Maury-Hess, S., J. Crancer and M. Brester. "Textbook Selec-
      tion for Associate Degree Nursing Programs (An Evaluative
      Study)," J NURS EDUC 18(1) (January 1979): 11-16.

      In order to determine if there is a need to select text-
      books geared to associate degree nurses, a survey of
      associate degree programs was conducted. The coordinators/
      directors responses were mixed. Textbooks currently used
      demonstrated preference for one medical surgical and one

pediatric text. The Flesch Formula analysis demonstrated the medical surgical text had a higher readability level than the pediatric text. Higher satisfaction was reported with the lower readability text. (34)

1293   Montag, M. "Looking Back: Associate Degree Education in Perspective," NURS OUTLOOK 28(4) (April 1980): 248-50.

The goal of associate degree nursing education was to prepare technicians not professionals. Lengthening of programs, increasing clinical hours and incorporating leadership courses have served to dilute rather than strengthen associate degree programs. (5)

1294   _____. COMMUNITY COLLEGE EDUCATION FOR NURSING. New York: Blakiston Division, McGraw-Hill Book Co., 1959.

Final report of a five year study of the Cooperative Research Project in Junior and Community College Education for Nursing. Provides developmental and evaluative data from seven junior-community colleges and one hospital school of nursing that created nurse technician programs. (4)

1295   Montag, M. and R.L. McManus. THE EDUCATION OF NURSING TECHNICIANS. New York: G.P. Putnam's Sons, 1951.

Describes a plan for the education of nurse technicians and faculty to teach nurse technicians. The community college was recommended for nurse technician preparation because of its purpose, its location, and the variety of curricular offerings.

1296   "SREB In Final Stages of Implementing Projects Based on Curriculum Study," AM J NURS 79(3) (March 1979): 394.

Reports the award of $2.5 million in grants to schools of nursing in the Southern Regional Educational area for the development of RN completion programs, continuing education programs for faculty development, graduate programs, and associate degree programs. (0)

1297   Vaughn, J.C. "Educational Preparation for Nursing-1982," NURS HEALTH CARE 4 (October 1983): 460-64.

Update of nursing education statistics from the National League for Nursing annual survey of state approved schools of nursing in the 56 jurisdictions of the United States. Data on admissions, graduations, enrollments, school closings, new schools, and changes in existing schools are reported. (0)

1298   Whelan, E. "Increasing Clinical Proficiency: A Summer Clinical Course," NURSE EDUC 7(5) (Autumn 1982): 28-31.

A mini course offered at a community college sought to increase students clinical skills, improve their organization of
nursing care for groups of three to five patients and improve
use of the nursing process. Students who took this elective
summer course demonstrated improved clinical performance in
subsequent nursing courses. (10)

1299 Williamson, J.A. "Crisis in Academic Nursing." THE NURSING
      PROFESSION: A TIME TO SPEAK. Edited by N.L. Chaska. New
      York: McGraw-Hill Book Co., 1983, pp. 63-69.

      The time is ripe for realigning professional education.
      Changes in content and focus are proposed. Leadership within
      academic institutions and for the profession at large should
      be restricted to doctorally prepared nurses. Unless we move
      to solve the whole problem we will simply move from one crisis
      to another. (2)

      See 1339.

                              Baccalaureate

1300 Ackerman, A.M., K.B. Partridge and H. Kalmer. "Effective
      Integration of Health Education into Baccalaureate Nursing
      Curriculum" J NURS EDUC 20(2) (February 1981): 37-44.

      Provides a model for integrating appropriate content and
      processes within the baccalaureate curriculum which will
      prepare students for the role of health educator. (33)

1301 _____. "Health Education in Baccalaureate Nursing Cur-
      riculum: Myth or Reality?," J NURS EDUC 21(1) (January
      1982): 15-22.

      Teaching is an essential role of nursing. A survey of 200
      baccalaureate school catalogs revealed minimal attention to
      content and methods explicitly designed to meet this learning
      need. A lack of agreement on what was encompassed in
      health education and what expectations were appropriate for
      baccalaureate students was found. More attention needs to
      be directed toward assuring curricular content in this area.
      (5)

1302 Adams, D.E. "Agency Staff Facilitate Student Learning," NURS
      OUTLOOK 28(6) (June 1980): 382-85.

      Recounts experiences of a baccalaureate degree program in
      the creation of staff facilitator positions to strengthen
      community health experiences. It was felt that such a re-
      lationship assisted in bridging the gap between education
      and service. (0)

1303 Ames, S.A. "Primary Care in Baccalaureate Education--Some
      Thoughts From an Adult Health Perspective," J NURS EDUC
      23(3) (March 1984): 117-19.

Since some 90 percent of the population need ambulatory health services and only 10 percent require care in the acute care facilities, it is reasonable to prepare baccalaureate nursing students in primary care. Perhaps a two track approach, one in acute care and one in primary care, should be offered to teach generalist content. (2)

1304 Anderson, N.E. "The Use of The Seminar as a Teaching Technique with Senior Undergraduate Nursing Students," J NURS EDUC 19(2) (February 1980): 20-25.

Provides an exploration of the definition and usefulness of the seminar technique in undergraduate education. (12)

1305 Baker, C.M. and G.G. Mayer. "One Approach to Teaching Cultural Similarities and Differences," J NURS EDUC 21(4) (April 1982): 17-22.

Cultural background affects one's language, values, goals, perceptions and expectation of others. The need to understand cultural diversity in the health provider role was recognized and a course developed in a baccalaureate nursing program to teach the concept of culture and its application to professional nursing practice. Students prepared reports which reflected the values of one of four cultural groups. (1)

1306 Banks, J. "Use of a Day Care Center for Implementing Primary Prevention by a Basic Nursing Program," J NURS EDUC 22(2) (February 1983): 70-73.

The development and threading of primary care are presented as it was integrated into the baccalaureate nursing program at Howard University. Clinical experiences at a day care center provided an opportunity for students to apply primary care skills. (7)

1307 Barrett, J.E. "Values Clarification As A Teaching Strategy in Nursing," J NURS EDUC 17(2) (February 1978): 12-18.

A values clarification course was offered in a baccalaureate nursing program to present value conflict issues in an effective manner to promote student understanding of their feelings and values. Student participation and interaction were directed toward understanding values in the practice of nursing. (10)

1308 Brock, A.M. "Impact of a Management-Oriented Course on Knowledge and Leadership Skills Exhibited by Baccalaureate Nursing Students," NURS RES 27(4) (July/August 1978): 217-21.

An experimental one month management course was found to significantly increase the knowledge of leadership concepts and demonstration of leadership behaviors in the sample group. (12)

1309 Calkin, J.D. and M.W. Gulbrandsen. "Nursing Practice De-
      cisions in Emergencies: A Course and How It Was Designed,"
      J NURS EDUC 17(9) (November 1978): 30-37.

      Describes the planning process used to design a program to
      assist students in establishing priorities in the clinical
      settings and dealing with emergency and crisis care. This
      three credit course with an optional one credit laboratory
      experience is offered early in the junior year to foster early
      skill development. (19)

1310 Camooso, C., M. Greene, J. Hoffman, J. Leuner, C. Mattis,
      E. Ptaszynski, P. Reiley, S. Silver, M.E. Winfrey and J.
      Winland. "Preventive Health Practices of Generic Bacca-
      laureate Nursing Students," NURS RES 29(4) (July/August
      1980): 256-57.

      A questionnaire was administered to 530 generic nursing
      students to assess application of preventive health practice
      to their personal life. Findings indicated students did not
      internalize these concepts. Experiences with illness in the
      family and high GPA scores positively influenced attitudes
      toward health. (6)

1311 Clemen, S., D.G. Eigsti and S. McGuire. "The Extended Ex-
      perience: Operationalizing the Ideal," J NURS EDUC 17(9)
      (November 1978): 5-13.

      In order to prepare students for the realities of community
      health nursing, an extended experience elective was offered
      at the University of Michigan. Students selecting this as
      a concentrated area of study spent an additional half day in
      clinical for ten weeks in which they explored the larger area
      of community health services beyond home visits. (0)

1312 Cronin-Stubbs, D. and J.J. Mathews. "A Clinical Performance
      Evaluation Tool for a Process-oriented Nursing Curriculum,"
      NURSE EDUC 7(4) (July/August 1982): 24-29).

      A criterion-referenced evaluation tool was developed to
      provide consistency in evaluation across the junior and senior
      years of a baccalaureate curriculum. Examples are provided
      which utilize the nursing process as an organizing framework.
      Level of competency is determined for general critical objec-
      tives. (9)

1313 Culang, T.G., S.L. Josephson, M.T. Marcus and M.L. Vezina.
      "Implementation of a Campus Nursing and Health Information
      Center in the Baccalaureate Curriculum, Part II," J NURS
      EDUC 19(5) (May 1980): 11-14.

      The development of a nursing clinic facilitated faculty
      and students' identification with primary care and the role
      of nursing in health promotion and maintenance. Development,
      implementation, and evaluation of the clinic as a teaching
      resource are discussed. (0)

1314   Damen, J. "Implementation of a Campus Nursing Health Infor-
       mation Center in the Baccalaureate Curriculum, Part III,"
       J NURS EDUC 19(5) (May 1980): 15-19.

       An independent study project in conjunction with clinical
       experiences in a nursing clinic helped students develop a
       sense of self-confidence and importance in evaluating health
       care needs of a community. (10)

1315   Dear, M.R. and M.F. Keen. "Role Transition: A Practicum for
       Baccalaureate Nursing Students," J NURS EDUC 21(2) (February
       1982): 32-37.

       A seven week course was begun for senior nursing students
       at Johns Hopkins University in 1978 for the express purpose
       of promoting transition from student to graduate nurse role.
       Both theoretical and clinical components were included.
       Faculty and students rated this as a positive experience which
       increased self-esteem, confidence, and self-worth in meeting
       the challenges of staff nursing. (2)

1316   Denny, E.O. and J.A. Denny. "A Comparison of Mental Health
       Nursing Education in the United Kingdom and the Psychiatric
       Component of a Baccalaureate Program in the United States,"
       J NURS EDUC 18(1) (January 1979): 42-49.

       Differences in psychiatric programs for nurses in the United
       Kingdom and those in the United States include: the focus on
       specialization versus generalization, entrance requirements,
       length of clinical component, content and source of guide-
       lines for content. Different education and practice struc-
       tures are described and compared. (5)

1317   Derwinski, B., B. Gohsman, N. Sowan and R. Tombre. "Fostering
       the Research Attitude," J NURS EDUC 18(7) (September 1979):
       23-26.

       Quality patient care requires baccalaureate graduates who
       are committed to the benefits of research in nursing practice.
       The need to prepare these nurses within required course work
       is necessary. Faculty at Montana State University at Billings
       describe their approach to teaching a research course. (5)

1318   Donabedian, D. "Teaching Clinical Public Health Nursing in
       a Collaborative Medical Center-Nursing School Program," J
       NURS EDUC 18(8) (October 1979): 4-8.

       Lack of clinical placement opportunities in public health
       agencies led to the utilization of outpatient departments
       within a large university hospital. Students in a pilot
       project made home visits and assumed responsibility for five
       to seven patients under faculty supervision. (0)

1319   Everson, S.J. and A.R. Mealey. "Baccalaureate Nursing Students
       as Leaders in Geriatric Groups," J NURS EDUC 17(7) (Septem-
       ber 1978): 17-26.

       A geriatric setting was chosen to teach group dynamics and
       leadership to nursing students. What began as an unpleasant
       student experience turned into a very successful one in terms
       of attainment of learning objectives and development of
       positive attitudes toward the aged. (5)

1320   Feeley, E. and J. Tarr. "Alternative Leadership Experiences
       for Senior Students in an Acute Care Setting," J NURS EDUC
       18(2) (February 1979): 25-28.

       The use of peer leadership and leadership of junior students
       by senior students were found effective methods in helping
       the students develop their own leadership style. These
       methods were helpful in increasing self esteem and effective-
       ness as well as developing helping, guiding relationships
       within the leadership role. (6)

1321   Fouts, J. "A Survey of Obstetrical Teaching Strategies in
       Baccalaureate Schools of Nursing," J NURS EDUC 19(7) (Sep-
       tember1980): 18-26.

       A survey of baccalaureate nursing programs in the United
       States was conducted to determine obstetrical and gyneco-
       logical content and experiences. Most programs presented
       content in block fashion in the junior year and provided
       inpatient and outpatient experiences. (1)

1322   Graham, B. and C. Gleir. "Health Education: Are Nurses Really
       Prepared?," J NURS EDUC 19(8) (October 1980): 4-6.

       Describes a three course sequence designed to provide bacca-
       laureate nursing students with the knowledge and skills needed
       to teach health education. Too many programs assume that
       students can teach by virtue of their knowledge. Greater
       attention needs to be directed toward preparing nurses for
       this vital professional role. (3)

1323   Haukenes, E. and M. Mundt. "The Selection of Clinical
       Learning Experiences in the Nursing Curriculum," J NURS
       EDUC 22(9) (November 1983): 372-75.

       A model is proposed which provides for the purposeful and
       systematic selection of clinical learning experiences for
       baccalaureate nursing students. Three factors are proposed
       which will assist in making experiences responsive to the
       social context of nursing. These are the (1) nature of nur-
       sing as understood by the profession and given faculty, (2)
       health needs of populations in given societies, and (3) the
       nature of the educational environment. (7)

1324   Hawkins, J.W. "Selection of Clinical Agencies for Bacca-
       laureate Nursing Education," J NURS EDUC 19(8) (October
       1980): 7-17.

       A survey of faculty in 65 baccalaureate programs in the
       United States and Puerto Rico sought information on the
       characteristics of clinical agencies which are desireable
       for and those that are necessary for successful attainment
       of program objectives. Compromise was found in the selection
       of agencies for clinical learning. Faculty need to reexamine
       clinical placements to assure congruence in this vital aspect
       of nursing education. (6)

1325   Himmelberger, A.H., J. Vermillion, J.A. Beal, M. Edmonds,
       L. Glover, C. Kneut, and C. Peterson. "Curriculum Revision:
       Evaluation of Prerequisite Courses in a Baccalaureate
       Nursing Program," NURSE EDUC 7(6) (Winter 1982): 7-12.

       A committee at Boston University undertook the task of eval-
       uating prerequisite courses to the baccalaureate program.
       Changes in prerequisites are described. (6)

1326   Jeffers, J.M. and M.G. Christensen. "Using Simulation to
       Facilitate the Acquisition of Clinical Observational
       Skills," J NURS EDUC 18(6) (June 1979): 29-32.

       An approach was successfully used to facilitate the develop-
       ment of observational skills of senior nurses in a leadership
       course. A two hour class utilized simulated client situations
       in audiovisual presentations. Faculty identified a smoother
       transition and greater observational acuity following the
       presentation. Feedback was considered essential to use of
       the audiovisual approach. (10)

1327   "Johns Hopkins School to be Resuscitated," AM J NURS 83(5)
       (May 1984): 700.

       Johns Hopkins School of Nursing will be opened in Fall, 1984
       in conjunction with Johns Hopkins University and offer a
       Bachelor of Science in Nursing Degree program. (0)

1328   Kim, H.S. "Critical Contents of Research Process for an
       Undergraduate Nursing Curriculum," J NURS EDUC 23(2) (Feb-
       ruary 1984): 70-72.

       In 1972, NLN charged all types of nursing programs to
       provide educational opportunities for students to learn to
       interpret research, understand its methods and significances,
       assess its findings and adopt those of value. Problems have
       arisen among nurse educators in delineating the knowledge and
       skill competency level for baccalaureate education. A concep-
       tual typology is proposed to assist in this process. (5)

1329   Kjervik, D.K. "Influencing Sex Role Opinions of Undergradute
       Nursing Students," J NURS EDUC 18(8) (October 1979): 43-49.

A course was developed at the University of Minnesota School
of Nursing to provide an opportunity for students to examine
their own beliefs about sex role behaviors and explore change
strategies. (13)

1330 Leddy, S. "Is That New Baccalaureate Program Feasible? or
      Necessary?," NURS OUTLOOK 27(6) (June 1979): 406-10.

      Provides guidelines for establishing a baccalaureate program
      with emphasis on early planning and use of feasibility
      studies. (0)

1331 Merritt, S.L. "Learning Styles Preferences of Baccalaureate
      Nursing Students," NURS RES 32(6) (November/December 1983):
      367-72.

      A study of basic and RN learners found no differences in
      student preferences for learning attributable to age and pro-
      fessional employment experience using Kolb's Learning Style
      Inventory. Differences in preference between the two groups
      were found for the conditions and modes of learning as defined
      by the Canfield Model. (23)

1332 Olson, E.M. "Baccalaureate Students' Perceptions of Factors
      Assisting Knowledge Application in the Clinical Laboratory,"
      J NURS EDUC 22(1) (January 1983): 18-21.

      Students in this study perceived selected learning factors
      as contributing to transfer of learning from classroom to
      clinical laboratory. The implications for nursing education,
      nursing service, and nursing research are discussed. (20)

1333 Ostmoe, P.M., S.R. Powell, L.M. Roskoski and C.A. Watson.
      "Nursing Electives in a Baccalaureate Program," NURS OUTLOOK
      26(8) (August 1978): 508-12.

      A decision to offer nursing electives posed many unantici-
      pated problems. Concerns for philosophy, objectives, faculty
      needs and budget were reviewed after three semesters. A
      faculty forum was useful in problem solving. (11)

1334 Pardue, S.F. "Blocked-and Integrated-content Baccalaureate
      Nursing Programs: A Comparative Study," NURS RES 28(5)
      (September/October 1979): 305-11.

      A study of the differences in student performance in blocked
      and integrated curricula revealed no significant difference
      in critical thinking abilities of students in the two pro-
      gram types. Blocked content program students scored signifi-
      cantly higher on state board examinations. (56)

1335 Quiring, J.D. and G.T. Clay. "Is Baccalaureate Education
      Based on a Patchwork Curriculum?," NURS OUTLOOK 27(11)
      (November 1979): 708-13.

Fifty-three catalogs from baccalaureate curricula were examined. Diversity in terms of general education and science requirements were noted. Generally 43 percent of the course work was in nursing, although the organizational frameworks varied. One needs to question what the content needs are within the lower division course work before the upper division nursing content can be outlined. (6)

1336   Ramphal, M. "Rethinking Diploma School and Collegiate Education," NURS OUTLOOK 26(12) (December 1978): 768-71.

The ideal nursing educational program requires collaboration between service and practice. Many practices of the diploma school may well be appropriate today and educators should not overlook these aspects in designing baccalaureate programs. (0)

1337   Rinke, L.T. "Involving Undergraduates in Nursing Research," J NURS EDUC 18(6) (June 1979): 59-64.

A description of a research project designed and implemented by a group of senior baccalaureate nursing students in an elective research course is presented. (7)

1338   Ronald, J.S. "Computers and Undergraduate Nursing Education: A Report on an Experimental Introductory Course," J NURS EDUC 18(9) (November 1979): 4-9.

An elective course entitled "Implications of Computer Technology for Nursing," was taught at State University of New York at Buffalo to assist students to develop a basic understanding of the computer and explore applications to the health care delivery system. Marked changes were noted in students' attitudes toward the computer following the course. (20)

1339   Rosenkoetter, M. and M. McSweeney. "Perceptions of Nurse Educators Regarding ADN and BSN General Education," WEST J NURS RES 5(2) (Spring 1983): 165-77.

Report of a survey to determine whether AD and BS nursing education administrators perceive a difference in the importance of the non nursing, general education component of ADN and BSN programs. (18)

1340   Ruffing, M.A. "Community Health Nursing in an Urban Day Care Center," J NURS EDUC 18(8) (October 1979): 21-26.

Community health nursing practice has expanded to include a variety of distributive care settings. Use of infant-toddler day care centers at Ohio State University provided students the opportunity to learn primary care skills in preventive/ health maintenance settings. (6)

1341   Seigel, H. "Baccalaureate Education and Gerontology," J NURS EDUC 18(7) (September 1979): 4-6.

Explores the need for gerontology content and clinical
experiences in baccalaureate programs which foster positive
attitudes toward the aged and includes knowledge of the
elderly. (4)

1342   Shelton, B.J. "Research Components in Baccalaureate Programs
        of Nursing," J NURS EDUC 18(5) (May 1979): 22-33.

A study of NLN accredited baccalaureate nursing programs
assessed the extent to which nursing programs are offering
research course work. Variations were found between colleges
and universities and within geographic regions. (17)

1343   Shine, M.S., M.C. Silva and F.S. Weed. "Integrating Health
        Education into Baccalaureate Nursing Education," J NURS
        EDUC 22(1) (January 1983): 22-27.

A funded project at George Mason University provided for
the identification of health education competencies and content appropriate for baccalaureate nursing students. Thirty-
two health education competencies and eighteen health education content areas were identified. These were integrated
within the curriculum and leveled by year and course. (4)

1344   Spruck, M. "Teaching Research at the Undergraduate Level,"
        NURS RES 29(4) (July/August 1980): 257-59.

A survey of 286 NLN accredited baccalaureate nursing
programs found that 164 programs (62%) required a research
course. Of the 164 programs, 70 percent also required completion of a research project and 69 percent included
actual data collection. (9)

1345   Suess, L.R., B.J. Schweitzer and C.A. Williams. "Nursing
        Students Experiment with Reality," NURSE EDUC 7(2) (March/
        April 1982): 28-33.

Students at the University of Connecticut School of Nursing
engaged in an elective summer program designed to increase
competence in dealing with work experiences. Three area
hospitals were utilized during the summer between junior and
senior years. Reality shock was experienced as school values
conflicted with bureaucratic realities. (4)

1346   Swendsen, L.A. "Self Instruction: Benefits and Problems,"
        NURSE EDUC 6(6) (November 1981): 6-9.

Self instruction provides a means of educating nurses in
times of diminishing resources, expanding knowledge and increased diversity among students. A survey of NLN accredited
baccalaureate nursing schools found that faculty support self
instruction and find it frees faculty time. (2)

1347 Thomas, B. and M.M. Price. "Research Preparation in Bacca-
      laureate Nursing Education," NURS RES 29(4) (July/August
      1980): 259-61.

      A study of 205 NLN accredited baccalaureate nursing programs
      sought to clarify the level of research taught within under-
      graduate programs. Respondents indicated emphasis of consumer
      rather than participant role objectives. The more pro-
      fessionally oriented the faculty, the less support was found
      for participant role objectives. (5)

1348 Tollett, S.M. "Geriatric and Gerontology Nursing Curricular
      Trends," J NURS EDUC 21(6) (June 1982): 16-23.

      A study of 570 nursing students in 12 baccalaureate programs
      revealed that the amount of geriatric content in the cur-
      riculum was not related to students´ attitudes toward the
      elderly. Nursing curricula should focus on the stresses
      of aging and the consequent adaptations of the elderly in
      order to foster more positive attitudes toward this growing
      group of health consumers. Well aged clients as well as
      institutionalized individuals should be considered within
      clinical experiences. (11)

1349 VanBree, N.S. "Undergraduate Research," NURS OUTLOOK 29(1)
      (January 1981): 39-41.

      A course structured to foster positive attitudes of students
      toward research required student projects. These projects
      were of high quality and contributed to students becoming
      informed consumers of research, able to assess the value of
      research done by others, and apply the results when appro-
      priate. (8)

1350 Voight, J.W. "Physical Assessment Skills in the Curriculum:
      A Pilot Project and Follow-up," J NURS EDUC 19(2) (Feb-
      ruary 1980) : 26-30.

      In evaluating the suitability of introducing physical
      assessment content in the sophomore year of a baccalaureate
      nursing program, student feedback recommended that skills be
      taught when ready to be used and that opportunities for
      regular use and role modeling be provided. (0)

1351 Watson, J. "How To Select Clinical Agencies for Clinical
      Experiences in Baccalaureate Nursing Education," J NURS
      EDUC 18(2) (February 1979): 29-35.

      Characteristics of agencies should be examined in selecting
      clinical learning experiences which foster attainment of
      program objectives. General characteristics, standards of the
      agency, client care standards, adequacy of learning experience,
      position of nurses in the agency and physical facilities

allow faculty to seek out appropriate agencies and when necessary compromise with full information of necessary versus
desired characteristics. (19)

1352 Zettiniq, P. and N.M. Lang. "Utilization of Quality Assurance
      Concepts in Educational Evaluation," NURSE EDUC 6(4) (July/
      August 1981): 24-28.

      A course evaluation tool was developed for a senior level
      leadership course utilizing a quality assurance framework.
      The evaluation tool contained outcome, structure and process
      components and provided useful data for course revisions. (7)

BSN Completion

1353   "A Nursing 79 Guide: Where To Go To Get Your BSN
            Degree, Part I," NURS 79 9(11) (November 1979):
            79-86.

              Lists BSN degree programs by state. Explores
          common misconceptions of registered nurses re-
          garding the nature of BSN degree programs that cause
          academic shock. Describes what registered nurses
          can expect, guidelines for coping, and important
          questions that should be asked in selecting a pro-
          gram. (0)

1354   Alward, R.R. and S.B. Swanson. "A Student
            Leadership Experience for the Experienced
            RN," NURS OUTLOOK 28(8) (August 1980): 498-
            500.

              RN students in a baccalaureate completion
          program report on rewarding experience of
          assuming leadership responsibilities in con-
          ducting a senior citizens health fair. (6)

1355   Baldwin, S. "Yesterday and Today," J CONT EDUC
            NURS 9(2) (March/April 1978): 22-24.

              The personal experiences of a nurse who re-
          turned for a bachelor of science in nursing degree
          reveals that the elective courses were growth
          producing and helped to relieve the difficulties
          of returning to school. (3)

1356 Borgman, M.F. and C.L. Ostrow. "An Advanced Placement Program
      for Registered Nurses," J NURS EDUC 20(5) (May 1981): 2-6.

      An advanced placement program for registered nurses at West
      Virginia University considers recognition of need, conceptual
      framework, philosophy of teaching-learning and faculty-student
      collaboration in planning and evaluation to individualize
      instruction for this unique group of learners. (1)

1357 "Cal State Launches Off-Campus Program for the Working RN,"
      AM J NURS 82(6) (June 1982): 893, 904.

      An external degree baccalaureate program in nursing for
      working RNs was launched by the California State University
      Consortium. Supported by the Kellogg Foundation, this state-
      wide nursing program will utilize self-paced instruction,
      modules and other nontraditional learning options to increase
      accessibility for RNs seeking a bachelor's degree. The New
      York Regents External Degree Program may be used in total or
      in part to meet degree requirements. (0)

1358 Cowart, M.E. and J.M. Burge. "Evaluation by Jury," NURS
      OUTLOOK 27(5) (May 1979): 329-33.

      In an attempt to provide more flexibility for students to
      accelerate or move more slowly through a baccalaureate cur-
      riculum, a team of faculty formed a jury by which to assess
      attainment of competency in nursing courses. This method was
      found particularly effective with registered nurse students.
      (0)

1359 Dieterle, J.A. "Clinical Validation of Psychiatric Nursing
      Skills," J NURS EDUC 22(9) (November 1983): 392-94.

      Registered nurse graduates of diploma programs are unable
      to transfer nursing credits obtained in hospital programs.
      Knowledge of theory is measureable by a variety of instruments.
      Clinical applicability of this knowledge is more difficult to
      measure. A clinical evaluation procedure for validating
      psychiatric nursing skills was found effective at Purdue
      University. (0)

1360 Dobbie, B.J. and N. Karlinsky. "A Self-Directed Clinical
      Practicum," J NURS EDUC 21(9) (November 1982): 39-41.

      RN students in a baccalaureate nursing program are allowed
      to select clinical learning activities focusing on teaching-
      learning, management or clinical nursing practice. Collabora-
      tive planning between student, faculty and institutional per-
      sonnel allow for the planning of individualized experiences.
      (3)

1361   Durham, J.D. "Assessing Nurses´ Prior Learning: Nursing Edu-
       cation´s Challenge of the 80´s." CURRENT ISSUES IN NURSING.
       Edited by J. McCloskey and H. Grace. Scranton, PA: Black-
       well Scientific Publications, 1981, pp. 207-17.

       A variety of methods for assessing experiential learning
       are discussed and applied to nursing programs for registered
       nurse students. Contrary to the beliefs of many nurse educa-
       tors, these assessment tools are more valid than teacher-made
       tests and subjective measurement methods currently utilized to
       grant advanced standing. (29)

1362   Erickson, H. "Coping With New Systems," J NURS EDUC 22(3)
       (March 1983): 132-35.

       A course was designed to facilitate registered nurse stu-
       dents in adapting to growth producing changes within a bacca-
       laureate completion program. (15)

1363   Fritz, E.L., K. Kisker and I. Ladson. "Computer Exams for
       RNs," AM J NURS 81(11) (November 1981): 2057.

       Computer based simulations are used at Ohio State University
       to measure clinical decision-making skills. These simulations
       allow RN students to complete the program more quickly. Other
       instructional alternatives for RN students are described. (0)

1364   Galliford, S. "Second Step Baccalaureate Programs in Nursing,"
       NURS OUTLOOK 28(10) (October 1980): 631-35.

       A survey of 442 BSN programs revealed that 318 offer some
       type of advanced placement and/or testing options for RNs. In
       addition, 146 offer second step BSN programs of which 51 per-
       cent are NLN accredited. A listing of the 146 second step
       programs are given by state. (8)

1365   Garvey, J. "An Alternative Baccalaureate Curriculum Plan for
       RNs," J NURS EDUC 22 (May 1983): 216-19.

       Eighty percent of the professional nursing membership is
       prepared below the baccalaureate degree. A need exists to
       design B.S.programs that address their unique needs. An
       alternative curriculum requires identification of content and
       skills within existing generic programs that are common to all
       nursing programs as well as content and skills unique to bac-
       calaureate education. A pretest is suggested to establish
       differences in competencies on entrance and a post test to
       assure similarity of learning outcomes on completion of
       an alternative program. (7)

1366   _____. "Individualization of Instruction for RN Students
       Articulating Into BS(N) Degree Programs." Ed.D. Disserta-
       tion. Ann Arbor: University Press, 1979.

A survey of seven colleges and universities from the Northeastern area is reported. Philosophical acceptance of individualization of instruction was greater than practical application. While a few schools offered considerable variety of
method there was a general lack of learner involvement in
program planning, selection of learning experiences, faculty-
student collaboration, choice of method of evaluation and
pace. This left the schools highly structured and they
stressed competencies to a greater extent than the adaptation
of learning experiences to the needs and interests of the
learner. (102)

1367 Garvey, J., P. Castiglia and B. Bullough. "Models for the
      Baccalaureate Education of Registered Nurses." NURSING
      ISSUES AND NURSING STRATEGIES FOR THE EIGHTIES. Edited by
      B. Bullough, V. Bullough, and M.C. Soukup. New York:
      Springer Publishing Co., 1983, pp. 254-66.

      Three major models exist for registered nurse education.
      All use generic terminal objectives but vary in the process
      by which these objectives are obtained: (1) a generic bacca-
      laureate pattern uses the four year baccalaureate program as
      the model; (2) a direct articulation model uses the career
      ladder pattern in which candidates cycle through nursing know-
      ledge and skills more than once;and (3) an assessment model
      uses tests rather than course work as a basis for granting.

1368 Gross, L.C. and C.W. Bevil. "The Use of Testing to Modify
      Curricula for RNs," NURS OUTLOOK 29(9) (September 1981):
      541-45.

      Delineation of content for RNs within a generic nursing
      curriculum was followed by development of testing measures
      (with paper and pencil and performance) to assure program
      needs. Item analysis provided feedback to additional needs
      for content. (5)

1369 Hale, S.L. and B.T. Boyd. "Accommodating RN Students in Bac-
      calaureate Nursing Programs," NURS OUTLOOK 29(9) (September
      1981): 535-40.

      A project co-sponsored by George Mason University Depar-
      tment of Nursing and the Southern Regional Education Board of
      Nursing Curriculum Project utilized several one-week workshops
      to discuss learning needs and desires of RN students in bac-
      calaureate completion programs. A problem-solving approach
      was used to address issues which included admission, advanced
      placement, faculty attitudes, learner needs, and curriculum
      sequencing. Internal and external factors which influence cur-
      ricular design were explored. (7)

1370 Higgins, P.G. and K.M. Wolfarth. AM J NURS 81(11) (November
      1981): 2062-63.

RN students returning for the baccalaureate degree experience a form of reality shock. Strategies which made schooling
a positive experience are described and guidelines proposed
for RNs encountering similar anxieties. (3)

1371   Hillsmith, K.E.   "From RN to BSN: Student Perceptions," NURS
       OUTLOOK 26(2) (February 1978): 98-102.

       A survey of 76 RNs in BSN completion programs revealed re-
       jection of the technical/professional levels of nursing prac-
       tice, resentment of the ANA proposal, denial and anger toward
       further schooling. A baccalaureate degree is today what
       a high school diploma was years ago. It is therefore reason-
       able to require this as a minimum credential if nurses are to
       be regarded as professional. (5)

1372   Hoffman, S. and M.J. Madden.   "You Can Get There From Here,"
       J NURS EDUC 17(2) (February 1978): 28-31.

       Accommodation of registered nurse students in the Univer-
       sity of Minnesota School of Nursing was promoted through
       structural changes rather than curricular changes. A relevant,
       flexible and challenging program was created. (2)

1373   Luther, D.C. and M.J. Wolfe.   "Toward a Partnership in Learn-
       ing," NURS OUTLOOK 28(12) (December 1980): 745-50.

       A learning history guide was developed to foster students
       involvement in formulating their own plans for learning.
       Identification of learning needs and patterns of learning
       assisted in improvement of teaching and the learning environ-
       ment. (8)

1374   McBride, H.   "Flexible Process-An Alternative Curriculum
       Option: Part III," J NURS EDUC 18(9) (November 1979): 20-25.

       Part III of a three part series discusses the development
       and implementation of clinical evaluation within a flexible
       process nursing program for registered nurses at the Univer-
       sity of Texas School of Nursing at San Antonio. (3)

1375   McGrath, B.J. and T.J. Bacon.   "Baccalaureate Nursing Educa-
       tion for the R.N.: Why Is It So Scarce?," J NURS EDUC
       18(6) (June 1979): 40-45.

       Problems encountered by registered nurses seeking baccalaur-
       eate education in North Carolina are explored and the need
       for outreach programs with flexible time frames proposed.
       (17)

1376   Mooneyhan, E.L.   "The Demise of a Baccalaureate Program for
       Registered Nurses: Lessons Learned," NURS HEALTH CARE 4
       (April 1983): 192-97.

Retrospectively recounts problems encountered in a baccalaureate completion program that failed to receive NLN accreditation and proposes actions which may have prevented its
eventual closure. Provides guidelines for sound program
development. (7)

1377 Muzio, L.G. and J.P. Ohashi. "The RN Student--Unique Charac-
      teristics, Unique Needs," NURS OUTLOOK 27(8) (August 1979):
      528-32.

Identifies characteristics of RNs returning for the baccalaureate degree which requires alterations in the structure
and processes of current baccalaureate education to design
programs to fit the RNs rather than shaping RNs to fit the
program. Characteristics of adult learners include: experiential knowledge rather than knowledge attained through
sequenced logical thinking; difficulty verbalizing; need for
role change rather than role development; focus on problems
rather than subjects. Programs should be individualized and
shift focus from teaching and content to learning and process.
(25)

1378 Nayer, D.D. "BSN Doors Are Opening for RN Students," AM J
      NURS 81(11) (November 1981): 2056-64.

Describes various philosophical frameworks for baccalaureate
education for registered nurses either within a generic or
RN only program. A list of educational institutions offering
programs for registered nurses is provided by state. (7)

1379 Neuman, B. and M. Wyatt. "Prospects for Change: Some Evalu-
      ative Reflections From One Articulated Baccalaureate Pro-
      gram," J NURS EDUC 20(1) (January 1981): 40-46.

Describes a competency based baccalaureate program for
registered nurses at the Ohio University School of Nursing
which resocializes from the ministering role toward facilitating care, collaborating and coordinating. (11)

1380 Reed, F.C. "Education or Exploitation," AM J NURS 79(7)
      (July 1979): 1259-61.

A warning is in order for RNs seeking baccalaureate degrees.
An increase in poor quality programs is apparent and the best
route is recommended as the generic baccalaureate programs.
Characteristics of substandard, exploitative programs are provided to promote informed consumerism. (3)

1381 Reed, S.B. "Flexible Process--An Alternative Curriculum
      Option: Part I," J NURS EDUC 18(9) (November 1979): 10-14.

A flexible process plan at the University of Texas School of
Nursing at San Antonio offers registered nurse students a
sound curricular alternative. This first part of a three
part series describes the characteristics, planning and implementation of the program. (1)

1382   Schoffstall, C. and A. Marriner. "Assessing Need and Feasi-
       bility for an Outreach Baccalaureate Program for RNs," NURSE
       EDUC 7(2) (March/April 1982): 25-27.

       The process of conducting a feasibility study for an RN-BSN
       program at University of Colorado at Colorado Springs and an
       outreach program for RNs are described. Interest and demand
       for the program; assessment of credentials; availability of
       clinical, library and classroom facilities; and, determination
       of community support are determined. (0)

1383   Slaninka, S.C. "Baccalaureate Programs for RNs," AM J NURS
       79(6) (June 1979): 1095.

       A survey conducted by a coordinator of a new RN program
       revealed information about admission criteria, challenge
       exams, full and part time study and advanced standing prac-
       tices available for RN students in baccalaureate programs in
       the United States. Of 266 NLN accredited programs contacted,
       69 percent responded. The characteristics of this study
       sample are presented. (0)

1384   Tillotson, D.M. "Flexible Process—An Alternative Curriculum
       Option: Part II," J NURS EDUC 18(9) (November 1979): 14-19.

       Part II of a three part series describes a flexible process
       curriculum at the University of Texas School of Nursing at San
       Antonio. This part focuses on the development and implementa-
       tion of evaluation methods. (0)

1385   Van Meter, M. and J. Oberle. "A New Directory of BSN Prog-
       rams," RN (September 1983): 110, 111, 114, 116, 118, 120,
       122, 124, 125.

       Employment policies increasingly show preferences for bacca-
       laureate prepared nurses. More nurses are returning to
       schools and more schools are providing special programs for
       RN students. In three years the number of programs for AD and
       diploma graduates has risen from 48 to 304. A directory of
       these programs is given by state for the reader to begin
       screening schools. Nursing administrators and nursing direc-
       tors polled predicted by 1987 a good number of institutions
       will hire only BSN graduates. (0)

1386   Williams, R.M. "Teaching Employed RNs in BSN Programs," NURS
       HEALTH CARE 4(10) (December 1983): 573-75.

       Detailed description of methodology for using employment
       settings for clinical learning activities for registered nurse
       students. (5)

1387   Wu, R. "Granting Credit for Previous Learning," NURS OUTLOOK
       26(11) (November 1978): 707-12.

Traces the development of articulation of RNs into California State University at Los Angeles School of Nursing baccalaureate completion program from previously used blanket
credit and challenge examinations to currently used advanced
placement mechanisms. (4)

Career Mobility,

1388 American Nurses' Association. CAREER LADDERS; AN APPROACH TO
      PROFESSIONAL PRODUCTIVITY AND JOBS SATISFACTION. Kansas
      City, MO.: American Nurses' Association, Pub. NO. NS-27,
      1984.

      Resource for those charged with initiating and implementing
      career ladder programs within an organization. Provides the
      basis for defining a relationship that incorporates the in-
      dividual nurse's career objectives into the overall organi-
      zational goals, while simultaneously enhancing quality of
      patient care delivery.

1389 Bullough, B. "The Associate Degree: Beginning or End?."
      NURSING ISSUES AND NURSING STRATEGIES FOR THE EIGHTIES.
      Edited by B. Bullough, V. Bullough and M.C. Soukup. New
      York: Springer Publishing Co., 1983, pp. 225-34. Also in
      NURS OUTLOOK 27 (May 1979): 324-28.

      Associate degree programs are growing in number and although
      originally conceptualized as a terminal educational option
      they are in reality a career ladder option. Students in ADN
      programs plan to continue their education following gradua-
      tion. Testing of technically and professionally prepared
      nurses using the Care-Cure Scale did not produce a dichotomy
      based on educational preparation. (22)

1390 Bullough, B. and C. Sparks. "Baccalaureate vs. Associate
      Degree Nurses: The Care-Cure Dichotomy," NURS OUTLOOK 23
      (November 1975): 688-92. Reprinted in EXPANDING HORIZONS
      FOR NURSES. Edited by B. Bullough and V. Bullough. New
      York: Springer Publishing Co., 1977, pp. 257-65.

      Questions whether the conception of care vs. cure justifi-
      cation for community college vs. baccalaureate programs is
      valid based on interview study of directors and graduates.
      (17)

1391 Slavinsky, A.T. and D. Diers. "Nursing Education for College
      Graduates," NURS OUTLOOK 30(5) (May 1982): 292-97.

      Programs that prepare college students in basic and special-
      ized nursing are not new. Variety within current programs is
      discussed and frequently found misconceptions clarified. (6)

1392   Styles, M.M. and H.S. Wilson "The Third Resolution," NURS
       OUTLOOK 27(1) (January 1979): 44-47.

       The ANA supports increased accessibility to high quality
       career mobility programs which use flexible approaches in
       academic degree programs in nursing. The School of Nursing of
       the University of California at San Francisco moved to act on
       this resolution through the development of an AD to MS program.
       (8)

                              Continuing Education

1393   Abruzzese, R.S. "Budgeting for Continuing Education Depart-
       ments," J NY STATE NURS ASSOC 10 (2) (June 1979): 24-27.

       Inservice educators have in recent years become increasingly
       responsible for budgeting. Personnel costs, capital expen-
       ditures and supplies are typical budget breakdowns. Knowledge
       of institutional policies regarding expenditures within these
       areas is necessary for the role of inservice director. (5)

1394   Arney, W.R. "Evaluation of a Continuing Education Program
       and Its Implications," J CONT EDUC NURS 9(1) (January/Feb-
       ruary 1978): 45-51.

       An example is provided of an evaluation of a continuing
       education program using pretest/posttests and participant
       evaluation. Implications and application of study results
       are discussed. (4)

1395   Aroian, J., J. Cloutterbuck, J. Gilbert, M. Newton and P.S.
       Williams. "Renewal--A Positive Outcome of Faculty Evaluat-
       ing," NURSE EDUC 7(1) (January/February 1982): 33-36.

       A positive systematic plan is described which provided eval-
       uation of personal and professional development of nursing
       faculty. Self, student, peer and administrative input was
       utilized in assessing, developing, and enriching faculty
       development. (10)

1396   Belock, S. "Preparing a Reentry Program for Inactive RNs,"
       J NURS EDUC 22(4) (April 1983): 165-70.

       Describes the preparation, implementation, and evaluation
       of an individualized, self-paced study designed to prepare
       inactive registered nurses to return to active practice.
       The impetus for this program was a State Board of Nursing
       mandate (Vermont) which required that nurses who had been
       inactive for five or more years update their knowledge and
       skills to minimum level of competency commensurate with that
       of newly graduated nurses. (15)

1397   Benner, P. and J. Wruhel. "Skilled Clinical Knowledge: The
        Value of Perceptual Awareness," NURSE EDUC 7(3) (May/June
        1982): 11-17.

        Experience is more than the passage of time but the trans-
        formations gained through examination of preconceived notions
        or theories to practical situations. A systematic program
        for clinical knowledge development is necessary to increase
        job satisfaction and retention of experienced nurses. (16)

1398   Binger, J.L. "Perceived Learning Needs and Resources of
        Undergraduate and Diploma Program Directors," J NURS EDUC
        18(6) (June 1979): 3-5.

        A survey of program directors of associate, baccalaureate,
        and diploma nursing programs in eight Western states iden-
        tified learning needs in the areas of making decisions, main-
        taining a budget, grievance procedures, professional writing
        skills and writing for publication. Preferred methods of
        attending to learning deficiences were identified as continuing
        education workshops and the nursing literature. (0)

1399   Bomberger, A.S. and C.J. Kern. "MIC: A Self-Directed Learning
        Method for Nursing Staff," NURSE EDUC 7(4) (July/August
        1982): 30-31.

        A Mobile Inservice Cart was utilized to provide self-directed
        learning to hospital staff. Several factors contributed to
        the success of this project. Initially it was necessary to
        "sell" the new approach. The cart was announced by flier
        prior to its arrival and reintroduced to the staff on arrival.
        Location and length of time the carts were on the unit
        effective in introducing new knowledge, techniques and equip-
        ment. (3)

1400   Borovies, D.L. and N.A. Newman. "Graduate Nurse Transition
        Program," AM J NURS 81(10) (October 1981): 1832-35.

        A description of a six month practical guided experience
        for beginning staff in intensive care offered in Northern
        Virginia. Contains a 1:2 ratio of classroom to clinical prac-
        tice. Objectives from two modules are presented as well as
        a sample of the assessment tool. (6)

1401   Boyar-Naito, V. and C.M. O'Keefe. "An Experiment in Nursing
        Education Via Satellite," J NURS EDUC 18(5) (May 1979):
        59-64.

        PEACESAT (Pan Pacific Education and Communications by
        Satellite) offered a continuing education program in basic
        leadership skills to nurses in America Samoa via satellite.
        Regularly scheduled classes were followed by evaluation and
        two-way dialogue. The course was well received and nurses
        expressed interest in additional coursework. (0)

1402 Boyer, C.M. "Performance-Based Staff Development: The Cost-
      Effective Alternative," NURSE EDUC 6(5) (September/October
      1981): 12-15.

      A performance based staff development program provided a
      comprehensive approach to orientation, inservice, intensive
      care training and leadership development at Columbia Presby-
      terian Hospital. Learning contracts, self-learning packages,
      coaching and group interactions were the primary methods of
      instruction. This approach was judged cost effective and
      freed faculty from classroom activities. (10)

1403 _____. "The Answer Doesn't Always Come Prepackaged,"
      NURSE EDUC 3(2) (March/April 1978): 17-18.

      An instance of inappropriate inservice education is des-
      cribed in which failure to effectively use the expertise of
      the inservice educator led to anineffective learning program.
      The need for communication between administrator and nursing
      service educator is critical to effective teaching. Guide-
      lines are provided to assist the inservice educator in working
      with management. (5)

1404 Brykczynski, K., W.S. Hayes, L.D. Waters, et al. "Nursing
      Faculty Develop Primary Care Skills," NURS HEALTH CARE 2(10)
      (December 1981): 538-42.

      A faculty development in primary care project was undertaken
      by the Southern Regional Educational Board. The project en-
      tailed two three week summer sessions and a year of precepted
      practice with the goal of preparing faculty with basic concepts
      and skills in primary health care and the subsequent inte-
      gration of these skills into baccalaureate nursing programs.
      Twenty-three baccalaureate nurse faculty from eleven colleges
      and universities participated. The authors share the accom-
      plishments and frustrations of participating as students in
      this program. (2)

1405 Bush, T.A. and C.W. Lewis. "Continuing Education for Nurses:
      Perceptions and Performances," J CONT EDUC NURS 9(2) (March/
      April 1978): 10-13.

      A study of practicing nurses within three hospitals in
      central Illinois found the perceived need for voluntary con-
      tinuing education was overwhelming (92%). Slight variations
      were found in support based on age and basic nursing education
      program. (2)

1406 Butters, S., V. Feeg, K. Harmon and A. Settle. "Computerized
      Patient Care Data: An Educational Program for Nurses," NURSE
      EDUC 7(2) (March/April 1982): 11-16.

An educational program was designed to provide a full understanding of the capabilities of a computer system and competence in operating the terminals and printers in one institution which was converting to a computerized information system. Lesson plans for nursing department integration are
provided. (7)

1407 "CE Now Required for Licensure in 16 States," AM J NURS 82(11)
      (November 1982): 1668, 1675.

      Sixteen state boards of nursing require some or all of the
      registered nurses to fulfill a specified number of continuing
      education hours to qualify for relicensure. In 11 states con-
      tinued education is necessary for all registered nurses where-
      as in five states continued education is mandatory for nurse
      practitioners only. The provisions for valid content and home
      study vary from state to state. (0)

1408 "California Loses Two Key Academic Providers of CE," AM J NURS
      82(6) (June 1982): 910, 913.

      Decreasing enrollments and an ailing economy prompted the
      University of California at San Francisco and the Davis Campus
      to suspend offering continuing education to the nurses in Cali-
      fornia. Competition for staffing and mandatory continuing
      education requirements have encouraged hospitals to increase
      inservice offerings and private providers to sponsor courses.
      The quality and applicability to professional practice with-
      in these programs are questionable. (0)

1409 Carozza, V., J. Congdon and J. Watson. "An Experimental Edu-
      cationally Sponsored Pilot Internship Program," J NURS EDUC
      17(9) (November 1978): 14-20.

      In response to identified serious inadequacies in the
      clinical performance skills of new graduates, an internship
      program was developed at the University of Colorado. An eval-
      uation of the program identified positive and negative factors.
      (9)

1410 Clements, I.W. and P.L. Hayes. "Collective Bargaining Dilemma
      for Nurse Educators," NURSE EDUC 6(7) (December 1981): 13-16.

      An understanding of collective bargaining and the three
      major bargaining agents within higher education is necessary
      in order that nurse faculty may assume an active role in the
      governance of academic institutions. (34)

1411 Collins, M.B. "Continuing Education/Continuing Practice,"
      NURSE EDUC 6(5) (September/October 1981): 32-33.

      Continuing education for nurse educators and those in leader-
      ship roles should include a practice component whereas con-
      tinuing education for practitioners should focus on theoretical
      knowledge. (3)

1412 "Colorado OKs Mandatory CE Regs," AM J NURS 82(6) (June 1982):
      903.

      Regulations for mandatory continuing education was approved
      by the Colorado State Board of Nursing. Problems have been
      encountered by nurses in rural areas in meeting the 20 contact
      hours required every two years for relicensure.(0)

1413 "Continuing Education to Become Mandatory in Massachusetts in
      1982 Under New Law," AM J NURS 78(2) (February 1978): 183,
      185.

      As of January 1, 1982 registered nurses and licensed prac-
      tical nurses will be required to maintain continuing education
      for relicensure in the State of Massachusetts. The specific
      number of hours required have not yet been established, how-
      ever, they will begin with not more than five clock hours for
      the first renewal period and gradually increase. (0)

1414 Cooper, S.S. "Continuing Education: Yesterday and Today,"
      NURSE EDUC 3(1) (January/February 1978): 25-29.

      An historical overview of continuing education for nurses
      provides insight into current concerns regarding organizational
      structure, voluntary versus mandatory requirements, the systems
      of accreditation and documentation and the proliferation of
      learning opportunities and innovative teaching methodologies.
      (19)

1415 Cooper, S.S. and J. Murphy. "Continuing Education About Al-
      coholism," J CONT EDUC NURS 9(2) (March/April 1978): 14-18.

      A continuing education program initiated at the University
      of Wisconsin-Extension provided emergency room personnel and
      others with a better understanding of the disease process
      of alcoholism and modes of treatment as well as an opportunity
      to assess one's feelings regarding alcoholism and alcoholics.
      (0)

1416 Cooper, S.S. "Teaching by Telephone," NURSE EDUC 4(1) (Jan-
      uary/February 1979): 10-13.

      The Wisconsin Educational Telephone Network utilizes a four
      wire telephone hookup with two-way audio communication.
      Nursing courses have been offered through teleconference since
      1966 and have been judged effective in providing continuing
      education to nurses across the State of Wisconsin. Tapes are
      available with a list of suggested readings and are mailed to
      nurses who request them. (8)

1417 Curran, C.L. and C.A. Lengacher. "RN Re-entry Programs: Pro-
      grammatic and Personal Considerations," NURSE EDUC 7(3)
      (May/June 1982): 29-32.

A refresher/re-entry program at the University of San Francisco prepared registered nurses for employment in an acute-
care setting. The learner needs and learning atmosphere were
selected based on knowledge of adult learners. Personal considerations included previous nursing experience, self-concept,
and role strain. As more older nurses are seeking employment,
well developed programs will contribute to personal and pro-
essional success. (9)

1418   Curran, C.L. and C.A. Smeltzer. "Collaboration Not Competi-
         tion" A Model for Nursing Continuing Education," J NURS
         EDUC 20(6) (June 1981): 24-29.

A joint educational committee which combines the efforts of
inservice education programs and continuing education programs
would reduce duplication of effort and cost. A description
of one such model is described. (1)

1419   Donovan, M., P. Wolpert and J. Yasko. "Gaps and Contracts,"
         NURS OUTLOOK 29(8) (August 1981): 468-71.

Reports on an attempt to improve learning outcomes of continuing education programs through a structural contract which
served to solve problems related to new learning within the
practice setting. Evaluation of learning through paper and
pencil tests, and impact on patient care were determined.
Follow-up between four and six months following the program
revealed 56 percent of the workshop participants reached or
were in the process of reaching their contract goals and 19
percent surpassed their contract goals. (2)

1420   Edelstein, R.R.G. and M. Bunnell. "Determinants of Continuing
         Education," J CONT EDUC NURS 9(1) (January/February 1978):
         19-24.

A survey of nurses in seven institutions sought information
regarding preferences in continuing education offerings.
The majority of nurses did not prefer participatory models.
Identified determinants were: the need to do prestigious or
socially rewarding work; interest in increasing one's broad
knowledge base; special needs related to employing institution; education perceived as work; difficulty in giving large
sections of time to study; preferences for different teaching
models; and presence of a nuclear element who prefer involvement and participation. (7)

1421   Edmunds, L. "Teaching Nurses to Use Computers," NURSE EDUC
         7(5) (Autumn 1982): 32-38.

An inservice education program provided hands on experience
for nurses to familiarize them with computerized information
systems. A training guide with corresponding computer visual-
ization is presented as well as a description of the program.
A training room was utilized prior to using terminals on the
patient units. (0)

1422 Eichhorn, E. "Continuing Education: Can It Be Legislated?,"
      NURS FORUM 20(1) (1981): 102-8.

      The practicality and rationale of mandatory continuing edu-
      cation for nurses are questioned. Legislation is not the
      mechanism by which to assure quality in practice. (12)

1423 Freeman, L.H. and P.F. Adams. "A Way to Provide Continuing
      Education," NURS HEALTH CARE 5(1) (January 1984): 34-36.

      In 1978, the Kentucky Nurse Practice Act mandated continuing
      education for relicensure. A recount of the development of a
      continuing education program at the University of Louisville
      School of Nursing considers contact hours, cost concerns,
      policy development, marketing, and program evaluation. (1)

1424 Gerber, R. "The Mini-Workshop," NURS OUTLOOK 28 (2) (February
      1980): 126-27.

      The use of one to two hour sessions for workshops proved
      convenient and effective in teaching faculty the use of audio-
      visuals for instructive purposes. Increased use and increased
      variety of equipment used demonstrated the effectiveness of
      the approach. (0)

1425 Goddard, H. "Mandatory Continuing Education: An Ongoing De-
      bate."   CURRENT ISSUES IN NURSING. Edited by J. McCloskey
      and H. Grace. Scranton, PA.: Blackwell Scientific Publi-
      cations, 1981, pp. 303-16.

      Relates progress and problems in implementing mandatory
      continuing education programs as a requirement for relicensure.
      (17)

1426 Graham, L.E. and J.L. Masters. "Nursing Continuing Education:
      California to Texas via Teleconference," J NURS EDUC 21(2)
      (February 1982): 45-47.

      Teleconferencing is being used to provide high quality con-
      tinuing education to staff nurses in many small hospitals
      scattered over hundreds of miles in Texas. The program has
      been in place since 1978 and allows presentations by well-
      known highly respected nurse educators for minimum cost and
      maximum efficiency and satisfaction. (0)

1427 Gress, L.D. and Sr. R.T. Bahr. "Continuing Education: Self-
      Actualization, Ethnicity and Aging," J CONT EDUC NURS 9(2)
      (March/April 1978): 5-9.

      A description of the content, methodology and mode of deli-
      very of a continuing education course delivered to eight rural
      sites across the State of Kansas. The course described con-
      siders unique needs of aging individuals peculiar to their
      ethnicity. (4)

1428 Haymes, H. "Running a CE Program: Administrative Strategies,"
      NURS OUTLOOK 28(3) (March 1980): 183-86.

      A detailed account of administrative strategies provides
      helpful advice as to the conduct of continuing education pro-
      grams. (0)

1429 Herron, Sr. C. "Assessment of Learning Needs in a Community
      Nursing Setting," J NY STATE NURSES ASSOC 10(2) (June 1979):
      20-23.

      Dramatic changes are occurring in community health nursing.
      Changes in clientele and their needs are associated with early
      hospital discharge. In determining learning needs of the
      community health nurse, one must assess the organizational
      needs at staff, supervisory and local office levels. Assess-
      ment followed by evaluation creates a continuous cycle for
      professional growth. (0)

1430 Hipps, O.S. "Faculty Development: Not Just a Bandwagon,"
      NURS OUTLOOK 26(11) (November 1978): 692-96.

      A variety of recommendations are proposed whereby nursing
      faculty may engage in personal and professional development
      in three required areas, namely: the academic discipline of
      nursing, the actual practice of nursing, and the teaching of
      both. (11)

1431 Holloran, S.D. "Teaching Male Catheterization: An Application
      of Change Theory for an Entire Nursing Staff," NURSE EDUC
      7(1) (January/February 1982): 11-14.

      A change in policy whereby 437 nurses were prepared in the
      technical and psychological aspects of male catheterization
      occurred when budgetary reductions resulted in the elimination
      of the catheterization team. Program development, implemen-
      tation and evaluation were achieved with careful attention to
      the critical components of change theory. (4)

1432 Jones, F.M. "Certification for Continuing Education Programs."
      CURRENT ISSUES IN NURSING. Edited by J. McClosky and H.
      Grace. Scranton, PA.: Blackwell Scientific Publications,
      1981, pp. 347-53.

      Continuing education programs must improve practice to be
      of value. They should be planned collaboratively by nurse
      educators and nurse practitioners according to sound data
      based on nursing research. Consideration for the needs of
      adult learners is critical to worthwhile programs. (14)

1433 Kleinberg, D.A. and E.M. Sporing. "The Educational Prepara-
      tion of Newly-Appointed Primary Nurses," NURSE EDUC 6(7)
      (December 1981): 31-33.

Dissatisfaction with the orientation program for newly ap-
pointed primary care nurses led to restructuring of the
content and process of the program. (3)

1434   Kowalski, K.   "Continuing Education Nurse Practitioner Programs," J CONT EDUC NURS 14 (1983): 33-35.

A history of the accreditation of continuing education nurse
practitioner programs. Suggest that, as funding sources for
nursing education programs disappear, continuing education
programs to prepare nurse practitioners will become extinct.
(0)

1435   LaMonica, E.L. and J.F. Karshmer.   "Empathy: Educating Nursing
in Professional Practice," J NURS EDUC 17(2) (February
1978): 3-11.

Describes a staff development program used to assist nurses
to perceive and respond with empathy. It is recommended as
a baseline for nurse educators in schools and service institutions in designing programs in behavioral empathy. (36)

1436   Larocco, S. and D.F. Polit.   "A Study of Nurses' Attitudes
Toward Mandatory Continuing Education for Relicensure."
J CONT EDUC NURS 9(1) January/ Feburary 1978): 28-35.

A survey revealed nurses strongly favored continued education for nurses (95%), however, only 53 percent thought it
should be required for relicensure. Nurses felt that these
programs should be free and more programs should be available. (6)

1437   "Mandatory CE Controversy Subsides as California Board Revises
CE Regs," AM J NURS 81(3) (March 1981): 460, 480, 482.

Debate of issues on transfer of credit, mandatory CE and
CE approval were the focus of recent meetings of the California Board of Registered Nurses. (0)

1438   "Mandatory Continuing Education," AM J NURS 82(11) (November
1982): 1668.

Lists the required contact hours for registered nurses and
for nurse practitioners by state in sixteen states requiring
continuing education. (0)

1439   McCaffrey, C.   "Performance Check Lists: An Effective Method
of Teaching, Learning and Evaluating," NURSE EDUC 3(1)
(January/February 1978): 11-13.

A performance check list was used in conjunction with other
teaching methods to orient new nurses to a neurological unit.
The time spent in orientation did not decrease, however, a
marked improvement in learner performance was observed. Check
lists facilitated mastery and provided self-paced learning,
feedback and reinforcement. (0)

1440   McGill, C. and L. Molinaro. "Setting Up and Operating Out-
       reach Centers for Continuing Education in Nursing," J CONT
       EDUC NURS 9(1) (January/February 1978): 14-18.

       A report of the second phase of a series of activities
       designed to pilot test a regional plan to increase access-
       ability of continuing education for nurses. Specific steps
       in setting up and operating outreach centers in Texas are
       described as: establishing and clearing policies with admin-
       istration of sponsoring institutions; selecting outreach
       center personnel; selecting an advisory committee; plan pro-
       gram offering content; and evaluating the overall program. (4)

1441   Meisenhelder, J.B. "A First-hand View of the Unit Teacher
       Role," NURSE EDUC 7(2) (March/April 1982): 17-20.

       A unit teacher provides a cost effective method of providing
       inservice education. The unit teacher and head nurse function
       in equal status and form a balanced leadership team. The
       head nurse is accountable for quality patient care and the
       unit teacher is accountable for the competence of staff
       nurses. This method is most appropriate in large teaching
       hospitals. (0)

1442   Meleca, C.B., F. Schimpfhauser, J.K. Witteman and L. Sachs.
       "Clinical Instruction in Nursing: A National Survey," J
       NURS EDUC 20(8) (October 1981): 32-40.

       A report on an investigation of clinical teaching skills in
       nursing attempted to gather and assess broad-based information
       useful in the design and implementation of clinical teaching
       improvement programs. A framework for identifying and select-
       ing objectives, activities and plans for the enhancement of
       clinical instruction is provided. (20)

1443   Minehan, P.L., L. May and L. Deluty. "Training Bicultural
       Leaders," NURSE EDUC 6(4) (July/August 1981): 29-32.

       A bicultural leader training program at Beth Israel Hospital
       in Boston focused on the concept of biculturalism and promoted
       skills in recognizing and effectively handling conflict re-
       lated issues. The program enabled participants to organize
       similar programs in their institutions. The program attempted
       to prepare new graduates to constructively deal with conflict
       between values taught in school and present in the work place.
       Fourteen institutions were represented among the participants.
       (5)

1444   Morrish, M. "So You Want A Cushy Job...," AM J NURS 82(11)
       (November 1982): 1800.

       A staff development instructor describes job responsibil-
       ities and frustrations and offers guidelines for organizing
       work. (0)

1445   Murphy, M.L. and S.M. Hammerstad. "Preparing a Staff Nurse
       for Precepting," NURSE EDUC 6(5) (September/October 1981):
       17-20.

       A program for preceptors at Stanford University contains
       components of preparation, support and recognition. A defin-
       ition and description of the preceptor role is necessary.
       Selection criteria require realistic expectations in the
       areas of clinical skills, leadership assets, teaching abilities
       and affective qualities. (13)

1446   Murray, R. "The Clinical Nursing Practicum," J NY STATE
       NURSES ASSOC 10(2) (June 1979): 8-12.

       Rural community hospital nurses who participated in contin-
       uing education programs rarely had the opportunity to apply
       knowledge of new and advanced nursing modalities in their
       work sites. A request for clinical opportunities within the
       program led to the development of a clinical practicum at
       Mount Sinai Hospital School of Continuing Education. (0)

1447   Norman, E.M. and L. Hauman. "A Model for Judging Teaching
       Effectiveness," NURSE EDUC 3(2) (March/April 1978): 29-35.

       Provides a schematic design illustrating the purposes of
       nursing evaluation, an objective-centered appraisal form and
       a student appraisal of teacher effectiveness form. An overall
       evaluation program to assess faculty performance is necessary
       for improvement in teaching, learning, and the total cur-
       riculum.(50)

1448   O'Connor, A.B. "Continuing Education for Nursing's Leaders."
       THE NURSING PROFESSION: A TIME TO SPEAK. Edited by N.L.
       Chaska. New York: McGraw-Hill Book Co., 1983, pp. 156-65.

       Continuing education for nurse leaders must be reconcep-
       tualized based on role demands. Leaders of nursing frequently
       function as mediators in various areas and this aspect of
       professional practice must be renewed and strengthened through
       individualized professional development activities. (14)

1449   _____. "Diagnosing Your Needs for Continuing Education,"
       AM J NURS 78(3) (March 1978): 405-6.

       Self-assessment and identification of learning needs should
       precede selection of continuing education programs. Malcolm
       Knowles' approach is applied to the continuing education needs
       of nurses. (3)

1450   _____. "The Continuing Nurse Learner: Who and Why,"
       NURSE EDUC 5(5) (September/October 1980): 24-27.

       A survey of 843 nurses in continuing education courses
       revealed that the majority were diploma graduates who were
       employed full time. Greater clinical knowledge and personal
       enjoyment were identified as reasons for participating. (18)

1451 Olson, M. "Early Development of ANA Accreditation," J CONT
      EDUC NURS 14 (1983): 5-8.

      The historical development of the American Nurses' Associa-
      ion's National Accrediting Board (for continuing education).
      (3)

1452 Palmer, M.E. and E.S. Deck. "Assertiveness Education: One
      Method for Teaching Staff and Patients," NURSE EDUC 7(6)
      (Winter 1982): 36-39.

      Assertiveness is described as an attempt through verbal and
      non-verbal means to expect and provide respect for one's self
      and others. A practical approach to assertiveness training
      in staff nurses was structured to provide them with skills
      necessary to guide patients through the process of behaving
      assertively. (3)

1453 Pickard, M.R. and N. Burns. "Continuing Education for Rural
      Hospital Nurses," NURS OUTLOOK 27(6) (June 1979): 416-19.

      Placement of students in rural hospitals led to the identi-
      fication of needs for continuing education programs. Through
      a funded project, a program was initiated. Initially it was
      not well received, however, after beginning the project en-
      thusiasm grew. After three years, the program continues as
      a state funded project which carries instruction to 24 rural
      hospitals. (0)

1454 Puetz, B.E. "A Formative Evaluation of the Indiana Statewide
      Plan for Continuing Education in Nursing (ISPCEN)," J CONTIN
      EDUC NURS 9(1) (January/February 1978): 11-13.

      A survey of nurses in Indiana revealed that the majority
      were unaware of the goals of a statewide project to provide
      continuing education programs. Effective structures are
      necessary but can only be judged effective through periodic
      systematic evaluation. (0)

1455 Rinaldi, L. "Continuing Education Today: Perspectives and
      Issues," J NY STATE NURSES ASSOC 10(2) (June 1979): 5.

      Suggestions are given whereby the consumers of continuing
      education may apprise the quality of a given program and its
      appropriateness to individual learning needs. A distinction
      is made between CEUs which are institutional programs with-
      out any agency approval and contact hours issued by NYSNA and
      ANA which are agency approved. (0)

1456 Rockwell, V.T. "Managing a Continuing Education Program With
      a Staff of One," J NY STATE NURSES ASSOC 10(2) (June 1979):
      13-19.

      Several collaborative approaches are described which provide
      cost effective high quality continuing education programs for
      nurses in small rural hospitals. (4)

1457   Roell, S.M.   "Nurse-Intern Programs: How They´re Working,"
       NURSE EDUC 6(6) (November 1981): 29-31.

       A survey of forty-three institutions offering semi-structured,
       supervised orientation programs for nurse graduates revealed
       marked similarities among programs. It was found that these
       programs are efficient, effective methods of bridging the gap
       between education and service. (29)

1458   "SREB Coordinates Nursing Education Research Project," AM J
       NURS 78(4) (April 1978): 534, 552.

       A project called Nursing Research Development in the South
       was begun to stimulate research in nursing education. Clin-
       ical performance evaluation, including graduate follow-up;
       curriculum; laboratory and clinical teaching strategies; and
       faculty development are being studied by small research teams
       comprised of 78 nurse educators in 49 collegiate nursing pro-
       grams. (0)

1459   Schor, I.   "The Continuing Nursing Education and Adult Edu-
       cation Movements in The United States," NURS FORUM 20(1)
       (1981): 86-101.

       Traces the roots and development of continuing nursing
       education and adult education with particular focus on the
       twentieth century. Considers present and future needs. (31)

1460   Schroeder, D.M., M.M. Cantor and S.W. Kurth. "Learning Needs
       of the New Graduate Entering Hospital Nursing," NURSE EDUC
       6(6) (November 1981): 10-17.

       In an attempt to assess the learning needs of new graduates
       from various educational programs, nursing service educators
       developed a test instrument. No major areas were mastered by
       all graduates and content needs could not be predicted on the
       basis of the educational program. It was found that educa-
       tional programs do not have established criteria for the
       mastery of any factual content needed for safe and effective
       nursing care. (2)

1461   Seigel, H.   "Innovation in Orientation: A Community Health
       Learning Package," J NURS EDUC 21(5) (May 1982): 8-15.

       A self learning module using a tape presentation was found
       superior to the traditional orientation program for new staff
       nurses in a community health agency. (11)

1462   Shaffer, M.K. and Y.K. Moody. "A Model for Career Develop-
       ment," J NURS EDUC 19(8) (October 1980): 42-47.

       A career development program implemented at a Veterans
       Administration hospital was found effective in increasing
       personal and professional growth. (7)

1463 Sherer, B.K. and M.A. Thompson. "The Process of Developing
      a Learning Center in an Acute Care Setting," J CONTIN EDUC
      NURS 9(1) (January/February 1978): 36-44.

      A description of procedures and activities of staff develop-
      ment instructors and staff members in establishing a learning
      center for staff development in an acute care hospital set-
      ting. (5)

1464 Shockley, J. "A Multi-faceted Program for Continuing Educa-
      tion in Nursing," J NURS EDUC 20(3) (March 1981): 20-26.

      A model for providing a multifaced continuing education pro-
      gram is presented. A description of implementation of this
      program includes methods for providing nurses and the public
      in rural areas with information about current developments in
      health care delivery. (5)

1465 Smith, C.E. "Principles and Implications for Continuing
      Education in Nursing," J CONT EDUC NURS 9(2) (March/April
      1978): 25-28.

      An exploration of the learning needs of adults which focuses
      on life experiences, practicality, success, active participa-
      tion, time, climate and learning skills. This discussion was
      used to orient individuals planning and implementing continu-
      ing education programs in nursing in Southeastern Minnesota.
      (7)

1466 Smith, C.M. "Learning On Your Own for Credit," AM J NURS
      80(11) (November 1980): 2013-15.

      The Washington State Nurses' Association developed criteria
      by which to evaluate independent study projects. Guidelines
      for programs are presented. Four model independent study
      proposals are presented whereby nurses can obtain continuing
      education recognition points. (0)

1467 Sovie, M. "Investigate Before You Educate," NURSE EDUC 6(2)
      (March/April 1981): 17-22.

      Problems and needs of staff nurses require investigation
      and identification of causative factors prior to designing an
      appropriate solution. A systematic problem solving approach
      is necessary at all levels and may involve both education and
      management. (3)

1468 Sovie, M.D. "Fostering Professional Nursing Careers in Hos-
      pitals: The Role of Staff Development, Part 2," J NURS ADM
      13 (January 1983): 30-33.

      This is the second part of an article identifying staff
      development educators' potential influence on job satisfaction
      and retention of hospital nurses. Sovie presents the
      challenge of staff development for career advancement. She

gives practical suggestions for how to meet these challenges
and how to redistribute resources to help create "magnet"
hospitals which attract both patients and excellent practitioners. (1)

1469   "Survey Shows Slow but Strong Movement in States Toward Man-
        datory Continuing Education," AM J NURS 78(5) (May 1978):
        766, 802, 804, 808, 810.

        A state by state report of the status of mandatory contin-
        uing education reveals states are moving toward this require-
        ment. The number of credits vary and are graduated to in-
        crease slowly in numbers following passage of the requirement.
        (0)

1470   Sweeney, M.A. and P. Olivieri. "Driving Nurses to Research,"
        NURSE EDUC 3(4) (July/August 1978): 7-13.

        A workshop for baccalaureate faculty was found helpful in
        increasing knowledge, experience and positive attitudes toward
        the research process. This workshop stressed the interrela-
        tionships between statistics, research and computers and was
        oriented toward learning by doing. Post workshop evaluation
        revealed an increased involvement in research and computer
        related activities. (11)

1471   Swenar, C., D. Luginbuhl and C. Alger. " Preceptor Program:
        An Avenue to Increased Accountability and Quality Assur-
        ance," NURS ADM Q 7(3) (1983): 63, 65-67.

        A hospital preceptor program for new nurse employees is
        described. The goal is to provide a supportive orientation
        by providing new employees with the opportunity to practice
        with an experienced peer on a one-to-one basis. The program
        is individualized for each new employee and may last from one
        week to one month.

1472   "Telecommunications Network Used to Beam RN Refresher Course
        to Georgia Hospitals," AM J NURS 81(7) (July 1981): 1278,
        1285.

        A statewide refresher course in Georgia was taught by a
        variety of experts using telecommunications. This approach
        delivered high quality programs to seventy-two returning RNs
        in eleven hospitals. (0)

1473   "The New York State Nurses Association Continuing Education
        Program," J NY STATE NURSES ASSOC 10(2) (June 1979): 29-35.

        A statement of philosophy, background, development and over-
        view of the NYSNA Review and Approval System for continuing
        education programs. Criteria for approval are included. (5)

1474   "These Are the Steps One State Took for Mandatory CE," AM J
       NURS 78(5) (May 1978): 766, 810.

       Recounts the ten year process of establishing mandatory
       continuing education for nurses in the State of Florida. (0)

1475   "University of Utah Will Study Effects of Mandatory CE," AM
       J NURS 79(2) (February 1979): 203.

       A three year project undertaken by the University of Utah
       College of Nursing and supported by a U.S. Public Health
       Service Grant seeks to study the effects of mandatory contin-
       uing education on nursing practice and patient care. (0)

1476   Varveri, P.S. and B.J. Gould. "Meeting the Needs of Inservice
       Educators," NURSE EDUC 7(2) (March/April 1982): 34.

       A two county inservice education group was formed to share
       common problems and solutions. A formal organizational struc-
       ture and strong member support has proved effective in in-
       creasing knowledge and reducing duplication of effort. (0)

1477   Vitagliano, A. "Retreading an RN: A Midlife Kicker," AM J
       NURS 81(6) (June 1981): 1168-69.

       A nurse returning to practice after a sixteen year absence
       recounts her experience with a nurse refresher course. (0)

1478   Walljasper, D. "Games with Goals," NURSE EDUC 7(1) (January/
       February 1982): 15-18.

       Games are like simulations but allow for more creativity,
       competition and learning. Theoretical and practical aspects
       of developing games for learning are explored and an example
       of use of a game in inservice education described. (17)

1479   Wasch, S. "The Role of Baccalaureate Faculty in Continuing
       Education," NURS OUTLOOK 28(2) (February 1980): 116-20.

       Examines differences in approach required of faculty who
       teach in continuing education programs from those used in
       teaching undergraduate students. (7)

1480   "Where CE Is Now: Rules and Information," AM J NURS 78(5)
       (May 1978): 766, 792, 799, 802.

       Reports the rules for mandatory continuing education in
       California, Colorado, Florida, Iowa, Kansas, Kentucky, Mas-
       sachusetts, Minnesota, and New Mexico. (0)

1481   Wilson, J.S. "Bridging the Gaps in Communication Among
       Nurses: Uses of the Teleconference," J NURS EDUC 18(7)
       (September 1979): 13-15.

A teleconference support system is described which was used
to provide clinical consultation to psychiatric nurses enrolled in a year long continuing education workshop. Advantages
and disadvantages are identified. This method of providing
clinical supervision/consultation following didactic content
could be particularly appropriate for registered nurse students. (3)

1482   Wise, P. and S. Yoder. "Curriculum Development in Continuing
       Education: Option or Necessity?," NURS OUTLOOK 28(5) (May
       1980): 318-20.

       Continuing education programs in nursing usually lack con-
       ceptual frameworks. Such frameworks serve to organize in-
       tended learnings consistent with the philosophy of the parent
       institution. It clarifies program offerings, types of format,
       and level of specificity. (11)

1483   Zebelman, E., K. Braschel and E. Larson. "Helping Staff
       Nurses Use Learning Modules," NURS HEALTH CARE 4(4) (April
       1983): 198-99.

       Examines the frequency of use of Learning Modules by staff
       nurses. Modules required for clinical advancement were well
       used and nurses tended to complete all learning activities
       as well as tests associated with the modules. Respiratory
       and endocrine modules were frequently utilized. (4)

       See 1206, 1862.

                                Diploma

1484   Galarowicz, L.   "Closing a Diploma School: A Time for Flexi-
       bility and Creativity," NURS HEALTH CARE 4 (April 1983):
       188-91.

       Discusses the administrative considerations necessary in
       closing a school of nursing. Faculty and student scheduling
       issues are reviewed. Provisions and plans are discussed for
       relieving stress, defining expectations and anticipating pro-
       blems. (2)

1485   "Mass. General Ends Diploma Program, Three-Year Master's Pro-
       gram to Begin," AM J NURS 79(5) (May 1979): 842.

       Massachusetts General Hospital announces closure of its
       diploma program with the graduating class of 1981. Plans to
       offer a three year master's program for college graduates with
       no previous nursing education are incomplete. (0)

1486   Rhinehart, N.W. "Eulogy for a Diploma Nursing School," NURS
       FORUM 20(3) (1981): 250-51.

       An emotional treatment of diploma school closure in a gen-
       eralized sense. (0)

1487   Van Doren, J.A.   "Community Health Nursing in a Diploma Pro-
       gram? Yes!," NURS OUTLOOK 27(8) (August 1979): 533-35.

       A community health experience in a diploma program helped
       students to gain a better knowledge of community resources,
       strengthen their skills in discharge planning and continuity
       of care and increase their understanding of how family, home
       and community influences a client's response to illness and
       recovery. (0)

       See 1336·

                                 Doctorate

1488   American Nurses' Association.   DIRECTORY OF NURSES WITH
       DOCTORALDEGREES 1984.   Kansas City, MO.: ANA, 1984,
       Pub. No. G-143.

       Includes information on close to 3,500 nurses with earned
       doctoral degrees from a study conducted by ANA, as well as
       listings by state, doctoral preparation, and areas of re-
       search/academic interest.

1489   Downs, F.   "Doctoral Education in Nursing: Future Directions,"
       NURS OUTLOOK 26(1) (January 1978): 56-61.

       The numbers of nurses applying to doctorate programs in
       nursing are substantial. Consensus is necessary in both
       labeling and developing this degree to prevent further con-
       fusion in nursing credentials. High quality in these programs
       is critical to the future of nursing. (16)

1490   Gorney-Fadiman, M.J.   "A Student's Perspective on the Doctoral
       Dilemma," NURS OUTLOOK 29(11) (November 1981): 650-54.

       Exploring the availability of doctoral programs for nurses
       reveals a variety of programs both within and outside nursing.
       The DNS and DNSc like the EdD degree are occupational degrees.
       The PhD in nursing is most highly valued and most employable.
       Career goals and personal resources need to be considered in
       choosing a program. (22)

1491   Grace, H.K.   "Doctoral Education in Nursing: Dilemmas and
       Directions." THE NURSING PROFESSION: A TIME TO SPEAK.
       Edited by N.L. Chaska.   New York: McGraw-Hill Book Co.,
       1983, pp. 146-55.

       Doctoral programs to date have emphasized the preparation
       of nurse researchers. The needs for such programs continue
       to exist, however, attention should also be directed to the
       preparation of clinician-teachers and clinician-practitioners.
       Ideally programs should provide a common core with branching
       to specialization in the three areas. (11)

1492 _____. "The Development of Doctoral Education in Nursing:
        A Historical Perspective." THE NURSING PROFESSION: VIEWS
        THROUGH THE MIST. Edited by N.L. Chaska. New York: McGraw-
        Hill Book Co., 1978, pp. 112-23.

        A historical review of doctoral education for nurses iden-
        tifies three forms. Within the first form, nurses are pre-
        pared to function as teachers and administrators. The second
        form prepares scientists in disciplines related to nursing.
        The third form prepares doctorates in nursing. Within the
        third form research is emphasized. It is important that we
        do not lose sight of the clinical field within nursing doc-
        torate programs.(10)

1493 _____. "The Development of Doctoral Education in Nursing:
        An Historical Perspective," J NURS EDUC 17(4) (April 1978):
        17-27.

        Traces problems affecting nursing and the development
        of nursing education. Current models for doctoral education
        in nursing are described and future directions proposed. (8)

1494 Holzemer, W.L. "Quality in Graduate Nursing Education," NURS
        HEALTH CARE 3(10) (December 1982): 536-42.

        Three types of assessment techniques are discussed in rating
        the quality of doctoral programs in nursing. These are
        ratings, productivity measures and descriptors. Context,
        environment for learning and outcome measures are considered.
        Standards, criteria and indicators are defined and norm versus
        criterion referenced measurements discussed. (29)

1495 May, K.M., A.I. Meleis and P. Winstead-Fry. "Mentorship for
        Scholarliness: Opportunities and Dilemmas," NURS OUTLOOK
        (January 1982): 22-28.

        An examination of the use of mentorship and sponsorship for
        the scholarly development of doctoral students. Proper match-
        ing between novice and expert is critical to a good exper-
        ience. (45)

1496 Murphy, J.F. "Doctoral Education In, Of and For Nursing: An
        Historical Analysis," NURS OUTLOOK 29(11) (November 1981):
        645-49.

        Doctorally educated nurses were at one time primarily pre-
        pared in the field of education (1926-1959). During the second
        phase of development, nurses received doctorates in education
        as well as scientific disciplines related to nursing and the
        newly emerged doctorate in nursing programs (1960-1969).
        Currently, doctorate in nursing programs are the preferred
        degree, however, basic issues as to the content and focus of
        these programs have not been resolved. (15)

1497 Podjasek, J.H., J. Blank and M. Ingram. "PhD or DNS?"
      CURRENT ISSUES IN NURSING. Edited by J. McCloskey and H.
      Grace. Scranton, PA.: Blackwell Scientific Publications,
      1981, pp. 69-81.

      Traces the history of doctoral education in nursing programs
      prior to and after 1950. Describes the Ph.D. degree as the
      academic degree focusing on research and the DNS degree as the
      professional degree focusing on practice. The need for both
      preparations is apparent. (14)

1498 Schlotfeldt, R. "The Professional Doctorate: Rationale and
      Characteristics," NURS OUTLOOK 26(5) (May 1978): 302-11.

      Proposes a rationale and description of characteristics for
      programs of study leading to the doctorate in nursing as the
      first professional degree. Care is needed in admitting aca-
      demically qualified baccalaureate graduates, selecting highly
      professional faculty, and positing these programs in univer-
      sities that prepare other health care professionals. (25)

1499 "University Offers Doctor of Nursing as Entry Degree," AM J
      NURS 78(8) (August 1978): 1285, 1288.

      Case Western Reserve plans a three year program leading to
      a doctor in nursing for college graduates and students who
      have completed three years of a liberal education. The BSN
      program is being phased out, however, the master's and Ph.D.
      programs will be retained. (0)

                              Master's

1500 Diminno, M. and E. Thompson. "An Interactional Support Group
      for Graduate Nursing Students," J NURS EDUC 19(3) (March
      1980): 16-22.

      An opportunity for graduate students to obtain support and
      understanding on entry into the program was offered through an
      optional group experience. Within the group professional and
      personal issues were discussed and contributed to increased
      self-awareness. The structure provided for emotional release,
      problem solving, interpersonal learning both personally and
      professionally, and experience in group dynamics. (5)

1501 Edmundson, M.A., B.J. Jennings and K. Kowalski. "A Nurse
      Practitioner Program for Women's Health Care," AM J NURS
      80(10) (October 1980:) 1784-85.

      A description is provided of a women's health care nurse
      practitioner program at the University of Colorado School of
      Nursing. Theory and clinical components are provided during a
      sixteen week semester for graduates of all types of nursing
      programs from AD to MS. (0)

1502 Fitzpatrick, M.L. and B.R. Heller. "Teaching the Teachers to
      Teach," NURS OUTLOOK 28(6) (June 1980): 372-73.

      In recent years, the focus of graduate education in nursing
      has shifted from functional to clinical specializations. Pre-
      paration of nurses for teaching and administrative positions
      has been neglected. There is a need to strike a balance so
      that those who know the content of nursing may also know how
      to function as teachers and leaders. (12)

1503 Flynn, B.C., J. Bottschalk, D. Ray and E. Selmanoff. "One
      Master's Curriculum in Community Health Nursing," NURS
      OUTLOOK 26(10) (October 1978): 633-37.

      Describes how a master's degree program in community health
      nursing adjusted and strengthened its curriculum to respond to
      the changing nature of health care systems, community needs
      and the recommendations of the Milbank Memorial Fund Commis-
      sion. (11)

1504 Hannon, J. "Group Process--Success in One Graduate Nursing
      Program," J NURS EDUC 19(1) (January 1980): 46-52.

      A group process course in a graduate program was judged
      effective in developing competencies which were useful in
      understanding one's self and one's relationships to others.
      (19)

1505 Keller, M.L. and K.N. MacCormick. "From Graduate Students to
      Faculty: A Simulation," NURS OUTLOOK 28(5) (May 1980): 305-7.

      A group of graduate students in a curriculum development
      course chose to forego the lecture/discussion format in favor
      of undertaking an exercise in program development. They pro-
      ceeded to act as "faculty" and utilized periodic peer evalua-
      tions to judge effectiveness. (0)

1506 Kilmon, C., P. Rowell, and N. Whitman. "Clinical Objectives
      for Nurse Practitioner Students," J NURS EDUC 19(8) (October
      1980): 37-41.

      Provides a list of objectives which may be used to guide and
      evaluate skill attainment in a pediatric nurse practitioner
      program. (0)

1507 Matejski, M.P. "Preparing Nurses to Teach--The Charge and A
      Response," J NURS EDUC 19(9) (November 1980): 25-30.

      A course "Introduction to Teaching Methodologies in Nursing"
      was designed to meet the need for better preparation in teach-
      ing skills in a master's degree program. A description of the
      theoretical framework, structure, and conduct of the course
      are provided.(8)

1508 McLane, A.M. "Core Competencies of Master´s-Prepared Nurses,"
      NURS RES 27(1) (January/February 1978): 48-53.

      A Process Competency Scale was constructed which reflected a
      conceptual model of the multiple roles of the master´s-prepared
      nurses regardless of clinical concentration or functional role.
      A survey of deans and graduate students perceptions of master´s
      level competence led to the formation of a twenty-five item
      competency list which was considered core to all programs. (32)

1509 Murphy, N. "Training Professionals to Support and Increase
      the Competence of Young Parents," J NURS EDUC 17(7)
      (September 1978): 41-49.

      Describes the content, process, and reactions of graduate
      students to a training program in family health care which
      provided long term contact with a young family. (0)

1510 Murphy, S.A. "Approaches to Research in Graduate Education,"
      J NURS EDUC 23(3) (March 1984): 97.

      The amount of research being done by nurses relevant to
      clinical specialization and issues in graduate nurse education
      is less than might be expected as the numbers of nurses with
      advanced preparation increase. (0)

1511 "NLN Calls for Master´s Degree for NPs," AM J NURS 80(2)
      (February 1980): 194, 197.

      The NLN supports the education of nurse practitioners in
      graduate nursing programs to clarify the role of autonomy and
      independent decision makers. The variety of certificate
      training programs is confusing and controversial. (0)

1512 Nelson, J.K.N. and D.S. Davis. "Educating the Psychiatric
      Liaison Nurse," J NURS EDUC 18(8) (October 1979): 14-20.

      A Psychiatric Nurse Liaison track within the graduate pro-
      gram at Yale University School of Nursing prepares students as
      skilled psychiatric practitioners with strong research back-
      grounds to function as psychiatric nurse consultants. (27)

1513 Pardue, S.F. "The Who-What-Why of Mentor Teacher/Graduate
      Student Relationships," J NURS EDUC 22(1) (January 1983):
      32-37.

      A course in a three course sequence of the functional teach-
      ing major utilized a ninety hour practicum under the supervi-
      sion of an undergraduate faculty member. A sixty-seven item
      evaluation form was found helpful in identifying the role of
      the mentor and objectives of the experience. Satisfactions
      and dissatisfactions within the experience are presented. (4)

1514   Sherman, J.E., A.G. Miller, L.L. Farrand and W.L. Holzemer.
       "A Simulated Patient Encounter for the Family Nurse Practi-
       tioner," J NURS EDUC 18(5) (May 1979): 5-15.

       An alternative learning model for teaching primary health
       care management utilized simulated problems via a programmed
       instruction format. The small sample size of the participants
       precluded any firm conclusions as to the effectiveness of the
       method. (10)

1515   Siegel, H.J. and N. Elsberry. "Master's Preparation for Joint
       Practice," NURS OUTLOOK 27(1) (January 1979): 57-60.

       A master's degree program which prepares primary care nurse
       generalists for joint practice with primary care physicians
       requires realignment through mutual involvement, cooperation
       and resolution of differences. Mutual confidence is the crux
       of the relationship. (11)

1516   Stoner, M.H., N.L. Hokanson and M.A. Murphy. "The Real
       S.O.A.P. on a Core Curriculum," J NURS EDUC 18(8) (October
       1979): 50-55.

       A core curriculum for nurse practitioner students at the
       University of Colorado utilizes congruent principles upon
       which the Nursing Process, the Scientific Method and the
       Problem-oriented recording system are based. Students are
       taught to perform health evaluations for preventive, curative
       and restorative purposes. (0)

1517   Sullivan, G.C., D.L. Anderson and S.C. Houde. "The Master's
       Degree in Nursing: Controversy in Nomenclature," J NURS EDUC
       22(8) (October 1983): 344-47.

       A historical review of the development of academic titles at
       the master's level is presented. Nursing currently has too
       many titles and distinctions between the degrees are unclear.
       Degree titles should be restricted to the Master of Science
       in Nursing and Master of Nursing. (8)

1518   Sultz, H.A., O.M. Henry, L.J. Kinyon, G.M. Buck, and B.
       Bullough. "A Decade of Change for Nurse Practitioners,"
       NURS OUTLOOK 31(3) (May/June 1983): 137, 138, 140, 141, 188.

       The first in a series of three studies which provided longi-
       tudinal data on nurse practitioner programs and students; this
       study describes changes which occurred from 1973 to 1977 and
       from 1977 to 1983. Changes in program length, type of prepara-
       tion and specialty focus are reported. (0)

1519   _____. "Nurse Practitioners: A Decade of Change-Part II,"
       NURS OUTLOOK 31(4) (July/August 1983): 216-19.

Part two of a longitudinal study of nurse practitioner programs in the United States reports on changes in practice
between 1973 and 1980. The title "Nurse Practitioner" became
the preferred term, and preparation shifted from hospitals and
other facilities to colleges and universities. An increase in
use of nurse faculty over physician faculty and from physician
direction to nurse faculty direction occurred. Guaranteed
employment following graduation decreased as a requirement for
entrance. (0)

1520   Sultz, H.A., O.M. Henry, B.Bullough, G.M. Buck and L.J. Kinyon.
"Nurse Practitioners: A Decade of Change-Part III," NURS
OUTLOOK 31(5) (September/October 1983): 267-69.

A longitudinal study of nurse practitioners in the United
States compared programs in 1973 to programs in 1980. A marked
increase in master's degree programs and marked decrease in
certificate programs was found. Fewer nurses were specializing
in pediatrics and more in midwifery, maternity, family and
adult specialty areas. The number of programs in the northeast
increased by 1980 and the number in the south declined whereas
in 1973 these programs were equally distributed across the
country. (0)

1521   Ulin, P.R. "What Master's Students Want to Know," NURS OUTLOOK
26(10) (October 1978): 629-32.

A survey of students and graduates in a master's degree program in community health nursing found the nursing core did
not prepare them for the realities of community health nursing.
They identified the need for more preparation in physical
assessment, community development, coordination of multiple
human services as they relate to health, legal aspects of
health care, and the politics of health. (6)

See 1175, 1578.

Nontraditional

1522   Brower, H.T. "The External Doctorate," NURS OUTLOOK 27(9)
(September 1979): 594-99.

The number of external doctoral programs are increasing dramatically. These programs offer an opportunity for highly
motivated, self directed individuals and eliminates many of
the structural concerns of traditional education. Nurses
within these programs are usually able to focus more on nursing
and its interdisciplinary aspects than they can in traditional
non-nursing doctoral programs. (18)

1523   _____. "Potential Advantages and Hazards of Nontraditional
Education for Nurses," NURS HEALTH CARE 3(5) (May 1982):
268-72.

Widespread acceptance of nontraditional education attests to
its success in meeting educational needs of the public. These
programs provide both hazards and advantages for nurses. Exploration and inspection is necessary in choosing a program.
Twelve points are given by which a non-traditional program can
be assessed. (14)

1524 Kuramota, A. "The Status of Nontraditional Study," J CONT EDUC
      NURS 9(2) (March/April 1978): 29–32.

A description of the definition and characteristics of nontraditional study and its application to nursing education.
Research is required to determine and clarify the purposes and
goals of nontraditional programs in nursing. (7)

1525 Lenburg, C.B. (Ed.) OPEN LEARNING AND CAREER MOBILITY IN
      NURSING. St. Louis: C.V. Mosby, 1975.

Focuses on the recent emergence of nontraditional educational
programs in nursing in which the learners and learning are considered more important to the educational mission than traditional academic structures. Considers issues and problems related to career mobility in nursing and describes various
models currently in use.

1526 _____. "The External Degree in Nursing: An Alternative Ready
      for Adoption." CURRENT ISSUES IN NURSING. Edited by
      J. McCloskey and H. Grace. Scranton, PA.: Blackwell Scien-
      tific Publications, 1981, pp. 177–95.

Nontraditional educational programs in the United States have
gained a recognized place in academe. The New York Regents
Degree Programs in nursing offer nurses an opportunity to
obtain degrees by assessment rather than instructional methods.
Variations between total instruction and total assessment
models are described. (31)

1527 _____. "Expanding the Options Through the External Degree
      and Regional Performance Assessment Centers." NURSING ISSUES
      AND NURSING STRATEGIES FOR THE EIGHTIES. Edited by
      B. Bullough, V. Bullough and M.C. Soukup. New York: Springer
      Publishing Co., 1983, pp. 235–53.

The New York Regents External Degree Nursing Program is an
assessment program which combines adult education, competency-
based education, and objective assessment philosophies. A non-
instructional program, it relies on theory and performance
examinations administered at regional assessment centers to
validate learning. It is projected that this model will increase in importance in the 1980s in providing an alternative
educational program for the nursing profession. (23)

1528 Notter, L.E. and M.C. Robey. "Open Curriculum Practices,"
      NURS OUTLOOK 27(2) (February 1979): 116–21.

The earliest form of open curriculum practice was advanced
placement. A study of 601 programs offering open curricula
for nurses revealed that such practices are of recent origins
(approximately five years); that students for the most part
were the impetus to change; and that most programs consisted
of modification of an existing program. Multiple entry and
exit programs took longer to develop than advanced placement
programs. (5)

1529   Simms, L.M. "A Perspective: The External Degree as a Viable
       Model in Nursing," J NURS EDUC 17(2) (February 1978): 23-27.

       Discusses the success of undergraduate external degree pro-
       grams and proposes this as a viable structure for education of
       nurses at the master's degree level. (10)

1530   Thomas, B., C. Crowell, R. Lavonne and C. Ping. "Developing
       a Challenge System," NURS OUTLOOK 27(5) (May 1979): 338-43.

       ANA and NLN support open curriculum practice. More than
       seventy percent of the nursing programs give credit and exemp-
       tions from other institutions or through examination. The
       question arises as to the adequacy of measurement techniques.
       A myriad of questions must be addressed in developing valid
       paper and pencil and performance examinations. (11)

       See 1357, 1386, 1459, 1499.

Curriculum

                           Models/Theories

1531   Aroskar, M.A. "Ethics of Nurse-Patient Relationships," NURSE
       EDUC 5(2) (March/April 1980): 18-20.

       Identifies four models of ethical relationships: priestly,
       engineering, contractual and collegial. Discusses a curri-
       cular framework for teaching ethics in a nursing program and
       course objectives appropriate to nursing. (6)

1532   Artinian, B.M. and N. Anderson. "Guidelines for the Identifi-
       cation of Researchable Problems," J NURS EDUC 19(4) (April
       1980): 54-58.

       The most difficult task nursing students encounter in
       developing a research project is in the identification of the
       problem. Guidelines are proposed which provide a step-by-step
       sequence in problem clarification. (8)

1533   Borgman, M.F. and L.D. Jenab. "The West Virginia Plan: A Por-
       trait of Curriculum Development," J NURS EDUC 20(9) (November
       1981): 37-44.

The West Virginia curriculum plan was an early model of an
integrated nursing curriculum. Over time responsive modifications diverted it from its original mission. A structural
realignment is described which improved the current curriculum
and allowed for future modifications. (8)

1534   Brown, S.J. "The Nursing Process Systems Model, J NURS EDUC
        20(6) (June 1981): 36-40.

        Describes the Systems-Developmental-Stress Model which pro-
        vided the foundation for a Nursing Process Systems Model at
        Azusa Pacific College. The model was found useful in provid-
        ing structure, organization and direction in curriculum
        development. (9)

1535   Brusich, J. "Social Learning Theory as a Basis for Teaching
        Decisions," J NURS EDUC 19(5) (May 1980): 27-31.

        Social learning theory provides a guide to teacher decision
        making based on concepts of freedom of movement, need value,
        need potential and psychological situation. An illustration
        using this model is provided whereby students moved from unsat-
        isfactory to satisfactory behavior. (1)

1536   Burgess, G. "The Personal Development of the Nursing Students
        as a Conceptual Framework," NURS FORUM 17(1) (1978): 96-102.

        A person-oriented program in which the framework is expli-
        citly stated as the personal development of the student nurse,
        should replace subject oriented and process oriented curricula.
        The criteria for retention within this framework are evidence
        of competence and capacity for growth. (6)

1537   Chase, B.M. "Clinical Experiences Made Easy!," J NURS EDUC
        22(8) (October 1983): 347-48.

        Discusses the needs and concerns of instructors and students
        in planning clinical instruction. The use of a matrix describ-
        ing student behaviors and desired behaviors is proposed to
        facilitate evaluation of clinical performance. (0)

1538   Cizmek, C. and J. Holland. "Coping With Change During Curri-
        culum Revision," NURSE EDUC 4(2) (March/April 1979): 30-35.

        Describes the planning and implementation of change in one
        school adopting a new curriculum. The identification of con-
        flict within this process and appropriate and inappropriate
        methods of conflict resolution are presented. (8)

1539   "Commission Sums Up Findings in 18 Recommendations," AM J NURS
        83(9) (September 1983): 1253.

        A report of the recommendations of the National Commission
        on Nursing regarding nursing practice, nursing education, and
        nursing and the public. (0)

1540   Davis, J.H. and D.D. Williams. "Learning for Mastery: Indi-
        vidualized Testing Through Computer-managed Evaluation,"
        NURSE EDUC 5(3) (May/June 1980): 9-13.

        Seven components are identified as primary to the develop-
        ment, implementation and evaluation of an individualized learn-
        ing center. Models are presented and an example of the process
        provided. (11)

1541   DelBueno, D.J. "Competency Based Education," NURSE EDUC 3(3)
        (May/June 1978): 10-14.

        Competency based education is both a broad and a narrow con-
        cept with distinct features which stress learning rather than
        teaching. Four steps are required and include competency,
        knowledge, skills and options. Illustrations of these steps
        are provided. This approach is particularly appropriate for
        adult learners. (6)

1542   Derdiarian, A.K. "Education: A Way To Theory Construction in
        Nursing," J NURS EDUC 18(2) (February 1979): 36-47.

        Describes a model curriculum for graduate education which
        effectively addresses present nursing issues. (14)

1543   Goodwin, J.O. "A Cross-cultural Approach to Integrating Theory
        and Practice," NURSE EDUC 5(6) (November/December 1980):
        15-20.

        A general model for the nursing process is used to incorp-
        orate theory as a guide to nursing practice in a French school
        of nursing. Clinical applications are necessary in order that
        students might conceptualize theory as integral to the profes-
        sional role. (10)

1544   Hall, K.V. "Current Trends in the Use of Conceptual Frameworks
        in Nursing Education." J NURS EDUC 18(4) (April 1979):
        26-29.

        Deans and program directors were queried regarding the con-
        ceptual framework in their school of nursing. Although the
        survey revealed programs were utilizing conceptual frameworks,
        little communication was apparent between programs. Research
        and sharing are needed. (4)

1545   Hawkins, J.W., J.A. Thibodeau, and C.A. Daisy. "Graduate Edu-
        cation for Primary Care Practitioners Using a Nursing Model,"
        NURS HEALTH CARE 4(10) (December 1983): 564-67.

        Describes development of a nursing model curriculum, the
        rationale and limitations. (11)

1546 Hayter, J. "Educational Taxonomies Revisited," J NURS EDUC
      22(8) (October 1983): 339-42.

      A review of cognitive, affective, and psychomotor domains.
      Examples of levels of objectives within these domains are
      applicable to nursing education. (4)

1547 Herrington, J.V. and L.S. Houston. "Using Orem´s Theory: A
      Plan for All Seasons," NURS HEALTH CARE 5(1) (January 1984):
      45-47.

      Orem´s Self-Care Deficit Theory was found to be a very work-
      able framework for teaching nursing process at the University
      of Southern Mississippi School of Nursing. Understanding and
      interpreting by faculty in both classroom and clinical situa-
      tions were judged critical to student success and satisfaction
      with the model. (1)

1548 Hipps, O.S. "The Integrated Curriculum: The Emperor is Naked,"
      AM J NURS 81(5) (May 1981): 976-80.

      An analysis of integrated curricula concludes that the con-
      cept is not clearly defined nor does it appropriately prepare
      nurses for practice. A return to the medical model would not
      serve any useful purpose.   Further development is needed to
      clarify the content of nursing programs. (4)

1549 Jaffee, M. and M.K. Flanagan. "Specialist In An Integrated
      Curriculum: An Odyssey," J NURS EDUC 18(6) (June 1979):
      46-49.

      A description of the process of changing to an integrated
      curriculum and problems encountered. The authors note that
      students must be responsible for integration. Preliminary
      evaluation indicates graduates of an integrated curriculum are
      less adept at logical thinking than graduates of a traditional
      program. (4)

1550 Jones, E.W. "Advocacy-A Tool for Radical Nursing Curriculum
      Planners," J NURS EDUC 21(1) (January 1982): 40-45.

      Proposes and discusses the value of using advocacy as an
      organizing concept for a nursing curriculum. (7)

1551 Kilchenstein, L. "The Birth of a Curriculum: Utilization of
      the Betty Neuman Health Care Systems Model in an Integrated
      Baccalaureate Program," J NURS EDUC 23(3) (March 1984):
      126-27.

      Recounts a total curriculum revision process undertakenat
      the University of Pittsburgh School of Nursing utilizing the
      Neuman Model. Describes a curriculum design reflecting philo-
      sophical and conceptual aspects and includes course and level
      descriptions. (1)

1552 King, V.G. "A Confluent Approach to Nursing Education Through
      Group Process," NURSE EDUC 3(3) (May/June 1978): 20-25.

      An instructor describes her philosophy of education and com-
      bined learning theory. Application of this model requires a
      restructuring of the content and methodology of a course.
      Concern for students' feelings contributes to more individual-
      ized instruction. (10)

1553 Kintgen-Andrews, J. "Curriculum Building: Process and Pro-
      ducts," NURSE EDUC 7(6) (Winter 1982): 32-35.

      Curriculum development in nursing requires visualization of
      the conceptual framework as a support for the entire curri-
      culum building process. Although the philosophy was previ-
      ously regarded as the fountainhead for curriculum development,
      values per se have no place within the conceptual framework.
      (12)

1554 Knowlton, C.N., M. Goodwin, J. Moore, A. Alt-White, S. Guarino
      and H. Pyne. "Systems Adaptation Model of Nursing for Fami-
      lies, Groups and Communities," J NURS EDUC 22(3) (March
      1983): 128-31.

      A report of the application of Roy's General Systems Theory
      and Roy's Adaption Model to the development of a nursing curri-
      culum. Family, group, community, nursing and the health care
      system are referred to as man's suprasystems and proved diffi-
      cult concepts to develop. (9)

1555 Kotchek, L. "Physical Fact vs. Social Fiction," J NURS EDUC
      17(1) (January 1978). 3-7.

      Curricular weighting tends to focus more on the physical
      sciences and less on the social sciences. Nursing students
      reflect this emphasis and regard social patterns as unimpor-
      tant. Curricular revisions are suggested. (2)

1556 Kramer, M. "Philosophical Foundations of Baccalaureate Nursing
      Education," NURS OUTLOOK 29(4) (April 1981): 224-28.

      Baccalaureate nursing graduates are prepared to function in
      five roles: caregiver; managerial-leadership; health promotion
      and health supervision; teaching-counseling; and health and
      illness screening. Technical nurses are prepared in ADN pro-
      grams to function as care givers. Technical nurses are pri-
      marily engaged in planning and implementing nursing care while
      professional nurses assess and evaluate nursing care. The two
      preparations are needed, however, articulation is problematic.
      Career mobility is necessary and requires a rethinking of even
      fundamental nursing skills. (5)

1557 Krawczyk, R.M. "Well Persons: Their Importance to Nursing
      Education and Practice," NURS FORUM 28(3) (1979): 220-30.

Education

Since the majority of individuals are born healthy, nursing education should focus more on wellness and prevention of illness. A course at Boston College utilizes well families for clinical placements. Family visitations allow students to observe lifestyles of well families. (6)

1558   Levine, L.B. "Through The Looking Glass at the Integrated Curriculum," J NURS EDUC 18(7) (September 1979): 43-46.

The evolution of curricular change to integrated models was never well reasearched or evaluated. The mission of nurse educators to prepare well qualified practitioners requires research to determine the effectiveness of integrated curricular models. (0)

1559   Matejski, M.P. "A Framework for Nursing: A Concept for Practice," J NURS EDUC 18(5) (May 1979): 49-58.

A conceptual framework for professional nursing practice is presented which considers the influence of stress on the rhythmic patterns of individuals with medical surgical problems. (6)

1560   McDaniels, O.B. "Existentialism and Pragmatism: The Effect of Philosophy on Methodology of Teaching," J NURS EDUC 22(2) (February 1983): 62-66.

The teacher's basic philosophy influences her philosophy of education. An existential orientation ascribes to self-education. Students are encouraged to think for themselves and take responsibility for their own learning. A pragmatic orientation ascribes to the social function of education. Students are encouraged to problem solve. The structure and control of the learning environment varies based on the philosophy of the teacher. (19)

1561   McEvoy, M.D. and E.C. Egan. "The Process of Develping a Nursing Intervention Model," J NURS EDUC 18(4) (April 1979): 19-25.

A step-wise description of the model development process is presented and applied to care of a dying patient. (15)

1562   Moritz, D.A. "Primary Nursing: Implications for Curriculum Development," J NURS EDUC 18(3) (March 1979): 33-37.

Primary care conceptualizes the case method of assignment in which the care giver assumes twenty-four hour responsibility for client care, plans the care, communicates the needs for care to other care-givers and uses the head nurse as a resource person. The implications of primary nursing for curriculum develpment are explored. (3)

1563   Packer, J. "Curriculum Consistency," J NURS EDUC 18(4) (April 1979): 47-52.

A clear overall picture of the relationships of curriculum
to a philosophic position is necessary. Curriculum options,
goals and objectives, learning theories, teaching methods and
evaluation differ within the context of realistic, idealistic
and pragmatic philosophies. (17)

1564   Pinch, W.J. "Values Exploration: A Teaching Model," J NURS
       EDUC 18(8) (October 1979): 56-59.

Student values and attitudes toward sexuality influence
their ability to assess and plan nursing care effectively. A
model is presented to assess students values and attitudes.
Discussions with an awareness of personal attitudes were
directed toward increasing objectivity in clinical situations.
(4)

1565   Quiring, J. and G. Gray. "Organizing Approaches Used in Curri-
       culum Design," J NURS EDUC 21(2) (February 1982): 38-44.

Presents and discusses a variety of models used for organization of nursing curricula. A discussion of these models
concludes that no one approach is universally satisfactory. (18)

1566   Rawnsley, M.M. "Toward a Conceptual Base for Affective Nurs-
       ing," NURS OUTLOOK 28(4) (April 1980): 244-47.

Nursing requires a sensitivity to a wide spectrum of human
experiences. This affective domain of nursing can be learned
and implemented as a scientific process utilizing simulated
and actual patient experiences, individual and group supervision and self-paced learning packages. (17)

1567   Redman, B.K. "On 'Problems' With Integrated Curricula in
       Nursing," J NURS EDUC 17(6) (June 1978): 26-29.

The current use of integrated curricula reflect an incomplete definition and an incomplete development of the concept.
A structure for nursing intervention is missing. Norms for
measuring outcomes are unclear. Additional work is needed to
clarify this framework. (4)

1568   Reed, J.C. "Management: An Experimental Approach," J NURS
       EDUC 17(6) (June 1978): 20-25.

Confusion and repetition of content was identified in teaching the problem-solving process within an integrated curriculum. An experimental program provided an organized approach
which resulted in more effective learning outcomes. (3)

1569   Rhode, M.A. "Skill Acquisition in Nurse Midwifery Education,"
       J NURS EDUC 19(7) (September 1980): 27-35.

Describes a conceptual model to facilitate skill acquisition
in a nurse-midwifery curriculum. (8)

1570   Richard, E. and S.K. Ostwald. "A Model for Development of an
       Off-campus Rural Nurse Practitioner Program," J NURS EDUC
       22(2) (February 1983): 87-92.

       An off-campus rural adult nurse practitioner certificate
       program developed at the University of Minnesota proved success-
       ful in providing primary care services in rural Minnesota.
       Eighty-eight percent of the graduates remained employed in
       rural communities. Employers and patients reported satisfac-
       tion with the services provided. (5)

1571   Rothweiler, T.M. "Needs Assessment in Nursing Education,"
       NURSE EDUC 3(3) (May/June 1978): 18-19.

       A flow chart is suggested in conducting a needs assessment
       for building or revising a curriculum. A model for proceeding
       is provided and a clear time schedule recommended. (4)

1572   Roy, Sr. C. "Relating Nursing Theory to Education: A New
       Era," NURSE EDUC 4(2) (March/April 1979): 16-21.

       Explores the meanings of nursing theory and nursing education
       and assesses the relationship between the two. An example is
       provided by describing curricular relationships developed at
       Mount St. Mary's College. (16)

1573   Santora, D. "Conceptual Frameworks of Undergraduate and
       Graduate Nursing Programs." THE NURSING PROFESSION: A TIME
       TO SPEAK. Edited by N.L. Chaska. New York: McGraw-Hill
       Book Co., 1983, pp. 101-9.

       A review of conceptual frameworks of sixty-one schools of
       nursing in thirty-six states reveals adaptation is the most
       frequently identified framework. One-third of the study sample
       had either no conceptual framework or an ambiguous framework.
       (24)

1574   Sateren, J.L. and D.E. Westover. "Baccalaureate Preparation
       for Action-Practice Nursing," NURSE EDUC 3(5) (September/
       October 1978): 12-14.

       Describes a program to prepare nurses for an "action-
       practice." Such nurses are accountable to themselves and the
       consumer, risk takers, decision makers, and they deliver care
       interdependently with other health professionals. (3)

1575   Sculco, C.D. "Development of a Taxonomy for the Nursing Pro-
       cess," J NURS EDUC 17(6) (June 1978): 40-48.

       Provides a taxonomy of the nursing process to assist stu-
       dents and teachers differentiate the various levels of the
       process. Two situations are used to demonstrate complex and
       highly complex nursing behaviors. (18)

1576   Smith, C.E. "Planning, Implementing and Evaluating Learning
       Experiences for Adults," NURSE EDUC 3(6) (November/December
       1978): 31-36.

       Understanding of adult learning needs is required in the
       development of educational programs. Planning, implementing
       and evaluating processes are highlighted and a checklist pro-
       vided to serve as a practical tool in program development. (9)

1577   Smith, G.R. "Nursing Beyond the Crossroads," NURS OUTLOOK
       28(9) (September 1980): 540-45.

       Massive restructuring is required within the health care
       system in collaboration with politically influential clientele
       if nursing is to attain real autonomy in the future. Hypo-
       thetical situations are offered to illustrate desirable nursing
       futures and guidelines to action proposed.(11)

1578   Starck, P.L. "Practical Aspects of Conducting a Feasibility
       Study for Graduate Education in Nursing," J NURS EDUC 19(4)
       (April 1980): 33-38.

       Provides guidelines and time plans for conducting a feasi-
       bility study for a master's degree in nursing program. (11)

1579   Stein, K.Z. and D.G. Eigsti. "Utilizing a Community Data Base
       System with Community Health Nursing Students," J NURS EDUC
       21(3) (March 1982): 26-32.

       A community data based management system was found helpful
       in ordering large amounts of information about a community.
       This data base was found helpful in promoting baccalaureate
       nursing students conceptualization of the community as a
       client. A master list of categories for recording descriptive
       data about a community is presented. (8)

1580   Thomas, B. "Promoting Creativity in Nursing Education," NURS
       RES 28(2) (March/April 1979): 115-19.

       A study of creativity in student nurses in an "old" curri-
       culum as compared to an integrated curriculum found the "old"
       curriculum student more creative and beginning students more
       creative than advanced students. (23)

1581   Thomas, S.P. "How to Conduct an Assertion Training Course for
       Nursing Students: A Step-By-Step Plan for Instruction,"
       J NURS EDUC 21(3) (March 1982): 33-37.

       Assertiveness training should be incorporated into basic
       nursing programs rather than approached through continuing
       education. Faculty should first prepare themselves thoroughly
       prior to developing such a program. (11)

1582   Thompson, M.A. "A Systematic Approach to Module Development,"
       J NURS EDUC 17(8) (October 1978): 20-26.

Identifies fourteen steps in the systematic development of
learning modules. Provides a reading list of sources to use
in module development and describes pertinent information
about each source. (7)

1583   Turnbull, E.N. "Interdisciplinarism: Problems and Promises,"
       J NURS EDUC 21(2) (February 1982): 24-31.

       Although the utilization of interdisciplinary education in
       the health sciences would lead to more effective utilization
       of human resources, little progress in this direction has
       taken place. Factors and issues related to this approach are
       discussed. (29)

1584   Vito, K. O´R. "Moral Development Considerations in Nursing
       Curricula," J NURS EDUC 22(3) (March 1983): 108-12.

       An examination of the application of moral development
       theory to nursing curriculum theory. The traditional concerns
       for values and ethics focused on the development of moral
       integrity. Nursing education now needs to design and plan for
       more mature levels of principled thinking. (44)

1585   Voight, J.W. "Assessing Clinical Performance: A Model for
       Competency," J NURS EDUC 18(4) (April 1979): 30-33.

       The disadvantages of grading and the advantages of a com-
       petency based model are discussed. By identifying entry,
       developing, continuing, critical and exit behaviors, instruc-
       tors can better develop a cumulative file of student progress.
       (5)

1586   Wales, S.K. and V. Hageman. "Guided Design Systems Approach
       in Nursing Education," J NURS EDUC 18(3) (March 1979):
       40-45.

       The Guided Design System attempts to assist students in
       developing decision making skills as they learn specific con-
       cepts and principles. An application of this approach to
       nursing education is described. (4)

1587   Walker, L. and R. Nicholson. "Criteria for Evaluating Nursing
       Process Models," NURSE EDUC 5(5) (September/October 1980):
       8-9.

       Nursing process is a concept which is gaining increasing
       recognition as a guide to nursing practice. A variety of
       models exist which have between three and ten or more steps.
       Although the general purpose is the same, the usefulness of
       one model over another will depend on the realities of clinical
       practice. Five criteria are proposed by which to select an
       appropriate model. (8)

1588   Walkington, J.F. "A Systematic Approach to Developing a
       Patient Education Program," NURSE EDUC 7(5) (Autumn 1982):
       19-21.

A systematic approach is required in preparing patient
teaching materials. The involvement of staff and physicians
in program design and the development of an action model contribute to a sound program. An open heart teaching program is
illustrated. (2)

1589   Welch, L.B. and J.C. Slagle. "Does Integrated Content Lead to
       Integrated Knowledge," J NURS EDUC 19(2) (February 1980):
       38-40.

Before learners can integrate they need to learn facts and
specifics. They cannot absorb differentiated knowledge of
facts and specifics at the same time they integrate. An integrated curriculum should be organized to facilitate analysis
and application of specific content, concepts, and principles.
Examination of the order, structure, scope, and depth of nursing content within such a curriculum is essential. (5)

1590   Wu, R.R. "Designing a Curriculum Model," J NURS EDUC 18(3)
       (March 1979): 13-21.

The curriculum model used at California State University at
Los Angeles is used to illustrate proper curriculum design.
(11)

Content

1591   Andrews, S. and S.A. Hutchinson. "Teaching Nursing Ethics:
       A Practical Approach," J NURS EDUC 20(1) (January 1981):
       6-11.

       Ethics as a component of the nursing curriculum
       is a recent development. Learning in this area
       should focus on ethical dilemmas in nursing prac-
       tice and extend to all areas. Emphasis should be
       placed on the method of thinking and reasoning and
       not on the substance of the content. Examples are
       provided. (11)

1592   Armstrong, M.L. "Paving the Way for More Effective Computer
       Usage," NURS HEALTH CARE 4(10) (December 1983): 557-58.

The use of computer technology in health care and nursing
should be taught in schools of nursing. Faculty should be
prepared in computer usage in order to plan meaningful experiences for nursing students. (25)

1593   Beare, P.G. et al. "The Real vs Ideal Content in Master's
       Curricula in Nursing," NURS OUTLOOK 28(11) (November 1980):
       691-94.

A survey of sixty-five master's degree nursing programs
sought to identify actual versus ideal program content. Congruence was not evident. Change theory, communication theory

and group dynamics ranked highest in the ideal curriculum and
research methodology, nursing process and individual assessment
ranked highest in the actual curriculum. (8)

1594   Beare, P.G., C.J. Gray and H.F. Ptak. "Doctoral Curricula in
        Nursing," NURS OUTLOOK 29(5) (May 1981): 311-16.

        A study of doctoral programs in universities with NLN
        accredited baccalaureate and master's programs assessed what
        was considered essential content that either was or should be
        taught and expected behavioral outcomes. A core of content
        was identified by all, however, variations were noted in the
        number of credits required, core, cognate and language
        requirements. (10)

1595   Benoliel, J.Q. "Ethics in Nursing Practice and Education,"
        NURS OUTLOOK 31(4)(July/August 1983): 210-15.

        Reviews the evolution of social and institutional values as
        they impact on health care delivery in the United States.
        Nursing students need to learn ethical inquiry and analysis
        as strategies for identifying and responding to complex moral
        problems. Learning experiences should be provided which foster
        the student's ability to reason logically in making decisions
        of a serious ethical nature. (23)

1596   Bille, D.A. "The Kreb's Cycle in Braille," J NURS EDUC 23(2)
        (February 1984): 51.

        Clinical expertise alone should not be the focus of graduate
        education in nursing. Administrative and teaching skills
        should be taught; not as electives but within the core. (0)

1597   Bloch, B. and M. Hunter. "Teaching Physiological Assessment
        of Black Persons," NURSE EDUC 6(1) (January/February 1981):
        24-27.

        Understanding of variation in skin response in black and
        white pigmentations is essential to providing effective nurs-
        ing care. Content and assessment techniques are described as
        taught in a beginning level course at the University of
        Michigan. (4)

1598   Brandon, A.N. and D.R. Hill. "Selected List of Nursing Books
        and Journals," NURS OUTLOOK 32(2) (March/April 1984): 92-101.

        A list of current nursing publications primarily from the
        United States are presented and arranged in subject categories.
        (15)

1599   Buschmann, M.B.T., E.M. Burns and F.M. Jones. "Student Nurses'
        Attitudes Towards the Elderly," J NURS EDUC 20(5) (May 1981):
        7-9.

The growing number of elderly living in the community requires positive attitudes in nurses regarding the health care
needs of the aged. A course for junior students at the University of Illinois sought to promote positive attitudes. A
pre course assessment indicated that eighty-one percent of the
students were positively disposed toward the aged. (8)

1600   Cahall, J.B.   "Research: A Vital Component Throughout the
       Nursing Curriculum," J NURS EDUC 19(4) (April 1980): 19-27.

If nursing research is considered an integral part of nursing
practice, then it should be introduced in the first nursing
course and be present in each level. The author decribes an
experience in which sophomore nursing students prepare clinical research projects. (6)

1601   Castles, M.R.   "Teaching Research Methods in Schools of
       Nursing," J NURS EDUC 23(3) (March 1984): 120-21.

The generation of new knowledge through research has long
been a university goal. Nursing needs to focus on this goal
in order to reach professional stature. All nurses must learn
enough about the research process to become consumers of research and graduate education should extend this knowledge.
Specific course structures and content are suggested. (0)

1602   "Characteristics of Graduate Education in Nursing Leading to
       the Master's Degree," NURS OUTLOOK 27(3) (March 1979): 206.

The Council of Baccalaureate and Higher Degree Programs of
the National League for Nursing present a statement of the
clinical and functional aspects of study leading to the
master's in nursing degree. Professional accountability is
considered as it relates to the student and the consumer of
health services. (0)

1603   Clayton, G.M.   "Identification of Professional Competencies."
       THE NURSING PROFESSION: A TIME TO SPEAK. Edited by N.L.
       Chaska. New York: McGraw-Hill Book Co., 1983, pp. 121-33.

A survey of registered nurses and nurse faculty utilized a
questionnaire listing suggested entry-level competencies for
registered nurses. Congruence between nurse faculty and registered nurse groups were noted on all but two of the competen-
ies. (12)

1604   Colls, J.P.   "Preparing Women's Health Care Nurse Practi-
       tioners," J NURS EDUC 19(1) (January 1980): 41-45.

Describes the structure and process of a women's health
nurse practitioner program at UCLA. The program relies on
collaboration of medical and nursing faculty and utilizes a
variety of teaching strategies to support role development. (2)

1605   Cummings, D.   "What a Rural FNP Needs to Know," AM J NURS 78(8)
       (August 1978): 1332-33.

       A nurse practitioner suggests content needs for training
       programs preparing nurse practitioners. Programs should focus
       on the diagnosis and treatment of acute ear-nose-and-throat
       problems, respiratory problems, and chronic cardiac conditions.
       Prehospital management of coronary patients and knowledge of
       emergency care especially on an ambulance are recommended.
       Community health experience and emergency room experience help
       the practitioner develop independence. (0)

1606   Devlin, K. and S.C. Slaninka.   "Writing Across the Curriculum,"
       J NURS EDUC 20(2) (February 1981): 19-22.

       The general decline in writing skills is particularly impor-
       tant in nursing education because of the extensive communica-
       tion demands within the professional role. In an attempt to
       remedy this problem faculty at West Chester State College
       attended an intensive week-long writing workshop entitled
       "Writing Across the Curriculum." Curricular changes were
       implemented to increase emphasis on writing skills. Specific
       changes are discussed. (0)

1607   Dexter, P. and M. Applegate.   "How To Solve a Math Problem,"
       J NURS EDUC 19(2) (February 1980): 49-53.

       In response to an identified problem of students in deter-
       mining medication dosages, the faculty at Indiana University
       developed additional math content for their associate degree
       nurses. The planned program was effective in strengthening
       a curricular deficiency. (1)

1608   Donabedian, D.   "What Students Should Know About the Health
       and Welfare Systems," NURS OUTLOOK 28(2) (February 1980):
       122-25.

       A self instructional module within a community health course
       addresses the major governmental health and welfare programs.
       The history of public assistance and the social forces which
       have influenced the development of social insurance and tax
       supported assistance are presented. Students with faculty
       assistance assess eligibility of families within their clinical
       experience. (0)

1609   Donaldson, S.K.   "Let Us Not Abandon the Humanities," NURS
       OUTLOOK 31(1) (January/February 1983): 40-43.

       Nursing contains a unique humanistic perspective which
       should not be ignored in favor of scientific inquiry. The
       need for liberal education in nursing is stressed as well as
       the need for doctorally prepared individuals who can explore
       the humanistic as well as the scientific base. (10)

1610   Dreher, M.C.   "The Conflict of Conservatism in Public Health
       Nursing Education," NURS OUTLOOK 30(9) (November/December
       1982): 504-9.

       Public health nursing varies from other specialty areas not
       simply on the basis of practice setting but also in its focus
       on the health of the public and communities seen in perspective
       to a larger whole. Health problems and addressing conditions
       within the community are more central to the role than is car-
       ing for an individual in his/her home. (10)

1611   Dubin, L.F.   "Teaching Biomedical Science," J NURS EDUC 21(5)
       (May 1982): 38-42.

       The Yale University Master's Program for Non-Nurse College
       Graduates utilizes a condensed science course which includes
       cell biology, biochemistry, genetics, embryology, immunology,
       anatomy and physiology. This course is contained within
       ninety-two lecture hours and selected supplemental laboratory
       exercises. (18)

1612   Dunlop, D., L. Higgins and N. Ling.   "Crisis Intervention in
       Basic Nursing Education," J NURS EDUC 17(4) (April 1978):
       37-41.

       A crisis intervention course was provided to bridge the gap
       between healthy and acutely ill clients. Students spent a
       four week block in suburban hospital emergency rooms where
       each client is in a potential or actual crisis. Students ob-
       served, interviewed, gathered data, planned and implemented a
       course of intervention for a patient or other family members.
       Many positive outcomes were noted. (6)

1613   English, J., J. Crook and E. Feldman.   "The McMaster Univer-
       sity BScN Graduate: Manpower Distribution and Characteris-
       tics for Graduating Classes," J NURS EDUC 4 (April 1983):
       171-75.

       Considers the need for nursing curricula to emphasize needed
       roles which manpower demands. Manpower distribution and
       characteristics are reported for graduates from 1975 through
       1978. Areas of need for nurse manpower include: geriatrics,
       intensive care, labor and delivery and psychiatric nursing.
       (6)

1614   Fagin, C.   "Primary Care as an Academic Discipline," NURS
       OUTLOOK   26(12) (December 1978): 750-53.

       Primary care is not an academic discipline but an integral
       part of nursing in all its nursing aspects. It evolved from
       community health nursing and essentially forms the core of the
       generic discipline. Whereas in medicine primary care is con-
       sidered low status, in nursing it is a status preparation.

Promotion and maintenance of health, prevention of illness, care of persons during acute phases of illness, and rehabilitation or restoration of health defines not only nursing but also primary care. (10)

1615   Fleming, J. "Teaching Nursing Research: Content," NURSE EDUC 5(1) (January/February 1980): 24-26.

A research content guide is provided which distinguishes appropriate levels for baccalaureate, master's and doctoral programs. Each level should develop research knowledge and a spirit of inquiry. (7)

1616   Frazer, J., M. Albert, J. Smith and J. Dearnes. "Impact of a Human Sexuality Workshop on the Sexual Attitudes and Knowledge of Nursing Students," J NURS EDUC 21(3) (March 1982): 6-13.

A pre-post test format was used to evaluate changes in knowledge and attitudes toward human sexuality following a Human Sexuality Workshop for nursing students at the University of Oklahoma. Knowledge was found to increase significantly following the workshop. Attitudes changed significantly in some areas but not in others. (10)

1617   Gordon, I.T. and C.P. Green. "The Impact of Sex-Role Stereotyping on Health Care: A Nursing Education Workshop," J NURS EDUC 20(4) (April 1981): 9-16.

A three and one-half hour experiential workshop was conducted to encourage risk-taking and role-breaking behaviors in third year nursing students at the University of British Columbia. Workshop experience and content are discussed which increased students' awareness of sex-role stereotyping and its ramifications on nursing practice. (35)

1618   Guerin, D.H. "Do You Underestimate Your Students," J NURS EDUC 20(4) (April 1981): 17-21.

An experiment is described which was aimed at bridging the meaning between old and new learning. Students are assisted in identifying the need for new learning. Such an approach fosters early skill development and greater competence in clinical practice. (5)

1619   Hazzard, M.E. and M.L. Thorndal. "Patient Anxiety: Teaching Students to Intervene Effectively," NURSE EDUC 4(1) (January/ February 1979): 19-21.

Describes the integration of teaching the concept of anxiety and its clinical application within a fundamentals of nursing course. Students reported an understanding of anxiety and intervention techniques, increased ease in approaching anxious patients, and increased ability to perceive anxiety components in their own and their patients' behavior.(4)

1620 Hein, E.C. "Teaching Psychosocial Wellness in Family Community
      Health Nursing," NURSE EDUC 3(5) (September/October 1978):
      22-25.

      An interpersonal learning lab is described in which students
      learn psychosocial needs required for wellness over one aca-
      demic year. This experience took place after the sophomore
      year and sought to shift focus from illness to wellness and
      foster acquisition of professional role behavior. (7)

1621 Heit, P. "Educating the Nurse-Community Health Educator to
      Educate," J NURS EDUC 17(1) (January 1978): 21-23.

      Communication is an important vehicle of educating. Being
      able to utilize a variety of teaching methodologies, includ-
      ing lecture, role play, debate, demonstration, field trips, guest
      speakers, laboratory, projects, and buzz groups enhance the
      change agent role of the community health nurse educator. In
      addition, knowledge of group process will assist them in their
      leadership role. (5)

1622 Hill, L. and N. Smith. "Client Assessment: An Integrated
      Model," J NURS EDUC 20(9) (November 1981): 16-23.

      Physical assessment and psychological assessment are des-
      cribed within an integrated course which provides theory and
      clinical practice of a holistic concept. Criteria for evalua-
      tion of history taking are provided in an appendix. (1)

1623 Johnson, M.H. and J.B. Zone. "Concentrating on the Process of
      Learning While Teaching Clearly Defined Communication
      Skills," J NURS EDUC 20(3) (March 1981): 3-14.

      A group of faculty in an associate degree program identified
      student difficulties in therapeutic communication with psy-
      chiatric patients. A model is presented which was developed
      and found successful in strengthening this aspect of the curri-
      culum. (0)

1624 Jones, D.A. and M.A. Poulin. "Having It Both Ways," NURS
      OUTLOOK 31(2) (March/April 1983): 119-22.

      Describes the successful incorporation of clinical content
      in a program preparing nursing administrators. (5)

1625 Judd, J.M. "'Blood, Sweat and Tears,' Coordinating A Clinical
      Course," J NURS EDUC 22(7) (September 1983): 299-301.

      Discusses the responsibilities of a course coordinator in
      not only planning and implementing a course, but also in
      orienting new faculty and representing the course to outsiders.
      (0)

1626   Korup, V. "Trends in General and Psychiatric Nursing Education
        in Selected Foreign Countries," J NURS EDUC 19(1) (January
        1980): 26-32.

        A study of the psychiatric focus in nursing education pro-
        grams in selected English speaking nations found that there
        was little exposure to the theory and practice of psychiatric
        nursing. Lack of clearly defined behavioral objectives, lack
        of uniform standards, and lack of familiarity with objective
        methods of evaluation deterred psychiatric nursing from
        attaining professional status. (7)

1627   LaMonica, E.L. "The Nurse and The Aging Client: Positive Atti-
        tude Formation," NURSE EDUC 4(6) (November/December 1979):
        23-26.

        An experiential approach is described to assist care givers
        in developing understanding of the aging process. A personal
        experience rather than a cognitive approach is used to focus on
        consciousness-raising and positive attitudinal development.
        (27)

1628   Lane, G.H., K.M. Cronin and A.G. Peirce. "Teaching Diploma
        Students How To Utilize the ANA Quality Assurance Model," J
        NURS EDUC 21(9) (November 1982): 42-45.

        A planned experience in a diploma school of nursing provided
        theory and clinical application of the ANA Quality Assurance
        Model. Within this program students researched, developed
        outcome criteria and standards of care, identified discrep-
        ancies, and proposed solutions. This experience proved effec-
        tive in preparing students for practice. (1)

1629   Leonard, A. "Client Assessment," J NURS EDUC 18(5) (May
        1979): 41-48.

        A topical outline and description of clinical requirements
        are presented for a health assessment course. Classical
        assessment techniques of palpatation, percussion and ausculta-
        tion are described. (48)

1630   Lewis, S.M. "Pathophysiology Content in Baccalaureate Pro-
        grams," J NURS EDUC 20(2) (February 1981): 32-36.

        A survey of NLN accredited baccalaureate nursing programs
        in the United States was conducted to obtain a general per-
        spective of teaching techniques and their comparative effect-
        iveness in teaching pathophysiology. (0)

1631   Lynaugh, J.E. and B. Bates. "Physical Diagnosis: A Skill for
        All Nurses?" AM J NURS 74 (January 1974): 58-59. Reprinted
        in EXPANDING HORIZONS FOR NURSES. Edited by B. Bullough
        and V. Bullough. New York: Springer Publishing Co., 1977,
        pp. 276-78.

        Argues for including physical diagnosis in curriculum. (3)

1632   Magilvy, K. "Seminar In Communication With Deaf Clients:
       A Nursing Elective to Assist Students in Meeting the Needs
       of a Special Population," J NURS EDUC 20(2) (February 1981):
       23-25.

       An elective course taught sign language and practice in
       using sign language within the nursing role. It was well
       received by nursing students and admission was opened to the
       rest of the medical center campus. (0)

1633   Mallick, M.J. "Nursing Diagnosis and the Novice Student,"
       NURS HEALTH CARE 4 (October 1983): 455-59.

       Argues that nursing schools should teach techniques of nurs-
       ing diagnosis as a primary nursing role. Deficiencies in
       current taxonomies discussed. (58)

1634   Marten, M.L. "A University Program to Improve Nursing Care
       to the Aged," J CONTIN EDUC NURS 9(1) (January/February
       1978): 7 10.

       A model university based educational program is provided
       which is intended to increase knowledge and skills relevent
       to nursing care of elderly and chemically-ill persons who re-
       side in nursing homes. Components are described for inclu-
       sion in undergraduate, graduate, and continuing education pro-
       grams. Such programs seek to improve attitudes toward the
       aged chronically ill. (4)

1635   Mayer, G.G. and C.W. Peterson. "Theoretical Framework for
       Coronary Care Nursing Education," AM J NURS 78(7) (July
       1978): 1209-11.

       Provides a theoretical framework which serves as a basis
       for designing and teaching a basic course in coronary care
       nursing for registered nurses. Maslow's theory is related to
       a patient with a myocardial infarction. (3)

1636   McCormick, K.A. "Preparing Nurses for the Technologic
       Future," NURS HEALTH CARE 4(7) (September 1983): 373-78.

       Describes necessary adaptations of educational methods to
       prepare nurses for the changing health care environment.
       Emerging technologies are grouped as: drugs, devices; medical
       procedures; surgical procedures; organizational systems, in-
       cluding hospital information systems; and, supportive ser-
       vices. Historical phases of nursing practice in response to
       technology are traced. Current concerns focus on ethical
       practice and computer literacy. (21)

1637   Munhall, P.L. "Moral Development: A Prerequisite," J NURS
       EDUC 21(6) (June 1982): 11-15.

Principled moral thinking is the highest level of moral
development. A study of graduate nurses in public health
settings revealed ninety-five percent of the sample were at
the lower level of conventional reasoning. Nursing education
needs to address the development of increased moral consciousness regarding quality of life, justice, trust, dignity,
responsibility, and individual (human) rights. This requires
structuring teaching to allow for students to reason. (15)

1638   Murdaugh, C., M. Kramer and C. Schmalenberg. "The Teaching
       of Nursing Research: A Survey Report," NURSE EDUC 6(1)
       (January/February 1981): 28-35.

A survey of the degree of emphasis on the teaching of research in nursing schools revealed that minimal emphasis on
research is reflected in baccalaureate nursing programs. More
emphasis on research was noted in master and doctorate degree
programs. Schools should utilize the results of this survey
to guide the inclusion of research content. (4)

1639   Murdock, J.E. "Regrouping For an Integrated Curriculum,"
       NURS OUTLOOK 26(8) (August 1978): 514-19.

Faculty adjustments are described which accompanied a
change in curricular focus from a traditional to an integrated framework. The new curriculum proposed many problems
as faculty moved to a generalist rather than specialist orientation. (2)

1640   Murphy, N. "A Broader Pespective on Teaching Pediatric
       Nursing: Graduate Students´ Reactions," J NURS EDUC 19(2)
       (February 1980): 54-49.

Educational programs in the health fields need to address
problems of contemporary health and illness. A course is
described which considers environmental and socioeconomic
factors, common health services interventions, decision
making and alternative approaches in the health of children
and families. Such an approach was successful in broadening
the students´understanding of the total picture of conditions
and circumstances which affect health. (22)

1641   Natapoff, J.N., C.A. Moetzinger and J.M. Quarto. "Health
       Assessment Skills in the Baccalaureate Program," NURS OUT-
       LOOK 30(1) (January 1982): 44-47.

Physical assessment skills are being taught in baccalaureate
programs according to a survey of 300 NLN accredited programs.
The hours allocated to teaching this content varies from ten
to sixty class hours. It is necessary to clarify and stand-
ardize content in this area and assure faculty competence
within the expanded role. (14)

1642   Noble, M.A. "Teaching Clinical Research: Idealism Versus
       Realism," J NURS EDUC 19(2) (February 1980): 34-37.

Identifies the needs for skill in public relations as prerequisite for nurse educators attempting to participate in
clinical research. Barriers currently exist as practicing
nurses and physicians do not welcome nurses doing clinical
research and patients are too ill to be interviewed. It is
necessary to balance the ideal with existing practicalities.
(5)

1643   O'Grady, D.J. and E. Haukenes. "Teaching Research Methods to
       Undergraduates in Nursing--Learning By Doing," J NURS EDUC
       17(8) (October 1978): 48-52.

A research sequence is offered at the University of Cin-
cinnati School of Nursing in which senior baccalaureate students conduct research studies, report results in writing,
and present their findings orally. Group as well as individual work is required. (5)

1644   Sanders, S.H., J.S. Webster and E. Framer. "Analysis of
       Nurses' Knowledge of Behavioral Methods Applied to Chronic
       and Acute Pain Patients," J NURS EDUC 19(4) (April 1980):
       46-50.

A study demonstrated that nurses have inadequate understanding of behavioral methods except for decreasing negative behavior. There is a need for formal training which emphasizes
methods to increase positive behavior. (14)

1645   Smeltzer, C. "Teaching the Nursing Process--Practical Method,"
       J NURS EDUC 19(9) (November 1980): 31-37.

The need for consistency among faculty teaching nursing
process is stressed. Examples of the components are presented
and compared to components of problem solving. An example of
a nursing care is compared to nursing process and a patient
problem is utilized as an example for each step of the nursing process. (4)

1646   Sparks, S.M. "Letting The Computer Do The Work," AM J NURS
       78(4) (April 1978): 645-47.

The National Library of Medicine's on-line data bases provide a variety of information systems useful to practitioner,
educator, or researcher in nursing. MEDLINE, AVLINE, MeSH,
TOXLINE, CHEMLINE, EPILEPSYLINE, CANCERLIT, and CANCERPROJ are
described. (0)

1647   Strauss, M.B. "Quality Assurance and Nursing Education,"
       NURSE EDUC 3(2) (March/April 1978): 19-21.

In order to achieve quality nursing care, quality assurance
preparation must be provided in basic and graduate nursing
programs and in continuing education. Focus on this goal will
provide direction in the attainment of a valued standard
while promoting excellence in practice. (7)

1648   Stuart-Siddall, S. and J. Creech. "Mandatory CPR in Nursing
       School Curricula," J NURS EDUC 20(3) (March 1981): 45-48.

       A plea for mandatory CPR training for nursing students,
       this article presents a reasonable case for inclusion of CPR
       in the curriculum or as a requirement. A survey of bacca-
       laureate and associate degree programs in California revealed
       that thirty-two percent of the respondents were not teaching
       CPR. (0)

1649   Sweeney, M.A. B. Hedstron and M. O'Malley. "Process Evalua-
       tion: A Second Look at Psychomotor Skills," J NURS EDUC
       21(2) (February 1982): 4-17.

       A study designed to investigate the importance of psycho-
       motor skills in an undergraduate nursing program utilized a
       modified Q-Sort and Delphi technique by which selected faculty
       rated 291 skills as essential, bonus, graduate level or non-
       nursing skills. Less than one-half of the identified skills
       were judged essential. (20)

1650   Tyler, L.W. "Increasing Spatial Awareness in Undergraduate
       Nursing Students: A Viable Concept," J NURS EDUC 21(4)
       (April 1982): 12-16.

       Students need to understand concepts of spatial behavior,
       territoriality and personal space in care of clients. Client
       response to space invasion by the health care provider is
       explored and curricular implications discussed. (14)

1651   Ulin, P.R. "International Nursing Challenge," NURS OUTLOOK
       30 (November/December 1982): 531-35.

       Primary care is nursing's major focus. The preventive and
       curative aspects of health care are not limited to certain
       specialty areas but basic to the practice of nursing through-
       out the world. (16)

1652   Wald, F.S. "Terminal Care and Nursing Education," AM J NURS
       79(10) (October 1979): 1762-64.

       Hospices and similar services for the terminally ill are
       growing rapidly. Educational preparation of health profes-
       sionals in this field is lacking. Integration of theory and
       practice in caring for the terminally ill should be required
       in all health care programs. (7)

                              Nontraditional

1653   Blatchley, M.E., P.M. Herzog and J.D. Russell. "The Media
       Center: It's Great, But...," J NURS EDUC 17(1) (January
       1978): 24-28.

Orientation to the medical center, deadlines, records of time, selection of personnel, time spent in development of materials and extending the learning experience are discussed in relation to a self study program. (1)

1654 "Kellogg Foundation Awards Over $300,000 to N.Y. Regents to Complete Development of External BSN Program," AM J NURS 78(1) (January 1978): 10.

The New York Regents External Degree BSN Program development is nearing completion and allows nurses from around the nation and abroad to fulfill degree requirements without attending college. (0)

1655 Myers, L.B. and S.E. Greenwood. "Use of Traditional and Autotutorial Instruction in Fundamentals of Nursing Courses," J NURS EDUC 17(3) (March 1978): 7-13.

Compares the performance of students taught by traditional methods with that of students taught by a combination of traditional and autotutorial methods in a fundamentals in nursing course. Students receiving autotutorial instruction appeared to achieve better than those taught by traditional methods alone. (13)

1656 Shaffer, M.K. and I.L. Pfeiffer. "You Too Can Prepare Video-tapes for Instruction," J NURS EDUC 19(3) (March 1980): 23-27.

The preparation and use of a videotape to teach the nursing process application to home visits in community nursing are described. The use of videotapes were found a viable alternative to traditional teaching methods. (7)

1657 Tilden, V.P. and K.K. Porter. "Manifest and Latent Content in Communication: Genesis of an Instructional Module in Psychiatric Nursing," J NURS EDUC 17(4) (April 1978): 11-16.

Unable to identify useful teaching materials for manifest and latent content in communication, two instructors at the University of California at San Francisco School of Nursing developed a module and audiovisual instructional package. The faculty found such a modular approach freed faculty for more creative activities. (10)

Teaching Strategies

1658 Almore, M.G., H. Jay, S. Pinterich, J. Pryor and F.K. Richardson. "Regional Coordination of Clinical Experiences," NURSE EDUC 5(1) (January/February 1980): 15-17.

Increases in the number of nursing schools vying for limited clinical facilities prompted a collaboration effort between schools and health care institutions in Fort Worth, Texas.

Clinical coordinators met with clinical representatives and
preplanned student experiences two months prior to the
semester. (1)

1659   Arlton, D.M. and O.S. Miercort. "A Nursing Clinic: The
       Challenge for Student Learning Opportunities," J NURS EDUC
       19(1) (January 198): 53-58.

       In an effort to provide a controlled learning environment,
       the faculty at Metropolitan State College in Denver developed
       a faculty operated nursing clinic in a senior citizens center.
       A description of the development, use, operational aspects,
       difficulties encountered, and effectiveness of the clinic as
       a learning site are discussed. (0)

1660   Arnold, J. "Let's Discuss Teaching Strategies," J NURS EDUC
       17(1) (January 1978): 15-20.

       Students are now entering community colleges with deficien-
       cies in reading, writing, and arithmetic skills. The use of
       a variety of teaching strategies, including programmed
       materials, lecture discussions and student choice were utilized
       in an experimental study. Little difference between the
       three modes was noted in learning outcomes. (9)

1661   Atwood, A.H. "The Mentor in Clinical Practice," NURS OUTLOOK
       27(11) (November 1979): 714-17.

       An experiment in utilization of a master's prepared nurse
       clinician as a mentor to students and graduate nurses on an
       oncology unit proved cost effective, improved student learn-
       ing, and improved quality of care. (6)

1662   Baldwin, B.A., L. Goodykoontz and E.L. Stone. "Out of the
       Desk and Onto the Stage: An Experiment in Assertive Role
       Playing," J NURS EDUC 18(7) (September 1979): 38-42.

       A surprise role playing episode between the instructor and
       guest lecturers demonstrated aggressiveness, assertiveness,
       and passive behaviors. Students subsequently assumed three
       behaviors in planned classroom interactions which strengthened
       professional and personal assertive behaviors. (6)

1663   Bartscher, P.W. "Human Sexuality and Implications for Nurs-
       ing Intervention: A Format for Teaching," J NURS EDUC 22(3)
       (March 1983): 123-27.

       Patient concerns regarding sexuality are often viewed with
       discomfort by student nurses. A planned program using taped
       interviews assisted students in addressing sexual concerns of
       patients in a therapeutic manner. (12)

1664   Bauman, K. and A.K. Kunka. "Overhead Transparencies: The
       Overlooked Medium," NURSE EDUC 4(4) (July/August 1979):
       21-25.

Provides a nine-step systematic approach to developing
transparencies for instructional purposes. In times of decreasing educational funds, transparencies provide a rela-
tively uncomplicated, inexpensive, and potentially satisfying
support technique. (7)

1665 Bauman, K., J. Cook and L.K. Larson. "Using Technology to
      Humanize Instruction: An Approach to Teaching Nursing
      Skills," J NURS EDUC 20(3) (March 1981): 27-31.

A laboratory was designed at the University of North Carolina
at Chapel Hill for purposes of teaching psychosocial skills
for nursing practice. Practice in coordinating skills and
theoretical content in the laboratory is provided and rein-
forced by supervised clinical practice. (8)

1666 Becktell, P. "A Dragon in the Land," NURSE EDUC 5(2) (March/
      April 1980): 13-15.

An examination is provided which integrates principles of
relaxation within a paper and pencil test. Surprise, fantasy,
entertainment, and humor are injected into a story format.
Item analysis following use of this test demonstrated its
effectiveness in evaluating cognitive learning. (4)

1667 _____. "The Effect of Freedom on the Learning of Gifted
      Nursing Students," J NURS EDUC 20(9) (November 1981): 24-30.

A study was undertaken to demonstrate that gifted students
learn better when provided with a self paced program with
freedom from time and place requirements. Freedom had a
positive influence of measurable value on the gifted learner.
The sample group approached learning differently than their
less gifted classmates, however, they tended to deny their
uniqueness. (9)

1668 Bell, E.A. "Antidote for 'Reality Shock'," J NURS EDUC
      19(4) (April 1980): 4-6.

In response to expressed needs of new nurse graduates and
employing agencies, one associate degree program developed
an experience in team leading for senior level students. It
served to reinforce problem solving skills, encourage professionalism, and prepare more qualified nurses. (0)

1669 Benda, E. "Nursing Students Go To Camp," J NURS EDUC 19(9)
      (November 1980): 16-18.

Unable to find adequate clinical experiences to teach
health maintenance to children, one school utilized a summer
camp. Planned teaching programs provided a satisfactory
learning experience. (2)

1670 Berendt, H. "The Issue of Change: Its Relationship to
      Teaching Foreign Nurse Students," J NURS EDUC 19(1) (January
      1980): 4-7.

Foreign nurses are resistant to changes in nursing practice
due to their cultural orientation. Their attitudes toward
the mentally ill require attitudinal changes reflective of
modern psychiatric nursing practice which discards stereotyping. Teaching strategies were developed to assist students
in identifying the sources of their attitudes and developing
a more positive approach toward working with the mentally
ill. (8)

1671   Betz, C.L.   "Making Assignments Count," J NURS EDUC 22(3)
       (March 1983): 117-18.

       An assigned teaching project for a group of students
       adapted professional ideals to the working environment.
       Working collaboratively with nursing staff and each other,
       they developed an information booklet which was adopted for
       use on an oncology unit.

1672   Billings, D.M.   "Evaluating Computer Assisted Instruction,"
       NURS OUTLOOK 32(1) (January/February 1984): 50-53.

       A model is proposed for comprehensive evaluation of com-
       puter assisted instructional strategies. An issues based
       approach is used to focus on the relationship of nursing
       values to CAI, the needs of a broad audience and the acti-
       vities within CAI that contribute to teaching and learning.
       Such a model will assist in decision making relevant to con-
       tinued use. (11)

1673   Bradshaw, C.E.   "Concentrated Experiential Learning Labora-
       tories," J NURS EDUC 17(2) (February 1978): 32-35.

       A group experience utilized doing and feeling activities
       to help students to develop strategies for dealing with
       clinical situations. The response to this teaching strategy
       was so positive that additional programs were developed. (0)

1674   Bridges, M.J.   "Prison--A Learning Experience," AM J NURS
       81(4) (April 1981): 744-45.

       Lack of clinical teaching facilities in a psychiatric
       hospital led faculty at North Georgia College to utilize a
       prison for the clinical practicum in psychiatric nursing.
       The problems and benefits are described. Students demon-
       strated success in meeting program objectives as evidenced
       in their state board test scores. (5)

1675   Chamings, P.A. and B.J. Brown.   "The Dean as Mentor," NURS
       HEALTH CARE 5(2) (February 1984): 88-91.

       The authors recount the benefits of their relationship as
       mentor and mentee in which a two semester experience pro-
       vided the learner familiarity with the role of a dean. (12)

1676 Chapman, J.J. "Microteaching: How Students Learn Group
        Patient Education Skills," NURSE EDUC 3(2) (March/April
        1978): 13-16.

        Microteaching was found to be a useful instructional
        strategy in promoting process learning. Videotaped sessions
        of patient teaching by students focused on specific behavioral
        characteristics of the teaching learning process. Evaluation
        and feedback regarding appropriate behaviors were provided
        immediately after each microteaching segment. (18)

1677 Chavigny, K.H. "Hospital Epidemiology: A Challenge to Nurs-
        ing Education," NURSE EDUC 4(1) (January/February 1979):
        28-34.

        Provides behavioral objectives and methodologies for
        teaching student nurses infection control practices. (7)

1678 Christian, P.L. and L.S. Smith. "Using Video Tapes to
        Teach Interviewing Skills," NURSE EDUC 6(4) (July/August
        1981): 12-14.

        Video taping is used to support instruction in interviewing
        for family nurse practitioner students at the University of
        North Carolina at Chapel Hill. The effective integration of
        theory in the skill development of taking a medical and
        psycho-social history was demonstrated. Having a standard-
        ized behavioral checklist and providing a supportive envir-
        onment were found beneficial. (3)

1679 Clark, C.C. "Teaching Nurses Group Concepts: Some Issues
        and Suggestions," NURSE EDUC 3(1) (January/February
        1978): 17-20.

        Increases in student load and decreases in clinical place-
        ments led one teacher to restructure a course in group pro-
        cess. A variety of situations, including simulation, peer
        supervision, and group process recordings were utilized as
        well as innovative real-life clinical group experiences to
        assist students in meeting course objectives. (16)

1680 Clark, M.D. "Staff Nurses as Clinical Teachers," AM J NURS
        81(2) (February 1981): 314-18.

        Rush College of Nursing utilizes primary nurses for stu-
        dent teaching. Practitioner-teachers assume responsiblity
        for orienting the clincial teaching assistants and make
        periodic rounds of all students, assigned patients and
        teaching assistants. Staff nurses have been enthusiastic
        about assuming the TA role and find the relationship with
        the academic setting attractive. (0)

1681 Clarke, L.M. and M.E. Willmuth. "Art Therapy: A Learning
        Experience for Students in Nursing," J NURS EDUC 21(9)
        (November 1982): 24-27.

Student nurses in a psychiatric clinic experience portrayed their feelings in paints, drawing materials and clay. This art session depicted student anxiety in the clinical setting and allowed the students to express their concerns in less threatening ways. Furthermore, it encouraged productive discussion in clincial conferences. (2)

1682   Conners, V.L. "Teaching Affective Behaviors," J NURS EDUC 18(6) (June 1979): 33-39.

An interactional analysis technique was used for assessing and evaluating affective behaviors. The effectivess of behaviors becomes the criteria for correctness rather than "good" or "bad" techniques. Students gain insight into their behaviors through use of this technique which is useful in teaching and evaluating affective behaviors. (2)

1683   Coombe, E.I., B.J. Jabbusch, M.C. Jones, B.L. Pesznecker, C.M. Ruff and K.J. Young. "An Incremental Approach to Self-Directed Learning," J NURS EDUC 20(6) (June 1981): 30-35.

Learning experiences in the senior year should promote self-direction and self-confidence in preparation for the graduate nurse role. A workshop was designed at the University of Washington to facilitate entry into the community health field. Teaching strategies were changed from a pedagogic approach to those more appropriate for adult learners. (4)

1684   Cowart, M.E. and R.F. Allen. "Moral Development of Health Care Professionals Begins With Sensitizing: Thirty-three Sample Encounters," J NURS EDUC 21(5) (May 1982): 4-7.

Moral development requires sensitivity to human needs and suffering. Activities are suggested whereby student nurses may experience new unfamiliar realities of people in need, make sense of what they see and develop responsible ways of responding. (0)

1685   Craig, J.L. and G. Page. "The Questioning Skills of Nursing Instructors," J NURS EDUC 20(5) (May 1981): 18-23.

A self instructional module was designed to help instructors improve their oral questioning skills during post-clinical conferences. Through use of the module, instructors classified questions according to Blooms´ Taxonomy, generated questions at each level and evaluated questions asked during post-clinical conferences. (17)

1686   Crancer, J. and S. Maury-Hess. "Games: An Alternative to Pedagogical Instruction," J NURS EDUC 19(3) (March 1980): 45-52.

Demonstrates the utilization of a non-traditional approach, Keller's Personalized System of Instruction, Cognitive Style recognition and antithesis of Postman's Listing of traditional teaching outcomes within six games. These games were used for instructional purposes and provided an alternative teaching strategy. (6)

1687   Cunning, B.R. and C.M. Crowell. "Well Elderly Screening Clinics: A Community Clinical Experience in Health Assessment," J NURS EDUC 21(3) (March 1982): 38-48.

The University of Iowa found a beginning clinical experience in well aged clinics fostered an understanding of community, prevention, and health assessment as well as more positive attitudes towards processes of aging. (12)

1688   Davidhizar, R. "A Nursing Student Experience in a Psychiatric Activity Program," J NURS EDUC 18(7) (September 1979): 56-59.

Change in clinical placement from a long term psychiatric facility to an acute care psychiatric unit required adjustment in clinical goals. Clinical schedules for students were expanded to include responsibilities in taking charge of group activities which focus on group discussion, arts and crafts projects, occupational therapy projects and socialization and broadening of interests. (1)

1689   Davidson, M.E. and P.E. McArdle. "Peer Analysis of Interpersonal Responsiveness and Plan for Encouraging Effective Reshaping--Pair/Peer," J NURS EDUC 19(2) (February 1900): 8-12.

Self-perception was compared to perception of peers in a workshop intended to assist students in changing behavior. Affective behaviors were identified which contributed to professionalism and leadership skills. (3)

1690   Dick, D.J. "Teaching Health Assessment Skills: A Self-Instructional Approach," J NURS EDUC 22(8) (October 1983): 355-56.

A health assessment course using study guides, pre and post tests, performance check lists, video tapes, and surrogate patients proved effective in teaching health assessment skills. Student progressed at their own pace over a trimester and prepared a video tape of their health assessment for faculty evaluation. (0)

1691   DiRienzo, J.N. "Before Client Care-An Interactive Conference," J NURS EDUC 22(2) (February 1983): 84-86.

A change in preclinical conferences focused on problem identification and problem resolution. The teacher facilitated higher level thinking by creating an interactive rather than passive conference. It was noted that such an

approach decreased the teacher's active participation and
increases students' participation. Students demonstrated an
increased ability to function independently throughout the
clinical day and required less time in conferencing on the
units. (10)

1692 Donaldson, M.L. "Instructional Media as a Teaching Strategy,"
      NURSE EDUC 4(4) (July/August 1979): 18-20.

      The capabilities of human interaction and mediated instruc-
      tion as teaching strategies are discussed. Guidelines are
      provided for using mediated instruction in education. (15)

1693 Downs, F.S. "Teaching Nursing Research: Strategies," NURSE
      EDUC 5(1) (January/February 1980): 27-29.

      Baccalaureate level research should be taught through a
      didactic approach. Master's should actively involve students
      in the research process while doctoral level research should
      focus on more intense theory building and hypothesis testing.
      (0)

1694 Duane, N.F. "An Audiovisual Overview," NURSE EDUC 4(4)
      (July/August 1979): 7-9.

      Describes various audiovisual techniques useful in support-
      ing instructional programs. Suggestions for the proper pre-
      paration and use of transparencies, slides, recordings, films,
      and television are presented. (2)

1695 Evans, A.D., A.T. Ullom-Morse and C.M. Engle. "Speech Com-
      pression: Options for Speeding Nursing Education," J NURS
      EDUC 19(5) (May 1980): 20-26.

      A study of usage of compressed speech videotapes indicated
      students selected normal rate tapes more frequently. Some of
      the benefits of compressed speech were identified by students
      as: saved time, good for review, required their attention,
      and less boring. Sixty-eight percent indicated they liked
      compressed speech. (25)

1696 Faron, A. and C. Evans. "Communication Skills: An Adjunct to
      the Nursing Curriculum," J NURS EDUC 20(2) (February 1981):
      45-47.

      Triton College utilized mini-workshops to teach communica-
      tion skills to nursing students. A four month follow up
      found students had increased confidence in responding to
      patients, and increased ability in observing and interpre-
      ting patients body language. More than seventy percent of
      the students' demonstrated one hundred percent retention of
      theories and terms presented at the workshop. (8)

1697 Farrell, J.J. "Media in the Nursing Curriculum," NURSE EDUC
      6(4) (July/August 1981): 15-19.

      In selecting media, faculty need to go beyond the subject
      matter content and evaluate the appropriateness of material
      in relation to the philosophy and conceptual framework of the
      school. When conflict is noted, the message may be noted in
      an introduction, a change in sequence, or a post-viewing
      discussion. Particular attention should be directed toward
      examining the media's unspoken portrayal of the nurse. (15)

1698 Finley, B., K.K. Kim and S. Mynatt. "Maximizing Videotaped
      Learning of Interpersonal Skills," J NURS EDUC 18(1)
      (January 1979): 33-41.

      A study of the effectiveness of using videotapes for teach-
      ing interpersonal skills demonstrated that learner character-
      istics were important variables. Guidelines are presented
      for use of this teaching strategy. (13)

1699 Flynn, J.P., M.T. Marcus and J.C. Schmadl. "Peer Review: A
      Successful Teaching Strategy in Baccalaureate Education,"
      J NURS EDUC 20(4) (April 1981): 28-32.

      Since peer review is commonly used method of evaluating
      professional performance, it is important that students learn
      this process. A planned program is described which empha-
      sizes peer collaboration, increased achievement of client
      outcomes and heightened accountability through group problem
      solving. (4)

1700 Forsyth, D.M. "Assisting in the Development of a Slide Tape:
      A Learning Experience," J NURS EDUC 19(4) (April 1980):
      42-45.

      A graduate student describes her experiences in preparing
      a slide tape for instructional purposes. (7)

1701 Francis, M.B. "Need Community Experiences? Ask the Senior
      Citizens," NURS EDUC 3(2) (March/April 1978): 22-24.

      A community experience in a senior citizen apartment build-
      ing was found useful in promoting students' positive atti-
      tudes toward the well aged. This experience provided oppor-
      tunities in history taking, interviewing, health screening,
      health teaching, and making referrals for senior level nurs-
      ing students. (6)

1702 Friedman, W.H., J.M. Ganong and W.L. Ganong. "Workshopping,"
      NURSE EDUC 4(6) (November/December 1979): 19-22.

      Engagement, commitment, focus, disclosure, and reinforce-
      ment are five steps utilized in successful workshopping. A
      workshop design is presented which facilitates maximum parti-
      cipation. Individualizing the evaluation process is neces-
      sary. (4)

1703   Girard, N.L.   "A Game-Oriented Strategy for Teaching Surgical
       Terminology," NURSE EDUC 6(5) (September/October 1981): 16.

       A word game is presented which was utilized to teach under-
       standing of surgical terminology to nursing students. (0)

1704   Gordy, H.E.   "Crisis Aspects of Test Taking: How The Teacher
       Can Help," NURS HEALTH CARE 5(2) (February 1984): 100-105.

       An understanding of anxiety and stress related to test
       taking can be helpful to students in turning threatening
       events into growth producing experiences. (13)

1705   Griffith, J.W. and A.J. Bakanauskas.   "Student-Instructor
       Relationships in Nursing Education," J NURS EDUC 22(7)
       (March 1983): 104-7.

       A student and faculty member discuss the student-teacher
       relationship in nursing education. Principles facilitating
       interpersonal growth and learning are described within the
       context of a helping relationship. (12)

1706   Griffith, J.W.   "Team Teaching: Philosophical Considerations
       and Pragmatic Consequences," J NURS EDUC 22(8) (October
       1983): 342-44.

       Concern for interdisciplinary learning and the current
       preference for integrated curricula may be best met through
       team teaching. Potential benefits and problems are discussed.
       (7)

1707   Grosskopf, D.   "Textbook Evaluation and Selection in the Cur-
       riculum," NURSE EDUC 6(6) (November 1981): 32-35.

       A textbook selection group which includes student represen-
       tation is recommended to assure selection of textbooks which
       meet identified needs and goals within an educational program.
       (21)

1708   Haggerty, L. and E.C. Kidzma.   "Expectant Parents´ Classes:
       An Alternative Environment for Learning Health Maintenance,"
       J NURSE EDUC 19(2) (February 1980): 13-19.

       Describes the utilization of parents´ classes to teach bac-
       calaureate nursing students concepts of health maintenance of
       the pregnant family. Students followed a volunteer couple on
       a continuous basis. The experience proved to be an effective
       alternative clinical assignment which promoted professional
       autonomy. (2)

1709   Hair, B.B., A.D. Hollerbach and M.P. Spain.   "The GU Clinic:
       A Clinical Learning Experience," NURS HEALTH CARE 5(3)
       (March 1984): 165-66.

The utilization of a GU Clinic was found helpful in providing students with skills necessary for the collection of urine samples and catheterization. (0)

1710   Hall, B.A. and B.K. Mitsunaga. "Education of the Nurse to Promote Interpersonal Attraction," J NURS EDUC 18(5) (May 1979): 16-21.

Little research is evident in the literature which considers nurses liking and disliking patients. Although affective neutrality is basic to professional training, no research has indicated that attraction problems can be solved by intellectual processes. Guidance is necessary to help students understand behaviors different from their own. (15)

1711   Hartin, J.M. "Nursing Apprenticeship," NURS MANAGE 14(3) (1983): 28-29.

Describes a twelve-week summer work experience for nursing students who were within one year of completing their training. (6)

1712   Hassett, M. "Computers and Nursing Education in the 1980's," NURS OUTLOOK 32(1) (January/February 1984): 34-36.

Computer based education has many applications within nursing education. A glossary of terms is provided to familiarize faculty with this technology. It is predicted that computers will be highly visible in nursing education within the next decade. (25)

1713   Holm, K.J., G. Llewellyn, M. Ringuette, E. Pierce, L. Schaaf, J. Tarnon and V. Zasadney. "A Teaching-Learning Experience: Nursing Rounds," J NURS EDUC 17(4) (April 1978): 33-36.

Students developed ability in organizing and presenting data through participating in weekly nursing rounds. This approach allowed for integration of various aspects of patient care, sharing of experience, on-the-spot decision making and refinement of assessment skills. (3)

1714   Horacek, L.A. "Senior Students' Experience in Primary Nursing," J NURS EDUC 23(3) (March 1984): 122-23.

A primary nursing experience within the senior year provided the opportunity for students to envision themselves as graduate nurses, utilize problem solving and leadership techniques, and derive considerable satisfaction within the professional role. (3)

1715   Huckabay, L.M.D., N. Anderson, D.M. Holm and J. Lee. "Cognitive, Affective and Transfer of Learning Consequences of Computer-Assisted Instruction," NURS RES 28(4) (July/August 1979): 228-33.

A comparison of nurse practitioner students cognitive, affective and transfer of learning abilities following computer assisted instruction and lecture-discussion instruction demonstrated that both groups learned significantly. The computer assisted groups were, however, better able to transfer learning to case study situations. (30)

1716   Huckstadt, A.A.   "Work/Study A Bridge to Practice," AM J NURS
       81(4) (April 1981): 726-27.

A work/study program offered at Wichita State University during an eight week summer session indicated significant changes in positive self-concept, increased self-confidence, increased ability to praise others, and an increase in the belief that nursing should change occurred in student participants. Problems encountered are described. (3)

1717   Humphrey, P. and N.F. Woods.   "Involving Undergraduate Students in Faculty Research," J NURS EDUC 19(5) (May 1980):
       4-6.

In an attempt to introduce baccalaureate nursing students to research, the faculty at Duke University involved students in their research projects. It was found that when junior students participated in research they were more likely to identify needs for research in the practice sites during their senior year and were more likely to participate in the honors program which requires the student to conduct research. (1)

1718   Infante, M.   "Toward Effective and Efficient Use of the Clinical Laboratory," NURSE EDUC 6(1) (January/February 1981):
       16-19.

Supervision implies overseeing, managing, directing, and assessing whereas guidance implies supporting, stimulating and facilitating. Guidance requires availability based on need whereas supervision requires constant presence. Faculty need to guide not supervise students and should consider alternative teaching strategies for clinical learning which reduce the supervisory role. (4)

1719   Iversen, S.M.   "Microcounseling: A Model for Teaching the Skills of Interviewing," J NURS EDUC 17(7) (September 1978):
       12-16.

Utilizes pre-interview, interview, and post-interview to teach microcounseling. Students receive a brief explanation of the experience, a reading assignment, and a taped or live role play of correct and incorrect behavior. Following a week of preparation, a two to five minute interview with a fellow student acting as client is taped. An evaluation conference includes discussion of appropriate and inappropriate techniques as demonstrated on the tape. (6)

1720   Jackson, N.E. "The Statistically Simple Study: A Guide for
       Thesis Advisors," J NURS EDUC 22(8) (October 1983): 351-54.

       Common sources of unnecessary statistical complexity are
       described. The research process can be strengthened by expli-
       cit advanced planning which includes the development of opera-
       tional constructs, hypothesis specification, selection of sta-
       tistical procedures and estimation of sample size. (14)

1721   Jacobi, E.M. "The Proper Environment for Educational Advance-
       ment: Academic Freedom." THE NURSING PROFESSION: VIEWS
       THROUGH THE MIST. Edited by N.L. Chaska. New York: McGraw-
       Hill Book Co., 1978, pp. 124-28.

       The rapidity of change in knowledge and technology demands
       educating nurses for a future that is unknown. Providing
       academic freedom to explore and teaching them how to learn
       rather than what to learn can prepare them for the uncertain
       future. (15)

1722   Janzen, S. "Taxonomy for Development of Perceptual Skills,"
       J NURS EDUC 19(1) (January 1980): 33-40.

       Suggests a taxonomy for teaching perceptional skills in a
       mental health context. Imitation, prescription, proficiency
       development, integration and internalization are identified
       as the stages in the development of perceptual skills in human
       interaction. The classification is suggested as useful to
       nurse educators in planning, implementing and evaluating pro-
       grams in mental health assessment. (19)

1723   Jeglin-Mendez, A.M. "Burnout in Nursing Education," J NURS
       EDUC 21(4) (April 1982): 29-34.

       A restructuring of the teaching process utilized group pro-
       jects rather than individual projects. This resulted in sav-
       ings of time and energy and decreased burnout in both faculty
       and students. (1)

1724   Jernigan, D.K. "Testing-A Learning Not a Grading Process,"
       NURS OUTLOOK 28(2) (February 1980): 120-21.

       Describes the use of a pre test as an organizational format
       for a course. This method reduced anxiety and increased stu-
       dents motivation to learn. (0)

1725   Johnson, R. "Evolution of a Format for Physical Assessment
       Rounds in A Primary Care Program," J NURS EDUC 22(9) (Novem-
       ber 1983): 383-85.

       A description of the use of physical assessment rounds to
       assist students in integrating the motor and cognitive aspects
       of physical assessment. This program has existed for more
       than ten years and evolved from a physician precepted ex-

perience to a faculty controlled program. Seven one and one-half hour sessions focus on strengthening physical assessment of the heart, lungs, and abdomen. Post-conferences follow each session. Problematic issues are discussed. (6)

1726   Johnston, T. "Moral Education for Nursing," NURS FORUM 19(3) (1980): 285-99.

Moral decision making is critical to nursing practice. Educational programs should foster moral development and avoid imposing a specific moral position. Using dilemmas to assist in the development of moral reasoning is helpful, however, integration throughout the curriculum and other methodologies are needed. (6)

1727   Kammer, C.H. "Using Peer Groups in Nursing Education," NURSE EDUC 7(6) (Winter 1982): 17-21.

The University of Indiana School of Nursing utilizes peer groups for learning in an integrated community health and psychiatric-mental health nursing course. Faculty visit infrequently but are available as resource persons. (26)

1728   Kauffman, M. "On Developing Empathy: Sharing The Patient's Experience," AM J NURS 78(5) (May 1978): 860-62.

Students assumed a disability to increase awareness of how handicaps affect one's ability and self-concept. Student insights are shared. (0)

1729   Kishi, K.I. "Communication Patterns of Health Teaching and Information Recalls," NURS RES 32(4) (July/August 1983): 230-35.

An investigation of verbal communication patterns between health care providers and clients in a well baby clinic using Flander's Interaction Analysis System did not support the principle that higher direct influence results in higher student achievement. The study found little support to indicate that the teacher is a major source of influence on student learning. (29)

1730   Kramer, M., B. Holaday and B. Hoeffer. "The Teaching of Nursing Research—Part III: A Comparison of Teaching Strategies," NURSE EDUC 6(3) (May/June 1981): 18-28.

The third article in a three part series which focuses on the effectiveness of small peer group discussion versus modeling in producing quality research proposals, affecting students' attitudes toward research and the research role and changing subjects long range behavior with respect to research activity and training. The role modeling strategy produced higher quality research proposals. (22)

1731 _____. "The Teaching of Nursing Research--Part II: A
     Literature Review of Teaching Strategies," NURSE EDUC 6(2)
     (March/April 1981): 30-37.

     A test of the differential effectiveness of teaching nursing
     research using small group and modeling strategies. Research
     methods training is best accomplished when students have an
     opportunity to observe researcher-models and then practice the
     observed behaviors. (178)

1732 Krawczyk, R.M. "Peer Participatory Conferences: A Dynamic
     Method of Nursing Instruction." J NURS EDUC 17(8) (October
     1978): 5-8.

     Student presentations of a brief patient case study applying
     a weekly focal concept to a patient under their care served
     to enhance the clinical learning of students in a community
     health center.(8)

1733 Kruse, L.C., C.W. Hahn, J.A. Barry and J.E. Gay. "Utilization
     of a Media Instructional Support Staff in the Development
     of a Simulated Learning Experience: Medication Adminis-
     tration," J NURS EDUC 17(8) (October 1978): 27-35.

     The use of a self-instructional simulated medication experi-
     ence provides students with the opportunity to integrate and
     utilize previously learned skills and knowledge in preparing
     medications for a group of patients prior to clinical prac-
     tice. This experience provided a risk free situation for
     learning. (15)

1734 Kuhn, J.K. and N.F. Fasano. "Benefits of an Independent Study
     Course," NURS HEALTH CARE 5(3) (March 1984): 150-54.

     A two-credit independent study course offered in the last
     quarter of the senior year of a baccalaureate program assisted
     students in transition from student to graduate role and en-
     couraged creative behaviors. (6)

1735 LaMancusa, M. and L. Robberson. "Nursing Homes for the Ini-
     tial Clinical Experience," J NURS EDUC 20(2) (February
     1981): 4-8.

     Overcrowded acute care facilities required use of nursing
     homes for initial clinical experiences at the University of
     Nevada. Through use of the campus skills laboratories and
     careful planning, this alternative proved most satisfactory in
     meeting course objectives. (7)

1736 Lehrer, S.S. "The Professional Patient Session as a Technique
     for Teaching the Gynecological Examination to Nurse Prac-
     titioner Students," J NURS EDUC 19(5) (May 1980): 39-47.

     An introduction to the professional patient program proved
     effective in developing interpersonal communication skills in
     nurse practitioner students. (22)

1737   Levinson, R.M. "The Potentials of Cross Cultural Field Study:
       Emory´s Comparative Health Care Systems Program in London,"
       J NURS EDUC 18(9) (November 1979): 46-52.

       A summer program is described which provided a study of
       comparative aspects of the health care systems in England and
       the United States. A six week program in London provided
       classroom and experiential components. Term papers indicated
       that students were able to apply sociological perspectives in
       a comparative view of health care. (19)

1738   Lopez, K.A. "Role Modeling Interpersonal Skills With Beginning
       Nursing Students: Gestalt Techniques," J NURS EDUC 22(3)
       (March 1983): 119-22.

       A Gestalt approach was used to assist students in inte-
       grating concepts of effective nurse-patient interaction.
       Structured clinical experience utilized the contact functions
       of communication as described within Gestalt Therapy. Teacher
       modeling was found an effective method of initiating learning.
       (8)

1739   Lord, A.A. and R. Palmer. "Teaching Psychiatric/Mental Health
       Nursing Via the Contract for Learning Activities," J NURS
       EDUC 21(4) (April 1982): 23-28.

       Presents information and examples of contract for learning
       activities within a psychiatric mental health course. Stu-
       dents indicated if course was required or elective and what
       grade level they chose to work toward. Students experienced
       decreased anxiety and greater control using the contract for
       learning approach. (0)

1740   Martens, K.H. "Self-Directed Learning: An Option for Nursing
       Education," NURS OUTLOOK 29(8) (August 1981): 472-77.

       The use of a self-directed learning approach as a cul-
       minating experience for RN students allows the student to
       build upon previous learning in an individual manner. Con-
       tracts are developed by the student and they engage in selec-
       ted experiences under preceptor and faculty supervision.(5)

1741   Mason, D.J. "Health Fair: Providing a Learning Experience
       Through A Community Service Project," J NURS EDUC 21(6)
       (June 1982): 39-47.

       Describes the planning, implementation, and evaluation of a
       community health fair for older adults in a New York City com-
       munity. This project replaced the traditional community
       health course and provided baccalaureate nursing students the
       opportunity to utilize problem-solving and decision-making on
       the community level. (8)

1742   McCarthy, N.C. and D. Brett. "Learning Primary Preventive
       Intervention in the Day Care Center," NURSE EDUC 4(3)
       (May/June 1979): 12-14.

A clinical course offered to junior students at Boston College utilizes a day care center for preschool children. Within this setting, students apply principles of health maintenance, assess the environment and clients and prepare a
health teaching project. (6)

1743 McGoram, S. "On Developing Empathy: Teaching Students Self-
Awareness," AM J NURS 78(5) (May 1978): 859-61.

By introspection, self-awareness, anxiety and self-develop-
ment students are able to better observe and assess patients
needs. A topical outline of a psychosocial nursing course is
presented which moves the student from self-awareness to effective nursing intervention. (2)

1744 McKay, S.R. "A Peer Group Counseling Model in Nursing Education," J NURS EDUC 19(3) (March 1980): 4-10.

Use of a peer counseling group consisting of senior nursing
students to assist junior nursing students is reported. The
purpose of the group was to provide a supportive and trusting
atmosphere for students to share their concerns and effectively problem solve. Although the junior students reported
some advantages to these sessions, the senior students con-
sistently commented on the contributions of the experience to
their personal development. (19)

1745 McKenzie, C.M. "Use of the Small Group Teaching Strategy in
Classroom Teaching for Diverse Nursing Students," J NURS
EDUC 22(9) (November 1983): 400-401.

An overview of the small group Teaching Strategy. Instructors should be aware of the dynamics involved in this instructional method and in what situations it may facilitate
learning. (13)

1746 Memmer, M.K. "Television Replay: A Tool for Students to Learn
to Evaluate Their Own Proficiency in Using Sterile Technique," J NURS EDUC 18(8) (October 1979): 35-42.

The use of videotaping simulated dressing changes proved
effective in teaching sterile technique. The advantages of
this approach are described. (0)

1747 Mezey, M. and D.N. Chiamulera. "Implementation of a Campus
Nursing and Health Information Center in the Baccalaureate
Curriculum, Part I," J NURS EDUC 19(5) (May 1980): 7-10.

Lack of clinical facilities for encountering individuals
needing health promotion, health maintenance, screening and
management, led the faculty at Lehman College to develop a
nursing clinic. The development of the center is described.
(6)

1748 Miller, T. "Too Much Institution--Too Little Learning: An
      Experience in Teaching Community Health Nursing," J NURS
      EDUC 21(4) (April 1982): 4-11.

      An experimental project undertaken at the University of
      Arizona utilized a problem solving approach to assist students
      in assessing a community. Such an approach provided a more
      meaningful experience as students learned to problem solve
      and be innovative in dealing with health care in a community.
      (0)

1749 Mitchell, C.A. and B. Krainovich. "Conducting Pre and Post
      Conferences," AM J NURS 82(5) (May 1982): 823-25.

      A discussion of the basic characteristics and strategies
      utilized in pre and post-clinical conferences. Assignments
      should build on past knowledge and skills, promote continuity
      and integration and facilitate thinking processes. (3)

1750 Mitchell, J.J. "The Use of Case Studies in Bioethics Course,"
      J NURS EDUC 20(9) (November 1981): 31-36.

      A case study approach was found beneficial in teaching bio-
      ethics as students became sensitized to the cases, applied
      carefully constructed methodologies in decision making and
      broadened their understanding of different philosophical and
      theoretical perspectives. (1)

1751 Morris, L., L.G. Hitchcock, J. Kucera and K. Vernon.
      "Student-made,Student-played Games,"AMJ NURS 80(10)
      (October 1980): 1816-18.

      Four board games are described to facilitate learning of
      nursing knowledge. The enlarged heart, acid-base balance,
      cardiovascular drug game, and the hormone game are briefly
      described. (0)

1752 Moyer, R.L. "Faculty Supervisory Conferences: Dynamic Role
      Model for Creative Teaching of Nursing Students," J NURS
      EDUC 17(3) (March 1978): 3-6.

      Describes the utilization of faculty supervisory conferences
      as a teaching-learning strategy. Within these conferences,
      faculty present case studies from their practice for discus-
      sion and review by colleagues and students. (4)

1753 Murray, L.M. "A Comparison of Lecture-Discussion and Self-
      Study Methods in Nursing Education," J NURS EDUC 21(9)
      (November 1982): 17-23.

      A comparison of self-study and lecture discussion teaching
      strategies revealed that students receiving lecture discussion
      performed better in post test than students who studied the
      material alone. (15)

1754   Mutzebaugh, C.A. and A.L. Mueller. "Nursing Homes for Student
       Learning," NURSE EDUC 3(1) (January/February 1978): 14-16.

       Clinical experiences in nursing homes were utilized and
       found beneficial in teaching developmental aspects of aging,
       rehabilitation in chronic illness and techniques of remoti-
       vation and reality orientation. Rich opportunities for
       student learning were found in a variety of extended care
       facilities. (3)

1755   Norman, K.A. "How To Increase Clinical Learning Opportunities
       in a Psychiatric Nursing Setting," J NURS EDUC 18(4) (April
       1979): 5-15.

       Methods are suggested to maximize clinical learning.
       Awareness of personal values assists the student in developing
       clinical behaviors. Critical thinking and problem-solving
       opportunities form the basis for nursing practice regardless
       of setting. (14)

1756   Paduano, M.A. "Bring About Learning in the College Labora-
       tory," J NURS EDUC 17(6) (June 1978): 30-33.

       Diminishing opportunities for traditional clinical place-
       ments led one faculty group to videotape children's behavior
       to provide observational experience in the normal growth and
       development of infants and toddlers. This method proved
       highly successful. (2)

1757   _____. "Introducing Independent Study Into the Nursing
       Curriculum," J NURS EDUC 18(4) (April 1979): 34-37.

       An experiment in offering independent study nursing courses
       to marginal or failing students proved a positive experience
       in personal and professional growth. Active involvement and
       lack of competition increased motivation, self confidence
       and enthusiasm. (5)

1758   Page, G.G. and P. Saunders. "Written Simulation in Nursing,"
       J NURS EDUC 17(4) (April 1978): 28-32.

       Problem solving is critical to the study of nursing and the
       nursing process. It can be taught effectively and without
       risk using written simulations. The creation of written
       simulations provides clinical teaching and evaluation
       experiences which may not occur in the clinical setting. (6)

1759   Patterson, R.J. "She's Not Clumsy, She's Left-Handed," NURSE
       EDUC 6(6) (November 1981): 36-37.

       Instructional modifications in the cognitive and fixation
       phases of psychomotor skill learning will facilitate learning
       for left-handed individuals. (8)

1760   Perry, S.E.   "Teaching Strategy and Learner Performance,"
       J NURS EDUC 18(1) (January 1979): 25-27.

       Knowledge of performance improves learning. An experience
       with mastery learning in which students were to take a pre-
       test, correct their own test, read a learning module, and
       take the post test demonstrated that too much knowledge, i.e.
       having the answers prior to reading the module, interfered
       with learning. (9)

1761   Petrowski, D.D.   "The Term Paper Revisited," J NURS EDUC 17(7)
       (September 1978): 50-52.

       The benefits of writing a term paper can be substantially
       increased if the teacher assists the students during develop-
       ment. Required preliminary outlines, deadlines for partially
       completed work during the course of the semester, and con-
       ferences are suggested as well as other measures that will
       improve both quality and learning. (4)

1762   Plasterer, H.H. and N. Mills. "Teach Management Theory-
       Through Fun and Games," J NURS EDUC 22(2) (February 1983):
       80-83.

       A simulated game offered toward the end of a management
       course provided a link between theory and practice. Through
       participation in the game, students engaged in cognitive,
       reflective and interpretive behaviors which assisted in crys-
       tallizing learning. A description of the game is provided.
       (5)

1763   Pletsch, P.K. and E. Benda. "Intrapartum Practicum in Nursing
       Curricula," J NURS EDUC 18(9) (November 1979): 26-29.

       A comparison was made of students knowledge in intrapartal
       nursing care following students participation in tutorial and
       observational experiences. No significant difference was
       found in the mean scores on post test of the two groups. (6)

1764   Ptasynski, E.M. and S.M. Silver. "Experience in Posology,"
       J NURS EDUC 20(8) (October 1981): 41-46.

       Faculty must decide when to introduce the study of dosage
       calculations and what are the most effective methods for
       introducing and integrating these concepts. Early curriculum
       intervention appeared to effect higher achievement and suf-
       ficient time for demonstration of acquired skills. The use
       of a self-learning module with small group sessions had a
       positive learning effect. (3)

1765   Reakes, J.C.   "Behavior Rehearsal Revisited: A Multi-faceted
       Tool for the Instructor," J NURS EDUC 18(2) (February 1979):
       48-51.

Role playing was utilized in an outpatient mental health
clinic to facilitate the learning of assertiveness and problem
solving. Students found the experience helpful in understanding the therapy aspects of groups with specific clients.
(4)

1766 Regan, J.H. "Teaching Crisis Creatively," NURSE EDUC 7(3)
      (May/June 1982): 18-20.

A crisis situation is presented to students in order to
teach crisis intervention in nursing practice. A surprise
announcement of devastating impact to the students provides
an opportunity for the examination of the physical and psychological impact of crisis. (0)

1767 Ryan-Merritt, M. "A Teaching Strategy for Evaluating Asser-
      tive Behavior Change," J NURS EDUC 21(9) (November 1982):
      13-16.

Students in an assertiveness training course assumed roles
of asserter and antagonist in a video role play prior to instruction. Later in the program students viewed the tapes
and described how they would change their behaviors based on
new learning. It was suggested that video taping of real
clinical situations might be more beneficial. A self critique
form is presented. (10)

1768 Rynerson, B.C. "Community Nursing--A Psychosocial Learning
      Experience," J NURS EDUC 20(1) (January 1981): 12-17.

An alternative experience combined psychiatric nursing and
community health nursing in home visits that focused on psycho
therapeutic interactions. The planning and benefits of this
experience which expanded students' understanding of cultural,
environmental and societal influences on health and health
services are described. (3)

1769 _____ "Using Video Tapes to Teach Therapeutic Interaction,"
      NURSE EDUC 5(5) (September/October 1980): 10-11.

A video taping process is used to assist students in
developing interpersonal and empathy skills prior to psycho-
therapeutic intervention with clients. Within a five minute
tape, students practice basic response modes which are then
reviewed and discussed by the instructor and students involved
in the tape. Individual conferences throughout the clinical
experience continue to explore and refine their response
modes. (7)

1770 Schalenberg, C. "Making and Using Slides," NURSE EDUC 4(4)
      (July/August 1979): 12-15.

Well-prepared slides enhance instructional presentations.
Suggestions are provided for the effective preparation and use
of slides. (14)

1771   Scheffer, B.   "An Innovative Placement in Mental Health for
        Baccalaureate Nursing Students," J NURS EDUC 20(4) (April
        1981): 33-39.

        Clinical placements of nursing students at Eastern Michigan
        University utilized adult foster care homes to teach nursing
        care of the chronic mentally ill. The experience was judged
        satisfactory in not only meeting student needs but also in
        providing services to the community. (4)

1772   Schleutermann, J.A., W.L. Holzemer and L.A. Farrand.   "An
        Evaluation of Paper-and-Pencil and Computer-Assisted Simula-
        tions," J NURS EDUC 22(8) (October 1983): 315-23.

        A study using latent-image and computer-assisted clinical
        simulations within a graduate family nurse practitioner pro-
        gram found students showed no preference for one system over
        another. Both simulations were well received. Problems in
        utilizing these formats were explored. (17)

1773   Schroy, I.J.   "TA: A Useful Tool in the Teaching-Learning
        Process," J NURS EDUC 18(1) (January 1979): 28-32.

        Discusses the use of transactional analysis in nursing
        education to promote better understanding of the teacher and
        student. Identifies the parts of the personality as Parent
        Ego, Adult Ego, and Child Ego and how they interact in the
        learning process. (21)

1774   Seidl, A.H. and S. Dresden.   "Gaming: A Strategy to Teach
        Conflict Resolution," J NURS EDUC 17(5) (May 1978): 21-28.

        A simulation experience provided students with an oppor-
        tunity to synthesize theory and behavior related to conflict
        resolution in a complex organizational problem. One 50
        minute classroom session was utilized and allowed application
        of concepts learned in the course. Four small groups assumed
        roles in four different conflict situations related to the
        school environment. Long term effects of the experience were
        noted. (10)

1775   Shamansky, S.L.   "Characteristics Contributing to Attachment
        Behavior and Its Outcomes in Student Nurse-Family Relation-
        ship," J NURS EDUC 20(2) (February 1981): 26-31.

        Attachment behavior occurs in the faculty-student relation-
        ship and in student-client relationships. By demonstrating
        empathy and mutually determined interdependence in faculty-
        student relations faculty can role model a similar relation-
        ship for students to emulate in student-client interventions.
        (10)

1776   Shumaker, D.   "Community Health Education for Senior
        Citizens," J NURS EDUC 20(1) (January 1981): 37-39.

A senior level course in a diploma program focused on role
function of the nurse and provided experience in health teaching in a community setting. A fifteen to twenty minute presentation was planned based on the needs of elderly clients
in the selected setting. Both students and clients benefited
from the experience. (0)

1777 Smallegan, M.J. "Teaching Through Groups," J NURS EDUC 21(1)
      (January 1982): 23-31.

      Differences between effective and ineffective use of the
      group teaching methodology are presented and discussed. (0)

1778 Smith, C.E. "Learning from Sensations," J NURS EDUC 19(2)
      (February 1980): 31-33.

      Describes teaching approaches which enable nurses to iden-
      tify and prevent sensory overload and sensory deprivation in
      patients. (14)

1779 Smith, I.K., F. Margolius and G.R. Ross. "Development and
      Validation of A Trigger Tape On Therapeutic Communication,"
      J NURS EDUC 21(4) (April 1982): 42-47.

      A trigger tape, "Therapeutic Versus Non-Therapeutic Communi-
      cation," consisting of six situations which simulate nurse-
      patient interaction was used to teach nursing students
      therapeutic communication. The tapes proved highly success-
      ful in teaching fundamental concepts and complex behavioral
      skills. Students observed, thought, asked questions, prac-
      ticed and contrasted therapeutic and non-therapeutic communi-
      cation. (9)

1780 Sommerfeld, D.P. and J.R. Hughes. "How Independent Should
      Independent Learning Be?," NURS OUTLOOK 28(7) (July 1980):
      416-20.

      A description of a course of independent study used to fos-
      ter critical thinking and problem solving in senior nursing
      students of a baccalaureate program. Student-teaching inter-
      actions and seminars were considered valuable adjuncts to
      independent study. (4)

1781 Soukup, M.C. "Reality Shock Alleviation: Student Experience
      in a Preceptored Advanced Clinical Nursing Practicum."
      NURSING ISSUES AND NURSING STRATEGIES FOR THE EIGHTIES.
      Edited by B. Bullough, V. Bullough and M.C. Soukup. New
      York: Springer Publishing Co., 1983, pp. 266-75.

      A culminating experience in a baccalaureate nursing program
      seeks to diminish reality shock in the new nurse graduate by
      providing a concentrated clinical exposure under a nurse pre-
      ceptor. Informal and formal evaluation indicate success of
      this model in meeting its stated objectives. (7)

1782   Sparks, S.M. and G.E. Mitchell. "The National Medical Audio-
       visual Center," J NURS EDUC 17(1) (January 1978): 29-34.

       The National Medical Audioviosual Center (NMAC) is a federal
       agency consisting of four branches, namely: the Education
       Research and Evaluation Branch; Educational and Consultation
       Branch; Materials Development Branch; and Materials Utilizaton
       Branch. The mission of each branch is described and their
       significance as a resource to nursing faculty proposed. (0)

1783   Sparks, S.M. and L.W. Kudrick. "AV Line: An Audiovisual
       Information Retrieval System," J NURS EDUC 18(7) (September
       1979): 47-53.

       A description of the development of AVLINE (Audio-visuals
       On-LINE) is presented. This computer retrieval program
       provides information regarding available instructional
       materials in nursing and health science. The AVLINE is use-
       ful to faculty in identifying and selecting audiovisual
       materials for instructional purposes. (0)

1784   Spratlen, L.P. "School-based Hypertension Screening As a
       Clinical Unit Experience for Nursing Students," J NURS EDUC
       22(9) (November 1983): 386-89.

       A school based screening program is described which provides
       an alternative non-traditional setting for clinical learning
       which allows nursing students to integrate, synthesize and
       utilize clinical knowledge and skills. The health maintenance
       focus fostered role identification as an independent and res-
       ponsible health professional. (5)

1785   Spruck, M. "An Approach to Analysis of a Symptom: An Educa-
       tional Experience," J NURS EDUC 19(7) (September 1980):
       45-48.

       An innovative method of teaching history taking is described
       in which student teams act as nurse and patient. A "chief
       complaint" is selected and explored prior to role-playing.
       A 15 to 20 minute session is taped and observed by fellow
       students. (2)

1786   Steiner, M.J. and S. Rothenberg. "Teaching Home Health Care
       With Videotapes," NURSE EDUC 5(4) (July/August 1980): 5-7.

       Ohio State University utilizes video taped home visits in
       conjunction with other instructional methods to prepare
       students to provide health care in the home. The contents of
       these video tapes include: interviewing and assessment;
       teaching self-care; management of the disabled; supervision
       of health care; and, interdisciplinary collaboration. Such
       programs can be used for preservice, inservice, continuing
       education, evaluation of nursing care, program development,
       consumer participation and patient education. (11)

1787 Stewart, P.H. "Utilizing Slides in the Learning Experience,"
      NURSE EDUC 6(4) (July/August 1981): 9-11.

      Well selected media can enhance and facilitate the learning
      process. Awareness of the advantages and disadvantages of
      slides is critical to selection. A pre-program check list is
      provided to assist faculty in utilizing slides. (10)

1788 Stoia, J.P. "Nursing Instruction: Can Data Base Searching
      Enhance the Practice? - A Guide to the Novice User," J NURS
      EDUC 22(2) (February 1983): 74-79.

      MEDLINE and ERIC are two data bases which are useful though
      seldom used by nursing faculty for purposes of developing and
      improving instruction. There is little duplication between
      the two. MEDLINE contains bibliographic data from nursing and
      nursing education journals while ERIC consists mostly of
      educational reports, projects, research and unpublished papers.
      (5)

1789 Strauser, C.J. "An Internship With Academic Credit," AM J
      NURS 79(6) (June 1979): 1070-72.

      An internship program at the University of Florida College
      of Nursing and the Gainesville Veterans Administration Hos-
      pital provides new graduates a combined education-service
      program to help in the development of leadership skills and
      expertise in a selected area of nursing practice. This nine
      month program allows the intern to earn 12 academic credits
      which may be applied to a Master's Degree. Participants are
      under no obligation to continue employment at the VA following
      completion of the program. (0)

1790 Stuart-Siddall, S. "Backwoods Nursing," NURSE EDUC 6(3)
      (May/June 1981): 14-17.

      A Rural Clinical Nurse Placement Center supported by Cali-
      fornia State University provided a six week clinical exper-
      ience in a very rural to semi-rural area in Northeastern Cali-
      fornia. Registered nurse students from accredited schools of
      nursing across the State of California were recruited during
      their senior year. This experience showed some success in
      increasing the number of nurses working in rural areas. (0)

1791 Swanson, E.A. and C.W. Dalsing. "Independent Study: A Cur-
      riculum Expander," J NURS EDUC 19(9) (November 1980): 11-15.

      An independent study is described which involved the conduc-
      ting of a research project on nurse midwives in a foreign
      country. The personal and professional experiences of
      student and instructor are described. (17)

1792 Tarnow, K.G. "Working With Adult Learners," NURSE EDUC 4(5)
      (September/October 1979): 34-40.

Adults are goal directed learners who prefer problem-solving rather than subject centered approaches. The characteristics and learning style of the adult require a rethinking of the teaching-learning process. Effective methods are explored based on characteristics of the learning process and adult learning principles. (13)

1793 Tarpey, K.S. and S.P. Chen. "Team Teaching: Is It For You?," J NURS EDUC 17(2) (February 1978): 36-39.

In a time when faculty are pressured by increasing demands for updated professional knowledge and skills, team teaching may provide an answer. The advantages to faculty and learner are explored. (1)

1794 Taubenheim, A.M. "Integrating Maternity Content Through a Health Promotion," J NURS EDUC 22(9) (November 1983): 389-91.

"Preparation for Parenthood" classes at a nursing center provided the opportunity for nursing students to gain skills in lesson planning, teaching, utilizing resources and using group dynamics. (0)

1795 Taylor, S.W., M.S. Brodish and H.W. Brown. "Creative Learning Experiences for Student Nurses," J NURS EDUC 18(4) (April 1979): 16-18.

Students working with pregnant adolescents expressed cultural shock. (3)

1796 Tilden, V.P. and L. Gustafson. "Termination in the Student-Patient Relationship: Use of a Teaching Tool," J NURS EDUC 18(8) (October 1979): 9-13.

An experiential exercise is presented which was used to assist nursing students in terminating professional relationships in a therapeutic manner.(6)

1797 Ulione, M.S. "Simulation Gaming in Nursing Education," J NURS EDUC 22(8) (October 1983): 349-51.

Games used for instructional purposes are classified as either content games or process games. Both have a place in nursing education and can benefit students' motivation, cognitive learning, and affective learning. Content games impart information and process games promote problem solving ability. A proper fit between the games and the educational objectives is essential. (5)

1798 Valentine, N.M. and Y. Saito. "Video Taping is a Viable Teaching Strategy in Nursing Education," NURSE EDUC 5(4) (July/August 1980): 9-17.

Boston State College uses a systematic approach to the
selection, development and use of video tapes to support instruction. A variety of equipment is described and illustrated. Criteria for evaluation consider content, quality and
existing resources. (14)

1799 Vogt, R.B. "Enhancing Students' Experience Through The Use of
      Tape Recordings," J NURS EDUC 19(4) (April 1980): 51-53.

The use of tape recording in lieu of written care plans
proved a more effective learning experience. Students selected patients based on their learning needs, visited patients,
read charts, and thoroughly researched health problems prior
to taping. (0)

1800 Walters, C.R. "Using Staff Preceptors in a Senior Experience,"
      NURS OUTLOOK 29(4) (April 1981): 245-47.

A senior baccalaureate nursing course allows students to use
a rural hospital for clinical experiences to prepare for
transition into the graduate role. A faculty member travels
with the students and is on call in the hospital where they
practice under preceptor supervision. (3)

1801 Weisensee, M.G. "Education of the Nursing Students for Better
      Collaboration of Client, Nurse and Physician," J NURS EDUC
      17(1) (January 1978): 8-14.

A faculty member describes her experiences in an extended
care role in an internist's office. The needs for students to
gain experience in meeting the informational needs of clients
in regard to health maintenance is stressed. (9)

1802 Welborn, P. and D. Thompson. "Strategies for Dealing with
      Students Whose Clinical Performance is Unsatisfactory," J
      NURS EDUC 21(5) (May 1982): 26-30.

Clinical evaluation involves four phases: problem identification, data collection and supervising the student, discussing the problem with the student and resolving the
situation. Dealing with unsatisfactory student performance
is a difficult task, however, a planned strategy can lessen
the stress. (0)

1803 Welch, L.B. "Team Teaching: Is It Effective?" NURS FORUM
      28(4) (1979): 394-404.

Experience with team teaching at Western Connecticut State
College was viewed as a logical extension of the integrated
curriculum. Various areas of expertise are represented and
faculty share areas of strength with their colleagues. Faculty
cliques and confusion in messages to students were noted as
problem areas. (0)

1804 Wessell, Sr. M.L. "Learning About Interdisciplinary Collabor-
      ation," J NURS EDUC 20(3) (March 1981): 39-44.

In order to foster an understanding of the interdisciplinary
nature of health care delivery in acute care settings, an
experience was provided for students to spend a clinical day
with a health professional other than nursing. Students
selected individuals who after the day's experience agreed to
participate in an interdisciplinary seminar. This experience
was judged successful in helping students define the nature
of different health professions and methods to communicate in
nursing practice. (31)

1805 Wutchous, S.M., H.I. Thurston and M.C. Carter. "The Nurse
Educator and The Adult Dialysis Patient," NURS FORUM 19(1)
(1980): 68-83.

A pilot study used program instruction to teach dialysis
patients about renal failure. An evaluation of the project
indicated successful teaching and patient satisfaction. (25)

1806 Yeaw, E.M.J. "Problem Solving as a Method of Teaching Strategies in Classroom and Clinical Teaching," J NURS EDUC
18(7) (September 1979): 16-22.

A three part article examines research findings which
identify the characteristics of successful and unsuccessful
problem solvers, the teaching principles which facilitate use
of the problem solving approach in classroom teaching and
utilization of the problem solving approach in clinical
teaching. (9)

See 1034.

Evaluation

1807 Behm, R.J. and F.N. Warnock. "State Board Examinations and
Associate Degree Program Effectiveness," NURS RES 27(1)
(January/February 1978): 54-56.

A study conducted in Washington State sought to correlate
state board examination results with program effectiveness.
A small positive relationship was found. (10)

1808 Bell, D.F. "Assessing Educational Needs: Advantages and Disadvantages of Eighteen Techniques," NURSE EDUC 3(5) (Septem-
ber/October 1978): 15-21.

Data gathered from society, the organization and the
individual provides useful information for needs assessment
prior to planning educational programs. Eighteen techniques
for assessing needs are provided and analyzed and guidelines
for conducting a written survey are presented. (12)

1809 Bell, D.F. and D.L. Bell. "Effective Evaluations," NURSE EDUC
4(6) (November/December 1979): 6-15.

Provides definitions, descriptions, examples, and differences
between formative and summative evaluation. Use of both
components in determining program effects is necessary and
consistency in the process is necessary. (16)

1810   Benner, R.V. and P. Benner. "Follow Through Evaluation: A
       Resource for Curriculum Planning and Development," NURSE
       EDUC 4(5) (September/October 1979): 16-21.

Three levels of evaluation of program graduates arc described which lend input into the degree of success attained
in preparing students for nursing practice. Information
regarding employability, job stability, utilization, career
patterns, and professional contributions is useful in curricular decision making. (8)

1811   Bondy, K.N. "Criterion--Referenced Definitions for Rating
       Scales in Clinical Evaluation," J NURS EDUC 22(9) (November
       1983): 376-82.

A five point rating scale interfaced with labels and their
definitions is offered as a framework for clinical evaluation
of nursing students. Clinical behaviors and criteria for
competency may be applied to any professional behavior.
Diagnostic feedback is provided. (6)

1812   Breyer, F.J. "Setting Passing Scores," NURS HEALTH CARE 4(9)
       (November 1983): 518-22.

A pilot procedure is proposed which might be utilized in
setting a passing score on tests used to differentiate
examinees on a pass-fail basis.(13)

1813   "California Board Studies SBTP Exam for ´Adverse Impact´," AM
       J NURS 81(3) (March 1981): 460,462.

California´s Department for Consumer Affairs noted the
negative impact of the State Board Test Pool Examination on
minority, foreign-born, and other groups. The examination is
being reviewed for occupational relevance. (0)

1814   Camooso, C., M. Greene and P. Reilly. "Students Adaptation
       According to Roy," NURS OUTLOOK 29(2) (February 1981):
       108-9.

Three former graduate students relate their role adjustment
to Roy´s Adaptation Model. Role function, self concept,
independence and physiological adaptation are described in the
evolving role change. Support of faculty and peers was
judged critical to the change process. (5)

1815   Clark, T., M. Goodwin, M. Mariani, M.J. Marshall and S. Moore.
       "Curriculum Evaluation: An Application of Stufflebeams´
       Model in a Baccalaureate School of Nursing," J NURS EDUC
       22(2) (February 1983): 54-58.

This article presents a description of Stufflebeams'decision
making process. The process consists of four steps: context,
input, process and product evaluations. In the context
evaluation step, planning and objective decisions are made.
In the input evaluation step, structuring decisions are made.
Process evaluation determines implementing strategies, and
product evaluation determines recycling decisons: The
Catholic University of America used Stufflebeams'model to
evaluate their current program and made recommendations concerning its use. (4)

1816   Curran, C.L. and A.E. Mattis. "Construction of a Reliable
       Instrument to Measure Attitudes," NURSE EDUC 3(6) (November/
       December 1978): 6-8.

       Attitudes may be measured through direct questioning, direct
       observation, or use of an attitude scale. Six steps are de-
       scribed in constructing an attitude scale. An illustration of
       attitude scale construction is provided. (5)

1817   Dachelet, C.Z. "The Critical Incident Technique Applied to
       the Evaluation of the Clinical Practicum Setting," J NURS
       EDUC 20(8) (October 1981): 15-31.

       A study was conducted to evaluate the specific characteris-
       tics of clinical settings and the preceptor-student inter-
       actions using a critical incident technique. The strengths
       and weaknesses of the technique are discussed. (5)

1818   Dean, N.R. "Effect of Free Time the Day Prior to Mastery
       Testing on Nursing Students' Scores," NURS RES 28(1) (Jan-
       uary/February 1979): 40-42.

       In response to student requests for free time the day pre-
       ceding the examination for purposes of study, a study was
       conducted to measure the effects on test outcomes. No signi-
       ficant differences were found in test results between students
       who engaged in clinical learning activities and those who
       were free to study the day prior to the examination. (4)

1819   Dean, P.R. and T.A. Edwards. "A Multidimensional Approach to
       Evaluation," J NURS EDUC 21(2) (February 1982): 18-23.

       A Curriculum of Attainments Program at Florida State Univer-
       sity utilized a multidimensional evaluation process known as
       the jury evaluation. Each jury was composed of specialists
       in nursing practice as well as faculty and assessed the
       attainment of terminal competencies on an individual basis.
       Future plans include mobilizing this process for purposes of
       evaluating registered nurses across the State of Florida. (2)

1820   Demetrulias, D. and L. McCubbin. "Constructing Test Questions
       for Higher Level Thinking," NURSE EDUC 7(5) (Autumn 1982):
       13-17.

By examining objectives, teaching strategies and measurement
instruments, nurse educators can consciously control the
difficulty level of test items and ensure balance of questions
between lower and higher order thinking. Examples of test
items are provided for each of Bloom's cognitive levels. (13)

1821   Dodd, M.J. "A Longitudinal Study in The Use of Credit/No
       Credit for Grading of Clinical Courses," J NURS EDUC 17(3)
       (March 1979): 14-21.

       A study of utilizing credit/no credit grading over satis-
       factory/unsatisfactory grading provided information regarding
       the advantages and disadvantages as perceived by faculty and
       students. (12)

1822   Fowler, G. and B. Heater. "Guidelines for Clinical Evalua-
       tion," J NURS EDUC 22(9) (November 1983): 402-4.

       A discussion of the issues surrounding clinical evaluation
       and the presentation of guidelines which may prevent legal
       actions. Academic requirements for graduation and standards
       for student performance evaluation should be clearly stated.
       Students should be informed of unsatisfactory performance
       before a dismissal process is initiated. (14)

1823   Gennaro, S., P. Thielen, N. Chapman, J. Martin and D.C.
       Barnett. "The Birth, Life and Times of a Clinical Evalua-
       tion Tool," NURSE EDUC 7(1) (January/February 1982): 27-32.

       Subjectivity and lack of consistency in clinical performance
       evaluations led a group of faculty to develop a new clinical
       evaluation tool. Although improvement was noted, further work
       in increasing objectivity, improving inter-rater reliability
       and attending to discrepancies between clinical and theoretical
       knowledge was found warranted. (7)

1824   Gould, E.O. "Satisfactory/Unsatisfactory Grading in the
       Evaluation of Clinical Performance in Nursing: Its Effect
       on Student Motivation as Perceived by Nursing Students," J
       NURS EDUC 17(8) (October 1978): 36-47.

       A study of senior nursing students found no significant
       difference in motivation in students who are graded with a
       satisfactory/unsatisfactory system and those who are graded
       with a letter grade in clinical evaluations as perceived by
       students. Statistical evidence was found which indicated
       higher levels of motivation under satisfactory/unsatisfactory
       grading as perceived by the sample group. (59)

1825   Gustafson, D.D. "Student Peer Evaluation: A Successful Adap-
       tation for Observed Home Visits," J NURS EDUC 19(2)
       (February 1980): 4-7.

Utilization of a faculty-student evaluation team for home
visits in a community health experience was well received by
students and introduced them to the peer review process they
would encounter following graduation. (4)

1826   Hassell, J., C.E. Davis and V. Larson. "Evaluation by Objec-
       tives: Teaching Students to Evaluate Faculty," NURS FORUM
       21(1) (1984): 15-18.

       Proposes a criterion-referenced instrument for students
       evaluation of teacher effectiveness. Such an instrument is
       more valid, reliable and objective than norm-referenced
       instruments. (11)

1827   Hautman, M.A. "Assessment: One Factor in Effective Client
       Teaching," NURS FORUM 28(4) (1979): 405-14.

       Determining patients' readiness to learn, level of communi-
       cation and reading level are essential prior to initiating
       patient teaching. The success of the teaching effort relies
       on understanding the physical and psychological status of the
       patient. (8)

1828   Hitchens, E.W. "Evaluation: The Griffiti Technique," J NURS
       EDUC 18(3) (March 1979): 46-47.

       A Graffiti technique used in course evaluation proved helpful
       in promoting open discussion of class behavior problems. (2)

1829   Huckabay, L.M. "Cognitive and Affective Consequences of For-
       mative Evaluation in Graduate Nursing Students," NURS RES
       27(3) (May/June 1978): 190-94.

       An experimental study using formative evaluation demon-
       strated that students cognitive and affective development was
       significantly greater than in the control group. (20)

1830   _____. "Cognitive-Affective Consequences of Grading
       Versus Nongrading of Formative Evaluations," NURS RES 28(3)
       (May/June 1979): 173-78.

       In comparing groups of students taught by means of forma-
       tive evaluation with grades, formative evaluation without
       grades, and lecture discussion, the group taught by formative
       evaluation without grades scored highest on the amount of
       cognitive learning. There were no significant differences
       among groups in affective behavior.(23)

1831   Jacobs, A.M., G. Fivars and R. Fitzpatrick. "What The New
       Test Will Test," AM J NURS 82(4) (April 1982): 625-28.

       Describes the development of test items for the new State
       Board Test Pool Examination using the critical incident tech-
       nique. (11)

1832   King, E.C. "Constructing Classroom Achievement Tests," NURSE
       EDUC 3(5) (September/October 1978): 30-36.

       The process of constructing classroom achievement tests
       requires the defining of objectives, construction of a table
       of specifications, writing test items and writing test direc-
       tions. Examples are provided to assist nursing instructors
       build better teacher-made tests. (6)

1833   _____. "Determining and Interpreting Test Validity,
       Reliability, and Practicality," NURSE EDUC 4(3) (May/June
       1979): 6-11.

       Provides information regarding selection and development of
       tests, interpreting test results, and utilizing test results
       to make informed decisions regarding the educational process.
       (10)

1834   Kirchhoff, K.T. and W.L. Holzemer. "Student Learning and A
       Computer Assisted Instructional Program," J NURS EDUC 18(3)
       (March 1979): 22-30.

       A study measuring the effectiveness of a computer assisted
       instructional program found that students perception of the
       degree of dullness of learning on the computer was the highest
       predictor and inversely related to learning. (13)

1835   Koehler, M.L. "Evaluating a Curriculum," J NURS EDUC 21(1)
       (January 1982): 32-39.

       A major curriculum change at California State University at
       Long Beach was evaluated using faculty and student perceptions
       and state board results. These evaluations revealed serious
       shortcomings not the least of which was an increased failure
       rate on state board examinations.(3)

1836   Kruse, L.C. and D.M. Fager. "Development and Implementation
       of a Contract Grading System," J NURS EDUC 21(5) (May 1982):
       31-37.

       A grade contract was used at the University of Iowa School
       of Nursing in a final core course. It was felt that such a
       system enhanced the sharing of learning experiences and know-
       ledge gained and increased students' self-direction and
       creativity.(10)

1837   Lee, L.A. "An Investigation of the Effects of Clinical Experi-
       ence on Cognitive Gains," J NURS EDUC 18(7) (September 1979):
       27-37.

       A comparative study of sophomore nursing students found sig-
       nificant differences in test results of high achievement versus
       low achievement students. Clinical experiences following
       classroom theory presentations had no significant effect on
       student performance on teacher constructed tests. (26)

1838   Loustav, A., M. Lentz, K. Lee, M. McKenna, S. Hirako, W.F.
       Walker, and J.W. Goldsmith. "Evaluating Students´ Clinical
       Performance: Using Videotape to Establish Rater Reliability,"
       J NURS EDUC 19(7) (September 1980): 10-17.

       A study demonstrated that training sessions using a student-
       patient videotaped situation improved rater reliability in
       clinical evaluation. The training sessions changed rating
       scores of younger faculty more than that of experienced fac-
       ulty. (9)

1839   MacAvoy, S. and L.B. Welch. "Tips on Test Construction," J
       NURS EDUC 20(3) (March 1981): 15-19.

       Provides suggestions for test construction identifying
       referencing, entering behaviors, preparing objectives, level-
       ing and item selections. (7)

1840   Marriner, A., T. Langford and L.D. Goodwin. "Curriculum
       Evaluation: Word Fact, Ritual, or Reality," NURS OUTLOOK
       28(4) (April 1980): 228-32.

       Too often evaluation efforts in schools of nursing fail to
       provide and be used for reality checks. The Stake Countenance
       Model is applied to an undergraduate nursing program and pro-
       vides a comprehensive evaluation model by which to judge pro-
       gram strengths and deficiencies. (3)

1841   Melcolm, N., R. Venn and R.B. Bausell. "The Prediction of
       State Board Test Pool Examinations Scores Within an Inte-
       grated Curriculum," J NURS EDUC 20(5) (May 1981): 24-28.

       A study of multiple variables and criteria for prediction
       of success on state board examinations revealed NLN Achievement
       Test scores are significant predictors and are constant across
       curricula and time in predicting student success on state
       board examinations. (9)

1842   Monninger, E. and J.T. Fullerton. "Establishing Standards
       for Clinical Preparation," NURS OUTLOOK 32(1) (January/
       February 1984): 28-33.

       A tool is provided which was used to collect information
       relevant to the clinical experiences of nurse practitioner
       students. A profile of patient population in practice sites
       was sought as well as knowledge regarding practice skills,
       independence of decison making and the relationship of clinical
       experience to course objectives. (0)

1843   Murphy, S.A. "Improving Teacher-Made Tests in an Integrated
       Curriculum," J NURS EDUC 18(9) (November 1979): 41-45.

       A project undertaken to improve teacher-made tests is des-
       cribed. Following the establishment of a theoretical frame-
       work, a plan of action was developed. Dialogues were arranged
       to gain faculty consensus on the value of testing. Inservice

programs on theories of evaluation and measurement and principles of item writing were presented in eight bimonthly
sessions. Evaluation of subsequent test items indicated
improved techniques.(11)

1844   Nelson, L.F. "Competence of Nursing Graduates in Technical,
       Communicative, and Administrative Skills," NURS RES 27(2)
       (March/April 1978): 121-25.

       Graduates of diploma, associate degree, and baccalaureate
       nursing programs rated their competency in technical, communi-
       cative and administrative skills and these ratings were com-
       pared to those provided by their immediate supervisors. (16)

1845   Olivieri, P. and M.A. Sweeney. "Evaluation of Clinical Learn-
       ing: By Computer," NURSE EDUC 5(4) (July/August 1980):
       26-31.

       A computer system offers a relatively inexpensive method by
       which faculty can learn about the clinical expertise of stu-
       dents and compare responses between students. Numerous advan-
       tages are described and examples provided. (4)

1846   Overstreet, L.P. "A Study of the Efficacy of Reinforcement
       Courses for Graduate Nurses on Success in Passing the State
       Board Test Pool Examination in Georgia," J NURS EDUC 22(1)
       (January 1983): 28-31.

       Within the State of Georgia, candidates failing State Board
       Examinations for the second time are required to take a rein-
       forcement course. A variety of reinforcement courses were
       offered and the authors undertook a study to determine if one
       course was more effective than others. No significant differ-
       ences were found. All reinforcement courses substantially
       raised the passing scores. Reinforcement or review courses
       prior to the first examination were recommended. (3)

1847   Portes, K.K. and C.M. Feller. "The Relationship Between
       Patterns of Massed and Distributive Clinical Practicum and
       Student Achievement," J NURS EDUC 18(8) (October 1979):
       27-34.

       A study of massed versus distributive clinical learning ex-
       periences demonstrated that advantages and disadvantages are
       present in both. Long term distributive experiences resulted
       in more enduring learning and were found appropriate for com-
       munity health nursing. Massed, concentrated learning increased
       students' ability to apply theory to medical-surgical patient
       care and appeared most appropriate for hospital settings. (5)

1848   Roy, A.L. "The Placement Process," NURSE EDUC 4(1) (January/
       February 1979): 14-18.

       A method of evaluation and placement of registered nurse
       students in an integrated baccalaureate curriculum is described.
       Within this approach instruction is individualized to adult

students without sacrifice of program objectives and philosophy.
Disadvantages were noted in terms of time expended and risk.
(3)

1849   Schoolcraft, V. and C. Delaney. "Contract Grading in Clinical
        Evaluation," J NURS EDUC 21(1) (January 1982): 6-14.

        In order to decrease subjectivity in clinical grading, one
baccalaureate nursing program adopted a contract system between
faculty member and student. Each grade level has specific
criteria which increases the consistency of grading and indi-
vidualizes the learning process. (3)

1850   Shaffer, M.K. and I.L. Pfeiffer. "Home Visit: A Gray Zone in
        Evaluation," AM J NURS 78(2) (February 1978): 239-41.

        Faculty at the University of Akron designed an evaluation
tool to be used in assessing independent home visits of senior
nursing students. The model focuses on students' abilities to
recognize their own strengths and weaknesses. An evaluation
graph is used and students and teachers cooperatively plan
remediation. (6)

1851   Smania, M.A., M.G. McClelland and J.C. McCloskey. "And Still
        Another Look at Clinical Grading: Minimal Behaviors," NURSE
        EDUC 3(3) (May/June 1978): 6-9.

        An attempt by new faculty to design a more objective clinical
evaluation instrument utilized a system of identified and
refined minimal behaviors. The process and product of faculty
growth in developing this project are described. (0)

1852   Smith, M.C. "Evaluation of a Master's Program by Graduates
        and Their Employers," J NURS EDUC 19(9) (November 1980):
        4-10.

        A survey of graduates and employers of graduates of the
University of Southern Mississippi master's program sought
information regarding the effectiveness of the curriculum in
preparing for practice. For the most part the curriculum was
judged effective. Leadership was identified as an area of
weakness and curriculum revision initiated. (4)

1853   Stamper, J., C. Huerta and J. Maville. "Evaluating for Ac-
        creditation: A Structural Approach," J NURS EDUC 22(2)
        (February 1983): 67-69.

        Three tools are presented which were used to provide a cur-
riculum evaluation framework in conjunction with a self study
report of an associate degree program. The conceptual framework, major threads and course objectives were identified and
relationships shown. (2)

1854   Stanton, M.P. "Objective Test Construction--A Must for
        Nursing Educators," J NURS EDUC 22 (8) (October 1983): 338-
        39.

Guidelines are presented for the construction of completion, true-false, matching, and multiple choice test items. (4)

1855   Stecchi, J.M., S.J. Woltman, C. Wall-Haas, B. Heggestad and M. Zier. "Comprehensive Approach to Clinical Education: One Teaching Team's Solution to Clinical Evaluation of Students in Multiple Settings," J NURS EDUC 22(1) (January 1983): 38-46.

A comprehensive clinical evaluation tool is presented which measures student achievement through the junior year coursework. This tool assisted in clarifying faculty and curriculum expectations and students assumed more responsibility for their learning. (0)

1856   Stein, R.F. "The Graduate Record Examination: Does It Predict Performance in Nursing Programs?" NURSE EDUC 3(4) (July/ August 1978): 16-19.

A study of the predictive value of Graduate Record Examination (GRE) scores on performance in graduate nursing programs, found GRE verbal scores were not significantly correlated with total graduate Grade Point Average (GPA). GRE quantitative scores were moderately predictive of graduate study performance. Other tests were recommended to more accurately assess readiness. (1)

1857   Sweeney, M.A., M. O'Malley and E. Freeman. "Development of a Computer Simulation," J NURS EDUC 21(9) (November 1982): 28-38.

Describes the development of a computerized test to evaluate nursing students' clinical competencies. Examples are given and problems with such a format explored. (6)

1858   Waltz, C.F. and W.C. McGurn. "An Approach to the Assessment of Programs in Nursing Education," NURS HEALTH CARE 4(10) (December 1983): 576-82.

The increased demand for evaluation of nursing programs requires a comprehensive evaluation framework for schools of nursing. Data collected relevant to attainment of program goals serve a variety of audiences from which decision making emanates. (4)

1859   Westwick, C.R. "Culture-Fair Testing," J NURS EDUC 17(1) (January 1978): 35-39.

Individuals develop different ways of thinking about the world based on cultural experiences. Attempts should be made in testing to remove cultural bias and promote better interpretation of test scores. (9)

1860   Williams, M.L. "Effects of Clinical Setting on Anxiety and Achievement in Psychiatric Nursing Education," J NURS EDUC 18(2) (February 1979): 4-14.

A study of second year students in a community college
associate degree program found the clinical practicum setting
in psychiatric nursing had an effect on the level of anxiety
at the time of the initial assignment. Anxiety levels decreased at the end of the course. Significant correlations
were found between anxiety levels and achievement as demonstrated on the NLN achievement tests. (16)

1861 Wolfle, L.M. and L.W. Bryant. "A Causal Model of Nursing
      Education and State Board Examination Scores," NURS RES
      27(5) (September/October 1978): 311-15.

      A study of 121 graduates of an associate degree nursing
      program sought to determine the relationship between perfor-
      mance on NLN achievement tests and State Board Examinations.
      It was found that the NLN scores proved good predictors of
      SBE scores in the areas of medical, surgical and obstetrical
      examinations but not good predictors of pediatric and psychi-
      atric areas.
      Ability and overall academic record were also found to be
      important predictors of both SBE performance and NLN perfor-
      mance. (19)

      See 987, 1181, 1209, 1273, 1358, 1447, 1521, 1537.

Entry Into Practice

1862 "Alabama Nurses Take Positions On Entry, Employment Standards,
      CE," AM J NURS 80(2) (February 1980): 198.

      The BSN degree as required for entry into professional
      nursing practice was endorsed by the House of Delegates of
      the Alabama State Nurses Association and a study is underway
      to plan implementation. Legislation is being sought to re-
      quire continuing education for relicensure. A set of Recom-
      mended Employment Standards for Registered Nurses in employing
      agencies was passed. (0)

1863 American Nurses' Association. "First Position on Education
      for Nursing," AM J NURS 65 (December 1965): 106-11.

      The American Nurses' Association's position on nursing
      education argues that: education preparatory to licensing
      for the practice of nursing should be conducted in institu-
      tions of higher education. Preparations for beginning profes-
      sional nursing practice should be within baccalaureate degree
      in nursing programs and preparation for technical nursing
      practice should be within associate degree nursing programs.
      Assistants who provide health services should be prepared
      through short, intensive programs within vocational institu-
      tions.
      Historical development of nursing and nursing education is
      used to support these positions. (0)

1864 _____ EDUCATION FOR NURSING PRACTICE IN THE CONTEXT OF
THE 1980's. Kansas City, MO.: American Nurses' Association,
1983.

Confirms the ANA's position on educational preparation for
nursing practice with the baccalaureate degree as the minimum
requirement for professional nursing practice and the
associate degree as the minimum requirement for technical
nursing practice. Grandfathering of currently registered
nurses is supported.

1865 "ANA Commission Schedules Briefing on Entry Issues," AM J NURS
80(2) (February 1980): 198.

Recommendations from national and state forums will be presented at a briefing planned by the ANA Commission on Nursing
Education. Reports on career mobility, titles and entry level
competencies for two categories of nurses will be discussed as
they relate to entry into practice. (0)

1866 Anderson, N.E. "The Historical Development of American
Nursing Education," J NURS EDUC 20(1) (January 1981): 18-36.

Reviews the evolution of nursing education in respect to the
current focus on baccalaureate education as a requirement for
entry into professional nursing practice. (39)

1867 "BSN Exam Plan Sparks Maryland Debate Over Entry," AM J NURS
83(8) (August 1983): 1119, 1208, 1209.

Maryland's Governor ordered the Board of Nursing to develop
a certification examination for BSN graduates. The Maryland
Association of Associate Degree Directors saw this action as
preceding legislative or executive action concerning entry
level. The impact of such an action on associate degree
programs is explored. (0)

1868 Buckeye State Nurses Association. "The Entry Into Practice
Issue." NURSING ISSUES AND NURSING STRATEGIES FOR THE
EIGHTIES. Edited by B. Bullough, V. Bullough and M.C.
Soukup. New York: Springer Publishing Co., 1983, pp. 197-
204.

Argues that there is insufficient data to demonstrate that
graduates of baccalaureate degree programs render better
nursing care than diploma graduates. Ohio lacks a responsible
statewide plan to insure a sufficient number of baccalaureate
degree programs to meet the health needs of the state. Based
on these facts, the Buckeye State Nurses Association supports
the current practice that ADN, diploma and baccalaureate programs prepare graduates for basic registered nurse practice
and opposes legislation which limits licensure of registered
nurses to baccalaureate program graduates. Furthermore, they
reject the professional/technical dichotomy and support programs which vary in length, level of complexity, degree of
responsibility, and area of practice. (32)

1869   Bullough, B.   "The Entry Into Practice Resolution," PED NURS
        (September/October 1979): 25-28.

        Examines the entry into practice resolutions in an histori-
        cal and political context. Discusses variations and conflicts
        in interpretation of entry into practice resolutions. Such
        concerns as who will be designated registered nurse, career
        ladder needs and provision for "grandfathering" are explored.
        Arguments for and against passage are presented. (12)

1870   Christy, T.E.   "Entry Into Practice: A Recurring Issue in
        Nursing History," AM J NURS 80(3) (March 1980): 485-88.

        Recounts the problems of differentiating levels of nursing
        education by title at the turn of the century and compares
        current problems which appear similar. Discusses the need for
        clarification and the impediments grandfathering will per-
        petuate in terms of levels of practice and titling. (15)

1871   "CNA Supports Baccalaureate for Entry With Push for Increase
        in Available Programs," AM J NURS 79(5) (May 1979): 838,
        845.

        The California Nurses Association supports the baccalaureate
        degree in nursing for entry into professional nursing practice
        but will not move to require this until accessibility of pro-
        grams is assured. Aggressive action is supported to increase
        the numbers of baccalaureate programs in the state. (0)

1872   "Concept of Grandfather Clause Explained in Background Paper,"
        AM J NURS 79(10) (October 1979): 1694, 1696-98.

        A review and discussion of the legislative actions involved
        in grandfathering. The requirement of the BS(N) for entry
        into professional nursing practice intends to grandfather
        practicing nurses. Theoretically it is attractive, however,
        practically it is not likely to occur. (0)

1873   "Degree Timetable Set for Indiana RNs," AM J NURS 80(1) (Jan-
        uary 1980): 28.

        The House of Delegates of the Indiana State Nurses Associa-
        tion mandated the development of a timetable for the require-
        ment of the baccalaureate degree in nursing for entry into
        professional nursing practice. All currently licensed nurses
        will be grandfathered within the timetable. (0)

1874   "Diploma Schools Fight N. J. Board Over Rule Change," AM J
        NURS 83(3) (March 1983): 343, 455.

        Describes the resistance to institution of the baccalaureate
        in nursing degree requirement for entry into professional
        nursing practice in the State of New Jersey. (0)

1875 Fondiller, S.H. THE ENTRY DILEMMA: THE NATIONAL LEAGUE FOR
      NURSING AND THE HIGHER EDUCATION DEPARTMENT, 1952-1972 WITH
      AN EPILOGUE TO 1983. New York: National League for Nursing,
      1983.

      An exploration of the challenges and responses of the
      National League for Nursing over the first twenty years of its
      existence.

1876 Grace, H. and J. McCloskey. "The 1985 Resolution: Implica-
      tions for Graduate Education." CURRENT ISSUES IN NURSING.
      Edited by J. McCloskey and H. Grace. Scranton, PA.: Black-
      well Scientific Publications, 1981, pp. 160-69.

      The 1985 proposal increases the need for higher education
      for preparing adequate numbers of faculty to teach. This then
      impacts on gradute nursing education for the period of growth
      which may ultimately result in too many highly prepared nurses
      with inadequate numbers of positions similar to dilemmas
      previously encountered in the field of education. (13)

1877 Hawkins, J.W. "Toward the Future: Graduate Education for
      Professional Nursing Practice," J NURS EDUC 19(4) (April
      1980): 39-41.

      Supports the need to provide basic nursing education at the
      graduate level with pre professional preparation at the bac-
      calaureate level. Such a structure is present in other
      professional education programs and independence as a profes-
      sion requires similarity in this respect. (12)

1878 Lynaugh, J. "The Entry Into Practice Conflict: How We Got
      Where We Are and What Will Happen Next," AM J NURS 80(2)
      (February 1980): 266-70.

      A review of the social context of nursing provides insight
      into current professional issues. The timing appears good for
      society to accept nursing as a profession. (21)

1879 Lysaught, J.P. AN ABSTRACT FOR ACTION. New York: McGraw-Hill
      Book Co., 1970.

      A report of the National Commission on Nursing and Nursing
      Education of a study which sought to propose recommendations
      for the improvement of health care through the improvement of
      nursing and nursing education. Three areas of focus within
      this study include: nursing roles and functions; nursing
      education; and nursing careers.

1880 McClure, M.L. "Entry Into Professional Practice: The New York
      Proposal." THE NURSING PROFESSION: VIEWS THROUGH THE MIST.
      Edited by N.L. Chaska. New York: McGraw-Hill Book Co.,
      1978, pp. 93-99.

Issues surrounding implementation of the New York Proposal
which requires the baccalaureate degree for professional
nurse licensure are clarified. Such issues as an insufficient
number of nurses presently prepared at this level; lack of
availability of educational programs for registered nurses;
the quality of baccalaureate programs; and other issues are
discussed. (8)

1881   McGriff, E.P. "If Not the 1985 Resolution, Then What?" NURS
        OUTLOOK 28(6) (June 1980): 365.

An alternative to the 1985 proposal is offered in which
baccalaureate prepared nurses take a separate and different
licensing examination than AD and diploma graduates. This
would prepare an "Independent Nurse (I.N.)" and cause less
disruption to the present system. (0)

1882   "NAACOG Board Unanimously Endorses BSN for Entry," AM J NURS
        80(2) (February 1980): 192.

Although fifty-nine percent of NAACOG members are diploma
school graduates, they support the BSN degree as required for
entry into professional nursing practice provided that:
licensed nurses are not penalized financially or professionally; the concepts of nursing practice are clarified;
BSN programs are available in sufficient numbers and accessible; and career mobility is established. (0)

1883   "NLN Reaffirms its BSN Stance Despite ´Technical Nursing´
        Rift," AM J NURS 83(7) (July 1983): 985, 994-95.

An attempt to rescind the National League for Nursing´s
position on baccalaureate education in nursing as a requirement for entry into professional nursing practice was defeated
despite the presence of a large delegation of diploma school
supporters. (0)

1884   National Advisory Council on Vocational Education. "The Edu-
        cation of Nurses: A Rising National Concern - Position
        Paper." Issue Paper No. 2, May 1980. Reprinted in NURSING
        ISSUES AND NURSING STRATEGIES FOR THE EIGHTIES. Edited
        by B. Bullough, V. Bullough and M.C. Soukup. New York:
        Springer Publishing Co., 1983, pp. 205-15.

Official response of the National Advisory Council on Vocational Education to the ANA position. Supports continuation
of all four routes to a career in nursing. The 1985 Proposal
according to this group is not in the best interest of the
nation nor the profession. Contains an appendix which includes reactions of the National Student Nurses Association;
American Association of Community and Junior Colleges; American Health Care Association; National Federation of Licensed
Practical Nurses; National Association for Practical Nurse
Education and Service, Inc.; American Vocational Association;
and National League for Nursing. (0)

1885   National Commission for the Study of Nursing and Nursing
       Education, J.P. Lysaught, Director. AN ABSTRACT FOR ACTION:
       APPENDICES. New York: McGraw-Hill Book Co., 1971.

       An extension of the first volume, AN ABSTRACT FOR ACTION,
       this volume contains further exploration of data findings of
       a study which sought to improve nursing and nursing education
       which would ultimately improve health care.

1886   "Participants at Entry Into Practice Meeting Agree on Bacca-
       laureate; Disagree on Terminology," AM J NURS 78(4) (April
       1978): 535, 560, 562, 565.

       Although participants in an entry into practice meeting
       agreed on the baccalaureate requirement, disagreement was
       expressed on whether the dichotomy between professional and
       technical should be labeled "kinds" or "levels" of nursing
       practice. Further discussion of this issue considered the
       lack of differentiation between nursing personnel within the
       practice areas. An educational dichotomy without a practice
       differentiation is useless. (0)

1887   "PNA Reaffirms BSN for Entry," AM J NURS 80(1) (January 1980):
       40.

       A task force will be appointed to study resources, accessi-
       bility, necessary support systems, financial aid programs and
       projects impact on health care delivery as Pennsylvania moves
       to enact the baccalaureate degree in nursing as required for
       entry into professional nursing practice. (0)

1888   Partridge, R. "Education for Entry Into Professional Nursing
       Practice: The Planning of Change," J NURS EDUC 20(4) (April
       1981): 40-46.

       Describes the evolution of education for nursing practice in
       light of the proposed entry into practice resolution. Major
       arguments and planning for change are discussed. (34)

1889   Pisani, J. "The Nursing Challenge: Eliminating the Two-step
       Backward Syndrome." NURSING ISSUES AND NURSING STRATEGIES
       FOR THE EIGHTIES. Edited by B. Bullough, V. Bullough and
       M.C. Soukup. New York: Springer Publishing Co., 1983,
       pp. 190-96. Also in J NY STATE NURSES ASSOC (December
       1978): 26-30.

       We live in an academic world. Nursing needs the 1985 Pro-
       posal in order to secure the credentials necessary to present
       nursing as a credible profession worthy of an independent
       political view. (0)

1890   Pohlman, K. and N. Mosca. "Should Nursing Implement the 1985
       Resolution?" CURRENT ISSUES IN NURSING. Edited by J. Mc-
       Closkey and H. Grace. Scranton, PA.: Blackwell Scientific
       Publications, 1981, pp. 149-59.

Although some nineteen state nurses associations are actively exploring the entry into practice, New York State is
the only one to have passed the resolution. The Goldmark
Report, Ginsberg Report, and Brown Report all stress the need
for higher education in nursing. Arguments for and against
the resolution are thoroughly discussed. (23)

1891 "Professional Practice of Nursing Calls for BSN Preparation,
NLN Board Says," AM J NURS 82(3) (March 1982): 358.

The Board of Directors of the National League for Nursing
passed a position statement requiring the baccalaureate degree
for entry into professional nursing practice. Support for
all four types of nursing education continues. (0)

1892 "Regional Forums on 'Entry Into Practice" Scheduled for May,"
AM J NURS 79(3) (March 1979): 416.

Forums were planned in Kentucky, Oregon, Michigan and
Washington, D.C. to discuss and plan for the implementation of
the ANA Resolution to require the baccalaureate degree in
nursing for entry into professional nursing practice by 1985.
(0)

1893 Schoen, D. "A Study of Nurses' Attitudes Toward the BSN
Requirement," NURS HEALTH CARE 3(7) (September 1982): 382-87.

Several studies reviewed indicate that the rank and file of
nurses do not support the 1985 Proposal. A survey was conducted of nurses in Illinois which supported the findings of the
previous studies. Nurses with baccalaureate degrees and who
belong to professional organizations were most likely to support the entry into practice resolution and nurses with baccalaureate degrees and intending to work full time in the
future were most likely to support the baccalaureate degree as
a requirement for supervisory positions. (9)

1894 "Specialty Organizations Support Move to BSN," AM J NURS 80(4)
(April 1980): 582, 629, 630.

Reports on support and movement toward support of various
specialty nurses associations for requirement of the baccalaureate degree for entry into professional nursing practice.
There is little opposition to the basic premise, however,
opinions differ on the timing, categories, and grandfathering.
(0)

1895 "Stand on BSN Taken by 34 State Associations," AM J NURS 80(4)
(April 1980): 628.

Controversies are being encountered in most states as they
move toward requiring the baccalaureate degree for entry into
professional nursing practice. Education and career mobility
opportunities and funding are problem areas needing resolution.
There is more acceptance each year, however, the logistics of
implementation are problematic. (0)

1896   Sweeney, J.   "An Associate Degree Educator Supports The Entry
       to Practice Resolution," NURSE EDUC 5(5) (September/October
       1980): 28-29.

       The nursing profession is fraught with confusion and a poorly
       defined educational system.   Current structures serve to con-
       fuse the public and frustrate nurses.   Acceptance of the Entry
       Into Practice resolution is necessary to ameliorate these
       problems. (8)

1897   Wood, J.H.   "RN-BSN Education: Helping RNs Make Tough Deci-
       sions," NURSE EDUC 7(1) (January/February 1982): 37-38.

       A one day workshop focused on assisting registered nurses in
       decision making relevant to seeking the baccalaureate degree.
       Values clarification, prevailing curriculum patterns, univer-
       sity resources and strategies for success were discussed to
       assist students in selecting programs best suited for their
       needs. (12)

       See 1060, 1289, 1374, 1375, 1379, 1381, 1382, 1498, 1848.

       For various education issues see: 591, 592, 593, 594, 595, 596,
       597, 598, 599, 600, 602, 603, 604, 606, 607, 608, 609, 610, 614,
       615, 616, 617, 618, 619, 620, 914, 916, 917, 918, 919, 920, 921,
       922, 923, 1636, 1721, 1857.

NURSING RESEARCH/NURSING THEORY

1898   Abraham, I.L. and S. Schultz, II. "Univariate Statistical
        Models for Meta-analysis," NURS RES 32(5) (September/October
        1983): 312-15.

        Says application of univariate models to nursing is question-
        able and comments on paper by O'Flynn in 1982 issue of NURSING
        RESEARCH (31:314-16). Says O'Flynn comments and analysis
        were well taken but paper contained major inaccuracies and
        violations of parametric and stochastic assumptions. (19)

1899   American Nurses' Association. ISSUES IN RESEARCH: SOCIAL,
        PROFESSIONAL, AND METHODOLOGICAL. Kansas City, MO.:
        American Nurses' Association, Pub. No. D-44, 1974.

        Six papers from the 1973 ANA Council of Nurse Researchers
        Program Meeting, addressing social responsibilities, relation-
        ships, and legal concerns of researchers, human rights and
        ethical concerns, and philanthropic assistance for research.

1900   _____. ISSUES IN EVALUATION RESEARCH. Kansas City, MO.:
        American Nurses' Association, Pub. No. G-124, 1976.

        A collection of papers presented at the 1975 ANA Conference
        on evaluation and quality assurance by nursing leaders and
        nationally known researchers.

1901   _____. RESEARCH IN NURSING: TOWARD A SCIENCE OF HEALTH
        CARE. Kansas City, MO.: American Nurses' Association, Pub.
        No. D-52, 1976.

        A publication prepared by the ANA Commission on Nursing
        Research for the general public demonstrating the range of
        unique interests that nurses have in the study of people with
        health care problems and the contributions nurses are making
        to research in health care.

1902   _____. RESEARCH PRIORITIES FOR THE 1980's: GENERATING A
        SCIENTIFIC BASIS FOR NURSING PRACTICE. Kansas City, MO.:
        American Nurses' Association, Pub. No. D-68, 1981.

        Definition of nursing research and directions for nursing
        research identified by the ANA Commission on Nursing Research.
        Includes priorities and examples.

1903   _____. NEW INVESTIGATOR FEDERAL SECTOR GRANTMANSHIP
        PROJECT: FINAL REPORT. Kansas City, MO.: American Nurses'
        Association Pub. No. D-75, 1983.

Summary of steps taken in 1981-83 cooperative project (ANA/
U.S. Public Health Service) which offered new investigators
agency staff review prior to formal application of research
proposals.

1904 Artinian, B.M. "Conceptual Mapping: Development of the
      Strategy," WEST J NURS RES 4(4) (Fall 1982): 379-93.

      Conceptual mapping is a strategy which will facilitate the
      research to adequately conceptualize the research problem
      both before and during the analysis phase. The conceptual map
      represents the theory that can be tested in a correlational
      or experimental research design. (18)

1905 Atkinson, L.D. and M.E. Murray. UNDERSTANDING THE NURSING
      PROCESS, 2nd Ed. New York: Macmillan Publishing Co., 1983.

      Explanations for formulating nursing diagnoses, goals, care
      plans and evaluations are provided. One clinical example is
      followed throughout to demonstrate the application of the
      process to a specific patient, and illustrations help explain
      the main concepts.

1906 Atwood, J.R. and B.P. Gill-Rogers. "Metatheory, Methodology,
      and Practicality: Issues in Research Uses of Roger's
      Science of Unitary Man," NURS RES 33(2) (March-April 1984):
      88-91.

      This is a response to Suzie Kim's article in NURS RES 32
      (1983): 89-91. Rogers has developed general principles but
      uses vague terminology, leaves relationships unclear, and
      provides formulations that cannot be tested. (19)

1907 Bailar III, J.C. "Research Quality, Methodologic Rigor,
      Citation Counts, and Impact," AM J PUBLIC HEALTH 72(10)
      (October 1982): 1103-4.

      Editorial comment on the measurement of the quality of re-
      search using citation indexes. (1)

1908 Ballard, S. and R. McNamara. "Quantifying Nursing Needs in
      Home Health Care," NURS RES 32(4) (July-August 1983): 236-41.

      The Health Status Score measuring deficits in daily acti-
      vities and nursing problems proved to be the best predictor of
      the quantity of nursing service and total agency service re-
      quired. (15)

1909 Benedikter, H. FROM NURSING AUDIT TO MULTIDISCIPLINARY AUDIT.
      New York: National League for Nursing, Pub. No. 20-1673,
      1977.

An update of the original 1973 publication. Nursing audit
is a retrospective evaluation of nursing care based upon documentation of that care in the patient's medical record. This
pamphlet indicated procedure for audit and the methodology of
evaluating it. It can be a valuable research tool.

1910   Bergstrom, N., B.C. Hansen, M. Grant, R. Hanson, W. Kubo, G.
        Padilla and H.L. Wong. "Collaborative Nursing Research:
        Anatomy of a Successful Consortium," NURS RES 33(1)
        (January-February 1984): 20-25.

        The Tube feed consortium group was composed of seven inves-
        tigators from four different geographic locations. One member
        served as principal investigator and chairperson. Major ad-
        vantages included large number of subjects studied in short
        time; data collection permitted wider generalization, and
        there was mechanism for direct replication. (5)

1911   Binger, J.L. and L.M. Jensen. LIPPINCOTT'S GUIDE TO NURSING
        LITERATURE: A HANDBOOK FOR STUDENTS, WRITERS AND RESEARCHERS.
        Phildadelphia: J.B. Lippincott, 1980.

        Suggestions and techniques for using a library, surveil-
        lance techniques for maintaining currency, and preparation and
        submission of journal articles; annotated listing of major
        nursing periodical literature and a listing of major reference
        and resource works.

1912   Bradley, J.C. "Nurses' Attitudes Toward Dimensions of Nursing
        Practice," NURS RES 32(2) (March/April 1983): 110-14.

        One hundred ninety-six nurses from nine NLN schools in Con-
        necticut utilized instrument based on 28 objectives repre-
        senting five constructs. Six meaningful dimensions of nursing
        behaviors or functions were identified which should help in
        developing a specific role behavior that constitute nursing.
        (20)

1913   Brown, J.S., C.A. Tanner and K.P. Padrick. "Nursing's Search
        for Scientific Knowledge," NURS RES 33(1) (January-February
        1984): 26-32.

        Through an analysis of research in four time periods from
        1952-53 to 1980, investigators report nursing research has
        increased substantially in amount, became more clinically
        focused, demonstrated greater theoretical orientation, became
        more sophisticated.(19)

1914   Bruer, J.T. "Methodological Rigor and Citation Frequency in
        Patient Compliance Literature," AM J PUBLIC HEALTH 72(10)
        (October 1982): 1119-23.

        An exhaustive bibliography which assesses the methodological
        rigor of the patient compliance literature, and citation data
        from the Science Citation Index (SCI) are combined to deter-
        mine if methodologically rigorous papers are used with greater

frequency than substandard articles by compliance investigators. There are low, but statistically significant, correlations between methodological rigor and citation indicators
for 138 patient compliance papers published in SCI source
journals during 1975 and 1976. The correlation is not strong
enough to warrant use of citation measures as indicators of
rigor on a paper-by-paper basis. The data do suggest that
citation measures might be developed as crude indicators of
methodological rigor. There is no evidence that randomized
trials are cited more frequently than studies that employ
other experimental designs. (50)

1915   Carpenito, L.J. (Ed.) NURSING DIAGNOSIS: APPLICATION TO
       CLINICAL PRACTICE. Philadelphia: J.B. Lippincott Co., 1983.

       Forty-three categories of nursing diagnoses are presented
       with treatments. Focus is on human responses to illness
       rather than on illness itself. Argued that these are the
       problems nurses can and should treat.

1916   Chinn, P.L. ADVANCES IN NURSING THEORY DEVELOPMENT. Rock-
       villc, MD.: Aspen Systems Corp., 1982.

       A collection of articles contributed by nurse researchers,
       educators, and theoreticians reflecting the idea of applica-
       tion of theory. Chapters address four areas of concern:
       development of nursing knowledge, development and application
       of nursing theory, concepts of individual health, and social
       concepts.

1917   Chinn, P.L. and K.J. Maeona. THEORY AND NURSING: A SYSTEMATIC
       APPROACH. St. Louis, MO.: C.V. Mooby Co., 1983.

       Stresses the importance of thorough understanding of nursing
       theory. Uses examples and analogies to clarify complex ideas.
       Compares and analyzes various definitions of theory and the
       purpose for which theory is constructed. Includes a helpful
       glossary and bibliography.

1918   Chiriboga, D.A., G. Jenkins and J. Bailey. "Stress and Coping
       Among Hospice Nurses: Test of an Analytic Model," NURS RES
       32(5) (September/October 1983): 294-300.

       Tested an analytic model of stress that included social and
       predisposing conditioning factors, stress appraisals, coping
       strategies, social resources, and adaptive status. Stress
       appraisals and coping strategies proved to be the best pre-
       dictors of adaptive status. (34)

1919   Clark, P.E. and M.J. Clark. "Therapeutic Touch: Is There
       Scientific Basis for the Practice," NURS RES 33(1) (January-
       February 1984): 37-41.

After critically reviewing literature on topic of therapeutic touch, authors conclude that well designed, double
blind studies have not indicated that therapeutic touch is
helpful. Current practice of therapeutic touch is empirically
little more than practice of placebo. Considerations for
further research are presented. (26)

1920   Cronenwett, L.R. "Helping and Nursing Models," NURS RES 32(6)
       (December 1983): 342-46.

       Concept of helping has been somewhat ignored in theory and
       research in nursing. Examines some of the recent theories on
       helping and the implication of these theories and findings for
       future development. (30)

1921   Dagenais, F. and A.I. Meleis. "Professionalism, Work Ethic,
       and Empathy in Nursing: The Nurse Self-Descriptive Form,"
       WEST J NURS RES 4(4) (Fall 1982): 407-22.

       One alternative for nursing research is to select an in-
       strument developed for studies of other non-nurse groups and
       proceed to establish its validity, reliability, and usefulness
       to nursing research. This paper examines the Nurse-Self Des-
       cription Form. (29)

1922   Damrosch, S.P. and E.R. Lenz. "The Use of Client-Advisory
       Groups in Research," NURS RES 33(1) (January-February 1984):
       47-49.

       Nursing research can be seen as an interaction between re-
       search and subject; this paper describes one means by which
       nurse researchers can exercise an advocacy role by involving
       selected clients as colleagues in various stages of clinical
       research projects. (7)

1923   Davitz, J.R. and L.L. Davitz. EVALUATING RESEARCH PROPOSALS
       IN THE BEHAVIORAL SCIENCES: A GUIDE. New York: Teachers
       College Press, 1977.

       Intended as a guide to those writing their first independent
       research proposal.

1924   Dempsey, P.A. and D. Arthur. THE RESEARCH PROCESS IN NURSING.
       New York: Van Nostrand Co., 1981.

       A textbook for nurse researchers. Includes the usual
       topics but has somewhat heavier emphasis on historical re-
       search than most. Summary tables compare the key features of
       major experimental designs.

1925   Derdiarian, A.K., and A.B. Forsythe. "An Instrument for
       Theory and Research Development Using the Behavioral Systems
       Model for Nursing: The Cancer Patient," NURS RES 32(5)
       (September/October 1983): 260-66.

Derdiarian Behavioral System Model is an instrument to
measure and describe the perceived behavioral changes of the
cancer patient within the Johnson Behavioral System Model. (5)

1926   Downs, F.S. and J.W. Fleming (Eds.). ISSUES IN NURSING
       RESEARCH. New York: Appleton-Century-Crofts, 1979.

       Volume represents a diversity of opinion on nursing research
       by seven contributors. In addition to the two editors, there
       are chapters by Susan Gortner, Virginia S. Cleland, Joanne S.
       Stevenson, Carolyn A. Williams and Jeane Hayter. Each chap-
       ter has its own notes and references.

1927   Eichelberger, K.M., D.H. Kaufman, M.E. Rundahl and N.E.
       Schwartz. "Self-care Nursing Plan: Helping Children to
       Help Themselves," PED NURS 6(3) (May/June 1980): 9-13.

       Orem's self-care theory applied to children. (2)

1928   Engel, G.L. "The Biomedical Model: A Procrustean Bed?,"
       MAN AND MEDICINE 4(4) (1979): 257-75.

       Engel, a physician, is critical of the medical model of
       health care and calls for a psychosocial model more akin to
       the nursing model. Encourages a system approach. (13)

1929   Erickson, H., E.M. Tomlin and M.A.P. Swain. MODELING AND ROLE
       MODELING: A THEORY AND PARADIGM FOR NURSING. Englewood
       Cliffs, NJ: Prentice-Hall, 1983.

       Draws upon the authors' own clinical experiences and re-
       search to provide a scientifically based, culturally sensitive
       perspective, and focuses on the concepts of holism, self-care
       strengths, and client control.

1930   Evaneshko, V. and M.A. Kay. "The Ethnoscience Research Tech-
       nique," WEST J NURS RES 4(1) (Winter 1982): 49-64.

       Ethnoscience research, developed by anthropologists, have
       implications for nursing since rather than answering questions
       such as "how much" or "how often," the "what" and "why" of
       cultural behavior are important. (19)

1931   Fagin, C.M. "The Economic Value of Nursing Research," AM J
       NURS 82(12) (December 1982): 1844-49.

       Nursing research has demonstrated several ways in which
       health care costs could be reduced. This article picks three
       areas: all R.N. staff, influencing patient care practices,
       and alternatives to hospitalization to show what research
       has said about what can be done to lower costs. Argues that
       nursing research is underfunded but has a high payoff. (51)

1932   Fawcett, J. "Hallmarks of Success in Nursing Research," ADV
       NURS SCI 7(1) (October 1984): 1-11.

Finds significant progress has been made in the last few
years in establishing nursing as a scholarly discipline.
Three major current problems remain: (1) elimination of obstacles to nursing research, (2) acceptance of multiple modes
of inquiry, and (3) utilization of research findings in the
clinical settings. (36)

1933   Fitzpatrick, J.L. and A.L. Whall. CONCEPTUAL MODELS OF
       NURSING: ANALYSIS, EVALUATION AND APPLICATION. Englewood
       Cliffs, NJ: Prentice-Hall (Brady), 1983.

       Analysis and evaluation of major nursing models, including
       Nightingale, Orlando, Levine, Peplau, Henderson, Widenback,
       Johnson, Neuman, Orem, Fitzpatrick and a new life perspective
       rhythm model.

1934   Fontes, H.M. "An Exploration of the Relationships Between
       Cognitive Style, Interpersonal Needs, and Eudaimonistic
       Model of Health," NURS RES 32(2) (March-April 1983): 92-96.

       Health in the eudaimonistics (or self actualization) model
       measured by Personality Orientation Inventory (POI) was the
       major focus of study. Hypothesized that moderation and
       balance would be correlates of eudaimonistic health. Study
       did not yield support for hypothesis. (30)

1935   Fox, D.J. and I.R. Leeser. READINGS ON THE RESEARCH PROCESS
       IN NURSING. New York: Appleton-Century-Crofts, 1981.

       Book is organized into two main sections: one on structure
       and functions of research in nursing and one which includes
       research in the clinical areas of nursing and in the nursing
       role. Selected samples of nursing research are provided.

1936   Fox D.J. FUNDAMENTALS OF RESEARCH IN NURSING, 4th Ed.
       Norwalk, CT.: Appleton-Century-Crofts, 1982.

       Purpose is to provide reader skills necessary to plan and
       carry out research studies. Organized into five sections:
       nature of research, research planning, process of data collec-
       tion, process of data analysis, and writing up report.

1937   Fox, R.N. and M.R. Ventura. "Small Scale Administration of
       Instruments and Procedures," NURS RES 32(2) (March-April
       1983): 122-25.

       The importance of pre testing and trial administration is
       emphasized. (11)

1938   Fuller, E.O. "Preparing an Abstract of a Nursing Study,"
       NURS RES 32(5) (September-October 1983): 316-17.

       Explains what should be included in an abstract of a study.
       (0)

1939 Gadow, S. "Toward a New Philosophy of Nursing," NURS LAW AND
      ETHICS 1 (October 1980): 1-2, 6.

      A brief summary of her concept of existential advocacy.

1940 Gaut, D.A. "Development of a Theoretically Adequate Descrip-
      tion of Caring," WEST J NURS 5(4) (Fall 1983): 313-24.

      Through a semantic analysis of the words care/caring, the
      author then went to the literature on caring, and arrived at
      an action description of caring that could be justified as
      both conceptually and theoretically adequate. (23)

1941 George, J.B. (Compiler). NURSING THEORIES: THE BASE FOR PRO-
      FESSIONAL NURSING PRACTICE, 2nd Ed. Englewood Cliffs, N.J.:
      Prentice-Hall, 1985.

      The second edition expands its list of theorists to sixteen
      and relates the work of each to the nursing process of asses-
      sing, diagnosing, planning, implementing and evaluating.
      An overview of the work of each of these important theorists,
      and shows the student how to apply each theory into real
      clinical practice.

1942 Goodwin, L.D. "The Use of Power Estimation in Nursing Re-
      search," NURS RES 33(2) (March-April 1984): 118-20.

      Explains the value of calculating a power estimate in con-
      junction with developing the design for a study. (8)

1943 Gorenberg, B. "The Research Tradition of Nursing: An Emerging
      Issue," NURS RES 32(6) (December 1983): 347-49.

      Nursing research has not been limited to the scientific
      method, both observation and experimental research have been
      used and the nursing tradition of research has continued to
      evolve to meet changing demands. Question is not what re-
      search method but what questions to ask and how best to answer
      them. (21)

1944 Gortner, S.R. "Research in Nursing: The Federal Interest and
      Grant Program," AM J NURS 73 (1973): 1052-55.

      Discusses the need for nursing research in all areas of
      nursing practice and nurse education. (13)

1945 _____. "The History and Philosophy of Nursing Science
      and Research," ADV NURS SCIENCE 5 (1983): 1-8.

      A brief historical review of research in nursing. Author
      believes that future contributions of nursing science will be
      in the provision of an interface between the biological and
      social sciences.

1946 Haughey, B.P. "Holter Monitoring: A Method for Nursing Re-
      search," NURS RES 32(1) (January/February 1983): 59-60.

Describes Holter electrocardiography, a longterm monitoring
of patient's ECG while the person is engaged in routines of
daily living. Procedure provides for high speed analysis of
the recorded ECG data, correlation of symptoms and activities
with arrhythmic episodes, and documentation of abnormal beats
and rate changes in a permanent record. (12)

1947   Haussman, R., K. Dieter and S.T. Hegyvary. MONITORING QUALITY
       OF NURSING CARE: PART III PROFESSION REVIEW FOR NURSING: AN
       EMPIRICAL INVESTIGATION. Hyattsville, MD.: U.S. Department
       of Health, Education and Welfare, 1977. DHEW Publication
       No. HRA 77-70.

       A report of the third phase of a study performed under con-
       tract with Division of Nursing to develop quality-monitoring
       methodology. Includes a literature review.

1948   Hayter, J. "Institutional Sources of Articles Published in
       13 Nursing Journals, 1978-1982," NURS RES 33(6) (November/
       December 1984): 357-61.

       Identifies institutions in which scholarly productivity is
       occurring. However, only thirteen nursing journals were
       analyzed as a data base. (5)

1949   Henderson, V. THE NATURE OF NURSING. New York: Macmillan,
       1966.

       Conceptualization of nursing recognized in many subsequent
       definitions. Historical significance.

1950   Hinshaw, A.S. and J.R. Atwood. "A Patient Satisfaction In-
       strument: Precision by Replication," NURS RES 31(3) (May/
       June 1982): 170-75.

       Patient Satisfaction Instrument (PSI) developed over a
       series of five clinical and administrative studies over eight
       year period involving 600 patients, primarily medical-
       surgical in patients and out patients. Overall the PSI has
       acceptable levels of validity and reliability with refinements
       indicated to be used by others. (15)

1951   Hinshaw, A.S., R.M. Gerber, J.R. Atwood and J.R. Allen. "The
       Use of Predictive Modeling to Test Nursing Practice Out-
       comes," NURS RES 32(1) (January/February 1983): 35-42.

       A middle range, multivariate practice model was constructed
       to test impact of perioperative teaching program on multiple
       patient outcomes. A quasiexperimental causal modeling
       approach was used. (32)

1952   Holm, K. "Single Subject Research," NURS RES 32(4) (July-
       August 1983): 253-55.

Single subject research models permit documentation of individual responses and help prevent important information from being lost. (17)

1953 Holmstrom, L.L. and A.W. Burgess. "Low Cost Research: A Project on a Shoestring," NURS RES 31(2) (March-April 1982): 123-25.

With ingenuity, much can be accomplished for free, by barter, or a small budget. This often means a greater time commitment by researcher but the advantage is intellectual autonomy, freedom to study what you want without being subjected to others' funding decisions. (2)

1954 Hymovich, D.P. "The Chronicity Impact and Coping Instrument: Parent Questionnaire," NURS RES 32(5) (September/October 1983): 275-81.

The Chronicity Impact and Coping Instrument: Parent Questionnaire is designed to measure (1) parent perceptions of the impact of chronic disorder on the family, and (2) how parents cope with the difficulties they encounter as a result of their child's condition. (4)

1955 Infante, M.S. CRISIS THEORY: A FRAMEWORK FOR NURSING PRACTICE. Englewood Cliffs, N.J.: Reston Publishing Co., Prentice-Hall, Inc., 1982.

Recasts the basic content of nursing practice into the crisis theory model. Presents an overview of crisis theory and related holistic health concepts.

1956 Johnson, D.E. "The Behavioral System Model for Nursing." CONCEPTUAL MODELS FOR NURSING PRACTICE, 2nd Ed. Edited by S.C. Roy and J.P. Riehl. New York: Appleton-Century-Crofts, 1980.

Johnson's behavioral system is an example of the balance model. Humanity is referred to as a behavioral system comprised of patterned, repetitive, and purposeful ways of behaving. Human behaviors are formed into an organized and integrated functional unit. Human health is implicitly expressed as the state of behavioral system balance and dynamic stability. It is not the nature of properties or state of a person that is central to his or her health and existence, but it is the system of behaviors as parts of an organized and integrated whole.

1957 Kelly, M.A. NURSING DIAGNOSIS: GUIDELINES FOR CLINICAL APPLICATION. Norwalk, CT.: Appleton-Century-Crofts, 1984.

Explores the development and use of nursing diagnosis (with practical guidelines on assessment for nursing diagnosis,

stating a nursing diagnosis, and clinical recording of information relative to a particular client´s nursing diagnosis);
and lists the most current (1982) accepted nursing diagnostic
category titles.

1958   Kerr, J.A.C. "An Overview of Theory and Research Related to
       Space Use in Hospitals," WEST J NURS RES 3(4) (Winter 1982):
       395-405.

       Examines the theoretical frameworks developed about space
       use in hospitals and the empirical studies lending support to
       these theories. (24)

1959   Kim, H.S. "Use of Roger´s Conceptual System in Research:
       Comments," NURS RES 32(2) (March/April 1983): 89-91.

       There are difficulties in translating principles within the
       Roger´s framework of unitary man to empirical studies. Argues
       that the model has to be tested more since it is much too
       abstract as it is.(4)

1960   _____. THE NATURE OF THEORETICAL THINKING IN NURSING.
       Norwlk, CT.: Appleton-Century-Crofts, 1983.

       In some eight chapters, the author examines nature of
       theoretical thinking in nursing. The concluding chapter deals
       with Issues in Theoretical Development. Four pages of notes
       and references plus index are included at end. Each chapter
       has its own references.

1961   Kim, M.J. and G. McFarland. POCKET GUIDE TO NURSING DIAGNOSIS.
       St. Louis: C. V. Mosby Co., 1984.

       Includes all nursing diagnoses, along with etiologies and
       defining characteristics approved at the Fifth National Con-
       ference on Classification of Nursing Diagnoses.

1962   Kim, M.J., G. McFarland and A.M. McLane. CLASSIFICATION OF
       NURSING DIAGNOSIS: PROCEEDINGS OF THE FIFTH NATIONAL CON-
       FERENCE. St. Louis: C.V. Mosby Co., 1984.

       A compilation of the papers presented at the Fifth National
       Conference on nursing diagnoses, along with valuable supple-
       mental information. The conference approached the development
       of nursing diagnosis classification systems from two different
       tracks: examinations of new nursing diagnoses (supported by
       clincial and research data), and a theorists´ framework.

1963   King, I.M. A THEORY FOR NURSING: SYSTEMS, CONCEPTS, PROCESS.
       New York: John Wiley, 1981.

       A conceptualizing of the nursing system as comprised of
       dynamic interacting systems. Within the dynamic interacting

personal, interpersonal, and social systems, nursing occurs
as actions, reactions, and interaction through which information is shared, relationships are created between the nurse
and the client, and goals and means for attaining the goals.

1964   Kishi, K.I. "Communication Patterns of Health Teaching and
       Information Recall," NURS RES 32(4) (July/August 1983):
       230-35.

       Investigates verbal communication patterns between health
       care provider and client using Flanders Interaction Analysis
       System. (29)

1965   Krueger, J.C., A.H. Nelson and M.O. Walanin. NURSING RESEARCH:
       DEVELOPMENT, COLLABORATION AND UTILIZATION. Germantown:
       Aspen Systems, 1978.

       Report of a six year project funded by Division of Nursing,
       H.E.W. and conducted by Western Interstate Commission on
       Higher Eucation. Aim was "to investigate feasibility of in-
       creasing nursing research activities through a regional
       effort," and this is a favorable report.

1966   Lancaster, J. and W. Lancaster (Eds.). THE NURSE AS A CHANGE
       AGENT: CONCEPTS FOR ADVANCED NURSING PRACTICE. St.Louis:
       C.V. Mosby Co., 1982.

       A compilation of twenty-eight essays organized around theme
       that professional nurses have a responsibility to understand
       the organization in which they practice and a responsibility
       to modify, adapt, and change the organization in order to
       enhance the quality of care.

1967   Larson, E. "Health Policy and NIH: Implications for Nursing
       Research," NURS RES 33(6) (November/December 1984): 352-56.

       The structure and functions of the National Institutes of
       Health explained. Proposal to establish an Institute of
       Nursing discussed. (23)

1968   Lebacqz, K. "Pediatric Drug Investigation: Current Ethical
       Guidelines." CLINICAL PHARMACOLOGY. Edited by B.L. Mirkin.
       New York: Year Book Medical Publishers, 1978, pp. 279-97.

       Provides a perspective on the ethical requirements for con-
       ducting research using children as subjects. Points out that
       the first ethical principle that governs the conduct of re-
       search with human subjects is that of justice.

1969   Leininger, M.M. CARE: THE ESSENCE OF NURSING AND HEALTH.
       Thorofare, N.J.: Slack, Inc., 1984.

       Examines the phenomenon of care from individual, group,
       family, community, and worldwide perspectives. Includes chap-
       ters on philosophical, theoretical, historical and motivational
       aspects.

1970 _____. QUALITATIVE RESEARCH METHODS IN NURSING. Orlando,
     FL.: Grune & Stratton, Inc., 1985.

     Offers insights about the nature, purpose, and significance
     of qualitative research methods for nurse researchers as well
     as the differences between qualitative and quantitative re-
     search methods. Special emphasis is placed on the emerging
     trend toward using qualitative research methods to advance
     humanistic and scientific knowledge about nursing and the
     health care field. Some of the methods presented include
     philosophical, ethnographic, historical, ethnonursing, ethno-
     science, grounded theory, phenomenological, descriptive, life
     history, clinical, audiovisual, and drawing methods. Multiple
     authors.

1971 Leslie, F.M. "Nursing Diagnosis: Use in Long-term Care," AM
     J NURS 81(5) (May 1981): 1012-14.

     Nursing diagnoses are more relevant in long-term care than
     medical diagnoses according to a one year study in Maryland.
     Medical and nurses diagnoses are compared. (0)

1972 Lindeman, C.A. THEORY AND RESEARCH AS BASIC TO NURSING PRAC-
     TICE. Kansas City, MO.: American Nurses' Association,
     1984.

     The importance of nursing research for the profession, the
     role of theory, the ethical issues and the future of nursing
     research are discussed in this position paper.

1973 Lindsey, A.M. "Phenomena and Physiological Variables of
     Relevance to Nursing, Review of a Decade of Work, Part I,"
     WEST J NURS RES 4(4) (Fall 1982): 343-64.

     Nursing research, published in nursing journals over the
     last ten years, was reviewed to identify and those studies in
     which physiological phenomena and variables were examined by
     nurse researchers. A classification scheme was developed to
     group the phenomenon studies. (74)

1974 _____. "Phenomena and Physiological Variables of Relevance
     to Nursing, Review of a Decade of Work, Part II," WEST J
     NURS RES 5(1) (Winter 1983): 41-63.

     This continuation deals with phenomena studied primarily
     related to the individual's environment and in which some
     aspect of a therapy or procedure was investigated. (81)

1975 Loomis, M.E. "Resources for Collaborative Research," WEST J
     NURS RES 4(1) (Winter 1982): 65-74.

     Report on the Conduct and Utilization of Research in Nursing
     Project (CURN) as it involved a collabortive research program.
     Describes the clinicians and researchers who were members of
     the team and nursing departments that were able to support

this research development. (20)

1976 Ludemann, R., C.M. Rorack and G.M. Bartol. "Commentaries on
      the article by Holly Skodol Wilson on 'Teaching Research in
      Nursing'," WEST J NURS RES 4(4) (Fall 1982): 373-76.

      A commentary.

1977 Malinski, V.M. ROGERIAN THEORY: CONCEPTS AND APPLICATIONS.
      Englewood Cliffs, NJ: Prentice-Hall (Brady), 1985.

      Following Roger's Model of Unitary Human Beings, this text
      explores its practical application in the clinical setting
      as well as the types of research that have been done to test
      it. Begins with a description of the model itself, theory
      development, and research approaches followed by nine studies
      of the model's applications.

1978 McCown, D.E. "Moral Development in Children, PED NURS 10(1)
      (January/February 1984): 42-44.

      Our complex society confronts us with many moral issues,
      such as nuclear war, abortion, racial equality, sexual promis-
      cuity and test-tube babies. Thus, children and adults may
      need assistance to make moral decisions that reflect the prin-
      ciples of justice and respect. Nurses can assist families to
      recognize their children's developmental levels of moral
      thought and to promote their moral decision-making abilities.
      (11)

1979 Melnyk, K.A.M. "The Process of Theory Analysis: An Examina-
      tion of the Nursing Theory of Dorothea E. Orem," NURS RES
      32(3) (May/June 1983): 170-74.

      Orem's self care model has been used as a theoretical base
      in developing academic curricula and as a classification scheme
      for nursing research. Concludes that her theory is very
      limiting to nursing, and would restrict nursing to much less
      than it now does. (8)

1980 Metzger, B.L. and S. Shultz, II. "Time Series Analysis:
      An Alternative for Nursing," NURS RES 31(6) (November/Decem-
      ber 1982): 375-78.

      In Time Series analysis observations occur in temporal
      order, different than in classical inferential statistics.
      Examines various data sets for this kind of research and
      explains its value. (10)

1981 Milio, N. PROMOTING HEALTH THROUGH PUBLIC POLICY. Philadel-
      phia: F.A. Davis, 1981.

      Conceptual framework for evaluating health effects of public
      policy.

1982   Miller, S.R. and P. Winstead-Fry. FAMILY SYSTEMS THEORY IN
       NURSING PRACTICE. Englewood Cliffs, NJ: Reston Publishing
       Co. (Prentice-Hall, Inc.), 1982.

       Describes Bowen's family system model as it relates to
       nursing practice.

1983   Mooney, M.M. "The Ethical Component of Nursing Theory," IMAGE
       12(1) (February 1980): 7-9.

       Briefly examines four nursing theories to determine their
       ethical components. (21)

1984   Munhall, P.L. "Nursing Philosophy and Nursing Research, In
       Apposition or Opposition," NURS RES 31(3) (May/June 1982):
       176-78.

       Research paradigms guide and perpetuate nursing practice
       and the linguistic components of the paradigm should demon-
       strate contextual and syntactical parallelism with beliefs
       and values of the discipline. If they are in conflict, alter-
       native paradigms should be explored. (3)

1985   National Institute of Health. ISSUES IN RESEARCH WITH HUMAN
       SUBJECTS: A SYMPOSIUM. Bethesda, MD.: U.S. Government
       Printing Office, 1980.

       A conference with presentations from the United States and
       the United Kingdom on clinical and ethical administrative
       problems in the conduct of clinical research. Also a dis-
       cussion on international standards of clinical research.

1986   Neuman, B. THE NEUMAN SYSTEMS MODEL: APPLICATION TO NURSING
       EDUCATION AND PRACTICE. Norwalk, CT.: Appleton-Century-
       Crofts, 1982.

       A compilation of presentations of the Neuman Health-Care
       Systems Model and description of its use in nursing education,
       administration, and a variety of practice areas.

1987   Newman, M.A. THEORY DEVELOPMENTS IN NURSING. Philadelphia:
       F.A. Davis, 1979.

       A theory of health based upon Roger's model of unitary man.
       Includes a six fold synthesis which posits disease at one
       end and non disease at the other. Time and space as the
       basis of life processes are regarded as having a complementary
       relationship.

1988   Notter, L. ESSENTIALS OF NURSING RESEARCH, 3rd Ed. New York:
       Springer Publishing Co., 1983.

       Gives a straightforward, systematic, and pragmatic approach.

1989   O'Flynn, A.I. "Meta-Analysis," NURS RES 31(5) (September/
       October 1982): 314-16.

Meta-analysis is the integration of findings, the analysis of analyses using statistical approaches. Various techniques for performing meta-analysis are examined.

1990   Oiler, C. "The Phenomenological Approach in Nursing Research," NURS RES 31(3) (May/June 1982): 178-81.

Phenomenology represents the effort to describe human experience as it is lived. It is proposed that it contains elements which are readily accessible to nurses as methods. For example, "phantom limb pain" in amputation is a categorization or classification not a description. (20)

1991   Orem, D.E. NURSING: CONCEPTS OF PRACTICE, 2nd Ed. New York: McGraw-Hill, 1980.

A version of a functional model of health. Health is conceptualized in relation to self care deficits which are expressed as deficiencies in any one of the self care foci identified in three categories of universal, developmental, and health deviation self care types. Health is a state of wholeness or integrity of the person in terms of his or her capacity to provide self care. Health is thus attained by sufficient and satisfactory self-care actions responding to varying demands for attention to self.

1992   Patton, M.Q. UTILIZATION-FOCUSED EVALUATION. Beverly Hills: Sage Publications, 1978.

Some 12 chapters dealing with both practical and theoretical aspects of utilization focused evaluation. Each chapter contains both a review of the relevant literature and actual case examples to illustrate a major point or points. Book assumes that evaluation research ought to be useful although much that passes for evaluation research is not. Book tries to distinguish between useful and not useful.

1993   Putt, A.M. GENERAL SYSTEMS THEORY APPLIED TO NURSING. Boston: Little, Brown and Co., 1978.

Systems theory utilizes terms like input, throughput and output, evaluation, feedback and control, and can be used to teach the nursing process: assessment, planning, intervention, and evaluation and is of value to the professional nurse. Several contributors besides Putt.

1994   Riehl, J.P. and C. Roy (Eds.). CONCEPTUAL MODELS FOR NURSING PRACTICE, 2nd Ed. New York: Appleton-Century-Crofts, 1980.

Discusses theory and models and reviews the history of nursing models in education, research, and service. Includes the basic theory of system, developmental, and interaction models from which most nursing models are derived.

1995   Roberts, S.L. PHYSIOLOGICAL CONCEPTS AND THE CRITICALLY ILL PATIENT. Englewood Cliffs, NJ.: Prentice-Hall, 1985.

Develops a nursing approach to family using a variety of theory building approaches. Utilizes nursing models to examine and reformulate existing theory and to derive psychiatric mental health nursing approaches. Also presents nursing knowledge which has been developed in practice to reassess existing psychiatric mental health theory. Contains theoretical perspectives, basing a family approach upon a nursing model, reformulation of existing theory using a nursing model, reformulation of existing theory using inductively derived nursing knowledge, and nursing approach based upon inductively derived knowledge.

1996   Rogers, M.E. "Nursing: A Science of Unitary Man." CONCEPTUAL MODELS FOR NURSING PRACTICE. Edited by S.C. Roy and J.P. Riehl. New York: Appleton-Century-Crofts, 1980.

Rogers conceptualizes a person as continually renewing his or her patterns of life toward increasing complexity and negetropy. The patterns of life process are seen as manifested through a person's mutual, simultaneous interactions with the environment in the forms of helicy, resonancy, and complementarity. The ever expanding and contracting human field is in the process of interchange with the environmental field in a reciprocal fashion. Such interchange is based on the homeo dynamic principles of complementarity, helicy, and resonancy. A person adopts these forms of interactive exchange of energy. Increasing complexity in organization and patterning is the law of human developmental process. Health is expressed as the process of life in its totality.

1997   Roy, C. Sr. INTRODUCTION TO NURSING: AN ADAPTATION MODEL, 2nd Ed. Englewood Cliffs, NJ.: Prentice-Hall, 1984.

Demonstrates each step of the nursing process according to the Roy Adaptation Model and then applies the Model to general and specific clinical situation.

1998   Roy, S.C. and S.L. Roberts. THEORY CONSTRUCTION IN NURSING: AN ADAPTATION MODEL. Englewood Cliffs, NJ.: Prentice-Hall, 1981.

A person is perceived as an adaptive system receiving inputs identified as stimuli from the external environment and as generated by the self, processing them by internal and feedback processes inherent in an individual's ever changing ability, and producing outputs as either adaptive or ineffective responses. Adaptation has a positive connotation, a state of all systems go, a green light in specific relation to what is happening to the person at a given moment. Roy's human response to stimuli uses four basic modes: physiological, self concept, role function, and interdependence.

1999   Sexton, D.L. "Some Methodological Issues in Chronic Illness Research," NURS RES 32(6) (November/December 1983): 378-80.

The case of Chronic Obstructive Pulmonary Disease (COPD)
issue to illustrate selected methodological issues that may
have wider application for nursing research. (10)

2000 Shelley, S.I. "The IDIR Model for Faculty Research with
      Students," WEST J NURS RES 5(4) (Fall 1983): 301-8.

      Instructor Directed Research Model is useful in teaching
      students research and at the same time can lead to publica-
      tion for the instructor and students. Commentaries by Bonnie
      Bullough, Moira Mansall, Jean Watson and response by author,
      pp. 308-12. (3)

2001 Smitherman, C. NURSING ACTIONS FOR HEALTH PROMOTION.
      Philadelphia: F. A. Davis, 1981.

      Analyzes and synthesizes existing information for nurses
      interested in a non medical based model of nursing practice.

2002 Stetler, C.B. MASSACHUSETTS GENERAL HOSPITAL, DEPARTMENT OF
      NURSING, NURSING RESEARCH IN A SERVICE SETTING. Englewood
      Cliffs, NJ.: Prentice-Hall, Inc., 1984.

      Examines the role of research within the health care set-
      ting, and presents a model for the integration of research
      into health care services.

2003 Stevens, B.J. NURSING THEORY: ANALYSIS, APPLICATION, EVALUA-
      TION. Boston, MA.: Little, Brown and Co., 1984.

      Updated edition of a popular text provides criteria for
      evaluating nursing theories, describes trends, pinpoints
      common themes, and analyzes the construction and development
      of nursing theories. Building upon that foundation, author
      then gives an overview of individual nursing theories and
      their implications for nursing practice. The theories dis-
      cussed are categorized and explained according to their sub-
      ject matter, principles, and methodologies.

2004 Sweeney, M.A. and P. Olivieri. AN INTRODUCTION TO NURSING
      RESEARCH: RESEARCH, MEASUREMENT, AND COMPUTERS IN NURSING.
      Philadelphia: J.B. Lippincott, 1981.

      Aimed at undergraduates, the first part of the book is
      devoted to importance of nursing research and gives an over-
      view of the research process. Twenty percent of the text is
      spent on instruction in computer usage.

2005 Trussel, P.B., A. Brandt and S. Knapp. USING NURSING RE-
      SEARCH: DISCOVERY, ANALYSIS, AND INTERPRETATION. Gaithers-
      burg, MD.: Aspen Systems Corp., 1981.

      Suggested techniques, locating citations, abstracts and
      reports of scientific inquiry.

2006   Walker, L.O. and K.C. Avant. STRATEGIES FOR THEORY CONSTRUC-
       TION IN NURSING. Norwalk, CT.: Appleton-Century-Crofts,
       1983.

       Argues that nurses consciously decided to design and test
       theory in order to professionalize. Gives some basic back-
       ground for theory construction.

2007   Wandelt, M.A. and D.S. Stewart. SLATER NURSING COMPETENCIES
       RATING SCALE. New York: Appleton-Century-Crofts, 1975.

       The Slater Nursing Competencies Scale, an eighty-four item
       scale to identify actions performed by nursing personnel as
       they provide for patients, is followed by a twenty-two page
       Cue sheet, instructions for use of the scale, standards of
       measurement and rating, tests of the scale, measurement
       for evaluation, and experience of others with the scale.
       An appendix provides a fold-out copy of the scale in a size
       convenient for use.

2008   Werley, H.H. and J.J. Fitzpatrick (Eds.). ANNUAL REVIEW OF
       NURSING RESEARCH, VOL. I, 1983. New York: Springer Publish-
       ing Co., 1984.

       Chapter nine by Rosemary Ellis, "Philosophic Inquiry," deals
       with some of the research theory, particularly the subsection
       on "Ethics" pages 215-216 and that on "Philosophy of
       Nursing Education" pages 216-218. (40)

2009   Wiley, K. "Effects of a Self Directed Learning Project and
       Preference for Structure on Self-Directed Learning Readi-
       ness," NURS RES 32(3) (May/June 1983): 181-85.

       Concluded that neither preference for structure nor conduc-
       ting an SDL project contributed significantly to the variance
       in post test SDL readiness, but interaction of these two
       variables did.   Persons who prefer low structure benefit
       from SDL teaching more than those who prefer high structure.
       (25)

2010   Wilson, H.S. "Teaching Research in Nursing: Issues and
       Strategies," WEST J NURS RES 4(4) (Fall 1982): 365-73,
       response to commentaries by author, p. 377.

       A brief historical sketch of the teaching of research
       methods in nursing is followed by a discussion of discrepan-
       cies between where we wish to be and where we are, after
       which the author offers some guiding principles to minimize
       these discrepancies. (14) (1)

2011   _____. RESEARCH IN NURSING. Menlo Park, CA.: Addison-
       Wesley, Co., 1984.

       Includes a chapter about placing nursing research in a
       theoretical context. Primarily a how to book about research,
       rather than a theoretical or critical discussion of research.

2012   Wooldridge, P.J., M.H. Schmitt, J.K. Skipper, Jr. and R.C.
       Leonard. BEHAVIORAL SCIENCE AND NURSING THEORY. St. Louis:
       C.V. Mosby, Co., 1983.

       Reviews and updates the approach of the Yale theorists
       of the 1960s. Distinguishes practice theory from social
       science theory. Insists theory should be empirically
       tested before application. Probably the most scientific
       of the extant works on nursing theory.

2013   Wright, W. THE SOCIAL LOGIC OF HEALTH. New Brunswick, NJ.:
       Rutgers University Press, 1982.

       Social theory of health--health used as an evaluative
       criterion for judging social institutions.

2014   Wysocki, A.B. "Basic Versus Applied Research: Intrinsic and
       Extrinsic Considerations," WEST J NURS RES 5(3) (Summer
       1983)· 217-24.

       As nursing moves from a practice oriented base to a scien-
       tific one, the issues of basic versus applied research
       increases in significance. Both, however, are complementary
       and the one does not exclude the other. (22)

2015   Yura, H. and M.B. Walsh. THE NURSING PROCESS: ASSESSING,
       PLANNING, IMPLEMENTING, EVALUATING, 4th Ed. Norwalk, CT.:
       Appleton-Century-Crofts, 1983.

       First edition appeared in 1967; this is fourth edition and
       update. Includes chapters on development of nursing process,
       theoretic framework, component, application and future of
       nursing process; appendices include national and international
       codes for nurses, standard of nursing practice, selected
       observations made using four senses, and bibliography.

See: 260, 623, 645, 945, 1035, 1096, 1218, 1317, 1328, 1337,
1342, 1344, 1347, 1349, 1458, 1470, 1510, 1532, 1543, 1600,
1601, 1638, 1642, 1643, 1693, 1717, 1730, 1731, 1858, 1912,
1984.

PROFESSIONAL ISSUES

General

2016 Abbott, A. "Professional Ethics," AM J SOC 88(5) (March
      1983): 855-85.

      Through comparative analysis, this paper establishes five
      basic properties of professional ethics codes: universal dis-
      tribution, correlation with intraprofessional status, enforce-
      ment dependent on visibility, individualism and emphasis on
      colleague obligations. After discussing traditional explana-
      tions of these properties from the functionalist and monopo-
      list perspectives, the paper adds a third perspective, re-
      lating ethics directly to intra- and extraprofessional status.
      A final section analyzing developments in professional ethics
      in America since 1900 specifies the interplay of the three
      processes hypothezied in the competing perspectives. (149)

2017 Brooten, D., L. Hayman and M. Naylor. LEADERSHIP FOR CHANGE:
      A GUIDE FOR THE FRUSTRATED NURSE. Philadelphia: Lippin-
      cott, 1978.

      Discusses changes that have been effected in nursing by
      individuals and groups. Identifies areas in which change has
      not yet occurred, and reviews the nature of change with an
      emphasis on the problem-solving model.

2018 Bullough, B. and V. Bullough. "The Professionalization of
      Nursing." EXPANDING HORIZONS FOR NURSING. Edited by B.
      Bullough and V. Bullough. New York: Springer Publishing
      Co., 1977, pp. 345-52.

      Examines the effects of professionalism upon nursing. (11)

2019 Chaska, N. (Ed.). THE NURSING PROFESSION: VIEWS THROUGH THE
      MIST. New York: McGraw-Hill, 1978.

      Collection of essays on contemporary issues. Emphasis is
      on issues related to the professionalization of nursing.

      Contains: 925, 933, 934, 943, 952, 955, 956, 962, 965, 1131,
      1492, 1721, 1880, 2323.

2020 Davis, F. (Ed.) THE NURSING PROFESSION: FIVE SOCIOLOGICAL
      ESSAYS. New York: John Wiley & Sons, Inc., 1966.

Five important essays that have shaped many of the subsequent analyses of nursing are published together. William Glaser's essay is on nursing leadership and policy; Anselm Strauss' is on the structure ideology of American nursing; Hans O. Mauksch's is on nursing organization; Esther Lucile Brown's is on patient care, and a three author essay by Fred Davis, Virginia Olesen, and Elva Waik Whittaker is on collegiate nursing education.

2021   deSantis, G.   "Power, Tactics and the Professionalization Process," NURS HEALTH CARE 3(1) (January 1982): 14-17, 24.

Using the Freidson model of professionalization the author points out the importance of power in the professionalization process. (7)

2022   Diers, D.   "Nursing Reclaims Its Role," NURS OUTLOOK 30 (September/October 1982): 459-63.

The definition and interpretation of the nursing profession to the public is essential if nursing is to be understood and valued. (0)

2023   Fitzpatrick, M.L.   PROLOGUE TO PROFESSIONALISM. Englewood Cliffs, NJ.: Prentice-Hall (Brady), 1983.

Designed to provide historical background for understanding the state of the nursing profession, this volume explores the development of nursing education, professional organizations, nursing practice, and credentialing in nursing.

2024   Humphrey, C.   "Introduction: Mandate for Nurses: Involvement in Health Policy." THE EMERGENCE OF NURSING AS A POLITICAL FORCE. New York: National League for Nursing, Pub. No. 41-1760, 1979, pp. 1-10.

Discusses the importance of nurses being involved in the decision making process for health policy issues, and provides specific suggestions for becoming politically involved. (10)

2025   Mauksch, I.G. and M.H. Miller.   IMPLEMENTING CHANGE IN NURSING. St. Louis: C.V. Mosby Co., 1981.

Social change in nursing; work explains how nurses can introduce change effectively into their own work setting.

2026   Molloy, J.T.   THE WOMAN'S DRESS FOR SUCCESS BOOK. New York: Warner Books, Inc., 1977.

Reports research which intends to help women make substantial gains in business and their social lives by revolutionizing clothes buying habits.

2027   Newton, L.H.   "In Defense of the Traditional Nurse," NURS OUTLOOK 29 (June 1981): 348-54.

Traditional nurse model is a worthy one, well founded in the hospital tradition and should be maintained. (0)

2028   Partridge, K.B.   "Nursing Values in a Changing Society," NURS OUTLOOK 26 (June 1978): 356-60.

Nursing's problems result from a rejection of feminine values and the neglect of basic physical care skills as nurses attempt to emulate other professions. (12)

2029   Poulin, M.A.   "Accountability: A Professional Imperative," CAN NURSE 73 (February 1977): 30-33.

Looks at four barriers to professional development: medical dominance, women's role, political naivete, and low visibility and how to overcome these. (4)

2030   Puetz, B.   NETWORKING FOR NURSES.   Rockville, MD.: Aspen Publications, 1983.

Discusses the fundamental concepts of networking and provides information on how to start and use networks to advance nursing careers.   Focuses on female nurses networking with one another and with other members of the health care team.

2031   Safier, G.   CONTEMPORARY AMERICAN LEADERS IN NURSING: AN ORAL HISTORY.   New York: McGraw-Hill Book Co., 1977.

Although nursing as a profession has undergone profound changes since World War II, neither the changes themselves nor those persons instrumental in bringing them about have received sufficient public recognition or scholarly attention. The book presents a number of American nursing leaders who gave account of their careers through the medium of oral history.

2032   Seigel, H.   "Up The Down Staircase in Nursing Education: An Analysis of the Nurse Educator as a Professional," J NURS EDUC 23(3) (March 1984): 114-17.

An examination of the historical status of nursing as a profession and the current status of nurse educators on six criteria of a profession suggests that nursing is advancing in respect to professionalism. (17)

2033   Styles, M.M.   ON NURSING: TOWARD A NEW ENDOWMENT.   St. Louis C.V. Mosby Co., 1982.

Makes distinction between professionalism and professionhood.   Points out that professionalism in nursing will be achieved only through the professionhood of its members.

2034   Turner, J.T. (Ed.)   VIOLENCE IN THE MEDICAL CARE SETTING: A SURVIVAL GUIDE.   Gaithersburg, MD.: Aspen Systems Corp., 1984.

Describes how staff members can protect themselves, their
patients, and visitors from the physical and emotional effects
of violent outbreaks. Covers basic security applications;
techniques for use by nonsecurity health care personnel; and
survival techniques to use when dealing with violence in hospitals, clinics, physicians' offices, pharmacies, and nursing
homes.

2035 Whitman, M. "Toward a New Psychology for Nurses," NURS OUT-
      LOOK 30(1) (January 1982): 48-52.

      Provides an historical background for the strides nurses
      have made and are making in improving their professional con-
      ditions. Education, politics, and research are identified as
      areas in which nurses have begun to change conditions and
      evaluate their practice on their own terms. (3)

2036 Winslow, G.R. "From Loyalty to Advocacy: A New Metaphor for
      Nursing," HASTINGS CENTER REPORT 14(3) (June 1984): 32-40.
      [12-1982]

      Historical essay; traces the stance of the profession as it
      moves from valuing caring obedience to a value for autonomy
      and patient advocacy. (63)

Collective Bargaining/Unionization

2037 Accord, L.G. "Protection of Nursing Practice Through Collec-
      tive Bargaining," INT NURS REV 29(5) (September/October
      1982): 150-52.

      Provides an historic overview of collective bargaining and
      the nursing profession. At present the ANA represents more
      than 110,000 nurses for collective bargaining. It is argued
      that unless control is through the professional associations,
      nurses will be dominated by other unions. (3)

2038 Alutto, J.A. "The Professional Association and Collective
      Bargaining: The Case of the American Nurses' Association."
      ADMINISTERING HEALTH SYSTEMS. Edited by Arnold, et al.
      Chicago: Aldine Publishing Co., 1971.

      Traces the history of the American Nurses' Association as it
      relates to collective bargaining and analyzes the problems of
      nurses in the collective bargaining arena. Characteristics of
      professional workers and nurses in particular present problems
      for any major collective bargaining effort. Although pub-
      lished in 1971, this analysis still offers insights.

2039 American Nurses' Association. ANA'S ECONOMIC & GENERAL WEL-
      FARE PROGRAM: ORGANIZING THE LOCAL UNIT. Kansas City, MO.:
      ANA, 1975, Pub. No. EC-133.

The ANA Commission on Economic and General Welfare presents guidelines for organizing nurses for collective action, including initial contacts with nurses, organization of the unit, and the election to determine exclusive representation.

2040 _____. ANA's ECONOMIC & GENERAL WELFARE PROGRAM; A HISTORICAL PERSPECTIVE. Kansas City, MO.: ANA, 1981, Pub. No. EC-143.

The ANA Commission on Economic and General Welfare presents a fifty year overview of the development and growth of ANA's economic and general welfare program for nurses.

2041 _____. ANA's ECONOMIC & GENERAL WELFARE PROGRAM: THE GRIEVANCE PROCEDURE. Kansas City, MO.: ANA, 1984, Pub. No. EC-132.

The ANA Cabinet on Economic and General Welfare discusses the grievance procedure, including a definition and guidelines for determining whether a complaint is a grievance.

2042 Anderson, B. "Labor Contracts and Negotiations," New York: National League for Nursing, Pub. No. 52-1805 (1979): 69-74.

Written from the administrator's viewpoint. Provides background history on labor negotiations and contracts as well as information on how to prepare for a strike. Discusses Public Law 93-360 and the responsibilities of the National Labor Relations Board. (0)

2043 Beason, C. "Nursing's Labor Relations Crisis," RN 42 (February 1979): 21-33.

Deals with the conflict and unhappiness with various groups of nurses over the ANA as collective bargaining agent. ANA's own structure prevented effective collective bargaining. (0)

2044 Beletz, E.E. "Nurses Participation in Bargaining Units," NURS MANAGE 13(10) (October 1982): 48-58.

Describes nurses' participation in bargaining units. Notes that some nursing professionals still believe that collective bargaining is incompatible with professionalism, and the availability of a collective bargaining program or a negotiated labor agreement does not in itself make collective bargaining effective from an employee's perspective. (22)

2045 _____. "Organized Nurses View Their Collective Bargaining Agent," SUPERVISOR NURSE 11 (1980): 46.

Notes that although nurses are the largest group of health care providers, they have not been able to achieve significant power. Suggests that if health care managers continue to exclude the professional model in collective bargaining, greater militancy among nurses will occur. (15)

2046   Bloom, J.R., C.A. O'Reilly and G.N. Parlette. "Changing
       Images of Professionalism: The Case of Public Health
       Nurses," AM J PUB HEALTH 69(1) (January 1979): 43-46.

       Reports the results of a survey of eighty nine public
       health nurses in a California county which explored reasons
       for the growing support of unionism and the trend towards
       militancy among nurses. Older nurses were found to be less
       likely to advocate collective bargaining and striking. Youn-
       ger nurses believe that unionism and militancy are compatible
       with professionalism. (15)

2047   Bloom, J.R., G.N. Parlette and C.A. O'Reilly. "Collective
       Bargaining by Nurses: A Comparative Analysis of Management
       and Employee Perceptions," HEALTH CARE MANAGE REV 5(1)
       (Winter 1980): 25-33.

       Discusses models of management and the expectations of both
       management and nurses in collective bargaining. (16)

2048   Boyer, J.M., C.L. Westerhaus and J.H. Coggeshall. EMPLOYEE
       RELATIONS AND COLLECTIVE BARGAINING IN HEALTH CARE FACILI-
       TIES. St. Louis: C.V. Mosby Co., 1975.

       Discusses legislation affecting personnel in hospitals,
       nursing homes and other health facilities. Includes guide-
       lines for nurses regarding unionization.

2049   Carrington, B.W. "Collective Bargaining: A Personal Profes-
       sional Experience and an ACNM Imperative," J NURSE MIDWIFE
       26(2) (March/April 1981): 23-26.

       Summarizes how a specific group of certified nurse-midwives
       (CNMs) became part of a collective bargaining unit, and dis-
       cusses the implications of unionization for nurse midwives.
       Provides suggestions to help CNMs study collective bargaining
       on a regional basis. (2)

2050   Cohen, A.G. "Labor Relations in the Health Care Industry:
       A View of the Effects of Unionization of Professional Regis-
       tered Nurses on Hospitals," HOSPITAL TOPICS 60(6) (November/
       December 1982): 33-39.

       Advocates the need for collective bargaining among nurses
       in the context of a health care system that has escalating
       requests for service and greatly increased costs. Discusses
       the conflict between economic realities and the fact that
       individuals consider health care to be a "right." (22)

2051   Cohn, K. "San Jose Nurses Stay Out," UNION W.A.G.E. 69
       (March/April 1982): 1-2.

       Reports on the 1982 nurses strike in San Jose, California
       and discusses the issue of comparable worth. (0)

2052   Colangelo, M.   "The Professional Association and Collective
       Bargaining," SUPERVISOR NURSE 11(9) (September 1980): 27-32.

       Examines the status of nursing and the context in which the
       main body of its practice occurs. Describes factors hindering
       and favoring collective bargaining for nurses and suggests
       some guidelines for the future. Suggests that the nursing
       profession should pay less attention to trying to achieve true
       "professional status" and more to control of its own practice.
       (36)

2053   "Collective Bargaining is ´Unwanted Child´ at ANA, Staff
       Charges," RN 42(1) (January 1979): 16,19.

       Discusses collective bargaining by the employees of the
       American Nurses´ Association. Reports that the employees´
       union charges that ANA management does not view the associa-
       tion as a labor organization. (0)

2054   Crooks, E.   "Nurses´ Associations and Collective Bargaining:
       Wave of the Past?," RN 42(4) (April 1979): 83-88.

       Discusses problems which occur when nurses´ associations
       represent staff nurses in collective bargaining. Associations
       are often charged with conflict of interest because membership
       in ANA and its state bodies is open to all RNs regardless
       of managerial or staff status. Suggestions are provided for
       removing management nurses from contact with collective bar-
       gaining activities. (0)

2055   DeGraw, D.K.   "Mini on the Scene: Seattle, Washington. Role
       of the Nurse Administrator in Labor Negotiations," NURS ADM
       Q 6(2) (Winter 1982): 50-56.

       Provides suggestions for negotiation preparations on the
       part of nurse administrators. (9)

2056   Dolan, A.K.   "The Legality of Nursing Associations Serving
       As Collective Bargaining Agents: The Arundel Case," J HEALTH,
       POLITICS, POLICY AND LAW 5(1) (Spring 1980): 25-54.

       Examines the legality of nursing associations serving as
       collective bargaining agents. A federal case ruled that
       because some state nursing associations are dominated by
       supervisors, they are inappropriate collective bargaining
       agents for nonsupervisory nurses. A review of the literature
       in this area indicates that nursing leaders are more interes-
       ted in pursuing what they consider a "professional" route to
       improving the status of nurses, and that they are not
       especially interested in collective bargaining for the staff
       nurse. (108)

2057   Douglas, J.M.   "Issues in Collective Bargaining for Nurses,"
       New York: National League for Nursing, Pub. No. 23-1874
       (1981): 1-17.

Compares the attitudes of nurses and college teachers
towards collective bargaining. Focuses on professionalism vs.
unionization. Examines the economic and collective bargaining
implications of nursing being a "female profession." (0)

2058   Easterling, J.F. "Autonomy, Professionalism and Collective
       Bargaining," MICH NURSE 56(2) (March/April 1983): 6-7.

       Discusses how collective bargaining agreements through state
       nursing associations can provide mechanisms for handling nurse
       practice concerns. (8)

2059   Emanuel, W.J. "Nurse Unionization is Dominant Theme,"
       HOSPITALS (April 1, 1981): 121.

       The dominant issue in nurse relations with hospitals is the
       interplay between professionalism and unionization. Emanuel
       discusses the issue of collective bargaining by nurses from
       the hospital's perspective. (29)

2060   Emerson, W.L. "Appropriate Bargaining Units for Health Care
       Professional Employees," J NURS ADM (September 1978): 10-15.

       Recent NLRA decision has raised complex questions and issues
       regarding what constitutes appropriate health care profes-
       sional units and which persons be included in them. At time
       of writing RNs are allowed to bargain separately from other
       health care groups; so are MDs. (24)

2061   Emerson, W. "The American Nurses' Association and Collective
       Bargaining," IMPRINT 24 (April 1977): 55, 57, 67.

       ANA is representing an increasing number of nurses in bar-
       gaining. In the future physicians and nurse bargaining units
       probably will work together closely on areas of mutual concern
       and as salary inequities are eliminated, professional issues
       will dominate. (0)

2062 Feldstein, P.J. HEALTH ASSOCIATIONS AND THE DEMAND FOR
      LEGISLATION: THE POLITICAL ECONOMY OF HEALTH. Cambridge,
      MA.: Ballinger, 1977.

       Analyzes the goals and behavior of several health associa-
       tions, including the American Nurses' Association. Explores
       why, despite the large membership of the ANA, nurses' wages,
       function and roles have been determined by physicians and
       hospitals.

2063   Flanagan, L. COLLECTIVE BARGAINING AND THE NURSING PROFES-
       SION. Kansas City, MO.: American Nurses' Association, Pub.
       No. D-72E, 1983.

       Provides an overview of nursing's involvement in collective
       bargaining and focuses on union activity in hospitals. Notes

that by using the collective bargaining process, nurses can
begin to control factors which influence the quality of nursing practice. (137)

2064   Gideon, J.   "The American Nurses´ Association: A Professional
       Model for Collective Bargaining," J HEALTH HUMAN RESOURCE
       ADM 2(1) (August 1979): 13-27.

       Outlines the structure and function of the American Nurses´
       Association in the context of how health care institutions are
       affected by the National Labor Relations Act of 1974. Con-
       tends that nurses have a need for collective bargaining, and
       that the ANA will continue to meet the main needs of nurses.
       (9)

2065   Guy, J.   "Professional Standards--Mandatory Issues for Bar-
       gaining," MICH NURSE 53(9) (October 1980): 4-5.

       Emphasizes that consideration of obstacles to safe and
       therapeutic practice should be addressed by collective bar-
       gaining. (0)

2066   Ibbotson, P.   "Collective Bargaining: A Tool for Professional
       Growth," MICH NURSE 54(1) (January 1981): 24.

       Discusses how collective bargaining provides a tool to gain
       power in the work environment. (0)

2067   Jacox, A.   "Collective Action: The Basis for Professionalism,"
       SUPERVISOR NURSE 11(9) (September 1980): 22-24.

       Discusses collective bargaining as a basis for profes-
       sionalism and examines the roles of collective bargaining and
       administration in a hospital. Emphasizes that both labor and
       management share the goal of delivering a high quality of
       professional service. The importance of a unified nursing
       community is noted, and nurses are warned not to affiliate
       with labor unions comprised of non-nurses. (3)

2068   Jones, B.   "The Right to Strike," NURS MIRROR 149(9) (August
       30, 1979): 12.

       Discusses whether or not a nurse should face proceedings for
       professional misconduct if he/she participates in a strike.
       (0)

2069   Katz, B.F.   "Why Nurses Form Unions," NURS LAW & ETHICS 1(2)
       (February 1980): 1-2, 6.

       Provides an overview of the history and development of labor
       unions for nurses. Considers bargaining subjects, grievances,
       patient care issues, and the issue of professionalism and
       unions. (12)

2070   Kluge, E.W.   "The Profession of Nursing and the Right to
       Strike," WESTMINSTER INST REV 2 (Fall 1982): 3-6.

Author argues that with some qualifications, nurses do have the right to strike.

2071 Krause, E.A. POWER AND ILLNESS: THE POLITICAL SOCIOLOGY OF HEALTH AND MEDICAL CARE. New York: Elsevier, 1977.

Discusses control over work in the health care field and illustrates nursing's struggle against the hierarchy. Provides a debate about professionalization and unionization. Identifies inadequacies in how the American health care system treats the poor and minority groups.

2072 Kruger, D.H. LABOR MANAGEMENT ISSUES FOR THE FUTURE. New York: National League for Nursing, Pub. No. 20-1801, 1979, pp. 1-12.

Six major issues affecting employer-employee relations are discussed: (1) autonomy, (2) specialization, (3) demographic changes, (4) collective bargaining issues, (5) economic environment, and (6) better-educated professional labor force. (0)

2073 LaViolette, S. "Collective Bargaining Given Funding, Priority Boost by ANA Delegates," MODERN HEALTH CARE 10(7) (July 1980): 48.

Reports that there is an increase of support of collective bargaining by nurses in local bargaining units and that the American Nurses' Association is giving collective bargaining a higher priority and a larger budget than it has in the recent past. (0)

2074 Levenstein, A. "Professionals and Collective Bargaining. The Art and Science of Supervision," SUPERVISOR NURSE 11(0) (October 1980): 15-16.

Summarizes reasons for increasing unionization of nurses and notes that many nurses have come to realize that there is not an inherent contradiction between professionalism and unionization. (0)

2075 Lorenz, F.J. "Nursing Administration and Undivided Loyalty," NURS ADM Q 6(2) (Winter 1982): 67-74.

Discusses the necessity of drawing a clear distinction between supervisors and staff nurses for purposes of collective bargaining. Examines the issue of whether state nurses' associations representing RNs are violating the National Labor Relations Act when their governing boards are comprised of nursing management personnel. (11)

2076 Millar, S. "A Nursing Assessment of Unions," HEART-LUNG 10(1) (January/February 1981): 24-26.

Summarizes the reasons for the existence of nurses' unions and discusses the benefits and liabilities of unionizing. (6)

2077   Muyskens, J.L. "Nurses´ Collective Responsibility and the
       Strike Weapon," J MED PHIL 7 (1982): 101-12.

       Right to strike and the duty to strike are examined in terms
       of collective responsibility of nurses. (2)

2078   Nousianen, T. "Story of a Strike," INT NURS REV 31(6)
       (November/December 1984): 184-86.

       In the summer of 1983 the Finnish Nurses Federation, a
       nursing organization in membership with the Union of Health
       Professions (TEHY) and within the Confederation of Salaried
       Employees (TVK) of Finland found themselves in dispute with
       the employers (KSV). A limited strike, supported by all poli-
       tical parties and the majority of members of parliament. The
       strike resulted in an increase in salaries. This is an ac-
       count of events. (0)

2079   Numerof, R.E. and M.N. Abrams. "Collective Bargaining Among
       Nurses: Current Issues and Future Prospects," HEALTH CARE
       MANAGEMENT REV 9(2) (Spring 1984): 61-67.

       Collective bargaining has made substantial progress in the
       health care industry in recent years, and the nursing staffs
       have been the primary focus of much of the organizational
       activity. Nurses are better educated than in the past and
       desire more autonomy; this creates discontent. (37)

2080   "Occupational Health Nurses and Collective Bargaining: A
       Statement by the American Association of Occupational Health
       Nurses, Inc.," OCCUP HEALTH NURS 28(9) (September 1980):
       30-31.

       Notes that in 1949 the members of the American Association
       of Occupational Health Nurses voted against collective bargain-
       ing, and that as of 1980 this stand remains unchanged. Sum-
       marizes the pros and cons of unionization. (0)

2081   O´Rourke, K.A. NURSE POWER-UNIONS, AND THE LAW. Bowie, MD.:
       Robert J. Brady Co., 1981.

       Provides nurses with basic facts about the law and the col-
       lective bargaining processes. Encourages nurses to unionize
       and emphasizes that there is no conflict between profession-
       alism and unionism. Includes a sample contract. (156)

2082   Ponak, A.M. "Unionized Professionals and the Scope of Bar-
       gaining: A Study of Nurses," INDUSTRIAL AND LABOR RELATIONS
       REV 34(3) (April 1983): 396-407.

       Reports the results of a study which examines the scope of
       negotiations of unionized professional nurses. The central
       question examined is how professional collective bargaining
       goals are differentiated from more traditional bargaining
       matters such as wages and hours. (37)

2083 Rothman, W.A. STRIKES IN HEALTH CARE ORGANIZATIONS. Owings
      Mills, MD.: National Health Publishing, 1983.

      Study of strikes in health care examines the history, impact
      on operations, legal and ethical issues, professional perspec-
      tives of nurses and physicians, and concludes with a guide to
      contingency planning in the event that a strike should occur.

2084 Rothwell, S. "Professionalism--Unionism--and the Future of
      Nursing," AARN NEWSLETTER 37(8) (1981): 1-3.

      Examines the consequences of parallel development in profes-
      sionalism and unionism in nursing, and considers future possi-
      bilities for strengthening the nursing profession in Canada.
      (2)

2085 Rotkovitch, R. "Do Labor Union Activities Decrease Profession-
      alism?," SUPERVISOR NURSE 11(9) (September 1980): 16-18.

      Criticizes collective bargaining for nurses and believes that
      when nurses unionize there is a loss of professionalism which
      diminishes the nurse's self-image, his/her public image, and
      ultimately causes a deterioration in the nurse's professional
      practice. (7)

2086 Rutkowski, A.D. and B.L. Rutkowski. LABOR RELATIONS IN HOSPI-
      TALS. Gaithersburg, MD.: Aspen Systems Corp., 1984.

      Discusses labor relations from a management standpoint.
      Covers legal responsibilities, grievances, and what management
      can and cannot do in election campaigns, strikes, and decerti-
      fication campaigns. Actual cases implementing basic labor re-
      lations theories are examined.

2087 Sain, T.R. "Effects of Unionization," NURS MANAGE 15(1)
      (January 1984): 43-45.

      Discusses the changes that middle managers must make when
      the people they supervise become unionized. Provides sugges-
      tions for cooperative union/management relationships. (0)

2088 Sorrel, L. "Comparable Worth," OFF OUR BACKS 12 (June 1982):
      11. Also in WOMEN STUDIES ABSTRACTS 11(3) (1982-83): 30.

      Discusses the California Nursing Association's efforts to
      win pay for nurses comparable to that of pharmacists (who go
      through comparable training). (0)

2089 Telesco, M. "Let's Say 'Yes' to Unions!," RN (November 1978):
      29-30, 32-33.

      Conditions under which nurses work is up to them but the
      most effective way of controlling work conditions is through
      unions. (0)

2090 "To Cut Costs Hospitals Try to Take Back RNs Health Benefits,"
      AM J NURS 84(4) (April 1984): 529, 548, 550.

      Reports that hospitals are attempting to shift health insur-
      ance costs to their employees. Includes information about
      health benefits from various state nursing associations. Dis-
      cusses how unions are fighting attempts to decrease nurses'
      benefits. (0)

2091 Wells, D. "A Study of Nurses' Attitudes to Different Forms
      of Collective Action," NEW ZEALAND NURS FORUM 7(1) (1979):
      4-5.

      Reports the results of a study which examined New Zealand
      nurses' attitudes to various forms of collective bargaining.
      It was found that the majority of nurses would be prepared to
      take action involving a withdrawal of their services from some
      clinical areas. (0)

2092 Zimmerman, A., V. Cleland and M. Leininger. "Taft-Hartley
      Amended: Implications for Nursing," AM J NURS 75 (February
      1975): 284-96.

      Reports repeal of the long standing exemption on non profit
      hospitals from the requirement that they do collective bar-
      gaining with employees. This development is significant in
      the development of collective bargaining for nurses. (8)

      See 384, 864, 982, 1410, 2058.

Wages/Benefits

2093 Alessi, D.J. PROVING SEX-BASED WAGE DISCRIMINATION UNDER
      FEDERAL LAW. Kansas City, MO.: American Nurses' Association,
      Pub. No. D-721, 1983.

      Discusses how judicial interpretation of the Equal Pay Act
      of 1963 has made it difficult for women to prove that they
      have been the subjects of wage discrimination. Considers how
      the decision in the case County of Washington v. Gunther has
      made it easier for women to prove such discrimination. (258)

2094 American Nurses' Association. REPORT OF THE SURVEY OF SALA-
      RIES OF REGISTERED NURSE FACULTY IN NURSING EDUCATION PRO-
      GRAM, JANUARY 1976. Kansas City, MO.: American Nurses'
      Association, Pub. No. D-61, 1977.

      Comprehensive report by ANA showing the median and percen-
      tage distributions of annual salaries by type of position,
      academic rank, highest educational preparation, service, ex-
      perience, responsibility, type of nursing program, geographic
      locations, and size of enrollment.

2095 "ANA Files Sex-Bias Charge vs. The State of Illinois," AM J
      NURS 84(2) (February 1984): 257.

Reports that the ANA has joined the Illinois Nurses Association in a complaint filed with the Equal Employment Opportunity Commission against the State of Illinois. The ANA is
charging that Illinois has intentionally discriminated against
women by failing to rectify pay inequities. (0)

2096   Beyers, M., R. Mullner, C.S. Byre and S.F. Whitehead. "Re-
       sults of the Nursing Personnel Survey, Part 3: RN Salary and
       Fringe Benefits," J NURS ADM 13(6) (June 1983): 16-20.

       Analyzes and interprets the results of the American Hospital
       Association's 1981 Nursing Personnel Survey. Discusses wage
       and fringe benefits that responding hospitals offered to full-
       time registered nurses. Reports that most studies of nurse
       job satisfaction indicate that salaries are less important to
       registered nurses than other factors. (16)

2097   Blaker, G. "Some of Us Are More Equal Than Others," CAN NURSE
       76(5) (May 1980): 6.

       Discusses equal pay for work of equal value and cites an
       example involving nurses who were paid nine percent less than
       male hospital technicians.(0)

2098   Brett, J.L. "How Much Is A Nurse's Job Really Worth?," AM J
       NURS 83(6) (June 1983): 876-81.

       An analysis of comparable worth as it applies to nurses. (18)

2099   "Comp Worth Study: 'Nurses Really Underpaid'," AM J NURS 84(2)
       (February 1984): 256-57.

       Reports that the Illinois Commission on the Status of Women
       has found that state-employed nurses and other female state
       employees in Illinois are earning far less than male employees
       in comparable jobs. Includes a chart which compares salaries
       for several job classifications. (0)

2100   del Bueno, D.J. A FINANCIAL GUIDE FOR NURSES: INVESTING IN
       YOURSELF AND OTHERS. Boston: Blackwell Scientific Publica-
       tions, 1981.

       Provides information about finding various types of nursing
       positions and about consulting, lecturing, starting a private
       practice, getting published, and making financial investments.
       (0)

2101   Diers, D. "Nursing Reclaims Its Role," NURS OUTLOOK 30(8)
       (September/October 1982): 459-63.

       Discusses how nurses must define and interpret their profes-
       sion to the public in order to be understood and valued.
       Nurses are refusing to stay invisible, controllable, patron-

ized, and underpaid, but they face many obstacles, partly
because to the untrained eye, what nurses do looks fairly easy
and also because nursing is economically invisible. Provides
a comparison of nurse and physician and salary trends. (0)

2102 Dittmar, C.C. RETIREMENT INCOME ISSUES FOR WOMEN AND REGIS-
      TERED NURSES. Kansas City, MO.: American Nurses' Associa-
      tion, Pub. No. D-72F, 1983.

      Explores elements of social security and private policies
      for nurses. Examines proposals for reforms to correct in-
      adequacies in retirement benefits for nurses. Discusses
      economic status of aged women and factors affecting retirement
      income levels. (33)

2103 _____. SALARIES OF REGISTERED NURSES. Kansas City, MO.:
      American Nurses' Association, Pub. No. D-72B, 1982.

      Discusses current earnings of registered nurses, salary
      trends, and occupational comparisons. Includes charts which
      show average annual salaries of registered nurses employed in
      selected nursing positions. (38)

2104 Donovan, L. "Survey of Nursing Incomes--Part 2. What In-
      creases Income Most?," RN 43(2) (February 1980): 27-30.

      Focuses on education, experience, and specialized skills and
      how they affect the income of the nurse. Reports that nearly
      two-thirds of nurses (regardless of experience level) res-
      ponding to a salary survey had annual earnings between $10,000
      and $15,000, a level which is considered entry level by most
      other professions. Emphasizes that the most significant
      finding of the survey is the lack of impact that experience
      has on earnings. (0)

2105 Edmunds, M.W. "Rectifying Salary Problems," NURSE PRACT 4(1)
      (January/February 1979): 36, 40.

      Discusses the problem of the nurse practitioner who brings
      more revenue into the practice in which she works than is
      reflected by the salary she receives. A case study is pre-
      sented and some practical suggestions for solving the problem
      are provided.(8)

2106 Friss, L.O. "Work Force Policy Perspectives: Registered
      Nurses," J HEALTH POLITICS, POLICY LAW 5(4) (Winter 1981):
      696-719.

      Notes that lack of equal pay for comparable work is an im-
      portant factor in the decline of the number of registered
      nurses who work in hospitals. Describes the network which
      determines how nurse salaries are decided, provides com-
      parisons with other groups such as policemen, teachers, and
      laborers. (51)

2107 Hicks, M. "NAPNAP Membership Survey 1981: PNP Salaries,
      Functions, and Distribution," PED NURS 8(2) (March/April
      1982): 111-12.

      Provides a brief report about information gathered from a
      1981 survey of pediatric nurse practitioners. (0)

2108 Johnson, J. "Comparable Worth: A Sleeping Giant," NURSE PRACT
      9(9) (September 1984): 11.

      Legislation proposing equal pay for women is being con-
      sidered by Congress. Regulations allowing medicare patients
      to use HMOs have been issued.(0)

2109 McKibbin, R.C. NURSING IN THE 80s: KEY ECONOMIC AND EMPLOY-
      MENT ISSUES. Kansas City, MO.: American Nurses' Associa-
      tion, Pub. No. D-72A, 1982.

      Discusses the impact of the general economic situation on
      nurses and nursing; changes in the health delivery system;
      salaries of registered nurses; the demand for nurses, career
      ladders; and reimbursement for nursing services. (31)

2110 _____. ECONOMIC AND EMPLOYMENT ISSUES IN NURSING EDUCATION.
      Kansas City, MO.: American Nurses' Association, Pub. No.
      D-72C, 1983.

      Considers economic aspects of elements of nursing education
      that are problematic. Explores the concept of demand in terms
      of employment opportunities for nurses as well as demand for
      education in nursing. Discusses the current and future occu-
      pational outlook for nurses. (35)

2111 Moskowitz, S. "Strategies for Ending Wage Discrimination in
      Nursing," NURS ECON 2(1) (January/February 1984): 25-32.

      Discusses litigation under federal and state anti-dis-
      crimination statutes, collective bargaining and new state
      legislation as ways of ending wage discrimination in nursing.
      (27)

2112 "News: House Tackles Pay Equity Issue: Kennedy To Introduce
      Legislation," AM J NURS (January 1983): 7, 32.

      Job worth issue--equal pay bill introduced.(0)

2113 "Nurses' Shrinking Pay Raises: A Recap of 1982," AM J NURS
      84(4) (April 1984): 530-31.

      Reports that pay raises for nurses were minimal from August,
      1982 to August, 1983 with starting salaries for staff nurses
      increasing only 2.9 percent over the previous year. Includes
      a chart which compares salaries of several hospital employee
      groups. (0)

2114 "Nursing Faculty Salaries Inching Up, Says AACN," AM J NURS
      84(4) (April 1984): 530-31.

      Reports that nursing faculty received an average of 4.5 per-
      cent increase in the 1983-84 academic year. Includes a chart
      of average salaries for academic ranks. (0)

2115 Pearson, L.E. "A Look at Fringe Benefits," NURS ECON 1(2)
      (September/October 1983): 138-42.

      Discusses benefits from both the employee and organization
      perspective. Warns that employers who offer exceptional
      benefits may have problems with turnover and the prospective
      working environment should be explored carefully. Discusses
      tax consequences of benefits for the self-employed nurse. (7)

2116 Player, J.M. "The Economic Importance of Nurses," NURS MANAGE
      13(11) (November 1982): 52-53.

      Summarizes why nurses should speak out loudly about economic
      issues such as salaries, benefits, practice climate, and pro-
      fessional stature. (7)

2117 Powell, P.J. "Fee for Service," NURS MANAGE 14(3) (March
      1983): 13-15.

      Discusses fee-for-service for nurses within the context of
      health care costs in the United States. Reports the results
      of a survey which was conducted among nursing associations
      and nursing specialty groups to determine current status of
      third-party reimbursement and fee-for-service around the
      country. (1)

2118 Robyn, D. and J. Hadley. "National Health Insurance and the
      New Health Occupations: Nurse Practitioners and Physician's
      Assistants," J HEALTH, POLITICS, POLICY AND LAW 5(3) (Fall
      1980): 447-69.

      Examines issues which could arise in formulating policy for
      nurse practitioners and physician's assistants. The develop-
      ment and expansion of the nurse practitioner and physician
      assistant professions are discussed, as well as their perfor-
      mance regarding the quality of health care provided and the
      impact on the cost of such care. Discusses national health
      insurance legislation, certification, and licensure, training
      subsidies, physicians' attitudes, and the potential impact of
      an increased supply of physicians on the careers of nurse
      practitioners.(43)

2119 Thaker, H.H. WAGE SETTING AND EVALUATION: ECONOMIC PRIN-
      CIPLES FOR REGISTERED NURSES. Kansas City, MO.: American
      Nurses' Association, Pub. No. D-72H, 1983.

      Provides nurses with an understanding of the factors that
      affect their wages. Discusses demand, supply and prices,

and encourages nurses to develop strategies that will help
raise their compensation to a level that reflects their worth.
(27)

2120   Weingard, M. "Establishing Comparable Worth Through Job
       Evaluation," NURS OUTLOOK 32(2) (March/April 1984): 110-13.

       Provides an historical overview of the concept of comparable
       worth and how nurses are affected by job segregation and wage
       discrimination. Suggests a strategy for establishing compar-
       able worth in nursing. (27)

       See 866, 1215, 2189.

Job Satisfaction/Dissatisfaction

2121   American Academy of Nursing Task Force on Nursing Practice in
       Hospitals. MAGNET HOSPITALS ATTRACTION AND RETENTION OF
       PROFESSIONAL NURSES. Kansas City, MO.: American Nurses'
       Association, 1983.

       An empirical study sponsored by the American Academy of
       Nursing which identified "magnet" hospitals known for their
       excellence. The magnet hospitals were studied in order to
       identify the factors in hospital organization and nursing
       service that attracted and retained professional nurses on the
       staff. The nurse administrators were strong persons, but they
       used participative management styles. Nurses reported that
       they had autonomy to carry out good patient care. Salaries
       were competitive. Nursing care was considered important in
       the magnet hospitals and the image of the individual nurse was
       good.

2122   Benner, P. and R.V. Benner. THE NEW YORK'S WORK ENTRY: A
       TROUBLED SPONSORSHIP. New York: Tiresias Press, Inc., 1979.

       Examines such problems as the retention of nurses in hos-
       pitals, the need for adequate skill training, and coping with
       organizational and professional change. Includes question-
       naires and interview protocols germane to the transition from
       school to work.

2123   Castiglia, P.T., L. McCausland and J. Hunter. "Blowout: An
       Alternative Conceptual Approach to Nursing Turnover." NURS-
       ING ISSUES AND NURSING STRATEGIES FOR THE EIGHTIES. Edited
       by B. Bullough, V. Bullough and M.C. Soukup. New York:
       Springer Publishing Co., 1983, pp. 55-70.

       Among reasons for leaving the job are lack of opportunities
       for advancement, family obligations, dissatisfaction with the
       organization, lack of control over standards of profession.
       Based on a study of nurses in Western New York. (14)

2124   Davitz, J. and L. Davitz. NURSES' RESPONSES TO PATIENTS'
       SUFFERING. New York: Springer Publishing Co., 1980.

Examines the significance of nurses´ perceptions of mental
anguish and physical pain. A concise report on the authors´
original six-year study.

2125 Duxbury, M.L., G.D. Armstrong, D.J. Drew and S.J. Henly.
      "Head Nurse Leadership Style With Staff Nurse Burnout and
      Job Satisfaction in Neonatal Intensive Care Units," NURS RES
      33(2) (March/April 1984): 97-101.

      Although head nurse structure itself has no relationships
      with satisfaction and burnout, it has effects in combination
      with other factors. NICU head nurses can promote competency
      and professional growth by displaying a leadership style that
      discourages the development of burnout and job dissatisfac-
      tion. (39)

2126 Fuszard, B. (Ed.) SELF-ACTUALIZATION FOR NURSES: ISSUES,
      TRENDS AND STRATEGIES FOR JOB ENRICHMENT. Rockville, MD.:
      Aspen, 1984.

      Examines the conflict between professional and institutional
      goals, and strategies to meet both through job enrichment by
      restructuring the work role of the professional nurse.

2127 Ginzberg, E. et al. "Nurse Discontent: The Search for Realis-
      tic Solutions," J NURS ADM 12(11) (November 1982): 7-11.

      Discusses the findings of a survey about graduate nurses´
      satisfactions and dissatisfactions with their jobs and
      careers; 49 percent of all respondents said that they would
      not choose nursing if they were starting a career again,
      and 44 percent would not advise a young person to study nurs-
      ing.(7)

2128 Joiner, C. and G.M. van Servellen. JOB ENRICHMENT IN NURSING:
      A GUIDE TO IMPROVING MORALE, PRODUCTIVITY AND RETENTION.
      Rockville, MD.: Aspen, 1984.

      Reviews literature about job enrichment, presents a model
      and strategies for redesigning the nurse´s role and carrying
      out the changes necessary for job enrichment.

2129 Kanungo, R.N. "Affiliation and Autonomy Under Stress,"
      PSYCHOLOGICAL REPORTS 46 (June 1980, Pt. 2): 1340.

      Reports about a study among 142 nurses which indicates that
      workers who experience a great deal of stress in their jobs
      show little desire for autonomy and responsibility, because
      increased job responsibility becomes a burden. (3)

2130 LeMaitre, G.D. "A Physician Speaks Out On Burnout," AM J NURS
      81(8) (August 1981): 1487.

Argues it is not physicians limiting nursing practice but
litigation-conscious nursing profession which won´t let nurses
do things physicians want them to do such as inflating the
esophageal balloon. (0)

2131 McConnell, E. BURNOUT IN THE NURSING PROFESSION: CAUSES,
      COSTS, AND COPING STRATEGIES. St. Louis: C.V. Mosby Co.,
      1982.

      Begins with an overview and historical perspective, and goes
      on to examine the physiology of stress, which nurses are at
      greater risk, the causes of burnout, its costs to the health
      care system, how to prevent burnout, and how to cope with it
      when it does occur.

2132 Parasuraman, S., B.H. Drake and R.F. Zammuto. "The Effect of
      Nursing Care Modalities and Shift Assignments on Nurses´
      Work Experiences and Job Attitudes," NURS RES 31(6) (Novem-
      ber/December 1982): 364-67.

      Examines how nursing job design relates to other work ex-
      periences of nurses and job attitudes other than satisfaction.
      Sample was 327 supervisors, nurses, and licensed practical
      nurses. (18)

2133 Rose, M. "Shift Work: How Does It Affect You?," AM J NURS
      84(4) (April 1984): 442-47.

      Discusses how shift work affects sleep, physiology and
      social and family life. Considers worker preference for fixed
      vs. rotating shifts and how job satisfaction and motivation
      are affected by shift work. (7)

2134 Sovie, M.D. "The Economics of Magnetism," NURS ECON 2(2)
      (March/April 1984): 85-92.

      A composite representation of a magnet hospital illustrates
      the findings of the study MAGNET HOSPITALS, ATTRACTION AND
      RETENTION OF PROFESSIONAL NURSES (McClure, Poulin, Sovie and
      Wandelt, 1983). Selected components of magnetism offer
      economic advantages that contribute to the hospital´s fiscal
      viability in the prospective pricing environment. These cost
      savings and benefits must be quantified by the nursing
      administration. (7)

2135 Thompson, L. "Job Satisfaction of Nurse Anesthetists," AANA
      J 49(1) (February 1981): 43-51.

      Examines the relative importance of six specific components
      of job satisfactions among nurse anesthetists in Pennsylvania.
      (29)

2136 Ventura, M.R., R.N. Fox, M.C. Corley and S.M. Mercurio. "A
      Patient Satisfaction Measures As a Criterion to Evaluate
      Primary Nursing," NURS RES 31(4) (July/August 1982): 226-30.

The Risser Patient Satisfaction Scale was used to evaluate the effectiveness of implementing the key concepts of primary nursing. Forty-six subjects from two units completed questionnaires. No significant differences obtained between the units on any of the subscales or total scores. (29)

2137   Vogt, J.F., J.L. Cox, B.A. Velthouse and B.H. Thames. RETAINING PROFESSIONAL NURSES: A PLANNED PROCESS. St. Louis, MO.: C.V. Mosby Co., 1983.

Presents creative and innovative approaches to keeping nurses in the profession and the work force. Explores the high turnover and dropout rate among nurses from financial, managerial, organizational, and professional viewpoints. Underscores the need for strategic planning as a basis for change. Examines retention from individual, supervisor, organization, and milieu perspectives.

2138   Wandelt, M.A., P.M. Pierce and R.R. Widdowson. "Why Nurses Leave Nursing and What Can Be Done About It," AM J NURS 81(1) (January 1981): 72-77.

A survey of 3,500 Texas nurses who have left nursing. In terms of rank order of explanation, salaries were most important reason for leaving. Other answers are also given, including lack of autonomy and recognition, quality of care et al.(0)

2139   Wolf, G.A. "Nursing Turnover: Some Causes and Solutions," NURS OUTLOOK 29(4) (April 1981): 233-66.

Explores causes of the high turnover rate of nurses and offers solutions to the problem. The primary reason for leaving has been identified as job dissatisfaction. Another problem identified is lack of nursing autonomy and professional recognition. (27)

See 83, 2094, 2095, 2099, 2100.

Women/Feminism

2140   Angel, G. and D.K. Petronko. DEVELOPING THE NEW ASSERTIVE NURSE: ESSENTIALS FOR ADVANCEMENT. New York: Springer Publishing Co., 1983.

Handbook instructs nurses, educators, and nursing managers in principles of assertiveness, offering practical advice, illustrated with case examples.

2141   Ashley, J.A. HOSPITALS, PATERNALISM AND THE ROLE OF THE NURSE. New York: Teachers College Press, 1976.

Discusses exploitation of nurses, the role of apprenticeship and paternalism in the hospital setting, and the myth of men and women and their roles in health care. Examines the systematic oppression of the nursing profession.

2142 _____. "Power in Structured Misognyny: Implications for the
      Politics of Care," ADV NURS SCI 2(3) (April 1980): 3-22.

      Shows how misogyny has been historically structured through-
      out human experience and interprets how structured misogyny
      affects current politics of health care. Notes that feminist
      thought advocates the nourishment and preservation of life,
      and emphasizes that nursing and all health care professions
      should share these goals. (19)

2143 Baumgart, A.J. "Nurses and Political Action: The Legacy of
      Sexism," NURS PAP 12(4) (Winter 1980): 6-16.

      Notes that organized nursing associations in Canada have
      begun to define themselves as political pressure groups having
      a direct, continuous, and active role in influencing health
      policy. Discusses the importance of nurses' awareness of the
      ways sexism contributes to their lack of political influence.
      (21)

2144 Bingham, S. MINISTERING ANGELS. ORADELL, NJ.: Medical
      Economics Co., Book Division, 1979.

      Provides a history of nursing as well as a description of a
      social revolution that has had a profound effect on women's
      role in today's society.

2145 Bowler, J.E., D.E. Hinkle and W.M. Wormer. "Do Women Aspire
      to the Same Administrative Positions as Men?," EDUC ADMIN
      Q 19(2) (1983): 64-81.

      Discusses the administrative aspirations of male and female
      faculty members in land grant universities. Includes pre-
      ferences for beginning-level positions and those ultimately
      sought. Refutes myths regarding women's administrative aspir-
      ations. (15)

2146 Buldt, B.W. "Sexual Harassment in Nursing," NURS OUTLOOK 30
      (June 1982): 336-43.

      Legal definition of sex harassment and what can be done
      about it. Includes a survey of 89 nurses. (22)

2147 Bullough, B. and V. Bullouogh. "Sex Discrimination in Health
      Care," NURS OUTLOOK 23 (January 1975): 40-45. Reprinted in
      EXPANDING HORIZONS FOR NURSES. Edited by B. Bullough and V.
      Bullough. New York: Springer Publishing Co., 1977, pp.
      293-306.

      Examines wage discrimination against women in nursing and in
      other health related occupations. (28)

2148 Bullough, V. THE SUBORDINATE SEX: A HISTORY OF ATTITUDES
      TOWARD WOMEN. New York: Penguin Books, 1974.

Historical background for many of the current problems faced by women. Traces societal attitudes towards women.

2149   Bullough, V.L. and B. Bullough. HISTORY, TRENDS, AND POLITICS OF NURSING. Norwalk, CT.: Appleton-Century-Crofts, 1984.

Includes four chapters on "Nurses as Women" and discusses such topics as how the profession of nursing has been influenced by being comprised primarily of the "subordinate sex," and how the women's movement has affected change in nursing.

2150   Chenevert, M. SPECIAL TECHNIQUES IN ASSERTIVENESS TRAINING FOR WOMEN IN THE HEALTH PROFESSIONS. St. Louis: C.V. Mosby, 1978.

Social and psychological conditions have made women afraid to express themselves - become chickens - and author indicates how to become an eagle. Inadequacies and injustices of the male dominated health care system are pointed out.

2151   Christopher, R. "Nursing Politics: Challenge to Socialist Nurses," HEALTH ACTIVISTS DIGEST 3(3) (Summer 1982): 15-24.

Discusses the conflict between the institution of nursing and the health care elite in the context of nursing professionalism and the sexual caste system in health care employment. Defends nursing as an institution in which women exercise power.

2152   Cleland, V.S. "To End Sex Discrimination," NURS CLIN NORTH AM 9 (September 1974): 563-71. Reprinted in EXPANDING HORIZONS FOR NURSES. Edited by B. Bullough and V. Bullough. New York: Springer Publishing Co., 1977, pp. 319-27.

Examines two streams of variables within the women's movement: social psychological ones and legal ones. (6)

2153   Connors, D.D. "Sickness Unto Death: Medicine as Mythic, Necrophilic and Iatrogenic," ADV NURS SCI 2(3) (April 1980): 39-51.

Uses inductive cross-disciplinary analysis to integrate 13 years of experience as a hospital nurse with the perspectives of sociology, philosophy, psychiatry, and political science. Illustrates how the medical profession perpetuates and lives out myths in order to insure its continued existence. Identifies women as targets of iatrogenic medicine. (27)

2154   "Court Rules Out Sex-Based Tables for Pension Plans," AM J NURS (September 1983): 1251, 1268.

News item. Reports Supreme Court decision outlawing discrimination against women in pension plans. (0)

2155   Cowan, C.E.   "Sexism by Nurses," LAMP 38(8) (August 1981):
       5-12.

       Examines sexism as perpetuated by nurses toward others and
       considers nurses' attitudes toward physical discipline as en-
       acted by husbands toward their wives. Discusses the nurse's
       perception of self and the nurse's attitude toward the female
       patient. (24)

2156   Daly, M.   GYNECOLOGY: THE METAETHICS OF RADICAL FEMINISM.
       Boston: Beacon Press, 1978.

       Presents an analysis of how women are (and have been through-
       out history) objects of attack by a patriarchal society.
       Identifies the role of the nurse in American gynecology as
       that of a token torturer. Encourages nurses to work towards
       changing the treatment of women by gynecologists.

2157   Donegan, J.B.   WOMEN & MEN MIDWIVES: MEDICINE, MORALITY AND
       MISOGYNY IN EARLY AMERICA. Westport, CT.: Greenwood Press,
       1978.

       Author considers the complex male-female relationships in-
       volved, showing how closely the history of midwifery is con-
       nected to the history of feminism.

2158   Ehrenreich, B. and D. English.   WITCHES, MIDWIVES, AND NURSES:
       A HISTORY OF WOMEN HEALERS. New York: The Feminist Press,
       1973.

       Focuses on two phases in the male takeover of health care:
       the suppression of witches in medieval Europe, and the rise
       of the male medical professor in 19th century America.

2159   Ehrenreich, B.   "Status Of Women As Health Care Providers in
       the United States," PROCEEDINGS OF THE INTERNATIONAL CON-
       FERENCE ON WOMEN IN HEALTH. Washington, D.C.: U.S.D.H.E.W.,
       1976, pp. 7-13.

       Discusses the subordination of women in the United States
       health industry and explores social factors which help per-
       petuate sexual division of labor and power. (42)

2160   _____.   FOR HER OWN GOOD: 150 YEARS OF THE EXPERTS ADVICE TO
       WOMEN. Garden City, NJ.: Anchor Press, 1978.

       Provides an historical overview of "experts" (primarily
       male) views on the nature of women. Traces how such indivi-
       duals have, over the years, claimed total knowledge of human
       biological existence and have passed judgment on the social
       consequences of female anatomy. Provides a framework for
       significant change in women's health care. (569)

2161   _____.   "The Purview of Political Action." THE EMERGENCE OF
       NURSING AS A POLITICAL FORCE. New York: National League for
       Nursing, Pub. No. 41-1760, 1979.

2162   Fitzpatrick, M. L.   "Nursing," SIGNS 2 (Summer 1977): 818-34.

Nursing as a women's profession and its impact and implications for nursing. (48)

2163   Friedan, B.   "Moving Into the Second Stage: An Interview with
       Betty Friedan," NURS OUTLOOK 29(11) (November 1981): 666-69.

Interview with Betty Friedan which emphasizes the value of
nursing in our society. Suggests that nurses take advantage
of being in demand and collectively demand salary increases,
flexible working hours, leaves, child care, and increased recognition and autonomy. (0)

2164   Greenleaf, N.P.   "Sex-segregated Occupations: Relevance for
       Nursing," ADV NURS SCI 2(3) (April 1980): 23-38.

Notes that the way nurses think and the way they come to
know their world and form self-images has been shaped by being
exposed to a male point of view. Discusses the androcentric
perspective in the context of theory construction in nursing.
(38)

2165   Grissum, M. and C. Spengler.   WOMANPOWER AND HEALTH CARE.
       Boston: Little Brown, 1976.

Focuses on issues, problems and barriers confronting women,
and especially women who are nurses. Discusses how the
socialization process of childhood helps perpetuate outmoded
roles for women and makes it difficult for women who become
nurses to break out of those roles and become autonomous
practitioners. Explores theories of change and the degree to
which women are willing to be change agents and risk-takers.

2166   Heide, W.S.   "Nursing and Women's Liberation: A Parallel," AM
       J NURS 73 (May 1973): 824-27.

Heide was President of NOW as well as a nurse and she writes
on how nurses can be leaders in bringing about a humanist
society as well as humanizing health care. (4)

2167   Huber, J. and G. Spitze.   SEX STRATIFICATION: CHILDREN, HOUSE-
       WORK, AND JOBS.   Orlando, FL.: Academic Press, Inc., 1983.

Based on an evolutionary theory of sex stratification, the
authors utilize data from a 1978 national probability sample
to test the effects of social factors on the division of
household labor, marital stability, and sex-role attitudes.
They show how the interaction of subsistence work and child
rearing has shaped female status in relation to male status.
Since the authors argue that current trends are likely to continue in this direction, their macro theory of sex-role
beliefs focuses on those macro variables that have changed
most recently; this study highlights women's employment as a
major independent variable (in contrast to the emphasis on
economic studies on spouses' relative wage levels).

2168   Hull, R.T.   "Dealing With Sexism in Nursing and Medicine,"
       NURS OUTLOOK 30 (February 1980: 89-94.

       Discusses positions that support sexism and how to deal with
       them. (22)

2169   Kasper, A.S.   "Some Observations on Nursing Service Today,"
       WOMEN AND HEALTH 7(2) (Summer 1982): 83-89.

       Notes that modern nursing service has been controlled by the
       medical profession, and that the nurse is undervalued mainly
       because her skills are associated with traditional female
       skills. Suggests that the 1985 Resolution makes nursing more
       hierarchical and unattainable for minority women. If minority
       women cannot afford to become "professional" nurses, the
       result will be that baccalaureate nurses will be mostly white
       and middle class, very much like the medical profession. (8)

2170   Larsen, J.   "The Effects of Feminism on the Nursing Profes-
       sion," ALBERTA ASSOC REGISTERED NURSEO 37(7) (July/August
       1981); 1-4.

       Discusses the role of women in Canadian society and how the
       role has influenced the development of the nursing profession.
       Encourages nurses to become politically aware and active. (6)

2171   Lewin, E. and V. Olesen (Eds.).   WOMEN, HEALTH AND HEALING.
       New York: Methuen, Inc., 1985.

       This collection of papers examines the current demographic,
       epidemiological, and social trends in women's health and as-
       sesses the likely impact of present trends on the health of
       women and their families. Some of the topics covered rep-
       resent highly developed issues which have been at the
       forefront of women's concerns for some time--such as abortion
       and the menopause; others represent a new departure into mat-
       ters such as the new technologies, the hidden division of
       labor in health care, and problems of public safety.

2172   Lorber, J.   WOMEN PHYSICIANS: CAREERS, STATUS, AND POWER.
       New York: Mathuen, Inc., 1984.

       Using the results of two surveys on American physicians,
       Lorber demonstrates that there is gender stratification and
       that through informal networks and "inner circles" men act to
       exclude women. Women have successful medical careers but, for
       the most part, they are not given the power or the authority
       to set standards or to make changes.

2173   Lovell, M.C.   "Silent But Perfect 'Partners': Medicine's Use
       and Abuse of Women," ADV NURS SCI 3(2) (January 1981):
       25-40.

       Provides an analysis of how the medical profession has cul-
       tivated and maintained the male dominant position over women.
       Discusses the physician's view and treatment of the nurse and

the relationship between the nurse and physician. Notes that throughout history nurses' silence has been imposed by physicians and that it is time for nurses to articulate their concerns. (45)

2174 _____ "The Politics of Medical Deception: Challenging the Trajectory of History," ADV NURS SCI 2(3) (April 1980): 73-86.

Discusses the relationships between medicine and nursing and between nurses, patients, and physicians. Charges that medicine has nurtured a symbiotic relationship in a deceitful, paternalistic, and sexist manner. (41)

2175 MacPherson, K.I. "Feminist Methods: A New Paradigm for Nursing Research," ADV NURS SCI 5(2) (January 1983): 17-25.

Discusses how the women's movement and the women's health movement have contributed to a new paradigm for nursing re- search which includes feminist theories. Encourages nurses to utilize feminist research methods in order to get beyond the sex biases which currently exist in most research on women's health issues. (35)

2176 Melosh, B. THE PHYSICIAN'S HAND: WORK CULTURE AND CONFLICT IN AMERICAN NURSING. Phildadelphia: Temple University Press, 1982.

Provides a history of the dilemmas facing women at work in the paid labor force. Explores the changing social contexts of nursing care and the responses of leaders and nurses on the job.

2177 Muff, J. (Ed.). SOCIALIZATION, SEXISM AND STEREOTYPING: WOMEN'S ISSUES IN NURSING. St. Louis: Mosby, 1982.

Discusses female development, sex-role socialization, sexual politics, discrimination, career choice and nursing stereo- types, physician-nurse conflict, and numerous other women's issues that affect nurses.

2178 Mulligan, J.E. "Some Effects of the Women's Health Movement," TOP CLIN NURS 4(4) (January 1983): 1-9.

Observes that until recently nurses have not, for the most part, been involved in women's health issues. Provides a his- tory of the feminist health movement begun in the early 1960s by women who established self-help clinics. Encourages nurses to become more involved in the feminist and women's health movement. (74)

2179 Nightingale, F. CASSANDRA: AN ESSAY. Westbury: Feminist Press, 1979. Introduction by M. Stark.

This was written in 1852, and later published privately.
Recounts Nightingale's feelings about the position of women
who were treated as school girls, their movements controlled,
their invitations supervised, et al. Women, like men, have
passion, intellect and morality.

2180   Nurses Network. "Collective Care Plan: Problem Statement
        For Nurses," HEALTH ACTIVISTS DIGEST 3(3) (Summer 1982):
        32-36.

        Discusses the economics of being a female nurse in the con-
        text of lower pay for women resulting from occupational seg-
        regation by sex. Encourages nurses to become politically
        aware and active. (0)

2181   O'Reilly, D.P. "Toward Autonomy of the Nursing Profession,"
        NURS LEADERSH 5(3) (September 1982): 18-22.

        Takes the position that the nursing profession has too long
        been viewed as only a support service with duties dictated by
        physicians and hospital administrators. The public image of
        the nurse is discussed in fiction, on film and in the media.
        (11)

2182   Pugh, E.L. "Florence Nightingale and J.S. Mill Debate Women's
        Rights," J BRITISH STUDIES XXI (1982): 118-38.

        Nightingale-Mill correspondence which falls into two periods,
        1860 and 1867, is essentially a debate on women's rights. One
        debate concerns terminology and hinges on the entire validity
        of the question of publicity for the women's movement then in
        its infancy, as well as the opening of the medical profession
        to women. The other focuses on differing perceptions of the
        role of women in political action. The exchange never became
        public during the lifetime of the participants. (86)

2183   Randolph, B.M. and C. Ross-Valliere. "Consciousness Raising
        Groups," AM J NURS 79(5) (May 1979): 922-24.

        Discusses the values to nurses of consciousness raising
        groups. Notes that change and growth in the nursing profession
        have been limited by sexual expectations of female roles, and
        it is emphasized that these roles should be challenged. (0)

2184   Roberts, S.J. "Oppressed Group Behavior: Implications for
        Nursing," ADV NURS SCI 5(4) (July 1983): 21-30.

        Argues that the style of leadership in nursing has evolved
        because nurses are an oppressed group which is controlled by
        societal forces. (33)

2185   Rowland, R. WOMEN WHO DO AND WOMEN WHO DON'T...JOIN THE
        WOMEN'S MOVEMENT. Boston, MA.: Routledge & Kegan Paul, 1984.

        Feminists and anti-feminists are compared.

2186   Sandelowski, M. "Women In Nursing." WOMEN, HEALTH AND CHOICE.
       Englewood Cliffs, NJ.: Prentice-Hall, 1981.

       The history of nursing, the nursing role and status are
       analyzed from a feminist perspective. (39) Additional refer-
       ences are provided.

2187   Sandroff, R. "Why Nurses Must Undermine the Medical Status
       Quo." RN 44 (September 1981): 33-35.

       This is an interview with Robert S. Mendelsohn, author of
       MALPRACTICE: HOW DOCTORS MANIPULATE WOMEN and CONFESSIONS OF A
       MEDICAL HERETIC. (0)

2188   Scott. H. WORKING YOUR WAY TO THE BOTTOM: THE FEMINIZATION
       OF POVERTY. Boston, MA.: Routledge & Kegan Paul, 1984.

       Author argues that the new poor are women and that they are
       invisible. She criticizes current research that permits this
       lack of visibility and stresses the need for a radical re-
       assessment of old economic assumptions which keep women "work-
       ing their way to the bottom."

2189   Simmons, R.S. and J. Rosenthal. "The Women's Movement and the
       Nurse Practitioner's Sense of Role," NURS OUTLOOK 29 (June
       1981): 371-75.

       Role perception of nurse practitioners leads to the conclu-
       sion that women's liberation movement has had a limited impact
       on nursing. (5)

2190   Smoyak, S.A. "Women/Nurses in 1982: How Are We Doing?," OCCUP
       HEALTH NURS 30(7) (July 1982): 9-13, 45.

       Comments that it was not until the women's movement in the
       1960s that questions were asked about the social, professional,
       and economic disparity between nurses and physicians. Paral-
       lels the work of women in the home (which is not reflected in
       the nation's statistics) with the work of women in hospitals
       (which is not billed separately as a professional fee). (0)

2191   Talbott, S.W. and C.N. Vance. "Involving Nursing in a Feminist
       Group-NOW," NURS OUTLOOK 29(10) (1981): 592-95.

       Discusses how two nurses successfully involved nurses and
       nursing in a National Organization for Women (NOW) national
       leadership convocation. Emphasizes that nurses provide an
       essential human service and that their contributions should
       become more visible in society. (3)

2192   Trandel-Korenchuk, D.M. and K. Trandel-Korenchuk. "Nursing
       Advocacy of Patients' Rights: Myth or Reality?, Part 1,"
       NURSE PRACT 8(3) (March 1983): 53, 55, 58-59. Part 2 NURSE
       PRACT 8(4) (April 1983): 37, 40-42.

An essay in two parts which examines the past and present
barriers to nurses functioning as patient advocates. The major
problem as the authors see it is the subordination of nurses
to physicians who have a monopoly power over decision making
in health care. The law supports this monopoly as evidenced
by the events of the Tuma case in Idaho. Tuma had her license
suspended for six months for giving a patient information about
chemotherapy and alternative possibilities. (33)

2193   Vance, C.N. "Women Leaders: Modern Day Heroines or Societal
       Deviants," IMAGE 11(2) (June 1979): 37-41.

       Discusses socialization and identity as powerful forces
       affecting women who try to exert strong leadership. Notes that
       nurses are ninety-eight percent women, and that to assume lead-
       ership they will have to end their isolation from social and
       poltical activity. (20)

2194   Watson, J. "Professional Identity Crisis--Is Nursing Finally
       Growing Up?," AM J NURO 01(8) (August 1981): 1488-90.

       Discusses problems with self esteem, achievement, and fear
       of success which characterize nurses and other women. Sugges-
       tions for overcoming these problems presented. (10)

2195   Wisniewski, S.C. "Achieving Equal Pay for Comparable Worth
       Through Arbitration," EMPLOYEE RELATIONS LAW J 8(2) (Autumn
       1982): 236-55.

       Examines the problem of sex stereotyping and notes that the
       earnings of women, relative to men, have not improved over the
       past two decades. Specific examples of recent Federal Court
       decisions in cases involving the Equal Pay Act are discussed.
       (25)

2196   Ziel, S. "The Androgynous Nurse Manager," J CONT EDUC NURS
       14(1) (January/February 1983): 27-31.

       Explains that the mixture of masculine and feminine charac-
       teristics of the androgynous nurse manager is useful in dealing
       with both the quantitative--analytical concerns (masculine) of
       the finance director and the public relations--quality concerns
       (feminine) of hospital administrators and patients. (3)

       See 254, 1119, 2056, 2070, 2096, 2101, 2146, 2180, 2203, 2206,
       2291, 2310.

Power and Politics

2197   American Nurses' Association. POWER: NURSING'S CHALLENGE FOR
       CHANGE: PAPERS PRESENTED AT THE 51ST CONVENTION, Honolulu,
       Hawaii, June 9-14, 1978.

Includes papers that explore the areas in which nursing is pursuing power as an instrument for change. Provides information about such topics as collective bargaining, expansion of nursing roles, nursing's potential for strength through the political process, and the roles of leaders within nursing. (173)

2198 _____. PROFESSIONALISM AND THE EMPOWERMENT OF NURSING. Kansas City, MO.: American Nurses' Association, Pub. No. G-157, 1983.

A collection of seven papers presented at the 1982 ANA Convention examining the need and means to empower professional nursing, and its potential for increasing the quality of health care.

2199 Bowman, R.A. and R.C. Culpepper. "Power: Rx for Change," AM J NURS 74 (June 1974): 1053-56. Reprinted in EXPANDING HORIZONS FOR NURSES. Edited by B. Bullough and V. Bullough. New York: Springer Publishing Co., 1977, pp. 339-44.

As nursing becomes more powerful it has the ability to change the rules under which it operates. (20)

2200 Burke, S. "Why Nursing Has Failed." THE EMERGENCE OF NURSING AS A POLITICAL FORCE. New York: National League for Nursing, Pub. No. 41-1760, 1979, pp. 57-64.

Suggests that nurses should become less virtuous and more realistic about the politics of health care and that nursing leaders have failed their profession by conformity and over-cooperation in the current health care system. Includes a plan for political action for nurses.

2201 Capuzzi, C. "Power and Interest Groups: A Study of ANA and AMA," NURS OUTLOOK 28 (1980): 478-81.

Notes that the ANA and the AMA have similar bureaucratic structures and similar size membership, but that there exist several differences that result in weaknesses in the ANA. Observes that nurses are the largest group of health care providers and that the ANA has the potential to be very influential and powerful. (32)

2202 Checkoway, B. "The Empire Strikes Back: More Lessons For Health Care Consumers," J HEALTH, POLITICS, POLICY AND LAW 7 (Spring 1982): 111-24.

An account describing how Health Systems Agency (HSA) local providers organized in response to the efforts of health care consumers' organization to provide information and generate publicity about local health care issues. The author concludes that health planning operates in an imbalanced political arena in which providers can mobilize powerful resources to defeat consumer action. (15)

2203 Dayani, E.C. "Professional and Economic Self-Governance in
      Nursing," NURS ECON 1(1) (July/August 1983): 20-23.

      Discusses professional and economic control of nursing prac-
      tice and proposes a model for self-governance in nursing.
      Nurses must educate the public and insurance companies about
      their independent and interdependent functions and the costs
      of such services. Notes that nurses are a cost-effective,
      underutilized resource in health care.(8)

2204 Donnelly, G.F., A. Mengal and D.C. Sutterly. THE NURSING
      SYSTEM: ISSUES, ETHICS AND POLITICS. New York: John Wiley,
      1980.

      Includes a section which discusses power, conflict, and
      collaboration in nursing. Considers the relationship between
      the nursing profession and the feminist movement.

2205 Dunn, A.M. "Nurse Activism in Oregon Politics," NURSE PRAC
      8(10) (November/December 1983): 54, 56, 80

      Recounts successful efforts of the Nurse Practitioner Special
      Interest group to obtain prescriptive privileges and third
      party reimbursement. (30)

2206 Edelstein, R.R. "Self Management in American Nursing," INTER
      NURS REV 26(3) (May/June 1979): 78-83.

      Suggests a plan for self-management by nurses. People in
      managerial roles would be elected for terms of office and
      nurses would have equal rights to shape their work days and to
      determine the policies that affect their working lives. (32)

2207 Garant, C.A. "Power, Leadership and Nursing," NURS FORUM
      20(2) (1981): 183-99.

      Provides a philosophical view of power and leadership in the
      health care professions and notes that power and nursing have
      had an ambivalent relationship. Observes that nursing is
      ninety-seven percent a woman's profession and as such, reflects
      the position of women in today's society. Discusses how nurses
      are circumventing physician control by moving into specialties
      where they can practice on their own. (62)

2208 Goldwater, M. "Political Power for Nurse Practitioners,"
      NURSE PRACT 9(11) (November 1984): 44-45, 49, 52.

      Legislative process and power of nurses discussed. Maryland
      experience used as example. (0)

2209 Halleran, C. "Power, Influence and Lobbying." THE EMERGENCE
      OF NURSING AS A POLITICAL FORCE. New York: National League
      for Nursing, Pub. No. 41-1760, 1979, pp. 19-26.

      Emphasizes the importance of political involvement for
      nurses. (0)

2210   Jordan, C.H.   "To Advance, We Must Unite," NURS OUTLOOK 29(8)
       (1981): 482-83.

       Discusses the importance of unity among the members of the
       nursing profession and suggests that if nurses were really
       unified, nearly all of the crucial problems in nursing could
       be solved. Focuses on the role of the American Nurses´ Asso-
       ciation in bringing nurses together. (0)

2211   Kalisch, B. and P. Kalisch. POLITICS OF NURSING. Philadel-
       phia: Lippincott, 1982.

       Encourages nurses to exercise their constitutional rights
       and become politically active in order to achieve a higher
       quality of working life for themselves and better health care
       at lower costs for the consumer.

2212   Kennedy, M.M. POWERBASE: HOW TO BUILD IT/HOW TO KEEP IT.
       New York: Macmillan Publishing Co., 1984.

       The author reviews the need for power, how to find it and
       how to use it. Attention is given to special power problems,
       such as sex and lifestyle, and ways to reduce others´ power-
       bases.

2213   Kupchak, Sr. B. "Do Nurses Enjoy Appropriate Levels of
       Power?," NURS SUCCESS TODAY 1(1) (January/February 1984):
       4-8.

       Reviews the concept of power and discusses the author´s
       beliefs that nurses have power to use. (0)

2214   Lieb, R. "Power, Powerlessness and Potential--Nurse´s Role
       Within the Health Care Delivery System," IMAGE 10(3)
       (October 1978): 75-83.

       Traces the role of women health care providers from the
       perspective of power and status roles historically assigned to
       women. Suggests that to achieve change in the health care
       delivery system nurses must communicate their concerns to
       health care consumers. Encourages nurses to recognize and
       exercise power. (78)

2215   Lockett, B.A. AGING, POLITICS AND RESEARCH: SETTING THE
       FEDERAL AGENDA FOR RESEARCH ON AGING. New York: Springer
       Publishing Co., 1983.

       Overview of the issues and events that influence both pub-
       lic and private support for research on aging in the United
       States. It tells the story of the forty year struggle that
       led to the creation of the National Institute on Aging, analyz-
       ing these events within a framework of an agenda-setting model,
       the changing demographic situation, and the poltical climate of
       the country.

2216 McFarland, D.E. and N. Shiflett. "The Role of Power in the
      Nursing Profession," NURS DIMENSIONS 7(2) (Summer 1979):
      1-13.

      Discusses the impact of power, authority, and control of
      nurses' careers and on the performance of nursing functions.
      Notes that power influences the ability of the profession to
      develop, grow and achieve its primary missions in patient care.
      (59)

2217 Moore, E. and D. Oakley. "Nurses, Political Participation,
      and Attitudes Toward Reforms in the Health Care System."
      NURS HEALTH CARE 4 (November 1983): 504-7.

      A sample of 153 nurses from the one congressional district
      in Michigan were questioned about their political participation
      and their attitudes about changes in the health care delivery
      system. Political participation as measured by voting was high,
      but only thirty percent had even contributed to a political
      campaign. Only moderate changes in the health care delivery
      system were supported. (23)

2218 Mundinger, M.O. AUTONOMY IN NURSING. Germantown, MD.: Aspen
      Systems Corp., 1980.

      Discusses criteria for development as a professional nurse.
      Several case studies illustrate the nursing process as the
      methodical way to identify, plan and evaluate effective nursing
      care. Challenges the traditional medical extension of the
      nurse practitioner, and suggests that often chronic illness is
      dealt with more effectively by nurse practitioners than by
      physicians.

2219 National League for Nursing. THE EMERGENCE OF NURSING AS A
      POLITICAL FORCE. New York: National League for Nursing,
      Pub. No. 41-1760, 1979.

      Discusses the following issues: (1) political action, (2)
      power, influence and lobbying, (3) financing health care,
      (4) nursing politics and trends, (5) politics of nursing re-
      search, and (6) economic forecast for health care.

      Contains: 2023, 2043, 2160, 2208, 2218.

2220 Roberts, M. "Economic Forecast for Health Care." THE EMER-
      GENCE OF NURSING AS A POLITICAL FORCE. New York: National
      League for Nursing, Pub. No. 41-1760, 1979, pp. 81-90.

      Discusses how the movement from quality through access to
      cost control and cost effectiveness (in health care) provides
      challenges for nurses in terms of new opportunities and new
      roles and environments.

2221 Sherwood, J. "Power and the Lobby," ALBERTA ASSOC REGISTERED
      NURSES NEWSLETTER 39(1) (1983): 12-15.

Discusses the amount of influence nursing associations have on the creation and changing of public policy. Provides suggestions for effective lobbying. (3)

2222   Stevens, B.J. "Power and Politics for the Nurse Executive,"
       NURS HEALTH CARE 1(4) (1980): 208-12.

Discusses sources of a profession's power and suggests political strategies to increase power in nursing. (4)

2223   Stevens, K.R. POWER AND INFLUENCE: A SOURCE BOOK FOR NURSES.
       New York: Wiley, 1983.

Focuses on the professional and personal sources of power that can enable the nurse to have a positive impact on health care. Identifies and describes power sources. Includes a discussion about the power of political activity.

2224   Wagner, D. "The Proletarianization of Nursing in the United
       States, 1932-1946," INT J HEALTH SERVICES 10(2) (1980):
       271-90.

Discusses the history of professional nursing in the United States, and notes that the traditional autonomy of private practice nursing was displaced by institutional nursing in hospitals and nursing homes. Contends that today's hospital nursing bears a strong resemblance to factory work. (55)

2225   Wieczorek, R.R. POWER, POLITICS, AND POLICY IN NURSING.
       New York: Springer Publishing Co., 1984.

Nineteen essays, some by leading figures in nursing, examine the structure of power in nursing and provide insights about how nurses can determine the direction of nursing education, research and practice.

See 39, 928, 983, 1032, 1049, 1051, 1194, 1220, 2021, 2080, 2100.

Image

2226   Alexander, J.W. "How The Public Perceives Nurses and Their
       Education," NURS OUTLOOK 27(10) (October 1979): 654-56.

A survey of 641 consumers indicated that the public believe nurses are better educated than they actually are. Most felt nurses need even more education and should be educated as professionals. Family units with higher income and more highly prepared wives were more inclined to want greater education for nurses. Respondents distinguished between practical and registered nurse preparation as to the amount of education required. (0)

2227   American Academy of Nursing. IMAGE-MAKING IN NURSING. Kansas
       City, MO.: American Nurses' Association, Pub. No. G-161,
       1983.

Papers and summary of discussion from the 1982 Annual Scientific Session of the American Academy of Nursing, on the images
of nursing, dissonant and ideal models, social and psychological perspectives, and on improving the public image of nursing.

2228   Aroskar, M.A. "The Fractured Image: The Public Stereotype of
       Nursing and The Nurse." NURSING IMAGES AND IDEALS. Edited
       by S.F. Springer and S. Gadow. New York: Springer Publishing
       Co., 1980, pp. 18-34.

       Thesis is that there are conflicts between public image of
       the nurse and the profession's own self-image. Suggestions
       are made for overcoming this public stereotype and the socio-
       logical context that perpetuates it.

2229   Baker, R. "Care of the Sick and Cure of Disease: Comment on
       'The Fractured Image'." NURSING IMAGES AND IDEALS. Edited
       by S.F. Springer and S. Gadow. New York: Springer Publishing
       Co., 1980, pp. 49-75.

       Comment on Aroskar.

2230   Bock, J. "Mirror, Mirror on the Wall: A Look at Nursing's
       Image Now and In The Future," CAN NURSE 76(3) (March 1980): 5.

       Discusses stereotypes in nursing and notes that the roots of
       the tendency of nurses to downgrade their own profession lie
       in the history of nursing. (0)

2231   Campbell, C. "Black Stockings and Bed Baths: The Public's
       Opinion of a Nurse," NURS MIRROR 152(4) (January 22, 1981):
       12.

       Provides a student's view of the public image of a nurse and
       what the public expectations are of the nursing profession. (0)

2232   Evans, D., T. Fitzpatrick and J. Howard-Ruben. "Improving the
       Image of Nursing: A District Takes Action," AM J NURS 83(1)
       (January 1983): 52-54.

       Reports how the Chicago Nurses' Association formed a "Task
       Force on Nurses' Image in the Media" in order to correct some
       myths and misconceptions about nursing. (0)

2233   Fernandes, R.C. "Let's Turn Off The Soap Opera Image of
       Nursing!," RN 43 (8) (August 1980): 77-78.

       Discusses the extent to which public opinion about nurses is
       formed by watching television. Encourages nurses to join
       together to work against offensive television programming. (0)

2234   Grosser, L.R. "Let's Take the Bedpan Out of the Public's Image
       of Nursing," AORN J 34(4) (October 1981): 589-94.

Analyzes the stereotyped public image of nurses and provides
a brief overview of the image of nurses in novels, television
and films. (7)

2235 Hinkley, C. "Nursing's Image," IMPRINT 28(3) (September 1981):
      41, 80-81.

Encourages nursing students to discard the notion that they
are helpless to effect change in their profession, and to become politically aware and involved in any proposed legislation
dealing with nursing. (0)

2236 Hott, J.R. "The Public Image of the Nurse on the Get-Well
      Card: To See Ourselves as Others See Us," IMPRINT 31(1)
      (February/March 1984): 45-58.

Discusses get-well cards that stereotype nurses in the context of the psychology of humor. Challenges greeting card
companies to develop cards that are humorous without capitalizing on negative, false images of nurses and other health
professionals. (2)

2237 Hughes, L. "The Public Image of the Nurse," ADV NURS SCI 2(3)
      (April 1980): 55-72.

Results of a historical study which examined the public
opinion of the nurse and the nursing profession during the
period 1896 to 1976. Notes that public opinion of the nurse
has had, and will continue to have, an effect on the ability
of the nursing profession to provide a unique service to the
public. (56)

2238 Hunt, J. "Do We Deserve Our Image?," NURS TIMES 80(9)
      (February 29, 1984): 53-55.

Discusses several stereotypical images of nurses and questions whether nurses perpetuate such images through their sub-
missiveness. Encourages nurses to assert themselves and to
educate the public about the profession of nursing. (11)

2239 Kalisch, B.J., P.A. Kalisch and J. Clinton. "How The Public
      Sees Nurse-Midwives: 1978 News Coverage of Nurse Midwifery
      in the Nation's Press," J NURS MIDWIFE 25(4) (July/August
      1980): 31-39.

Analyzes newspaper articles and photographs on the subject
of nurse midwifery that appeared in 1978. Suggests that there
is a need for a greater effort on the part of nurse-midwives
to communicate to the public who they are and what they do.
(8)

2240 Kalisch, B.J., P.A. Kalisch and M. Scobey. "Reflections On a
      Television Image: The Nurses' 1962-1965," NURS HEALTH CARE
      2(5) (May 1981): 248-55. Reprinted in NURSING ISSUES AND
      NURSING STRATEGIES FOR THE EIGHTIES. Edited by B. Bullough,
      V. Bullough and M.C. Soukup. New York: Springer Publishing
      Co., 1983, pp. 71-88.

      Analyzes a television program called "The Nurses" (CBS 1962-
      1965) and notes that the image of the nurse in this series was
      the strongest and most positive image on any series to feature
      nurses as regular characters. (7)

2241 Kalisch, B.J. and P.A. Kalisch. "Improving the Image of Nurs-
      ing," AM J NURS 83(1) (January 1983): 48-52.

      Discusses nursing's negative public image and the implica-
      tions of such negative opinion on the nurse's self image and
      the ability of nursing to attract quality students. Provides
      suggestions for monitoring the media. (5)

2242 Kalisch, P.A., B.J. Kalisch and E. Livesay. "The 'Angel of
      Death': The Anatomy of 1980's Major News Story About Nurs-
      ing," NURS FORUM 19 (1980): 212-41.

      Examines the media victimization of a nurse accused of mur-
      dering patients to collect bets.(0)

2243 Kalisch, P.A. and B.J. Kalisch. "Perspectives on Improving
      Nursing's Public Image," NURS HEALTH CARE (1) (July/August
      1980): 10-15.

      Discusses why nursing should be included in health care re-
      form and the role of the media in such reform. Concludes that
      a greater attention to the quality of public information about
      nursing is needed. (23)

2244 _____. "When Nurses Were National Heroines: Images of Nursing
      in American Film 1942-1945," NURS FORUM 20(1) (1981): 14-61.

      Illustrates through numerous examples how the image of nurs-
      ing in feature films produced during World War II reached the
      strongest and most positive expression of nursing ever seen by
      the viewing public. (10)

2245 _____. "The Image of Psychiatric Nurses in Motion Pic-
      tures," PERSPECT PSYCHIATR CARE 19(3-4) (1981): 116-29.

      Examines the stereotyped depiction of psychiatric nurses in
      films and notes that motion picture psychiatric nurses lack the
      nurturant behavior that most often typifies the image of the
      nurse. Provides specific examples of character portrayals of
      films. (3)

2246 _____. "Nurses on Prime-Time Television," AM J NURS 82
      (February 1982): 264-70.

After looking at prime time television shows from the 1950´s the authors conclude that the reality of contemporary nursing practice has found little or no echo in the largely fictional world of television broadcasting. (5)

2247 _____. "The Image of the Nurse in Motion Pictures," AM J NURS 82(4) (April 1982): 605-11.

Documents the nurse´s image in films released between 1930 and 1979 in whch nurses or nursing were a focus. Notes that nursing´s image reached a high point in 1940´s and a very low point in the 1970´s. Considers the influence of films on health consumers and policy makers. (0)

2248 _____. "The Image of Nurses in Novels," AM J NURS 82(8) (August 1982): 1220-24.

Reports the results of an analysis of 207 novels involving a nurse character. Notes that nursing´s image had an increased respectability in the early twentieth century, reached a pinnacle during the 1940´s and 1950´s, and fell back to the bottom during the 1960´s and 1970´s. (4)

2249 _____. "The Press Image of Community Health Nurses," PUBLIC HEALTH NURS 1(1) (March 1984): 3-15.

Using content analyses, 2,561 articles on community health nursing for the period 1978-1981 were coded for key message themes and compared with articles on other nursing subjects. Analysis of annual trends shows that community health nursing articles, while expanding on absolute numbers, constitute a declining proportion of nursing articles overall, and that the quality of information in current press coverage is diminishing. It is recommended that community health nurses embark on a concerted campaign to improve the quality of information carried in newspapers about their clinical specialty. (13)

2250 Kalisch, P.A., B.J. Kalisch and J. Clinton. "The World of Nursing on Prime Time Television," NURS RES 31(6) (November/ December 1982): 358-63.

An analysis of 320 episodes from twenty-eight series found nurses predominantly acting as a resource to other health professions, not using problem solving and evaluation skills, deficient in administration abilities, and remiss in providing physical comforting, engaging in expanded role activities, patient education, or scholarly endeavors. (24)

2251 Kalisch, P.A., B.J. Kalisch and M. Scobey. IMAGES OF NURSES ON TELEVISION. New York: Springer Publishing Co., 1983.

Documents the way in which nurses have been presented on television from the early days of broadcasting to the present. Provides an exhaustive and longitudinal examination of the problem, and is based upon a complete survey of all television programs that have ever featured nurses.

2252   Kennedy, C.W. and B. Garvin. "The Effect of Status and Gender
       on Interpersonal Relationships in Nursing," NURS FORUM 20(3)
       (1981): 275-87.

       Status and gender are two important factors which affect
       communication. Dominant and submissive roles are assumed.
       Understanding of professional communication can be enhanced by
       the examination of individual patterns and need for change.
       (29)

2253   Lee, A.A. "How Nurses Rate With The Public: How-and Where-The
       Handmaiden Image is Changing," RN 42(6) (June 1979): 36-39.

       Notes that whether or not an individual has been hospitalized
       recently influences his/her understanding of the professional
       value of nurses. Reports that people who have had recent hos-
       pital experiences are more likely to favor greater autonomy
       for nursing and that the handmaiden image is changing, (0)

2254   _____. "How Nurses Rate Nursing's Shopworn Image: How It
       Hurts You, How It Helps," RN 42(8) (August 1979): 42-47.

       Reports that results of a recent survey show that the stereo-
       type of the nurse as the handmaiden to the physician persists
       and that aggressive measures will be necessary to overcome such
       an image. (0)

2255   Marieskind, H.I. WOMEN IN THE HEALTH SYSTEM: PATIENTS, PROVI-
       DERS AND PROGRAMS. St. Louis: C.V. Mosby Co., 1980.

       View of women's health care historically and currently.
       Discussions consider key issues in the health and public
       health fields.

2256   Martin, S. "Women Together Are Strong," NURS MIRROR 153
       (September 23, 1981): 37-39.

       Discusses British health system from a feminist perspective
       and argues that improvement in status of nursing is linked to
       status of women in society. (0)

2257   McGrory, A. "Women and Mental Illness: A Sexist Trap?
       Part I," JPN AND MENTAL HEALTH SERVICES (September 1980):
       13-19.

       Women have often been stereotyped as mentally ill. This
       article gives the facts. Part II discusses sex role stereo-
       types and their effect on diagnosis and treatment of women
       with mental illness. (14)

2258   _____. "Women and Mental Illness: A Sexist Trap?
       Part II," JPN AND MENTAL HEALTH SERVICES 18 (1980): 17-22.

       Discusses women's high use of mental health services as
       compared to men. (22)

2259   Muff, J. (Ed. with 34 contributors). SOCIALIZATION, SEXISM,
       AND STEREOTYPING: WOMEN'S ISSUES IN NURSING. St. Louis:
       C.V.Mosby Co., 1982.

       Contributors discuss the problems of development and dis-
       crimination that face women, linking them to the problems of
       nurses, and seeking positive solutions. Exploring the forms
       sexism can take in nursing, along with its effects, the text
       provides coverage of female and nursing stereotypes, as well
       as social/psychological/political problems in nursing. Refer-
       ences follow each paper.

2260   Muff, J. "A Look At Images In Nursing," IMPRINT 31(1) (Feb-
       ruary/March 1984): 40-44.

       Examines nursing images and stereotypes and notes that the
       image problems of nurses come from the image problems of women
       in general. Emphasizes that in order to change nursing's
       image, nurses must change how they see themselves. (14)

2261   Newton, L. "A Vindication of the Gentle Sister: Comment on
       the Fractured Image." NURSING: IMAGES AND IDEALS. Edited
       by S.F. Spicker and S. Gadow. New York: Springer Publishing
       Co., 1980, pp. 34-41.

       Argues that the public stereotype of the nurse is "coherent,
       possible, and functional."

2262   O'Heath, K.A. "The Challenge: Nursing's Accurate Portrayal,"
       IMPRINT 31(1) (February/March 1984): 53-55.

       Discusses how nursing's image has been devastated by the
       media and nurses themselves who allow themselves to have a
       negative image. Considers the relationship between public
       image and self-image. (9)

2263   Pearson, A. "What The Public Thinks," NURS TIMES 79(8) (Feb-
       ruary 23, March 1, 1983): 18-19.

       Reports the results of a patient questionnaire which ex-
       plored how nursing is viewed by the general public. Notes
       that the public often rates a cheerful personality as more im-
       portant for a nurse than advanced education. (4)

2264   Salvage, J. "Changing The Image," INT NURS REV 30(6) (Novem-
       ber/December 1983): 181-82.

       Discusses the effects of nursing's negative public image
       which emphasizes "feminine" attributes while excluding the
       fact that nurses are well-educated and highly capable profes-
       sionals. (0)

2265   Storms, D.M. and J.G. Fox. "The Public's View of Physician's
       Assistants and Nurse Practitioners: A Survey of Baltimore
       Urban Residents," MEDCARE 17(5) (May 1979): 526-35.

Report about a study of public attitudes towards physician's assistants and nurse practitioners which found that the public regards the two groups of health workers as very similar. (52)

2266   Swansburg, R.C. "The Consumer's Perception of Nursing Care," SUPERVISOR NURSE (May 1981): 30-33. Reprinted in NURSING ISSUES AND NURSING STRATEGIES FOR THE EIGHTIES. Edited by B. Bullough, V. Bullough and M.C. Soukup. New York: Springer Publishing Co., pp. 105-14.

Reports and analyzes a Good Housekeeping poll in which nurses, physicians, and consumers rated each other. Other data is also given. (10)

2267   Woolley, A.S. "Nursing's Image on Campus," NURS OUTLOOK 29(8) (August 1981): 460-66.

Focuses on the attitudes of the faculty and administration towards nursing students and nursing faculty at a liberal arts college. Notes that individuals in the liberal arts have a traditional image of how nurses are educated and what they actually do. (8)

See 1132, 1134, 2286, 2338.

Men in Nursing

2268   Annas, G.J. "Male Nurses in the Delivery Room," HASTINGS CENTER REPORT 11(6) (December 1981): 20-21.

Summarizes the case of a qualified male registered nurse who was refused placement in the labor and delivery department of an Arkansas hospital (Backus vs. Baptist Medical Center, 510 F. Supp. 1191, 1981). The author contends that the court's ruling is overtly sexist. (0)

2269   Auld, M. "In Camera: Does Nursing Need More Men?," NURS MIR-ROR 147(24) (December 14, 1978): 16-17.

Includes interviews with several British nurses which explore why more men are not going into the nursing profession. (0)

2270   Benda, E. "When The Postpartum Nursing Student Is Male--A Challenge to Maternity Instructors," J NURS EDUC 20(4) (April 1981): 5-8.

Discusses the attitudes of the male student nurse which may influence his learning experience in a post-partum setting, and suggests that such a student requires support and encouragement from the instructor and his peers. (5)

2271   Blackford, N. and R. Devlin. "Male Midwives: Will They Be Denied a Chance?," NURS MIRROR 152(16) (April 16, 1981): 8-9.

Discusses the problems and difficulties encountered by male
midwives who attempt to practice in the United Kingdom.
Interviews with male midwives are included. (0)

2272   Bowman, M. "Female Chauvinists," NURS MIRROR 156 (14) (April
       6, 1983): 34-35.

       Summarizes the status of male nurses in the United Kingdom
       and notes that many female nurses have a chauvinistic attitude
       towards their male colleagues, and that the major source of
       discrimination against male nurses has been female nurses.(5)

2273   Cearns, E. "Male Midwives--Time To Allow Them Freedom to
       . Practice," MIDWIVES CHRON 95 (1132) (May 1982): 159-60.

       Reports about five years of training men at a midwifery
       school in England. (1)

2274   Ellis, S. "Nursing--A Question of Sex," NURS TIMES 74(45)
       (November 9, 1978): 1830-31.

       A male nurse in England shares his reasons for choosing the
       nursing profession. Includes the findings of a questionnaire
       designed to investigate public opinion on the subject of male
       nurses. (0)

2275   Greenlaw, J. "Delivery Rooms: For Women Only?," LAW, MED
       HEALTH CARE 9(6) (December 1981): 28-29, 40.

       Reviews the case of Backus vs. Baptist Medical Center which
       upheld the right of a hospital to prevent a qualified male
       nurse from working in its labor and delivery section, and com-
       ments that such a decision is an obstacle to professional
       nursing. (7)

2276   _____. "Legally Speaking: A Sexist Judgment Threatens
       All of Nursing," RN 45(7) (July 1982): 69-70.

       Commentary on Arkansas decision which permitted hospitals to
       ban male registered nurses from delivery room. (0)

2277   _____. "Mississippi University for Women vs. Hogan: The
       Supreme Court Rules on Female-Only Nursing School," LAW, MED
       HEALTH CARE 10(6) (December 1982): 267-68.

       An analysis of the July 1, 1982 U.S. Supreme Court decision,
       Mississippi University for Women v. Hogan ruling that "female
       only" admission policy of state supported nursing schools
       violated the equal protection clause of the fourteenth amend-
       ment. (21)

2278   Groff, B. "The Trouble With Male Nursing," AM J NURS 84(1)
       (January 1984): 62-63.

       The problems of dealing with patients and co-workers who
       think the only good nurse is a woman.(0)

2279   Gumley, C.J., J. McKenzie, M.B. Ormerod, and W. Keys. "Per-
       sonality Correlates in a Sample of Male Nurses in the
       British Royal Air Force," J ADV NURS 4(4) (July 1979): 355-
       64.

       Provides a review of the literature concerning male nurses.
       Refutes the stereotyped image often associated with the male
       nurse and notes that in the sample studied the majority of
       male nurses preferred general nursing to more technical and
       administrative positions. (5)

2280   Holt, F.X. "A Male Nurse is More than Muscle!," RN 45(9)
       (September 1982): 102-4.

       Argues that the majority of the problems which male nurses
       face are caused not by patients but by colleagues who are
       women. Cites examples of how the male nurse is stereotyped as
       being fit for only manual labor and psychiatric ward duty. (1)

2281   Johnston, T. "The Sexist in Nursing: Who is She?," NURS FORUM
       18(2) (1979): 204-5.

       Provides a male nurse's view of female sexism in nursing and
       notes that nurses are guilty of perpetuating the idea that
       nursing is a profession for women only. Observes that sexism
       is well entrenched in both nursing education and clinical
       nursing practice. (0)

2282   Jones, E.M. "The Vanishing Male Nurse," NURS MIRROR 149(8)
       (August 23, 1979): 28-29.

       Provides a brief overview of the history of men in nursing
       and observes the problems in educating the public and poten-
       tial male nurses to see nursing as a job for men. (4)

2283   Kantner, J.E. and R.C. Ellerbusch. "Androgyny and Occupa-
       tional Choice," PSYCHOLOGICAL REPORT 47 (December 1980,
       Part 2): 1289-90.

       Discusses the relationship between sex-role orientation and
       occupational choice and reports about a study involving male
       nurses and male teachers. No significant relationship between
       sex-role orientation and occupational choice was found. (5)

2284   Kennedy, S.L. "A Campaign for Men," NURS HEALTH CARE 2(2)
       (February 1981): 58.

       Encourages female nurses to reflect on discrimination
       against male nurses that comes from within the nursing pro-
       fession. (0)

2285   Laroche, E. and H. Livneh. "Regressional Analysis of At-
       titudes Toward Male Nurses," J PSYCH 113(First Half)
       (January 1983): 67-71.

Examines the relationship between sex demographic variables
of 174 respondents and acceptance of males in the nursing
profession. Implications of findings are discussed in light
of the minority role status of male nurses. (17)

2286   Lemin, B.   "Men in a Women's World," NURS MIRROR 155(21)
       (November 24, 1982): 32-34.

       Reports the results of an Australian survey designed to de-
       termine female patients' acceptance of visiting male nurses.
       Seventy percent of the respondents found the care given by
       male nurses fully acceptable. (0)

2287   Levine, I.   "The Image and The Reality: Machismo and The Male
       Nurse," NURS TIMES 79(21) (May 25, 1983): 50-51.

       Discusses the stereotyped image of the male nurse and argues
       that nursing's image and status will only be improved by com-
       bining "masculine" and "feminine" attributes. (0)

2288   Lewis, M.C.   "A Black Perspective: Afro American Men in Nurs-
       ing," NURS LEADERSH 4(3) (September 1981): 31-33.

       Provides an historical perspective for the Black male nurse
       through an explanation of African health culture. Concludes
       that a major change in the attitudes of the nursing profession
       as well as society will be necessary to improve the standing
       of the Black male nurse. (2)

2289   Lewis, P.   "Men in Midwifery: The Inside Story," NURS MIRROR
       158(12) (March 21, 1984): 17-18.

       Reports that in Great Britain the act which precluded men
       from training and practicing as midwives has been repealed.
       Explains the attitudes and experiences encountered by a male
       midwife and notes that acceptance by female midwives is essen-
       tial to the success of male midwives. (0)

2290   "Male Midwives," MIDWIVES CHRON 95(1135) (August 1982): 277.

       Summarizes the position of the Royal College of Midwives
       (RCM) on the question of male midwives. Discusses equal op-
       portunity for men in the profession of midwifery. (0)

2291   "Male Nurses: What They Think About Themselves--and Others,"
       RN 46(10) (October 1983): 61-63.

       Reports the results of an opinion poll of Oklahoma male
       nurses which showed that male nurses believe they are more
       professional, cope better with stress, understand administra-
       tion better, and are more promotable than female nurses. (0)

2292   Marks, L.N.   "Nursing Is Not a Women's Profession," RN 43(4)
       (April 1980): 81-86.

Calls for the elimination of sex typing and the image that
sex typing has brought about in the nursing profession. (10)

2293   Milliken, B. "Men and Women in Nursing: Do We Need Both?,"
       NZ NURS J 74(1) (January 1981): 21-24.

       Reports the results of a questionnaire about male and female
       nurse employment which was circulated among sixteen psychi-
       atric and psychopaedic hospitals in New Zealand. (3)

2294   Moore, J. "A Man's Job," NURS TIMES 78(10) (March 1982): 398.

       Reports about a survey in Great Britain regarding male mid-
       wives that found that most women would welcome male midwives.
       (0)

2295   Morton, A. "Are Men Starting A New Era In Nursing?," NURS
       MIRROR 156(13) (March 30, 1983): 9.

       Discusses the implication of British male nurses being al-
       lowed by law to train as midwives.(0)

2296   Nuttall, P. "PINC: Male Takeover or Female Giveaway," NURS
       TIMES 79(2) (January 12-18, 1983): 10-11.

       Discusses that in Great Britain nursing is still a female
       profession, but that it is dominated and led by men. Mobility
       of female vs. male nurses is discussed and it is noted that
       society expects female nurses to stay close at home and assume
       responsibility for elderly relatives. (2)

2297   Sharpe, D. "Male and Female Nurse Ratios in a Psychiatric
       Hospital," NURS TIMES 74(40) October 5, 1978): 1656.

       Discusses problems associated with complete integration of
       male and female nurses in psychiatric hospitals in Great
       Britain. (0)

2298   _____. "Male Nurses on Female Psychiatric Wards," NURS
       TIMES 75(41) (October 11, 1979): 1773-74.

       Discusses some of the specific problems faced by male nurses
       on female wards. (2)

2299   Snavely, B.K. and G.T. Fairhurst. "The Male Nursing Student
       as a Token," RES NURS HEALTH 7(4) (December 1984): 287-94.

       Test of Kanter's theory of tokenism using male nursing stu-
       dents. It was hypothesized that token students would feel
       isolated, performance pressure, and role entrapment. Male
       students did not. Explanations in terms of sex differences
       and the nurturing characteristics of nursing are suggested.(20)

2300   Tagg, P. "Male Nurses in Midwifery," NURS TIMES 77(43)
       (October 21, 1981): 1851-53.

Reports the results of a British survey about male midwives which showed that women in a maternity unit did not object to being cared for by a male nurse. (0)

2301   Trandel-Korenchuk, K.M. and D.M. Trandel-Korenchuk. "NAQ Legal Forum: Restrictions on Male Nurse Employment in Obstetric Care," NURS ADM Q 6(1) (Fall 1981): 87-90.

Summarizes the case of Backus vs. Baptist Medical Center and discusses the impact of the court's decision in that case on employment policies. (4)

2302   Vestal, C. "Men Nurses--Who Needs Them? Attitudes Toward Men in Nursing," IMPRINT 30(2) (April/May 1983): 55-59.

Provides an overview of attitudes toward men in nursing in the United States. Includes an historical basis for nursing as a man's profession, and describes the evolution of the profession of nursing as it is known today. Emphasizes that American culture has stereotyped nursing as a women's profession. Discusses attitudes found in nursing schools among faculty and students, most of whom are women. (18)

2303   Watson, C. "The Men Worry Me," NURS MIRROR 156(10) (March 9, 1983): 32.

Questions whether male nurses fully understand the experience of their female co-workers and whether it is in the best interests of nursing that they represent a female-dominated profession in national nursing organizations. (0)

2304   Wray, D.A. "Men In Nursing: A Continuing Struggle," IMPRINT 27(5) (December 1980): 20, 26.

Summarizes the history of men in nursing and their continuing struggle to be accepted by the nursing profession. Suggests that the problem is not with the male nurse, but rather with female nurses and public stereotyping of the nursing profession. (4)

2305   Yardley, B. "I'm In Charge!," NURS MIRROR 156(19) (May 11, 1983): 33-34.

Discusses the problems encountered by male nurses who are in charge of wards in terms of how they are perceived and treated by the public, the patients, and other hospital workers. (0)

Racial, Ethnic, or Sexual Minorities In Nursing,
Opportunities/Discrimination

2306   American Nurses' Association. AFFIRMATIVE ACTION PROGRAMMING FOR THE NURSING PROFESSION THROUGH THE AMERICAN NURSES' ASSOCIATION. Kansas City, MO.: American Nurses' Association, Pub. No. M-23, 1975.

A model affirmative action plan, selected ANA resolutions on
civil rights and minority nurses, and a historical perspective
on ANA's affirmative action program are included in this book-
let designed by the ANA Affirmative Action Task Force to provide direction and focus for state and district nurses' association.

2307   _____. CONTEMPORARY MINORITY LEADERS IN NURSING: AFRO-
        AMERICAN, HISPANIC, NATIVE AMERICAN PERSPECTIVES. Kansas
        City, MO.: American Nurses' Association, Pub. No. M-29, 1983.

        Statements by fifty-seven minority registered nurses on what
        they believe about nursing, followed by a biographical sketch
        of each of these nurse leaders.

2308   Branch, M.F. "Ethnic Minorities in Nursing," URBAN HEALTH
        6(5) (August 1977): 49-52.

        Reports that there is a critical shortage of ethnic minor-
        ities among registered nurses, and far too many minorities
        among the lower paying jobs, e.g. orderlies and practical
        nurses. It is suggested that nursing school entrance require-
        ments become more flexible and include nontraditional criteria
        such as an individual's ability to communicate with and be
        trusted by patients from ethnic groups with special customs
        and health needs. (15)

2309   Brown, V. "How To Succeed as a Minority Student in Nursing,"
        IMPRINT 30(2) (April/May 1983): 66-71.

        Reviews various solutions to the problem of minority student
        recruitment, and notes that such solutions place insufficient
        emphasis on what minority students can do to help themselves.
        Provides specific interventions that minority students can use
        to increase their success. (15)

2310   Bureau of Health Professions. MINORITIES & WOMEN IN THE
        HEALTH FIELDS. Washington, D.C.: DHHS Pub. No. (HRSA) HRS-
        DV 84-5, 1984.

        Update of report first prepared in 1974. Statistics on
        women and minorities in health occupations as well as students
        in health professions schools. Good reference work.

2311   Carrington, B.W. "Minority Recruitment," J NURSE MIDWIFE
        26(1) (January/February 1981): 1-2.

        Discusses the very low representation of ethnic minorities
        in American nurse-midwifery and recommends an increase in
        minority recruitment into the nurse-midwifery field. Notes
        that the majority of certified nurse midwives work with ethnic
        minority clients. (5)

2312   Castillo, M.H. "Hispanic Leadership Considerations in Nurs-
        ing," NURS LEADERSH 4(1) (March 1981): 14-18.

Discusses how Hispanics perceive leadership differently from Anglo-Saxons and how such perceptions affect the Hispanic nurse's leadership role. (8)

2313   Forrest, L. "Get Your Black Hands Off Me," RN 43 (8) (August 1980): 54-55.

Discusses how a psychiatric nurse came to terms with her patients' prejudice. (0)

2314   Meaux, C.A. "Breakthrough to Nursing," IMPRINT 29(5) (December 1982): 15, 64-67.

Notes that since 1963 the National Student Nurses' Association (NSNA) has actively sought to involve minority groups in the field of nursing, both as staff nurses and as administrators. Evaluates the impact of the NSNA's efforts. (1)

2315   _____. "Nursing Still Has Barriers," IMPRINT 30(1) (February/March 1983): 24.

Discusses the barriers in nursing to minorities of various sociocultural origins and emphasizes that minority students must continue to break down such barriers if nursing is ever to represent the entire population. (6)

2316   Salvage, J. " Suitable to Nurse?," NURS MIRROR 152(17) (April 23, 1981): 6-7.

Discusses homosexuality among nurses in England. Reports that although homosexuality is gradually becoming more acceptable, there is still a long way to go. (0)

See 1089, 1597, 1670, 1710, 1737, 1791.

Interprofessional Relationships

2317   American Nurses' Association. GUIDELINES FOR ESTABLISHING JOINT OR COLLABORATIVE PRACTICE IN HOSPITALS. Kansas City, MO.: American Nurses' Association, Pub. No. G-E-J, 1981.

Report of a demonstration project directed by the National Joint Practice Commission in four selected hospitals on successful alterations of the nurse-physician relationship in order to establish joint practice.

2318   Brown, B.S. "Practice Management: Competition and Collaboration after GMENAC," PED NURS 10(2) (March/April 1984): 153-54.

Medicine as a monopoly is analyzed. Services by nurse practitioners and clinicians are now offering some competition to medicine but collaboration is also possible. (7)

2319   Corless, I.B.   "Physicians and Nurses: Roles and Responsibili-
       ties in Caring for the Critically Ill Patient," LAW MED
       HEALTH CARE 10(2) (April 1982): 72-76.

       Argues that a revision of health care responsibilities would
       provide a higher quality of care to patients and improve
       nurse-physician relationships.   Includes a reformulation of
       roles, including giving nurses more responsibility. (21)

2320   Cruikshank, B.M.   "A Survey of Iowa Pediatricians Concerning
       Hiring of Pediatric Nurse Practitioners," PED NURS 6(3)
       (May/June 1980): 17-19.

       Use of a pediatric nurse practitioner appears, most likely
       among recent medical school graduates, those in multispecialty
       settings, with large practices and an interest in prevention.
       (7)

2321   Edmunds, M. (Ed.)   "Non-Clinical Problems: Nurse Practitioner-
       Physician Competition," NURSE PRACT 6 (March/April 1981):
       47, 49, 53-54.

       The GMENAC Report has predicted a physician surplus by 1990.
       This has increased a sense of competition between physicians
       and nurse practitioners.   Strategies for coping with this
       situation are discussed. (7)

2322   Friedman, F.B.   "A Nurse's Guide to the Care and Handling of
       MDs," RN 45 (March 1982): 39-42, 118, 120.

       Reports a survey of nurse- physician relationships. (0)

2323   Gunn, I.P.   "Nurse Anesthetist-Anesthesiologist Relationships:
       Past, Present and Implications for the Future," AANA J 43
       (April 1975): 129-39.

       Traces historical roots of nurse anesthetist-anesthesiolo-
       gists relationships, and discusses present problems with sug-
       gestions for solutions.(15)

2324   Hoekelman, R.A.   "Nurse-Physician Relationships: Problems and
       Solutions." THE NURSING PROFESSION: VIEWS THROUGH THE MIST.
       Edited by N.L. Chaska.   New York: McGraw-Hill, 1978, pp.
       330-35.

       Physician describes problems in nurse-physician relationship
       as he sees them, including sexism, and offers solutions.

2325   Kalisch, B.J.   "Of Half Gods and Mortals: Aesculapian Author-
       ity," NURS OUTLOOK 23 (January 1975): 22-28.

       Working against patient participation in the decision making
       process is a three pronged power base: the physician's exper-
       tise, the patient's faith in him (her), and the belief that
       the physician has almost mystical power. (17)

2326   Keenan, T., L. Aiken and L.E. Cluff. NURSES AND DOCTORS:
       THEIR EDUCATION AND PRACTICE. Cambridge, MA.: Oelgeschlager,
       Gunn and Haen Publishers, Inc., 1981.

       Report of conference on working relationships between
       medical and nursing faculties.

2327   Lee, A.A. "How Nurses Rate With the MDs: Still the Hand-
       maiden," RN 42 (July 1979): 21-30.

       Survey results. (0)

2328   Deleted.

2329   McGuire, M.A. "Nurse-Physician Interactions: Silence Isn't
       Golden," SUPERVISOR NURSE 11 (March 1980): 36, 38-39.

       Contends that nurses by their silence reinforce childish
       behavior in physicians and perpetuate the notion that nurses
       are servants. (0)

2330   Mechanic, D. and L.H. Aiken. "A Cooperative Agenda for Medi-
       cine and Nursing," NE J MED 307 (September 16, 1982): 747-50.

       Nurses primarily support and complement medical care. Ex-
       panded clinical responsibilities of nurses have freed physi-
       cians to perform medical functions that require their unique
       expertise and that tend to be more remunerative. There still
       exists a lack of communication between physicians and nurses.
       (18)

2331   Muldary, T.W. INTERPERSONAL RELATIONS FOR HEALTH PROFES-
       SIONALS: A SOCIAL SKILLS APPROACH. New York: Macmillan
       Publishing Co., 1983.

       Argues that better understanding of interpersonal behavior
       can improve patient care. Each section offers insights into
       the basic processes of human interaction. Case examples and
       illustrations provided.

2332   Murphy, P. "Deciding to Blow the Whistle," AM J NURS (Sep-
       tember 1981): 1691-92.

       A nurse reports an unsuccessful attempt to report a case of
       physician negligence that caused the death of a patient.
       She analyzes her attempt, and the act of "whistle blowing"
       in general. (2)

2333   Ritter, H.A. "Nurse-Physician Collaboration," CONNECTICUT
       MED 45 (January 1981): 23-25.

       Report on collaborative projects in four sites across the
       country which resulted in better patient care, fewer errors,
       less litigation, better satisfaction by both nurses and physi-
       cians. (2)

2334   Roth, C. "Nurses and Pharmacists: A Study of Consultation
        Patterns on Patient Units," NURS HEALTH CARE 3(8) (1982):
        438-42.

        Report of a study of consultation patterns of nurses.
        Nurses consulted pharmacists more often than physicians did.
        Most questions related to anti-infectives, analgesics and
        cardiovascular drugs. Even with clinical pharmacists avail-
        able nurses did most of the patient teaching about drugs. (10)

2335   Steel, J.E. "Putting Joint Practice Into Practice," AM J
        NURS 81(5) (May 1981): 964-67.

        The essence of a joint practice is the explicit determina-
        tion of mutual goals and the negotiation of roles or parts
        of each participant will assume. This can be described as
        taking place in three stages. (3)

2336   Stein, L.I. "The Doctor-Nurse Game." ARCHIVES OF GENERAL
        PSYCHIATRY 16 (June 1967): 699-703 Reprinted in NEW DIREC-
        TIONS FOR NURSES. Edited by V. Bullough and B. Bullough.
        New York: Springer Publishing Co., 1971, pp. 129-37.

        Classic description of the interaction pattern of physicians
        and nurses, particularly as it relates to advice given by
        nurses. Both participants in the game pretend that nurses do
        not give advice. (0)

2337   Thomstad, B., N. Cunningham and B. Kaplan. "Changing the
        Rules of the Doctor-Nurse Game," NURS OUTLOOK 23 (July
        1975): 422-27. Reprinted in EXPANDING HORIZONS FOR NURSING.
        Edited by B. Bullough and V. Bullough. New York: Springer
        Publishing Co., 1977, pp. 328-38.

        How to renegotiate the rules in traditional doctor nurse
        game. (1)

2338   Weiss, S.J. "Role Differentiation Between Nurse and Physician:
        Implications for Nursing," NURS RES 32(3) (May/June 1983):
        133-39.

        Aim of study was to determine whether a series of systematic
        dialogue sessions among nurses, consumers, and physicians
        would result in consensus regarding unique areas of nursing
        practice differentiated from medical practice and (2) areas of
        common practice. (22)

2339   Williams, R.A. and C.C. Williams. "Hospital Social Workers
        and Nurses: Interprofessional Perceptions and Experiences,"
        J NURS EDUC 21(5) (May 1982): 16-21.

        A study of interprofessional contact between nurses and
        social workers assessed the type and frequency of contact,

stereotyping images they held of each other, and the relationship between contact and stereotyping. Social workers reported more contact with nurses than nurses with social
workers. The greater the interprofessional contact the less
stereotyping occurred. (11)

See 142, 147, 792.

Substance Abuse

2340 American Nurses' Association. ADDICTIONS AND PSYCHOLOGICAL
      DYSFUNCTIONS IN NURSING: THE PROFESSIONS'S RESPONSE TO THE
      PROBLEM. Kansas City, MO.: American Nurses' Association,
      Pub. No. PMH-6, 1984.

      Analysis of health problems compromising nurses' abilities
      to function within professional practice standards, addressing
      professional nursing's responsibility, problems of impaired
      practice, program planning as social change, and prevention.

2341 Bissell, L. and R.W. Jones. "The Alcoholic Nurse," NURS OUT-
      LOOK (February 1981): 96-101.

      A study of 100 nurses recovering from alcoholism reveals
      that their disease pattern is similar to other women and went
      unchecked longer than it did in alcoholic physicians. (17)

2342 Elkind, A.K. "Nurses, Smoking and Cancer Prevention," INT J
      HEALTH EDUC 23 (1979): 92-101.

      Nurses' smoking behavior and its relationship to their views
      on cancer prevention was studied using the nursing staff of
      one hospital in England. Most nurses to some extent accepted
      that non-smoking is of value in preventing cancer. But
      smokers in general were less likely to accept the idea of a
      definite preventive value. (13)

2343 _____. "Nurses' Smoking Behaviour: Review and Implications,"
      INT J NURS STUDIES 17 (1980): 261-69.

      Studies of nurses' smoking behavior are reviewed: explana-
      tions for the behavior are examined, and implications discus-
      sed. (42)

2344 Fulton, K. "Drug Abuse Among Nurses: What Nursing Management
      Can Do!," SUPERVISOR NURSE (January 1981): 18-20.

      Describes problem and suggests actions for nursing adminis-
      trators. (0)

2345 Hillier, S. "Nurses Smoking Habits," POSTGRADUATE MED J 49
      (1973): 693-94.

Investigation of smoking habits of a group of student
nurses. Aim was to examine how social factors, in particular
job stress and social climate of the hospital setting influenced nurses to begin smoking or to change their pattern of
smoking. (0)

2346   Hillier, S., G. Hazan and M. Jefferies. A Study of the Rela-
        tionship Between Situational Stress and the Smoking Habits
        of Nurses in Three Selected Hospitals. Social Science Re-
        search Council Final Report as reported in A.K. Elkind,
        "Nurses´ Smoking Behaviour: Review and Implications," INT J
        NURS STUDIES (17) (1980): 261-69.

        This article looks at a worldwide picture of nurses´ smoking
        behavior. It offers explanations and examines implications
        for both health education and the nursing profession. (42)

2347   Jacobson, B. "Smoking Questionnaire: Warning Nursing Can
        Damage Your Health," NURS MIRROR 152 (1981): 16-18.

        An analysis of a survey published in June, 1980. The most
        common reason nurses gave for smoking was anxiety and stress
        related to the hospital environment. (4)

2348   Jaffe, S. "First-Hand Views of Recovery," AM J NURS 82 (April
        1982): 578-79.

        Interviews of ten recovering alcoholic nurses and six alco-
        holic patients are presented. (2)

2349   Jefferson, L.V. and B.E. Ensor. "Help for the Helper-Confront-
        ing a Chemically-Impaired Colleague," AM J NURS 82 (1982):
        573-78.

        A profile of the chemically impaired nurse, both alcohol and
        drug, with markers to identify the problem. Suggests ap-
        propriate intervention and treatment. (7)

2350   Tagliacozzo, R. and S. Vaughn. "Stress and Smoking in Hos-
        pital Nurses," AM J PUB HEALTH 72(5) (1982): 441-48.

        Focuses on smoking behavior of hospital nurses and the as-
        sociation between work related stress and smoking. Question-
        naires were mailed to the nursing staff of the University of
        Michigan Hospital. Smokers showed higher levels of physical
        and emotional stress than non-smokers. (40)

2351   "The Dependent Nurse," NURS TIMES (January 19, 1983).

        The Georgia Nurses Association and the Georgia Board of
        Nursing has established one of the first official programs for
        dependent nurses. It is the Impaired Nurse Program with
        emphasis on education, entry and rehabilitation for drug
        dependent nurses. (17)

        See 378, 386, 389, 391, 392.

Physical Fitness

2352   Brown, B.S. "Fitting Fitness Into Your Life," NURS ECON 1(2)
       (September/October 1983): 93-96.

       Discusses the importance of personal fitness programs, and
       describes criteria for establishing a program that meets in-
       dividual needs. (8)

2353   Lachman, V.D. STRESS MANAGEMENT: A MANUAL FOR NURSES.
       Orlando, FL.: Grune & Stratton, Inc., 1983.

       A guide for reducing stress.

2354   Rimer, B. and B. Glassman. "The Fitness Revolution: Will
       Nurses Sit This One Out?," NURS ECON 1(2) (September/October
       1983): 84-89, 144.

       Fitness is becoming big business, both inside and outside of
       health care institutions. Nurses can, and do, play a wide
       variety of roles, ranging from counseling patients to managing
       and owning self-supporting fitness enterprises. This article
       looks at the professional literature and at the experience of
       individual nurses in fitness. (27)

2355   Williams, A. "Hepatitis B Virus Vaccine," NURSE PRACT 8(9)
       (October 1983): 30, 32.

       Hepatitis B is a major public health problem. Complications
       of the disease can include a carrier state, chronic active
       hepatitis, cirrhosis and hepatocellular carcinoma. The de-
       velopment of hepatitis B virus vaccine has made active im-
       munization against HBV possible. Although studies are still
       in progress, the vaccine appears quite safe and remarkably
       free of side effects. Vaccination is recommended for indivi-
       duals who are at risk for exposure to infectious blood or body
       fluids from hepatitis B patients. (10)

International Nursing

2356   Brower, T. "A Look at China's Eldercare," GERIATR NURS 5(6)
       (July/August 1984): 250-53.

       China faces a growing challenge from an increasing number of
       elderly persons. Resources for the elderly are as yet scarce.
       (10)

2357   Brown, B.S. "Growing Up Healthy: The Chinese Experience,"
       PED NURS 9(4) (July/August 1984): 255-57.

       The Chinese emphasis on group strength and respect for
       authority is reflected in China's health care policies and
       pediatric health care practices. (3)

2358   Brown, M.S., M.M. McBride and M.K. Thompson. "Health Care in
       the Soviet Union," NURSE PRACT 9(4) (April 1984): 50-54.

Health care system of the Soviet Union described and discussed. (0)

2359   Brown, M.S., C.E. Burns and P.J. Hellings. "Health Care in
       China," NURSE PRACT 9(5) (May 1984): 39-42, 46.

       History and current status of Chinese health care. (0)

2360   Kelly, L.Y. "Other Worlds of Nursing," NURS OUTLOOK 30(1)
       (January 1982): 64.

       Comments on nursing in the Soviet Union. (0)

2361   Lowe, A.G. "The Counterpart System In International
       Nursing," PED NURS 9(4) (July/August 1983): 259-61.

       Introducing change while being sensitive to what is involved
       in dealing with counterparts in developing areas demand objec-
       tivity and cooperation. One approach used by an international
       nurse and potential change agent, herein presented, was the
       research method applied in a newborn nursery in Brazil. (4)

2362   Lukasik, C. "International Nursing With Project HOPE," PED
       NURS 9(4) (July/August 1983): 267-68.

       International nursing within the philosophy and programming
       of a private voluntary not-for-profit international health
       agency is described.(2)

2363   Mahler, H. "The Meaning of 'Health For All By The Year
       2000'," WORLD HEALTH FORUM 2(1) (1981): 5-22.

       The Director-General of the World Health Organization (WHO)
       explains the WHO target of "health for all by the year 2000."
       This goal is a difficult one. It will involve the reorienta-
       tion of the health care systems, industry, and world politics.
       A key element in the plan is the development of basic primary
       health care for all people. (3)

2364   Mathias, J. "Anesthesia in Developing Countries," AANA J 52
       (August 1984): 405-12.

       Present status of anesthesia in developing countries; work
       force, agents and equipment used, and problems related to
       culture. (24)

2365   Rorabaugh, M.L. "The Pediatric Nurse Practitioner in South-
       east Asia: A Personal Account," PED NURS 9(4) (July/August
       1983): 263-66.

       Nursing in South East Asia involves overcoming cultural bar-
       riers and tropical disease in an area overwhelmed by war,
       poverty, and shifting population. Aspects of preparation,
       risks, and benefits are common to nursing opportunities in
       other parts of the Third World. (2)

2366   Salzer, J.L. and N.A. Nelson. "Health Care of Ethiopian
       Refugees," PED NURS 9(6) (November/December 1983): 449-52.

       Providing health care for refugee children requires an
       understanding of their culture and its influence on their
       health care beliefs. The authors´ experience caring for
       Ethiopian refugee children illustrate the need to integrate
       cultural awareness into comprehensive health care. (3)

2367   Ulin, P.R. "International Nursing Challenge," NURS OUTLOOK
       30(9) (November/December 1982): 531-35.

       Removing primary health care from the central domain of
       nursing practice can be a serious deterrent to its acces-
       sibility, creating an offshoot of nursing instead of a solid
       discipline. (16)

Organizations

2368   American Academy of Nursing. PRIORITIES WITHIN THE HEALTH
       CARE SYSTEM: A DELPHI SURVEY. Kansas City, MO.: American
       Nurses´ Association, Pub. No. G-148, 1981.

       The American Academy of Nursing employed the Delphi method
       of soliciting and combining the opinions of experts to develop
       consensus on the relative importance of critical issues con-
       fronting nursing and the potential impact of the Academy in
       dealing with those issues.

2369   American Nurses´ Association. ONE STRONG VOICE: THE STORY OF
       THE AMERICAN NURSES´ ASSOCIATION. Kansas City, MO.:
       American Nurses´ Association, Pub. No. G-122, 1976.

       Comprehensive volume containing information about nursing
       in this country, from Revolutionary War days to the present.

2370   _____. HOUSE OF DELEGATES REPORTS 1978-1980. Kansas
       City, MO.: American Nurses´ Association, Pub. No. G-144,
       1980.

       Reports to the House of Delegates from all ANA commissions,
       divisions, committees and councils for activities during the
       1978-1980 biennium.

2371   _____. NURSING: A SOCIAL POLICY STATEMENT. Kansas City,
       MO.: American Nurses´ Association, Pub. No. NP-63, 1980.

       The ANA Congress for Nursing Practice presents a new descrip-
       tion of the scope of nursing practice. It offers a defini-
       tion of nursing and a description of the characteristics of
       specialization in nursing practice.

2372   _____. SUMMARY OF PROCEEDINGS. THE ´80´s: DECADE FOR
       DECISIONS. Kansas City, MO.: American Nurses´ Association,
       Pub. No. G-150, 1981.

An overview of 1980 ANA Convention events, a discussion
of actions taken by the ANA House of Delegates, and reports
to the House from ANA units.

2373 _____. ANA BYLAWS. Kansas City, MO.: American Nurses'
      Association, Pub. No. G-77, 1982.

      Bylaws as amended July, 1982. Booklet includes historical
      sketch and certificate of incorporation.

2374 _____. ANA CONVENTION '82: SUMMARY OF PROCEEDINGS.
      Kansas City, MO.: American Nurses' Association, Pub. No.
      G-162, 1983.

      Content of ANA's 1982 Convention in Washington, D.C.,
      "Nursing: A Force for the Nation's Health." Includes over-
      view, addresses, reports, organizational changes, considera-
      tion of bylaws, elections, summaries of business meetings...
      a significant historical record and reference work.

2375 Capuzzi, C. "Power and Interest Groups: A Study of ANA and
      AMA," NURS OUTLOOK 28 (August 1980): 478-82.

      Classifies professional organizations as special interest
      groups. Compares two such groups- the American Medical As-
      sociation and American Nurses' Association in an attempt to
      provide some answers to why certain interest groups are more
      powerful than others. (32)

2376 Fry, S.T. "The Social Responsibilities of Nursing," NURS
      ECON 1(1) (July/August 1983): 61-64, 72.

      This article describes the social responsibilities of nurs-
      ing according to the historical context of Victorian England
      and the social context of modern health care services. In
      discussing these responsibilities, the ANA's NURSING: A SOCIAL
      POLICY STATEMENT is explored in depth, and suggestions are
      made for communicating this statement of nursing's social
      responsibilities to the general public. (19)

2377 "News: Federation Votes New Name, Criteria," AM J NURS (August
      1981): 1430.

      Nineteen nursing organizations, including ANA voted to re-
      name themselves the "National Federation for Nursing Specialty
      Organizations." Formerly group was called the "Federation of
      Specialty Organizations and ANA." (0)

2378 Shamansky, S.L. "Nursing Is The Time For All Good Girls To
      Do What They Are Told To Do," PUBLIC HEALTH NURS 1(3) (Sep-
      tember 1984): 127-28.

      Editorial criticizing the ANA Social Policy Statement. (0)

2379   Steel, J.E. "The Social Policy Statement: Assuring A Posi-
       tive Future For Nurse Practitioners," NURSE PRACT 9(2)
       (February 1984): 15-16, 68.

       An essay about the ANA policy statement by a member of the
       task force who wrote it. Focus is on the nurturative, pro-
       tective, generative characteristics of nursing, and on the
       nurse´s direct relationship with the consumer. The statement
       calls for professional power over credentialing rather than
       public or state power. Article concludes with a call for all
       nurse practitioners to avoid organizing outside of ANA. (3)

2380   White, C.M. "A Critique of the ANA Social Policy Statement,"
       NURS OUTLOOK 32(6) (November/December 1984): 328-31.

       Argues that the ANA Social Policy Statement is too narrow.
       It fails to cover the role of nurses in health policy formu-
       lation and it underplays environmental concerns. (17)

       See 1903, 2038, 2039, 2040, 2371.

HEALTH CARE DELIVERY SYSTEM

The Delivery of Health Care, Health Policy,
and Economic Issues

2381 Aday, L.A., R. Anderson and G.V. Fleming. HEALTH CARE IN THE
      U.S.: EQUITABLE FOR WHOM? Beverly Hills, CA.: Sage Pub-
      lications, Inc., 1980.

      A detailed study of the availability of medical care to
      various populations throughout the United States.

2382 Ahmed, M.C. "Taking Charge of Change in Hospital Nursing Prac-
      tice," AM J NURS 81(3) (March 1981): 540-43.

      The successful experience of one nurse in trying to change
      and upgrade nursing practice on a fifty-one bed unit which she
      supervised. (2)

2383 Aiken, L. "Nursing Priorities for the 1980's: Hospitals and
      Nursing Homes," AM J NURS 81(2) (February 1981): 324-30.

      Nurses have the opportunities to help overcome the major
      problems experienced by hospitals and nursing homes in the
      delivery of safe, effective care. How they respond is criti-
      cal. Examines problems and possible responses. (28)

2384 Aiken, L.H. and S.R. Gortner (Eds.). NURSING IN THE 1980s:
      CRISES, OPPORTUNITIES, CHALLENGES. Philadelphia: J.B. Lip-
      pincott, 1982.

      Contains twenty-seven papers by thirty-three nurses and
      other members of the health care professions dealing primarily
      with economics and politics of health care.

2385 American Academy of Nursing. LONG-TERM CARE IN PERSPECTIVE:
      PAST, PRESENT, AND FUTURE DIRECTIONS FOR NURSING. Kansas
      City, MO.: American Nurses' Association, Pub. No. G-120,
      1976.

      Papers presented at the 1975 Scientific Session of the
      American Academy of Nursing. Includes consideration of shared
      control of the system among professionals, evaluation of care,
      economics and promotion of health as they relate to long-term
      care. Also includes a statement on long-term care.

2386 _____. NURSING'S INFLUENCE ON HEALTH POLICY FOR THE
      EIGHTIES. Kansas City, MO.: American Nurses' Association,
      Pub. No. G-134, 1979.

The concerns of the American Academy of Nursing are synthe-
sized in this monograph, which focuses on alternate care
models, payment for services of nurses, and women and power.
Proceedings of the annual meeting of the academy, September,
1978.

2387   _____. THE IMPACT OF CHANGING RESOURCES ON HEALTH POLICY.
        Kansas City, MO.: American Nurses´ Association, 1981.

Major papers presented at the 1980 Scientific Sessions of
the American Academy of Nursing. Seven papers included more
or less focused on the impact of changing reosurces on nursing. References for individual papers.

2388   _____ (L.H. Aiken, Ed.). HEALTH POLICY AND NURSING
        PRACTICE. New York: McGraw-Hill Book Co., 1981.

Seventeen papers by leaders in nursing analyzing a variety
of innovative health care and nursing practices. Included
are descriptions of nurse managed ambulatory care settings,
alternative birthing centers, and nursing practices in health
maintenance organizations, clinics, and hospitals. Proposals
for changes in nursing education to meet current needs are
presented. References follow each paper. (290)

2389   _____. FROM ACCOMMODATION TO SELF-DETERMINATION: NURSING´S
        ROLE IN THE DEVELOPMENT OF HEALTH CARE POLICY. Kansas City,
        MO.: American Nurses´ Association, Pub. No. G-153, 1982.

Five papers presented at the 1981 Scientific Session of the
American Academy of Nursing providing examples of how nurses
are building a body of knowledge and experience that can contribute significantly to shaping health care policy in this
country.

2390 American Medical Association. HEALTH POLICY AGENDA, PHASE I
        REPORT, VOL. I. Chicago, IL.: American Medical Association,
        1984.

American Medical Association sponsored report. This volume
reports the early planning phase of the study. The purpose
is to develop a long-range comprehensive health care policy
for the country.

2391 American Nurses´ Association. A NATIONAL POLICY FOR HEALTH
        CARE: PRINCIPLES AND POSITIONS. Kansas City, MO.: American
        Nurses´ Association, Pub. No. G-130, 1977.

Deals with certain specific aspects of national health
policy, including health planning, health manpower, quality
of health care services, health education, home care, aging
adults, mental health, and child health.

2392 American Nurses´ Foundation, Inc. THE HEALTH OF FAMILIES IN A
        CULTURE OF CRISIS. Kansas City, MO.: American Nurses´ Asso-
        ciation, Pub. No. FD-25, 1981.

W. K. Kellogg Foundation Fiftieth Anniversary Lecture in
which Maxene Johnston discusses what the challenge of today's
world poses for health professionals planning and developing
strategies for coping, adapting, and surviving in a changing
culture.

2393   Binder, J.   "Toward a Policy Perspective for Nursing," NURS
       ECON 1(1) (July/August 1983): 47-50.

       Explores several health policy perspectives in terms of
       their implications for nursing values, autonomy and roles.
       Advocates an integrated perspective for nursing which accepts
       the necessity of certain medical and technological advance-
       ments, but emphasizes the individual's right to health and the
       necessity for more preventive rather than curative/medical
       programs. (15)

2394   Brook, R.H., J.E. Ware, Jr., W.H. Rogers, E.B. Keeler, A.R.
       Davies, C.A. Donald, G.A. Goldberg, K.N. Lohr, T.C. Marthay
       and J.P. Newhouse. "Does Free Care Improve Adults' Health?
       Results from a Randomized Controlled Trial," NE J MED 309
       (December 8, 1983): 1426-34.

       In a study done by the Rand Corporation a sample of 3,958
       persons were followed to determine the outcomes of various
       health care financing situations for health. For most outcome
       measures there were no significant differences. For persons
       with poor vision and low income persons with hypertension free
       care resulted in a better outcome. (34)

2395   Browne, W.P. and L.K. Olson (Eds.). AGING AND PUBLIC POLICY:
       THE POLITICS OF GROWING OLD IN AMERICA. Westport, CT.:
       Greenwood Press, 1983.

       Editors Browne and Olson and nine other authors analyze aging
       programs and policies of recent decades. The overall theme is
       that although older Americans have emerged as a distinctive
       political force, the fragmentation of the special interest
       groups that affect to speak for them.

2396   Chen, M.K. and R.D. Buck. "Measuring the Health Care Needs of
       An Adult Population in California," MEDICAL CARE (April
       1981): 452-64.

       Assesses the health status of the black population in Alameda
       County, California. The data collected by the Human Population
       Laboratory in Berkeley show that black adults lost several
       useful life years per person unnecessarily as compared with
       the numbers of life years enjoyed by the white population in
       that county. (10)

2397   Conway, M.E. THE IMPACT OF CHANGING RESOURCES ON HEALTH
       POLICY. Kansas City, MO.: American Nurses' Association,
       1981.

Discusses how environment, energy, labor, and technology
are important in the context of the future of health care.

2398   Corning, P.A. THE EVOLUTION OF MEDICARE: FROM IDEA TO LAW.
       Washington, D.C.: U.S. Department of Health, Education and
       Welfare, Social Security Administration, Office of Research
       and Statistics, Research Report No. 29, 1969.

       Traces history of attempts to pass state and national health
       care insurance laws from 1912-1965. This history facilitates
       an understanding of the current medicare law.

2399   Davis, C.K. "The Federal Role in Changing Health Care Financ-
       ing, Part I," NURS ECON 1(1) (July/August, 1983): 10-19.

       First article in a two part series on the federal role in
       changing health care financing. As the federal agency respon-
       sible for Medicare and Medicaid, the Health Care Financing
       Administration is acutely aware of the increasing health care
       costs, factors contributing to that increase, and the federal
       expenditures for health services. A variety of plans for cost
       containment are discussed, including prospective payments to
       hosptials, restructuring of Medicare and Medicaid, health
       incentives, limiting the amount of insurance that are tax
       free, and encouraging HMOs. (2)

2400   Davis, K. NATIONAL HEALTH INSURANCE: BENEFITS, COSTS, AND
       CONSEQUENCES. Washington, D.C.: The Brookings Institution,
       1975.

       Describes the seven major national health insurance proposals
       that have been introduced in the Congress. Examines the dis-
       tribution of benefits, and costs associated with each of the
       insurance plans; and clarifies health care issues and choices.

2401   Driscoll, V.M. "Remedies for a Troubled Health Care System,"
       J NY STATE NURSES ASSOC 11(4) (December 1980): 15-22.

       Suggests that if the nursing profession would resolve its
       troubled nursing care system, society would be better able to
       deal with the country's troubled health care system. (0)

2402   Falkson, J.L. HMOs AND THE POLITICS OF HEALTH SYSTEM REFORM.
       Chicago: American Hospital Association, 1980.

       The evolution of the federal government's commitment to pre-
       paid health care in the United States in the 1970s is dis-
       cussed.

2403   Georgopoulos, B.S. (Ed.). ORGANIZATION RESEARCH ON HEALTH
       INSTITUTIONS. Ann Arbor, MI.: The Institute for Social
       Research, The University of Michigan, 1972.

       Twenty-two contributors review research on hospitals as
       complex organizations. The approach is social psychological.
       A classic in the field.

2404   Glaser, W.A. "For Profit Hospitals: American and Foreign
       Comparisons," HEALTH CARE MANAGEMENT REV 9(4) (Fall 1984):
       27-34.

       In other developed countries proprietary hospitals are dis-
       appearing. They are increasing in United States. Author is
       concerned about their impact on the quality of care. (29)

2405   Goad, S. and G. Moire. "Role Discrepancy: Implications for
       Nursing Leaders," NURS LEADERSH 4(2) (June 1981): 23-27.

       Role expectations of 240 baccalaureate graduates in primary
       and team nursing setting were examined to determine the con-
       cept of ideal nursing role and difference in ideal and percep-
       tion of real. (7)

2406   Jacox, A. "Significant Questions About IOM´s Study of Nurs-
       ing," NURS OUTLOOK 31 (January/February 1983): 28-33.

       Raises serious question concerning the extent to which nurs-
       ing´s viewpoint is adequately represented by the decision
       makers in the study advisory groups. Offers guidelines for a
       judicious review of the study findings. (16)

2407   Jonas, S. (Ed.) HEALTH CARE DELIVERY IN THE UNITED STATES,
       2nd Ed. New York: Springer Publishing Co., 1981.

       A non-technical description of how personal health services
       are organized and delivered.

2408   Kraegel, J.M. (Ed.). ORGANIZATION-ENVIRONMENT RELATIONSHIPS.
       Rockville, MD.: Aspen Systems, 1980.

       The fifth in a series of books on management, this volume
       focuses on organizational theory and characteristics of the
       organizational environment. The initial chapters offer an
       overview of theory.

2409   Lang, R.H. "Implementation of Comprehensive Service Systems
       for the Elderly and Chronically Ill," J HEALTH AND HUMAN
       RESOURCES ADM 4 (Spring 1982): 415-50.

       Develops a conceptual framework applicable to any human
       system which will make multiple funding streams and conflicting
       mandates work as a system for the people. (6)

2410   Lee, P.R., C.L. Estes and N.B. Ramsay. THE NATION´S HEALTH,
       2nd Ed. San Francisco: Boyd & Fraser Publishing Co., 1984.

       Overview of the current status of the health care delivery
       system as well as the current and emerging policy issues.
       Although there is a section on nursing, health care is most
       often conceptualized as medical care. Wide variety of essays
       by many well-known authors.

2411   Lutjens, L.R.   "The Name of This Game is Conflict," NURS
       MANAGE 14(6) (June 1983): 23-24.

       Describes modes of conflict resolutions and suggests that
       these should be taught to senior nursing students to prepare
       them for conflict they will experience on the job. (1)

2412   Macrae, N.   "Health Care International," THE ECONOMIST 29
       (April 28, 1984): 17-20, 25-26, 29-32, 35.

       Analysis of American, British and Japanese health care de-
       livery systems, with comparisons to other countries. (0)

2413   McKinley, J. (Ed.).   ISSUES IN THE POLITICAL ECONOMY OF HEALTH
       CARE.   New York: Methuen, Inc., 1984.

       The seven contributors--who include a biologist, sociolo-
       gists, political scientists, and two physicians--examine the
       relationships of capitalism to health care, in terms of its
       influence on the physical environment, the incidence of social
       diseases and the prevailing view of what constitutes health
       itself; and in terms of the consequences of the new medical-
       industrial complex it has created, such as the declining pro-
       vision of health care for the poor and disadvantaged, the grow-
       ing power of the pharmaceutical industry and the eroding con-
       trol of physicians over the delivery of health care.

2414   Mechanic, D.   FUTURE ISSUES IN HEALTH CARE: SOCIAL POLICY
       AND THE RATIONING OF MEDICAL SERVICES.   New York: Free
       Press, 1979.

       Argues that technological advances have made some types of
       care so expensive rationing is necessary.   Market and regula-
       tory approaches discussed. Shift in policy related to mental
       illness leading to deinstitutionalization discussed.

2415   _____.   HANDBOOK OF HEALTH, HEALTH CARE, AND THE HEALTH
       PROFESSIONS.   New York: Free Press, 1983.

       A revision of a well-known sociological book about the
       health care delivery system.   Chapters by thirty-four authors
       cover epidemiology, clinical issues, management of health care
       institutions, health care occupations, health and illness,
       psychosocial issues, and related topics.

2416   Mendelson, M.M.A.   TENDER LOVING GREED.   New York: Vintage
       Books, 1975.

       A critique of the nursing home industry.

2417   Milio, N.   "Ethics and the Economics of Community Health Ser-
       vices: The Case of Screening," LINACRE QUARTERLY 44
       (November 1977): 347-60.

       Looks at cost benefit of screening programs as well as
       alternatives. (45)

2418 _____. "Chains of Impact From Reaganomics on Primary Care
      Policies," PUBLIC HEALTH NURS 1(2) (June 1984): 65-73.

      Analyzes the effects of federal fiscal policy in the Reagan
      administration on primary care programs. A wide array of pri-
      mary care services became less available and accessible,
      thereby limiting their cost-savings potential and their effec-
      tiveness in supporting people's health. These program defi-
      cits, together with lowered living standards among large seg-
      ments of the population, resulted in rising rates of infant
      mortality in many states. (66)

2419 National League for Nursing. ORGANIZATIONAL BEHAVIOR-CONFLICT
      AND RESOLUTION. New York: National League for Nursing, Pub.
      No. 52-1509, 1974.

      Studies the elements of leadership in general and looks at
      the systems approach to problem solving and covers such sub-
      jects as organizational behavior, new roles in action, chang-
      ing patterns of health care, recommendations for task groups,
      and a comparison of several health insurance plans.

2420 O'Donnell, M.P. and T.H. Ainsworth (Eds.). HEALTH PROMOTION
      IN THE WORKPLACE. New York: John Wiley and Sons, 1984.

      Beginning with the concept of health promotion, the authors
      discuss program design, content (health assessment, nutrition,
      fitness, substance dependency, stress), administration, and
      the role and impact of external institutions.

2421 Penberty-Valentine, M. HEALTH PLANNING FOR NURSE MANAGERS:
      STRATEGIES FOR SUCCESS. Rockville, MD.: Aspen Systems Corp.,
      1984.

      Describes the health care system as it exists today, and
      examines the changes that can be expected. Details the proce-
      dures for strategic planning, long-range planning, institu-
      tional planning, and certificate of need review, plus shows
      you how to effectively plan.

2422 Porter-O'Grady, T. and S. Finnigan. SHARED GOVERNANCE FOR
      NURSING: A CREATIVE APPROACH TO PROFESSIONAL ACCOUNTABILITY.
      Rockville, MD.: Aspen Systems Corp., 1984.

      A management text focused on a participative administrative
      style.

2423 Prussin, J.A. and J.M. Prussin. HEALTH SERVICES AND THE
      ELDERLY. Owing Mills, MD.: National Health Publishing, 1982.

      Facts, figures, trend data, and policy approaches to the
      organization, delivery, and financing of health services for
      the elderly.

2424 Quick, J.D., M.R. Greenlick and K.J. Roghmann. "Prenatal
      Care and Pregnancy Outcome in an HMO and General Population:
      A Multivariate Cohort Analysis," AM J PUB HEALTH 71(4)
      (April 1981): 81-90.

      Factors related to infant mortality studied in an HMO and
      non HMO sample. Despite lower cost of care the HMO sample had
      comparable outcomes. (39)

2425 Roemer, M.I. AN INTRODUCTION TO THE U.S. HEALTH CARE SYSTEMS:
      HISTORICAL, DESCRIPTIVE, AND POLICY PERSPECTIVES. New York:
      Springer Publishing Co., 1982.

      Basic structure and operation of the U.S. health care system
      explained.

2426 Roemer, R., C. Kramer and J.E. Frink. PLANNING URBAN HEALTH
      SERVICES: FROM JUNGLE TO SYSTEM. New York: Springer Pub-
      lishing Co., 1975.

      Analysis and critique of the fragmentation in the health
      care delivery system. Basic study done in California but com-
      parative data from national and international studies used.

2427 "Role of State and Local Governments in Relation to Personal
      Health Services," AM J PUB HEALTH 71(1) (January 1981):
      Supplement.

      Issue is made up of papers from a 1980 conference on the
      role of state and local governments in providing health ser-
      vices. Primary ambulatory care is the focus of several papers,
      but hospital care is also included. Focus includes rural and
      urban settings.

2428 Rutkowski, A.D. and B.L. Rutkowski. LABOR RELATIONS IN HOSPI-
      TALS. Rockville, MD.: Aspen Systems Corp., 1984.

      Written from the management point of view, this work covers
      union dynamics, organizational campaigns, negotiations, legal
      trends, grievances, and arbitrations. It explains what to
      expect in a unionized hospital and how to plan for action.
      The authors also offer helpful guidelines for supervisors to
      use in communicating the wish to deal with personnel directly.

2429 Sasmor, J.L. "Dollars and Sense: Looking at Costs in Patient
      Care," AM J NURS 81(3) (March 1983): 546-47.

      Nurses have to measure cost as well as convenience for them
      in treating patients and use appropriate technology. Use of
      I.V. therapy is an example used. (0)

2430 Sexton, D.L. "Organizational Conflict: A Creative or Destruc-
      tive Force," NURS LEADSH 3(3) (September 1980): 16-21.

A survey of research into conflict resolution and suggestions on how to make conflict work for creative and fruitful ends. (20)

2431 Sidel, R. and V. Sidel. REFORMING MEDICINE, LESSONS OF THE LAST QUARTER CENTURY. New York: Pantheon (Random House, Inc.), 1984.

Presents an analysis of several efforts to reform health care in America. Each chapter written by an expert in a particular field.

2432 Starr, P. THE SOCIAL TRANSFORMATION OF AMERICAN MEDICINE. New York: Basic Books, Inc., 1982.

An account of the social and economic development of medicine in America. The development of the medical profession is traced from its infancy to one of independence in which private, solo practice was the dominant force. He explains how this led to growth of medical centers and insurance plans, et al., and how the structure incorporated built-in incentives to raise costs. Argues it may be too late to establish a vertical integration of medical care which he sees as the most efficient structure and sees the possibility of control being exercised by for profit corporations. The author is not an apologist for the medical profession, but neither does he accept the notion that the growth of scientific medicine was a capitalist plot.

2433 U.S. Department of Health and Human Services, Public Health Service. HEALTH-UNITED STATES 1982. Washington, D.C.: U.S. Government Printing Office, DHHS Pub. No. (PHS) 83-1232, 1982.

Annual report of the health status of the nation. Started in 1976, the 1982 report is the seventh. Good basic overview of health statistics.

2434 Veninga, R.L. "Resolving Role Confusion: A Source of Employee Conflict," HOSPITAL PROGRESS 62 (December 1981): 41-44, 54.

Though organization conflict is caused by many factors, any change that indicates an interest by management and which creates a humane and productive environment also diminishes disruptive conflicts. (15)

2435 Waitzkin, H. THE SECOND SICKNESS: CONTRADICTIONS OF CAPITALIST HEALTH CARE. New York: The Free Press, 1983.

A well researched radical critique of the American health care delivery system with the major focus on medicine. Analyzes alternative proposed solutions to the problems he outlines.

2436   Warner, K.E. and B.R. Luce. COST-BENEFIT AND COST-EFFECTIVE
       ANALYSIS IN HEALTH CARE: PRINCIPLES, PRACTICE, AND POTENTIAL.
       Ann Arbor, MI.: Health Administration Press, 1982.

       Presents two key tools of health care economic analysis--
       cost-benefit and cost-effectiveness analysis. It summarizes
       the economics background and the health care cost problems
       that spurred a growing interest in CBA-CEA and clarifies the
       differences between the two techniques while describing their
       methodology.

2437   Younger, J.B. "Theory Z Management and Health Care Organiza-
       tions," NURS ECON 1(1) (July/August 1983): 40-45, 69.

       Theory Z is the term proposed by William G. Ouchi for the
       style of management characteristic of successful business in
       Japan. The industrial success of Japan in recent years has
       attracted American interest in Japanese methods. American
       companies that have adopted Theory Z methods have also had
       compelling records of success. This article examines the
       characteristics of Z organizations and considerations related
       to American health care organizations. (7)

       See 660, 702, 823, 884, 885, 886, 888, 889, 890, 891, 892, 893,
       894, 895, 896, 898, 898, 900, 901, 902, 904, 905, 906, 907,
       908, 909, 911, 915, 1098, 1920, 1981, 2013, 2199.

Health Care for Members of Racial or Ethnic Minorities
and Poverty Populations, Transcultural Nursing

2438   Alvarez, R. et al. RACISM, ELITISM, PROFESSIONALISM: BARRIERS
       TO COMMUNITY MENTAL HEALTH. New York: Aronson, 1976.

       Examines racism in its personal, professional, institutional,
       and structural forms and discusses how racism affects community
       mental health.

2439   American Nurses´ Association. A STRATEGY FOR CHANGE. Kansas
       City, MO.: American Nurses´ Association, Pub. No. M-27, 1979.

       Three papers presented at a conference sponsored by the ANA
       Commission on Human Rights in June 1979 discuss the effects of
       ethnicity on the nurse and on his/her interaction with clients.

2440   Bahr, R.T. and L.D. Gress. "Course Description: The Nursing
       Process: Ethnicity and Aging," J GERONTOL NURS 6(4) (April
       1980): 210-13.

       Describes the objectives, content, methodology, and course
       requirements of a college course called "Ethnicity and Aging."
       Notes that such a course is important because knowledge of an
       individual´s culture, health beliefs, and practices is essen-
       tial to high quality nursing care. (2)

2441   Belle, D. (Ed.). LIVES IN STRESS: WOMEN AND DEPRESSION.
       Beverly Hills, CA.: Sage Publications, 1982.

       Reports on one of the first in-depth field studies of the
       causes and consequences of depression in women. Focusing on
       low income mothers with children, the authors use interviews
       to explore the relationship between a woman's life situations
       and her emotional well-being.

2442   Berk, M.L. and G.R. Wilensky. HEALTH CARE OF THE POOR ELDERLY:
       SUPPLEMENTING MEDICINE. Washington, D.C.: U.S. Department
       of Health and Human Services, National Center for Health
       Services Research, March 1, 1984.

       Using data from the National Medical Care Expenditure survey,
       it was found that the elderly poor who did not have supplemen-
       tary insurance in addition to Medicare use fewer services yet
       they have more health problems than the elderly group with
       supplementary insurance. (12)

2443   Branch, M.F. PROVIDING SAFE NURSING CARE FOR ETHNIC PEOPLE
       OF COLOR. New York: Appleton-Century-Crofts, 1976.

       Discusses cultural health traditions and implications for
       nursing care from the perspective of Latino-chicanos, American
       Indians, Asians, and Blacks. Focuses on epidemiology in health
       and disease and goals of nursing care for several ethnic
       groups.

2444   Brink, P.J. (Ed.). TRANSCULTURAL NURSING: A BOOK OF READINGS.
       Englewood Cliffs, NJ.: Prentice-Hall, Inc., 1976.

       Discusses cultural differences in the context of child rear-
       ing, language, value systems, and personality, and how under-
       standing of such variables can positively affect a nurse's
       ability to provide quality health care.

2445   Brown, H. "Breakthrough to Nursing: Equal Rights Nursing,"
       IMPRINT 26(4) (October 1979): 19.

       Stresses the need of minorities as registered nurses and
       encourages more nurses to adopt a holistic perspective, encom-
       passing concern about a patient's culture and how it affects
       his/her medical condition. (0)

2446   _____. "Breakthrough to Nursing: Ethnocentrism in Nursing,"
       IMPRINT 27(1) (February 1980): 26, 69.

       Discusses the implications of a nurse having an ethnocentric
       view of patients. Encourages awareness of ethnocentrism in
       order to eliminate cultural bias from nursing care. (0)

2447   Brown, J. and N.R. Ballard. "Prejudice and Discrimination in
       Nursing." CURRENT PERSPECTIVES IN NURSING: SOCIAL ISSUES AND
       TRENDS. Edited by B.C. Flynn and M.H. Miller. St. Louis:
       C.V. Mosby Co., 1980, pp. 223-38.

Examines the scope of prejudice and discrimination that
nurses direct toward minority group members and the poor.
Considers solutions that have been proposed to moderate such
discrimination and discusses the success of programs instituted
to modify the attitudes and behaviors of nurses. (44)

2448   Brownlee, A.T.   COMMUNITY, CULTURE, AND CARE: A CROSS-
       CULTURAL GUIDE FOR HEALTH WORKERS. St. Louis: C.V. Mosby
       Co., 1978.

       A cross cultural orientation to community health nursing.

2449   Bullough, V. and B. Bullough. HEALTH CARE FOR THE OTHER
       AMERICANS. New York: Appleton-Century-Crofts, 1982.

       A revised and retitled version of the book, POVERTY, ETHNIC
       IDENTITY AND HEALTH CARE first published in 1972. This work
       reviews the historical and current problems that the poor, the
       ethnic minorities, and the elderly have in finding reliable
       and affordable health care.

2450   Bullough, B. and V. Bullough. POVERTY, ETHNIC IDENTITY AND
       HEALTH CARE. New York: Appleton-Century-Crofts, 1972.

       Identifies inadequacies in the health care delivery system
       of the United States and how the poor and members of minority
       groups are most affected by such inadequacies. Proposes ideas
       for improving health care delivery.

2451   Committee for a Study of the Health Care of Racial/Ethnic
       Minorities and Handicapped Persons. HEALTH CARE IN A CON-
       TEXT OF CIVIL RIGHTS. Washington, D.C.: National Academy
       Press, 1981.

       Reports the results of a study which reviewed information
       about observable disparities in health care affecting minor-
       ities and handicapped persons. Discusses the extent to which
       race/ethnicity or handicaps affect whether and where people
       obtain health care and the quality of that care.

2452   Dobson, S. "Bringing Culture Into Care," NURS TIMES 79(6)
       (February 9, 1983): 53-57.

       Discusses why nurses should have a good understanding of
       how culture affects health status. Encourages sharing among
       nurses of cross-cultural nursing care studies. (10)

2453   Duncan, G.J., R.D. Coe, M.E. Corcoran, M.S. Hill, S.D. Hoffman
       and J.N. Morgan. YEARS OF POVERTY, YEARS OF PLENTY: THE
       CHANGING ECONOMIC FORTUNES OF AMERICAN WORKERS AND FAMILIES.
       Ann Arbor, MI.: Institute for Social Research, 1984.

The researchers have discovered that, contrary to popular
assumptions, the "poverty population" is constantly changing
over time. Several chapters explore the economic, social and
political implications of the findings about family composi-
tion changes and poverty.

2454   Dunham, A., J.A. Morone and W. White. "Restoring Medical
        Markets: Implications for the Poor," J POLITICS, POLICY
        AND LAW 7(2) (Summer 1982): 488-501.

Paper explores the implications of proposals to use health
maintenance organizations and vouchers to promote competition.
Authors conclude that, as they stand, pro-competitive proposals could cause a significant deterioration in the position
of the poor, especially if costs continue to rise, and that
their effects are likely to be exacerbated by problems with
implementation. (35)

2455   Folta, J. and E. Deck. A SOCIOLOGICAL FRAMEWORK FOR PATIENT
        CARE, 2nd Ed. New York: John Wiley and Sons, 1979.

Differentiates between "health care" and "medical care" and
defines "health care" as having an emphasis on quality as opposed to just duration of life. Discusses psychosocial concepts that assist nurses in the provision of quality health
care for all people, and includes information regarding health
and social class and ethnicity. Includes contributions from
forty authors.

2456   Gonzalez-Swafford, M.J. and M.G. Gutierrez. "Ethno-Medical
        Beliefs and Practices of Mexican-Americans," NURSE PRACT
        8(10) (November/December 1983): 29-30, 32, 34.

A summary of Mexican American health beliefs, practices, and
health care seeking behavior. (31)

2457   Grosso, C., M. Barden, C. Henry and M.G. Vieau. "Bridging
        Cultures. The Vietnamese American Family," MCN 6(3) (May/
        June 1981): 177-80.

Reports how a hospital made major adjustments to provide
patient centered care to a Vietnamese-American family. Discusses how expressed needs of a family can be accommodated by
application of principles of transcultural nursing. (2)

2458   Harwood, A. ETHNICITY AND MEDICAL CARE. Cambridge, MA.:
        Harvard University Press, 1981.

Provides a practical reference to basic sociocultural information pertinent to the provision of health services to
several major American ethnic groups.

2459   Henderson, G. and M. Primeaux. TRANSCULTURAL HEALTH CARE.
        Menlo Park, CA.: Addison-Wesley Publications Co., 1981.

Examines transcultural issues in health care by discussing
the sociocultural dimensions of health care as well as folk
medicine and patient care. Emphasizes that all health care
professionals need to be sensitized to the cultural aspects
of client care.

2460   Hicks, C. "Racism in Nursing," NURS TIMES 78(19) (May 12,
       1982): 789-91.

       Discusses the status of overseas nurses in Britain who were
       recruited from such areas as the Caribbean, Malaysia, and the
       Philippines, and how such nurses are subjects of racial
       chauvinism, condescension, fear and hostility. (1)

2461   Hodgson, C. "Transcultural Nursing: The Canadian Experience,"
       CAN NURSE 76(6) (June 1980): 23-25.

       Discusses the need for changes in nursing curricula to pre-
       pare nurses for transcultural health care. Provides examples
       of special knowledge needed to care for native Canadians.
       Provides a checklist for assessing one's "cultural awareness."
       (7)

2462   Horn, B. "Cultural Beliefs and Teenage Pregnancy," NURSE
       PRACT 8(8) (September 1983): 35, 38, 39, 74.

       The influence of cultural variables on teenage pregnancy is
       not clearly understood. In-depth interviews with 20 Native
       American Indians, 17 Black and 18 white teenage women in-
       dicated intercultural differences in beliefs about: (1) pre-
       vention of pregnancy, (2) significance of becoming a mother at
       an early age, and (3) kinds of support systems available to
       them within their social network. (21)

2463   Jones, E.E. and S.J. Korchin. MINORITY MENTAL HEALTH. New
       York: Praeger, 1982.

       Overviews concepts of ethnic psychology that are applicable
       to all minority groups and also discusses particular issues
       in each of several minority groups. Examines issues of inter-
       vention with minority populations.

2464   Kane, R.L., J.M. Kasteler and R.M. Gray (Eds.). THE HEALTH
       GAP: MEDICAL SERVICES AND THE POOR. New York: Springer
       Publishing Co., 1976.

       Ten articles focus on the barriers to health services and
       other poverty related problems. Comprehensive annotated bib-
       liography.

2465   Leininger, M.M. REFERENCE SOURCES FOR TRANSCULTURAL HEALTH
       AND NURSING (FOR TEACHING, CURRICULUM RESEARCH, AND CLIN-
       ICAL-FIELD PRACTICE). Thorofare, NJ.: Slack, Inc., 1984.

Bibliography of health-related cultural sources from transcultural nursing, anthropology, and other fields contributing
to cross-cultural health care. Includes specific references
on cultural illnesses, rituals, symbols, and other social and
cultural factors which influence health.

2466 Leininger, M. TRANSCULTURAL NURSING: CONCEPTS, THEORIES, AND
PRACTICES. New York: John Wiley and Sons, 1978.

Provides comprehensive and scholarly information about the
new subfield of transcultural nursing. Intended to help
nurses incorporate cultural concepts, theories, and research
findings into nursing care.

2467 Link, C.R., S.H. Long and R.F. Settle. "Access to Medical
Care Under Medicaid: Differentials by Race," J HEALTH,
POLITICS, POLICY AND LAW. 7(2) (Summer 1982): 345-65.

The Medicaid Program was designed to help correct for the
unequal access to medical care by income and race in pre-1965
America. Previous evaluations of the program have claimed
that on average the eligible poor have enjoyed considerable
gains in access, but that the benefits of Medicaid have not
been shared equally by Blacks and whites, however, between
1969 and 1976 all race, region, and health status groups of
nonelderly Medicaid recipients experienced increases in physician visits that far outpaced those of the entire nonelderly
U.S. population. By 1976 Blacks clearly achieved equality
with whites in Medicaid ambulatory care use. (23)

2468 Loss, L. "How Do You Cope With the Patient Who is Different?"
J PRACT NURO 28(7) (July 1978): 30-33.

Emphasizes the importance of being non-judgmental with all
patients, but especially with those who are in some way "different," e.g. physically or emotionally handicapped, homosexual, or addicted to drugs. (0)

2469 Luft, H.S. POVERTY AND HEALTH: ECONOMIC CAUSES AND CONSEQUEN-
CES OF HEALTH PROBLEMS. Cambridge, MA.: Ballinger Publishing Co., 1978.

Explores the interrelationship between poverty and health
problems. Discusses socioeconomic factors as a cause of poor
health as well as disability and social welfare. Suggests a
design of economic incentives to deal with health problems.

2470 Manuel, R.C. and M.L. Berk. "A Look at Similarities and Differences in Older Minority Populations," AGING (May/June
1983): 21-29.

This study argues that important sub-cultural differences
exist within the minority elderly population. Data are pre-

sented comparing the differences and similarities between
various components of the elderly minority population. The
study uses several data sources, to show differences in health
status access to care and expenditures for service by ethnic
status.

2471   Martinez, R.A. HISPANIC CULTURE AND HEALTH CARE: FACT, FIC-
       TION, FOLKLORE. St. Louis: C.V. Mosby, 1978.

       Provides a collection of readings about Hispanic health
       care beliefs and practices. Includes an overview of Hispanic
       cultural attitudes, focusing on the Mexican-American family,
       and explores the significance of societal influence on the
       health attitudes of Hispanics. Discusses Hispanic reactions
       to nurses, hospitalization, and the health care system.

2472   McKenna, M. "The Cultural Connection: Including Cultural
       Variations in Quality Nursing Care," WASH NURSE 12(3) (June
       1982): 4-7.

       Discusses concepts of illness, disease, and illness behavior
       and how a patient´s behavior is influenced by his/her culture
       and upbringing. Presents questions that a nurse may ask to
       elicit culturally specific beliefs. Considers the implica-
       tions for nursing of the incidence of selected diseases among
       ethnic groups. (27)

2473   Metress, J.F. MEXICAN-AMERICAN HEALTH: A GUIDE TO THE LITERA-
       TURE. Monticello, IL.: Council of Planning Librarians,
       1976.

       Provides 360 citations to books and journal articles which
       encourage health professionals to gain an understanding of
       the history, customs, and variations in the sociocultural
       patterns of Mexican-American culture.

2474   Mindel, C.H. and R.W. Haberstein. ETHNIC FAMILIES IN AMERICA:
       PATTERNS AND VARIATIONS. New York: Elsevier North Holland,
       1981.

       Provides information about patterned differences among
       ethnic groups found in the United States. Discusses the
       values, attitudes, lifestyles, customs, and rituals of indi-
       viduals who identify with specific ethnic groups.

2475   Morgan, J.N. and G.J. Duncan. FIVE THOUSAND AMERICAN
       FAMILIES--PATTERNS OF ECONOMIC PROGRESS, VOL. X: ANALYSES
       OF THE FIRST THIRTEEN YEARS OF THE PANEL STUDY OF INCOME
       DYNAMICS. Ann Arbor, MI.: Institute for Social Research,
       University of Michigan, 1983.

       The Institute for Social Research has done a major longitu-
       dinal panel study of 5,000 families to determine causes of

poverty and well being. Volume 1 covered the years 1968-1972. Yearly updates have followed, each focusing on different factors or taking a different approach. The 1983 volume includes interview data over a span of fifteen years.

2476   Orque, M.S., B. Bloch and L.S. Ahumada Monrroy. ETHNIC NURS-
       ING CARE: A MULTICULTURAL APPROACH. St. Louis: C.V. Mosby,
       1983.

       Authors and five contributors focus on the health care of
       people from selected ethnic origins: Filipino, Chinese, Japa-
       nese, and Spanish Americans, Blacks, South Vietnamese and
       American Indians. The history of each ethnic group, the cul-
       tural background, health and illness concepts, special nutri-
       tional factors, and unique needs are presented for each group.

2477   Richardson, L. "Breakthrough to Nursing: Caring Through
       Understanding, Part I," IMPRINT 29(1) (February 1982): 13,
       67, /1.

       Reports that the National Student Nurses' Association spon-
       sors a project to help nursing students become prepared to
       provide holistic nursing care to people of all cultural and
       ethnic backgrounds. Discusses transcultural nursing. (0)

2478   _____. "Breakthrough to Nursing: Caring Through Under-
       standing, Part II," IMPRINT 29(2) (April 1982): 21, 72-77.

       Discusses nursing care of ethnic populations and focuses on
       folk medicine in the Hispanic population. (10)

2479   Rudov, M.H. HEALTH STATUS OF MINORITIES AND LOW-INCOME GROUPS.
       Washington, D.C.: U.S. Department of Health, Education and
       Welfare, Pub. No. (HRA) 79-627, 1979.

       Examines health status of the disadvantaged from the follow-
       ing perspectives: (1) reproductive and genetic health, (2)
       acute disease conditions, (3) chronic disease conditions,
       (4) preventive health, and (5) utilization of health services.

2480   Ruffen, J.E. CHANGING PERSPECTIVES ON ETHNICITY AND HEALTH.
       Kansas City, MO.: American Nurses' Association, Pub. No.
       M-27, 1979, pp. 1-45.

       Describes changing perspectives on ethnicity and health care
       with a particular focus on the sociopolitical climate in-
       fluencing these perspectives. Offers recommendations for the
       improved delivery of health care to minority groups. (172)

2481   Smith, W.D. MINORITY ISSUES IN MENTAL HEALTH. Reading, MA.:
       Addison-Wesley, 1978.

Examines some of the major issues affecting the mental
health of minority groups in the United States. Emphasizes
that the health of minority groups must be examined in the
context of social, economic, education, and environmental
conditions.

2482   Snowden, L.R. REACHING THE UNDERSERVED: MENTAL HEALTH NEEDS
        OF NEGLECTED POPULATIONS. Beverly Hills, CA.: Sage Publi-
        cations, 1982.

        Illuminates concerns associated with the present inequit-
        able distribution of mental health services in the United
        States. Authors define the populations that are underserved,
        assess the specific service delivery problems facing them,
        and examine a wide variety of possible solutions.

2483   Spector, E. CULTURAL DIVERSITY IN HEALTH AND ILLNESS. New
        York: Appleton-Century-Crofts, 1979.

        Conceptual framework for considering cultural concepts pre-
        sented and specific customs, health beliefs, and folk remedies
        of the major ethnic groups are presented. Barriers to ade-
        quate health care for the poor and members of ethnic minority
        groups are also discussed.

2484   Tripp-Reimer, T., P.J. Brink and J.M. Saunders. "Cultural
        Assessment: Content and Process," NURS OUTLOOK 32(2)
        (March/April 1984): 78-82.

        Discusses how cultural assessment helps nurses meet their
        patients' needs, and provides examples of several assessment
        tools. Includes a table which compares the scope of nine cul-
        tural assessment guides. (15)

2485   Viers-Henderson, V. "The Nurse and Minority Health Problems
        in the United States," IMPRINT 30(2) (April/May 1983): 60--
        65.

        Observes that nurses of the future have an important role to
        play in improving health status of individuals of many socio-
        cultural origins. Discusses genetic, environmental and multi-
        factoral causes of illness for several ethnic groups. (9)

2486   Wilensky, G.R. and M.L. Berk. "Health Care, The Poor and The
        Role of Medicaid," HEALTH AFFAIRS (Fall 1982): 93-100.

        This study examines the thirty-five million poor and the
        near poor persons in 1977, their insurance coverage, health
        status, and their use of medical services. About 5 million
        poor and near poor persons had no insurance whatever through-
        out the year. When health status is used as a control, the
        uninsured poor use far fewer medical services than do the poor
        who have Medicaid coverage. There were also large differences
        in out-of-pocket costs with the Medicaid population incurring
        lower expenses than those who lacked any health insurance in
        1977.

See 1087, 1097, 1136, 1137, 1150, 1154, 1162, 1267, 1305, 2168, 2287.

Health Care for Gay or Lesbian Clients; Homosexuality

2487   American Medical Association, Council on Scientific Affairs. "Health Care Needs of a Homosexual Population," J AM MED ASSOC 248(6) (1982): 736-39.

Provides an overview of the physical and mental health care needs of gay men and lesbians. Includes a discussion of various definitions and theories of the origins of homosexuality. (8)

2488   Bachman, R. "Homosexuality: The Cost of Being Different," CAN NURSE 77(2) (February 1981): 20-23.

Notes that nurses come into contact with gay people in all areas of practice, and provides suggestions for dealing with homosexual patients. Suggests that each nurse explore his/her feelings about sexuality and provides a reading list of books about homosexuality. (11)

2489   Bath, R. and J. Skelchley. "Homosexuality: Treating Patients in General Practice," BRITISH MEDICAL J 283(6295) (September 26, 1981): 827-29.

Encourages health professionals to become better prepared to deal with homosexuality and discusses social support for homosexuals as it exists in Great Britain. (6)

2490   Brossart, J. "The Gay Patient: What You Should Be Doing," RN 42(4) (April 1979): 50-52.

Provides suggestions for changing staff behavior and attitudes towards homosexual patients and emphasizes that the nurse has a responsibility to create an atmosphere in which the homosexual patient is comfortable. (0)

2491   Bullough, V.L. "Homosexuality and the Medical Model," J HOMOSEXUALITY 1 (1974): 99-110. Reprinted in EXPANDING HORIZONS FOR NURSES. Edited by B. Bullough and V. Bullough. New York: Springer Publishing Co., 1977, pp. 91-101.

A brief history of how homosexuality came to be labeled an illness by the medical community and the implications of this kind of labeling. (23)

2492   Caulkins, S. "The Male Homosexual Client," ISSUES HEALTH CARE WOMEN 3(5-6) (September-December 1981): 321-40.

Suggests that nurses need to learn how to deal with their feelings about caring for homosexual patients. Presents an overview of the homosexual person which includes psychodevelopment, psychodynamics, family relationships, and health care. (39)

2493   Dardick, L. and K.E. Grady. "Openness Between Gay Persons and
       Health Professionals," ANNALS OF INTERNAL MEDICINE 93(1)
       (July 1980): 115-19.

       Reports the results of a study which was undertaken to as-
       certain what factors contribute toward being open with health
       professionals about one's sexual orientation and how this
       openness affects quality of care. (16)

2494   Fenwick, R.D. THE ADVOCATE GUIDE TO GAY HEALTH. Boston:
       Alyson Publications, 1982.

       Provides information about gay health for the layperson and
       health professional.

2495   Galloway, B. (Ed.). PREJUDICE AND PRIDE: DISCRIMINATION
       AGAINST GAY PEOPLE IN MODERN BRITAIN. Boston, MA.: Routledge
       & Kegan Paul, 1984.

       A report on the systematic, legal and social discrimination
       against gays in modern society.

2496   Irish, A.C. "Straight Talk About Gay Patients," AM J NURS
       83(8) (August 1981): 1168-70.

       Encourages health professionals to be accepting of a homo-
       sexual lifestyle and to not make conformity necessary for
       empathy. (6)

2497   Lawrence, J.C. "Homosexuals Hospitalization and the Nurse,"
       NURS FORUM 14(30 (1975): 305-17.

              Homosexuals and their entitlement to quality nursing
       care is discussed. Homosexual lifestyle, treatment of the
       homosexual in the general hospital, mental health care, and
       alternative treatments addressed. (10)

2498   Maurer, T. "Health Care and The Gay Community," NURS DIMEN-
       SION (Spring 1979): 83-85.

       Examines several areas of concern regarding the health prob-
       lems of gay people. Emphasizes a need for health profes-
       sionals to alter their attitudes toward homosexuality. (0)

2499   O'Donnell, M., V. Loeffler, K. Pollock and Z. Saunders.
       LESBIAN HEALTH MATTERS. Santa Cruz, CA.: Women's Health
       Collective, 1979.

       Consolidates information specific to lesbian health and
       identifies areas of health concerns that need further re-
       search. Discusses problems encountered by lesbians when
       dealing with the traditional U.S. health care system.

2500   O'Donnell, M. "Lesbian Health Care: Issues and Literature,"
       SCIENCE FOR THE PEOPLE (May/June 1978): 8-19.

Examines how the heterosexual bias and nuclear-family orientation of the present United States health care system affects lesbians. Encourages health professionals to educate themselves on the validity of lesbianism as a lifestyle. (42)

2501 Paul, W. and J.D. Weinrich (Co-Eds.), J.C. Gonsiorek and M.E. Hotvedt (Assoc. Eds.). HOMOSEXUALITY: SOCIAL, PSYCHOLOGICAL, AND BIOLOGICAL ISSUES. Beverly Hills, CA.: Sage Publications, Inc., 1982.

Prepared by a task force of the Society for the Psychological Study of Social Issues.

2502 Pogoncheff, E. "The Gay Patient: What Not To Do," RN 42(4) (April 1979): 46-50.

Discusses gay rights in the hospital and gives several examples of wrong behavior for nurses who deal with homosexual patients. (0)

2503 White, T.A. "Attitudes of Psychiatric Nurses Toward Same Sex Orientations," NURS RES 28(5)(1979): 276-81.

Attitudes of psychiatric nurses toward lesbianism as studied in a descriptive study. It showed a relationship between negative attitudes and different demographic variables such as religion and education. (18)

Standards of Care, Quality Assurance, Peer Review

2504 Ainsworth, T.H., Jr. QUALITY ASSURANCE IN LONG TERM CARE. Gaithersburg, MD.: Aspen Systems Corp., 1977.

Part I analyzes and explains the two parts of the Quality Assurance Program...current regulations for control mechanisms...accountability for the aged...and development of quality assurance methodologies. Part II is a self-instructional manual for implementation of a quality assurance pro= gram..complete with forms and instructions.

2505 Allbritten, D., B. Boland, P. Hubert and B. Kiernan. "Peer Review: A Practical Guide," PED NURS 8(1) (January/February 1982): 31-32.

Peer review can counter the isolation of everyday practice. The authors describe a peer review process that is adaptable to many practice settings. (5)

2506 American Nurses' Association. STANDARDS OF NURSING PRACTICE. Kansas City, MO.: American Nurses' Association, Pub. No. NP-41, 1973.

The ANA Congress for Nursing Practice defines basic standards for all types of practices in order to fulfill nursing's professional obligation to provide and improve nursing care.

2507   _____   A PLAN FOR IMPLEMENTATION OF THE STANDARDS OF
        NURSING PRACTICE. Kansas City, MO.: American Nurses' Asso-
        ciation, Pub. No. NP-51, 1975.

        The ANA Congress for Nursing Practice focuses on the ANA
        Model for Quality Assurance as a means of implementing the
        Standards of Nursing Practice.

2508   _____   GUIDELINES FOR REVIEW OF NURSING CARE AT THE LOCAL
        LEVEL. Kansas City, MO.: American Nurses' Association, Pub.
        No. NP-54, 1976.

        An aid for developing an evaluation system for quality of
        care, with emphasis on Professional Standards Review Organi-
        zations and procedures for developing and validating outcome
        criteria for the review of nursing care.

2509   _____. QUALITY ASSURANCE WORKBOOK. Kansas City, MO.:
        American Nurses' Association, Pub. No. NP-55, 1976.

        Includes workshop objectives, organizations and content,
        and a graphic presentation of the ANA Model for Quality As-
        surance. Includes selected bibliography.

2510   _____. STANDARDS FOR ORGANIZED NURSING SERVICES. Kansas
        City, MO.: American Nurses' Association, Pub. No. NS-1,
        1982.

        Standards developed by the ANA Commission on Nursing Ser-
        vices for departments or divisions of nursing in institutional
        settings, with specific criteria for evaluation.

2511   _____. PEER REVIEW IN NURSING PRACTICE. Kansas City, MO.:
        American Nurses' Association, Pub. No. NP-67, 1983.

        Covers social and historical contexts, guidelines, and prin-
        ciples of peer review, an essential element in nursing quality
        assurance.

2512   _____. NURSING QUALITY ASSURANCE MANAGEMENT/LEARNING
        SYSTEM. Kansas City, MO.: American Nurses' Association,
        1984.

        System jointly developed and published by ANA and Suther-
        land Learning Associates, Inc., provides printed materials
        and visual aids, effective, in-house, self-learning com-
        ponents; Useful in meeting requirements of external review
        agencies, in preparation of undergraduate and graduate nursing
        students for QA participation, and in management of Quality
        Assurance Programs in hospitals, long-term care settings, and
        community health agencies.

2513   Carter, J.H., M. Hilliard, M.R. Castles, L.D. Stoll and A.
        Cowan. STANDARDS OF NURSING CARE: A GUIDE FOR EVALUATION,
        2nd Ed. New York: Springer Publishing Co., 1976.

Text prepared by the nursing service department at St. Louis
University Hospital.

2514   Mullins, A.C., R.E. Colavecchio and B.E. Tescher. "Peer Re-
view: A Model for Professional Accountability," J NURS ADM
9(12) (1979): 25-30. Reprinted in NURSING ISSUES AND NURS-
ING STRATEGIES FOR THE EIGHTIES. Edited by B. Bullough,
V. Bullough and M.C. Soukup. New York: Springer Publishing
Co., 1983, pp. 115-130.

Describes the experience in a large university hospital in
implementing peer review for the classification, promotion
and ongoing evaluation of professional nurses. (5)

2515   Pena, J.J., A.N. Haffner, B. Rosen and D.W. Light (Eds.).
HOSPITAL QUALITY ASSURANCE, RISK MANAGEMENT, AND PROGRAM
EVALUATION. Gaithersburg, MD.: Aspen Systems Corp., 1984.

Provides information for improving efficiency and effectiveness of quality assurance programs while limiting risks to
patients and employees.

2516   Phanaeuf, M.C. THE NURSING AUDIT: SELF-REGULATION IN NURSING
PRACTICE, 2nd Ed. New York: Appleton-Century-Crofts, 1976.

A guide for nursing administrators and staff who wish to use
nursing audit as one method of quality control in hospitals
and other settings in which nursing is a basic service. It
asserts nursing responsibility and authority for nursing
measurement and control of the quality of nursing care as a
moral obligation.

2517   Sheridean, J.E., T.J. Fairchild and M. Kaas. "Assessing the
Job Performance of Nursing Home Staff," NURS RES 32(2)
(April 1983): 102-7.

Behavioral Anchored Rating Scales (BARS) were used to
measure job performance of nursing employees at four nursing
homes. BARS evaluation had convergent reliability with two
independent evaluations of same employees. There was a "halo"
effect in evaluation, resulting in little discriminant reliability between employees performance rating on different job
dimensions. BARS evaluation tended to cluster in upper half
of scale ranges. (25)

2518   Wandelt, M.A. and J.W. Ager. QUALITY PATIENT CARE SCALE. New
York: Appleton-Century-Crofts, 1974.

Grew out of the Slater Nursing Performance Rating Scale.
Included is the sixty-eight item Qualpacs, cue sheet, guidelines for using the scale, experiences of others in using the
scale, and development of Qualpacs (Quality Patient Care
Scale) along with result of testing.

Prospective Payment, Diagnostic Related Groups

2519   American Academy of Nursing. NURSING RESEARCH AND POLICY
       FORMATION: THE CASE OF PROSPECTIVE PAYMENT. Kansas City,
       MO.: American Nurses´ Association, Pub. No. G-164, 1984.

       A collection of eight papers examining the knowledge base
       underlying the central issue. Addresses philosophy and prag-
       matics, policy status and future projections, current models,
       nursing administration and clinical nursing, and quality of
       care.

2520   Caterinicchio, R.P. (Ed.). DRGs - WHAT THEY ARE AND HOW TO
       SURVIVE THEM - A SOURCEBOOK FOR PROFESSIONAL NURSING.
       Thorofare, NJ.: Slack, Inc., 1984.

       Discusses the impact being made by the DRG Prospective Hos-
       pital Pricing and Payment System on health care personnel.
       The transition to this new method of payment is opening a
       new era in cost-cutting incentives, and is challenging all
       health professionals to work with greater efficiency and cost
       effectiveness in the face of looming cutbacks.

2521   Curtin, L. and C. Zurlage (Eds.). DRGs: THE REORGANIZATION
       OF HEALTH. Chicago, IL.: Nursing Management Books, 1984.

       Forty health care professional contributors explain the cur-
       rent Federal regulations on prospective payment. Details of
       implementation as they relate to hospitals, community based
       care, and hospices are covered.

2522   Davis, C.K. "The Federal Role in Changing Health Care Finan-
       cing, Part II," NURS ECON (September/October 1983): 98-104,
       146.

       Part II in a series. Discusses prospective payment for
       Medicare, suggests consequences for nursing, and offers recom-
       mendations related to nursing service, research and education.
       (6)

2523   "Hospitals Must Cost Out Nursing Care Under Landmark Maine
       Law," AM J NURS (September 19830: 1251,1262.

       News item. Maine DRG rules include a requirement for an an-
       nual report of nursing service costs. This move praised by
       the journal because it will cost out nursing care. (0)

2524   Jones, K.R. "Severity of Illness Measures: Issues and Op-
       tions," NURS ECON 2(5) (September/October 1984): 312-17.

       The DRG-based prospective payment system (PPS) has been
       criticized for not adequately accounting for severity of ill-
       ness variations among patients. This could place certain
       types of hospitals at greater financial risk than others.
       There are several severity of illness measurement techniques
       that could be considered for PPS. (28)

2525   May, J.J. and J. Wasserman. "Selected Results from an Evalua-
       tion of the New Jersey Diagnosis-Related Group System,"
       HEALTH SERVICES RESEARCH 19(5) (December 1984): 547-59.

       The New Jersey Diagnosis Related Group (DRG) system is des-
       cribed and compared with the Medicare prospective payment
       system. Both systems are analyzed. (7)

2526   "Multi-Unit Systems, Getting Set for DRGs, See Staff Cuts
       Likely," AM J NURS 84(4) (April 1984): 529, 540, 542, 546.

       Discusses how multi unit providers are preparing for reim-
       bursement at a fixed rate based on a patient's diagnosis-re-
       lated grouping and how such reimbursement practices will af-
       fect nurse staffing. (0)

2527   Plomann, M.P. and F.A. Shaffer. "DRGs As One of Nine Ap-
       proaches to Case Mix in Transition," NURS HEALTH CARE 4
       (October 19830: 438-43.

       The 1983 Social Security Act established new payment limita-
       tions to hospitals. At the present time the payments are
       tied to DRGs (Diagnostic Related Groups). The authors dis-
       cuss other ways of setting up the payment mechanism. (4)

2528   Rosko, M.D. "The Impact of Prospective Payment: A Multi-
       Dimensional Analysis of New Jersey's SHARE Program," J
       HEALTH POLITICS, POLICY, LAW 9(1) (Spring 1984): 81-101.

       The SHARE Program, which set per diem prospective rates
       for New Jersey hospitals during the period 1975-1982 is evalu-
       ated. Analysis suggests that this program did contain hos-
       pital cost increases. However, the program threatened the
       viability of most inner-city hospitals. Indirect evidence
       suggests that there was cost-shifting in response to this
       program, which regulated payment for only Blue Cross and
       Medicaid patients. Structural features of this program and
       its successor, the New Jersey DRG Program, are analyzed; and
       implications for the Medicare prospective payment system are
       examined.

2529   Sanford, S. "President's Message: Prospective Payment: Get
       Out Your Baseball Mitt," HEART AND LUNG: THE JOURNAL OF
       CRITICAL CARE 13(5) (September 1984): 24a, 26a, 27a.

       The current changes in medicare reimbursement unfreeze the
       status quo and give nurses a chance to identify and be accoun-
       table for the care they give. (0)

2530   Shaffer, F.A. "A Nursing Perspective of the DRG World, Part
       1," NURS HEALTH CARE 5(1) (January 1984): 48-51.

       The new prospective payment plans using diagnostic related
       categories are explained and nursing implications are discus-
       sed. (2)

2531   Shaffer, F.A. (Ed.). DRGs: CHANGES AND CHALLENGES. New York:
       National League for Nursing, 1984.

       Contributors analyze the prospective payment legislation ac-
       cording to diagnostic related groups (DRGs) from a nursing
       point of view. Includes a ten part series published in NURS-
       ING AND HEALTH CARE plus other material.

2532   Short, T.L. and R.M. Coffey. "Diagnosis Related Groups vs.
       Disease Staging: Implications for Hospital Reimbursement,"
       U.S. Department of Health and Human Services, National Cen-
       ter for Health Services Research, November, 1984.

       Under the Federal Government's new Medicare prospective
       payment system a hospital is reimbursed a fixed price for each
       discharge depending on the disease category of the patient.
       The current method of disease classification used by the
       Medicare system is Diagnosis Related Groups (DRGs), which has
       been criticized for not distinguishing severity of illness
       differences adequately among patients within the same diag-
       nosis group. An alternative classification system is Disease
       Staging which was developed to assign a disease category and
       stage of severity to each patient.
       Results of this study suggest that the issue is balance of
       compensation. Reliance on medical classification alone might
       result in unacceptable reductions in reimbursement to teaching
       or large, surgically intensive institutions. Ideally, a sys-
       tem which captures medical diagnosis and severity of illness
       distinctions and at the same time allows payments by specific
       medically appropriate procedures would serve both to capture
       case-mix differences and to insure that appropriate treatments
       will be undertaken.

2533   Vanderzee, H. and G. Glusko. "DRGs, Variable Pricing, and
       Budgeting for Nursing Services," J NURS ADM 14(5) (May
       1984): 11-14.

       The traditional method of routine charges for nursing ser-
       vices is compared with a variable charge structure based on
       patient classification. (0)

2534   Willian, M.K. "DRGs--A Primer," NURS ECON 1(2) (September/
       October 1983): 135-37.

       Good basic explanation of the history and current status of
       DRGs (diagnosis related groups).(4)

2535   Young, D.A. "Prospective Payment Assessment Commission:
       Mandate, Structure, and Relationships," NURS ECON 2(5)
       (September/October 1984): 309-311.

       The Prospective Payment Assessment Commission was estab-
       lished in 1983 to make recommendations to Congress and the

garding updating and maintaining the new Medicare payment
system. The commission's legislative mandate requires, among
other things, evaluation of nursing resources. (2)

Consumerism, Self-Help, Self-Care

2536   Clark, C.C. ENHANCING WELLNESS. New York: Springer Publish-
       ing Co., 1983.

       A popular guide to physical and emotional health.

2537   Claus, K.E. LIVING WITH STRESS AND PROMOTING WELL-BEING.
       St. Louis: C.V. Mosby Co., 1980.

       Handbook on job-related stress. Discusses the "burnout
       syndrome" with the intensive care unit serving as the focus,
       presents fifteen independent Stress-Reduction Training Modules
       for Nurses, and provides practical strategies nurses can use
       to handle stress and provide better patient care.

2538   Corea, G. THE HIDDEN MALPRACTICE: HOW AMERICAN MEDICINE MIS-
       TREATS WOMEN AS PATIENTS AND AS PROFESSIONALS. New York:
       Harcourt Brace Jovanovich, 1977.

       Discusses how women have been barred from healing and how
       the male domination of medicine affects the health care of
       women. Comments on the impact of the women's health movement
       and notes that women must join together to regain control of
       their bodies.

2539   Cousins, N. THE HEALING HEART: ANTIDOTES TO PANIC AND HELP-
       LESSNESS. New York: W.W. Norton and Co., 1983.

       A book of comments on the health care delivery system oc-
       casioned by the author's heart attack. Cousins points out
       the importance of good doctor/patient relationships and argues
       that the patient's own strengths should be used in the healing
       process.

2540   Gartner, A. and F. Riessman (Eds.). THE SELF-HELP REVOLUTION.
       New York: Human Sciences Press, Inc., 1984.

       The rapidly growing self-help movement is described.
       Organized self-help groups are an important focus of the work.

2541   Hamilton, P.A. HEALTH CARE CONSUMERISM. St. Louis: C.V.
       Mosby Co., 1981.

       Health care issues as seen through the eyes of the consumer.
       Points out ways in which professionals can support and educate
       consumers so that they can participate more fully in main-
       taining and restoring maximum health at reasonable cost.

2542   Haug, M. and B. Lavin. CONSUMERISM IN MEDICINE: CHALLENGING
       PHYSICIAN AUTHORITY. Beverly Hills, CA.: Sage Publications,
       Inc., 1983.

Consumerism is increasing. Using a national survey of
medical consumerism the authors explore the manifestations of
this movement and its implication for health policy.

2543   Hill, L.L. and N.L. Smith. SELF-CARE NURSING.   Englewood
       Cliffs, NJ.: Prentice-Hall, 1985.

       Designed for health care professionals interested in learn-
       ing about self-care (wellness, holistic) theory, process, and
       application. Focuses very strongly on the application of the
       self-care process, as well as on modeling and the specific
       role of the nurse as a model of self care. Utilizes self-con-
       tracting as a mechanism for facilitating behavior change.

2544   Knowles, R.D.   A GUIDE TO SELF-MANAGEMENT STRATEGIES FOR
       NURSES. New York: Springer Publishing Co., 1984.

       Self-management involves exercising control over the way
       one thinks, feels, and behaves. Book shows how health profes-
       sionals can realize self-management on their own.

2545   National League for Nursing. CONSUMERISM AND HEALTH CARE.
       New York: National League for Nursing, Pub. No. 52-1727,
       1978.

       Considers the history of the consumer's voice in health
       care, comparing various bills of patients' rights and con-
       sidering pertinent legislation; the responsibility of the
       nurse to offer themselves as patient advocates and what
       advocacy entails; and the impersonal qualities of hospitaliza-
       tion.

2546   Pender, N.J. HEALTH PROMOTION IN NURSING PRACTICE. Norwalk,
       CT.: Appleton-Century-Crofts, 1982.

       Provides nurses with a conceptual framework for under-
       standing the many factors that affect the health behavior of
       individuals and families; and presents specific nursing
       strategies for providing prevention and health promotion ser-
       vices to clients.

2547   Romalis, S. (Ed.). CHILDBIRTH: ALTERNATIVES TO MEDICAL CON-
       TROL. Austin: University of Texas Press, 1981.

       A series of essays on childbirth. It is a political collec-
       tion in which all the contributors share an ideology, ex-
       plicitly or implicitly.

2548   Saucier, C.P. "Self Concept and Self-Care Management in
       School-Age Children With Diabetes," PED NURS 10(2) (March/
       April 1984): 135-38.

       Children's self concepts and self-care abilities are often
       presumed to be directly related. However, in this study of
       school-age children with diabetes, self-care management could

not be predicted by any single factor but instead was related
to the interaction of the child's age, self concept and participation in outside activities. (17)

2549   Scully, D.H.   MEN WHO CONTROL WOMEN'S HEALTH: THE MISEDUCA-
       TION OF OBSTETRICIAN-GYNECOLOGISTS.   Boston: Houghton Mif-
       flin, 1980.

       Report of a study of obstetrical-gynecological surgical
       residency training. Participant observer methodology used.
       Concludes that a significant number of operations are unneeded.
       Suggests reforms including changes in the payment mechanisms
       for physicians, stepped up use of nurse midwives, and a more
       well informed public.

2550   Shamansky, S.L., M.C. Cecere and E. Shellenberger (Eds.).
       PRIMARY HEALTH CARE HANDBOOK: GUIDELINES FOR PATIENT EDUCA-
       TION. Boston: Little, Brown and Co., 1984.

       Based on the belief that clients are the managers of their
       health, this handbook presents meaningful ways to promote
       health and encourage people to assume responsibility for their
       health.

2551   Smythe, E.E.M.   SURVIVING NURSING.   Menlo Park, CA.: Addison-
       Wesley Publishing Co., 1984.

       Specific coping strategies and practical stress reduction
       techniques; exercises, activities, and self-assessment tools;
       and problem-solving processes. Explains the principles and
       theories behind specific coping techniques and includes cur-
       rent supporting research, annotated bibliography, and resource
       section.

2552   Steiger, N.   SELF-CARE NURSING: THEORY AND PRACTICE.   Engle-
       wood Cliffs, NJ.: Prentice-Hall (Brady), 1985.

       Focuses on historical, philosophical and theoretical aspects
       of self-care. The importance of self-care in the clinical
       context; the components of health with specific assessment
       tools and substantive content to increase the individual's
       self-care ability; and the potential impact of self-care on
       nursing service, nursing education, and nursing research.

2553   Weiss, K. (Ed.).   WOMEN'S HEALTH CARE; A GUIDE TO ALTERNA-
       TIVES. Englewood Cliffs, NJ.: Reston Publishing Co. (Pren-
       tice-Hall, Inc.), 1983.

       A unique presentation of self-care techniques and alterna-
       tive medicine in areas of women's health care.

Environmental Issues

2554   Annas, G.J.   "The Case of Karen Silkwood," AM J PUBLIC HEALTH
       74(5) (May 1984): 516-18.

Presents a summary of the controversial Karen Silkwood case.
Silkwood was an employee of a plant fabricating plutonium fuel
pins and in November, 1974 she was contaminated with plutonium.
The result was a series of controversies which continued even
after her death which resulted from an auto accident which
her supporters say was caused by company officials, and which
both a movie and a book left unclear. This article summarizes
the information about her case. (6)

2555   Eisenbud, M. ENVIRONMENT, TECHNOLOGY AND HEALTH: HEALTH
       ECOLOGY IN HISTORICAL PERSPECTIVE. New York: N.Y.U. Press,
       1978.

       An examination of the contemporary environmental movement
       insofar as public health is concerned.

2556   Epstein, S.S., L.O. Brown and C. Pope. HAZARDOUS WASTE IN
       AMERICA. San Francisco: Sierra Books, 1982.

       Presents statistics related to overall problem, case studies
       of specific areas, and discusses laws and regulations now in
       effect. Argues problem is a major one for society.

2557   Levine, A.D. LOVE CANAL: SCIENCE, POLITICS, AND PEOPLE.
       Lexington, MA.: Lexington Books, D.C. Heath and Co., 1982.

       A classic sociologic case study that chronicles the strug-
       gle of citizens living in the Love Canal area of Niagara Falls
       with corporate bureaucracies. It follows their effort to at-
       tain resources necessary to move from homes poisoned by
       chemical waste.

       See 822.

Supply, Staffing, Manpower, Marketing Nursing Services

2558   "A.H.A. Nursing Manpower Study of Factors in Nursing Supply
       and Demand," AARN NEWSLETTER 37(3) (March 1981): 8-11.

       Documents the nature and extent of the current nursing shor-
       tage in Canada, identifies causes of the shortage, and recom-
       mends ways of dealing with the issue. (0)

2559   Aiken, L.H., R.J. Blendon, and D.E. Rogers. "The Shortage of
       Hospital Nurses: A New Perspective," AM J NURS 81(9) (Sep-
       tember 1981): 1612-18. Published simultaneously in THE AN-
       NALS OF INTERNAL MEDICINE 95(3) (September 1981): 365-75.
       Reprinted in NURSING ISSUES AND NURSING STRATEGIES FOR THE
       EIGHTIES. Edited by B. Bullough, V. Bullough and M.C.
       Soukup. New York: Springer Publishing Co., 1983.

       Analyzes data related to the shortage of nurses. Points out
       that supply of nurses has increased significantly since 1970.
       At the same time the intensity of nursing care has also in-

creased and hospital beds have decreased. Analyzes the relationship of wages to shortage. Proposes increasing nurses
wages to halt the substitution of nurses for other health
workers. Discusses deterrents to this proposal. (38)

2560 Aiken, L.N. "The Nurse Labor Market," HEALTH AFFAIRS 1(4)
      (Fall 1982): 31-40.

      Reports that the national shortage of nurses has subsided
      considerably, and that current shortages appear to be concen-
      trated primarily in large urban public hospitals. Provides a
      chart which illustrates the relation between nurses' relative
      incomes and hospital vacancy rates from 1960 to 1981. (18)

2561 Aiken, L. "Nursing's Future: Public Policies, Private
      Actions," AM J NURS 83 (October 1983): 1440-44.

      Reports major findings of the Institute of Medicine study of
      nursing economics, including the fact that there is no longer
      an overall shortage of nurses although there are geographic
      shortages and too few nurses with appropriate graduate pre-
      paration. Suggests federal government should support graduate
      nurse education and nursing research. Report also supports
      the cost effectiveness of nurse practitioners, the need for
      greater attention to gerontological nursing and the critical
      role of employers in dealing with nurse dissatisfaction and
      turnover. (21)

2562 Alley, L. "Nursing Shortage? Turnover? Maldistribution?"
      IMPRINT 29(4) (October/November 1982): 20-23.

      Discusses the problems of nursing shortages and high turn-
      over rates. High turnover rates result in a decrease in the
      quantity and quality of nursing care and in higher costs for
      the health care consumer. Identifies major sources of dissat-
      isfaction among nurses. (18)

2563 American Nurses' Association. NURSING STAFF REQUIREMENTS
      FOR IN-PATIENT HEALTH CARE SERVICES. Kansas City, MO.:
      American Nurses' Association, Pub. No. NS-20, 1977.

      The ANA Commission on Nursing Services describes steps to
      identify actual costs of providing nursing care and design a
      program to assure that nursing services delivered are approp-
      riate to consumer needs and that care provided is scientifi-
      cally and technologically sound.

2564 _____. GUIDELINES FOR USE OF SUPPLEMENTAL NURSING SERVICES.
      Kansas City, MO.: American Nurses' Association, Pub. No.
      NS-25, 1979.

      Guidelines developed by the ANA Commission on Nursing Ser-
      vices concerning use of temporary nursing personnel for those
      who use or administer supplemental nursing services.

2565 "Are We Wasting Nursepower? More Efficient Use of RNs Could
       Help Stem the Shortage," COST-CONTAINMENT 3(2) (January 27,
       1981): 3-6.

       Suggests that more efficient use of registered nurses could
       help reduce the shortage of professional nurses. Observes
       that when non-nursing activities are delegated to support
       personnel, time available for nursing care increases substan-
       tially. Recommends strategies for staff reorganization in
       hospitals. (0)

2566 Arnold, N. "Where Have All The Nurses Gone?" BRITISH MEDICAL
       JOURNAL 280(6208) (January 19, 1980): 199-201.

       Discusses the shortage of nurses in England. Notes that as
       a result of their struggle to establish professional status,
       many nurses have begun to work independent of the medical pro-
       fession. (3)

2567 Balzar, J. "The Florence Nightingale Shortage," CALIFORNIA
       JOURNAL: THE MONTHLY ANALYSIS OF STATE GOVERNMENT AND POLI-
       TICS 12(5) (May 1981): 167-70.

       Discusses the problem of unfilled nursing jobs in California
       and notes that one in five hospital nursing jobs in California
       is unfilled and that the shortage worsens each year. Reports
       that hospitals have begun hiring nurses to work with promises
       of bonuses and vacations. (0)

2568 Ciocci, G. "Capitalizing on the Hidden Job Market," NURSE
       PRACT 9(12) (December 1984): 31-33.

       Jobs for nurse practitioners are less obvious. The article
       describes some hidden job markets. (18)

2569 Curtin, L. "A Glut of Nurses?" NURS MANAGE 14(3) (March
       1983): 9-10.

       Emphasizes that there is not a critical shortage of nurses,
       but rather a critical shortage of nursing care because too
       many nurses are underemployed or misemployed. (0)

2570 _____. "A Shortage of Nurses--or The Sabotage of Nursing?"
       SUPERVISOR NURSE 12(4) (April 1981): 7.

       Argues that the current nursing shortage results from mal-
       distribution of nurses, misutilization of nurses´ talents,
       and mismanagement of the health care system. (0)

2571 Deane, R.T. and D.E. Yett. "Nurse Market Policy Simulations
       Using An Econometric Model," RESEARCH HEALTH ECON 1 (1979):
       255-300.

Discusses the labor market for professional nurses. Notes that nurses constitute the largest health manpower occupation requiring formal training and licensing, and that nursing is the largest almost exclusively female (paid) occupation. Comments on employment opportunity forecasts. (29)

2572   "Do You Think Nurses Are Leaving Nursing?" AORN J 31(4) (March 1980): 692, 694, 696-97.

Reports about shortages of nurses around the United States. Notes that only 70 percent of the 1.4 million registered nurses are currently working. Includes interviews with nurses who give their reasons for staying with or leaving the nursing profession. (0)

2573   Donovan, L. "The Shortage: Good Jobs Are Going Begging These Days, So Why Not Be Choosy?" RN 43(6) (June 1980): 21-27.

Discusses the nursing shortage and attributes a great deal of the shortage to registered nurses who have dropped out of nursing. Notes that despite the shortage, nursing salaries and benefits have remained uncompetitive with other career alternatives. A table is included which provides facts and figures about nursing employment and education. (0)

2574   Durbak, I. "How Uncle Sam White-washed the Nursing Shortage," RN 45(5) (May 1982): 45-47.

Discusses forecasting models developed by the federal government during the mid 1970's which were supposed to ac-curately predict registered nurse supply and demand. The government's predictions were inaccurate and the author warns nurses to be on guard because as current budget deficits worsen, it is likely that the crisis in nursing will be mini-mized further by the government. (4)

2575   Fagin, C.M. "The Shortage of Nurses in the United States," J PUBLIC HEALTH POLICY 1(4) (December 1980): 293-311.

Reports that a real nursing shortage exists and that it can be expected to worsen in the future if decreasing enrollments in nursing schools continue. Identifies reasons for the shor-tage and provides recommendations to increase the supply of nurses. (21)

2576   Feldstein, P.J. HEALTH CARE ECONOMICS. New York: Wiley, 1979.

Explores numerous aspects of the economics of health and includes a chapter which discusses the performance of the mar-ket for registered nurses and federal support for nurse training.

2577   _____. "The Market for Registered Nurses." HEALTH CARE ECONOMICS. New York: Wiley and Sons, 1983, pp. 417-43.

Investigates the performance of the registered nurses market
and explores whether there has been or is any justification
for federal subsidies to nursing education. (24)

2578 Fralic, M.F. "Nursing Shortage: Coping Today and Planning for
      Tomorrow," HOSPITALS 54(9) (May 1980): 65-67.

Explores why health care agencies are demanding more nurses
than ever before. Observes that because of declining enrollments and increasing, demand, the present shortage of nurses
is likely to continue. Offers suggestions for nursing management and hospital administration to follow in order to attract
and retain qualified nurses. (4)

2579 Greenleaf, N.P. "Labor Force Participation Among Registered
      Nurses and Women in Comparable Occupations," NURS RES 32
      (September/October 1983): 306-11.

Reports the results of a survey which compared labor force
participation of female nurses with women in comparable occupations. It was found that the presence of young children
at home keeps married teachers and others out of the labor
force but has no effect on married nurses. (27)

2580 Johnson, W.L. SUPPLY AND DEMAND FOR REGISTERED NURSES: SOME
      OBSERVATIONS ON THE CURRENT PICTURE AND PROSPECTS TO 1985,
      PART I. New York: National League for Nursing, Pub. No.
      19-1837, 1980, pp. 1-6.

Explores what is happening to the supply of nurses, discusses matching supply with demand, and considers which
policies and programs are indicated on the basis of projected
need. (8)

2581 _____. SUPPLY AND DEMAND FOR REGISTERED NURSES: SOME
      OBSERVATIONS ON THE CURRENT PICTURE AND PROSPECTS TO 1985,
      PART 2. New York: National League for Nursing, Pub. No.
      19-1838, 1980, pp. 1-8.

Discusses predictions of shrinking admissions to nursing
schools. Identifies factors influencing the severity of the
nurse shortage and provides recommendations for reversing the
trend. (6)

2582 _____. "Supply and Demand for Registered Nurses: Some Obser-
      vations on the Current Picture and Prospects to 1985, Part
      2," NURS HEALTH CARE 1(2) (September 1980): 73-79, 112.

Notes that it has been predicted that fewer students will be
applying to nursing schools in the coming years. Factors influencing the nurse shortage are identified, and suggestions
for reversing the trend are provided. (26)

2583 Johnson, W.L. and J.C. Vaughn. "Supply and Demand Relations
      and the Shortage of Nurses," NURS HEALTH CARE 3(9) (Novem-
      ber 1982): 497-507.

Analyzes two distinctly different perspectives of the nursing shortage, i.e. "reasoning from anecdotal materials," and
the "neoclassical economic theory." Discusses the wage rate
of registered nurses and provides a critique of the relative
wage theory. (30)

2584   Kalisch, B.J., P.A. Kalisch and J. Clinton. "An Analysis of
        News Flow on the Nation's Nurse Shortage," MEDICAL CARE
        19(9) (September 1981): 938-50.

        Analyzes characteristics of 1978 news coverage of the
        nation's nurse shortage by using data from national newspapers.
        Suggests that the public needs to be better informed about the
        causes of and possible solution to the nursing shortage. (8)

2585   Kalisch, P.A. and B.J. Kalisch. "The Nurse Shortage, the
        President, and the Congress," NURS FORUM 19(2) (1980): 138-
        64.

        Notes that the problem of nurse supply is an important ele-
        ment of the current national health crisis. Argues that the
        Carter administration was wrong when it concluded that no
        nursing shortage existed in 1980. (0)

2586   Kramer, M. REALITY SHOCK: WHY NURSES LEAVE NURSING. St.
        Louis: C.V. Mosby, 1974.

        Explores the problems encountered by young nursing graduates
        who have visions and skills of the future, but lack some of
        the knowledge needed to function in today's health care system.
        Discusses how such problems can be solved so that new nurses
        will not become disillusioned and leave the profession.

2587   Lee, A. "Government Report on Nursing Shows a Booming Profes-
        sion," RN 45(11) (November 1982): 19, 105-6.

        Reports on the 1982 government statistics on nursing employ-
        ment and notes that RNs are earning more and that there has
        been a dramatic increase in the number of RNs in the workforce
        over the previous three years. Projects that nursing will
        become a more associate degree dominated profession in the
        years to come. (0)

2588   Levine, E. "Nursing Supply and Requirements: The Current
        Situation and Future Prospects." NURSING PERSONNEL AND THE
        CHANGING HEALTH CARE SYSTEM. Edited by M.L. Millman. Cam-
        bridge: Ballinger Publishing Co., 1977, pp. 23-42.

        Examines existing evidence concerning the presence or ab-
        sence of a shortage of registered nurses and discusses four
        efforts at projecting nursing supply and requirements. (27)

2589   Lewis, E.N. and P.V. Carini. NURSE STAFFING AND PATIENT CLAS-
        SIFICATION: STRATEGIES FOR SUCCESS. Gaithersburg, MD.:
        Aspen Systems Corp., 1983.

Tells how to develop, implement, and to evaluate a staffing system. Covers staffing policy, position control, scheduling, and department budget development. Helps examine organizations in terms of accountability, autonomy, decentralization, and the process of change. Discusses contemporary issues and challenges of the nursing administrator vis-a-vis the medical staff.

2590 Link, C.R. and R.F. Settle. "Wage Incentives and Married Professional Nurses: A Case of Backward-bending Supply?" ECONOMIC INQUIRY 19(1) (January 1981): 144-56.

Investigates how increases in the supply of registered nurses can best be facilitated. Concludes that it is not likely that nurse shortages can be alleviated by wage incentives, and that perhaps the supply of nurses can substantially increased only through large investments in the training of new nurses. (19)

2591 _____. "Simultaneous-equation Model of Labor Supply, Fertility and Earnings of Married Women: The Case of Registered Nurses," SOUTHERN ECONOMIC J 47 (April 1981): 977-89.

Observes that except for teaching, more women have been attracted to nursing than to any other profession. In 1977 about one million female RNs were working as nurses and an additional 300,000 RNs were not in the labor force. Provides a three-equation simultaneous model of labor supply, fertility and market earnings for married professional nurses. (30)

2592 _____. "Financial Incentive and Labor Supply of Married Professional Nurses: An Economic Analysis," NURS RES 29(4) (July/August 1980): 238-43.

Reports results of an investigation to determine the extent to which the supply of nursing services would increase in response to higher nurse salaries and other inducements (such as child care services). It was found that higher wages probably would not be effective in providing more nursing services, but would actually have the opposite effect--that is, the registered nurses would reduce the number of working hours. (22)

2593 _____. "Labor Supply Responses of Married Professional Nurses: New Evidence," J HUMAN RESOURCES 14 (Spring 1979): 256-66.

Reports that it has been found that moderate increases in RN wages would attract many inactive nurses back to the labor force. Considers several potentially important influences on nurse labor supply such as nurse health and the structure of the nurse labor market, and concludes that an increase in the RN wage would lead to a much smaller increase in the supply of nurses than was previously indicated. (18)

2594   Logan, W. "The Migration of Nursing Personnel," INT NURS REV
       27(4) (July/August 1980): 119-22.

       Reports about a study designed by the World Health Organiza-
       tion which identifies patterns of physician and nurse migra-
       tion and suggests methods of changing those patterns. Accor-
       ding to the study, nurses are more inequitably distributed
       around the world than physicians. (4)

2595   Lum, J.L. "WICHE Panel of Expert Consultants Report: Imp-
       lications for Nursing Leaders," J NURS ADM 9(7) (July 1979):
       11-19.

       Discusses how the Western Interstate Commission for Higher
       Education (WICHE), Boulder, Colorado projected nursing re-
       quirements for the future using an analytic model. Includes
       projects and recommendations for educational preparation,
       distribution of nursing services, and practice which have im-
       plications for nursing administrators and nursing educators.
       (8)

2596   MAGNET HOSPITALS: ATTRACTION AND RETENTION OF PROFESSIONAL
       NURSES. Kansas City, MO.: American Nurses' Association,
       1983.

       Focuses on the reasons why nurses in some hospitals stay in
       their jobs and on the reasons for their job satisfaction.
       Discusses the influence of management style, quality of
       leadership, organizational structure, personnel policies, and
       quality of patient care on a hospital's ability to retain
       nurses.

2597   Maraldo, P. MANPOWER MALDISTRIBUTION. New York: National
       League for Nursing, Pub. No. 52-1755, 1979, pp. 69-75.

       Suggests that the problem of maldistribution is a problem of
       political perspectives of various vested interests and prior-
       ities determining how many nurses are needed and where they
       are needed. Emphasizes that if nurses do not become involved
       in defining the services they provide, the government will.
       (0)

2598   McTernan, E.J. and A.M. Leiken. "A Pyramid Model of Health
       Manpower in the 1980s," J HEALTH POLITICS, POLICY AND LAW
       6(4) (Winter 1982): 739-51.

       Argues that health manpower situation has changed dras-
       tically in the last twenty years from shortage to an impending
       oversupply. Implications of this change discussed. (18)

2599   Mejia, A. "Migration of Physicians and Nurses: A World Wide
       Picture," INT J EPIDEMIOLOGY 7(3) (September 1978): 207-15.

       Discusses the results of the World Health Organization's
       (WHO) Multinational Study of the International Migration of
       Physicians and Nurses. Reports that countries producing more

physicians and nurses than they can economically afford become donors of such manpower and those that produce fewer
than they can afford become recipients. (6)

2600   Moscovice, I. and M. Nestegard.   "The Influence of Values and
        Background on the Location Decision of Nurse Practitioners,"
        J COMMUNITY HEALTH 5(4) (Summer 1980): 244-53.

        Discusses results and implications of a study which examined
        the relationship between value systems of family nurse prac-
        titioners, background characteristics of family nurse practi-
        tioners and their spouses, and the decision of the family
        nurse practitioner about practice location. (16)

2601   Moses, E. and A. Roth.   "Nurse Power, What Do Statistics Re-
        veal About the Nation's Nurse?" AM J NURS 79 (October 1979):
        1745.

        Reports the results of a study about registered nurses which
        explores licensing status, family structure, family income
        levels, educational background, racial and ethnic background,
        employment status, and mobility. (0)

2602   "No Nursing Shortage, National Study Says," AORN J 37(4)
        (March 1983): 788-90.

        Summarizes a report of a National Academy of Sciences Com-
        mittee to Congress which concludes that no general nursing
        shortage exists, but that there are shortages in specific
        geographic areas and in specialty areas of nursing. (0)

2603   Novicky, D.   "The Nursing Shortage: A Long Term Dilemma,"
        CONNECTICUT MEDICINE 45(3) (March 1981): 148-49.

        Notes that a challenge for the 1980's will be to retain
        nurses currently in the work force and suggests that this will
        be difficult to do unless employers realistically examine
        their work environments and recognize that nursing is a physi-
        cally and emotionally demanding profession. (7)

2604   "Nurses Today--A Statistical Portrait," AM J NURS 82(3)
        (March 1982): 448-51.

        Summarizes a survey that indicates that as of November,
        1980, there were over 1.6 million RNs. Male RNs make up 2.7
        percent of the country's RNs, and males have a higher employ-
        ment rate than women (86 percent compared to 76 percent for
        women). (0)

2605   "Nursing Shortage Linked to Hospital Environment," HOSPITALS
        54(1) (January 1980): 18-19.

        Identifies dissatisfaction with jobs as the main cause of
        the nursing shortage. Notes that in metropolitan areas turn-
        over for staff nurses has reached 200 percent. (0)

2606 Personett, J.D. and M.A. Boyle. "Abuse, Poor Image Causes
       Shortage," MODERN HEALTH CARE 10(7) (July 1980): 92, 99.

       Identifies three major causes of the nurse shortage as:
       working conditions, physician-nurse relationships, and the
       image of the nurse. Recommends ways of reversing high nurse
       turnover. (0)

2607 Prescott, P.A., J.K. Janken, T.L. Langford and P. McKay.
       "Supplemental Nursing Services: How and Why Are They Used?"
       AM J NURS 83(4) (April 1983): 554-57.

       Data indicates that supplementary nurses are adequately
       oriented to the settings in which they work, their job perfor-
       mance is evaluated, they do not threaten the continuity of
       care, and their patient assignements are comparable to those
       of staff nurses. (5)

2608 Prescott, P.A. "Supplemental Nursing Services: How Much Do
       Hospitals Really Pay?" AM J NURS 82(8) (August 1982): 1208-
       13.

       In a survey of hospitals, study found that they paid between
       twenty-nine percent to sixty percent more per shift for tem-
       porary service than for a regularly employed staff nurse.
       None of this could be attributed to fringe benefits. Apparen-
       tly hospitals are paying more to attract some nurses rather
       than raise salaries across the board. Policy seems short
       sighted in terms of long term policy implications. (9)

2609 Price, J.L. and C.W. Mueller. PROFESSIONAL TURNOVER: THE
       CASE OF NURSES. New York: S.P. Medical and Scientific Books,
       1981.

       Reports that hospital nurses have more than three times the
       rate of teachers (a comparable profession) and explores
       reasons for such a high rate of turnover. Discusses the sig-
       nificance of high turnover from the perspective of hospitals,
       society, and the nursing profession. Provides eight recommen-
       dations to increase job satisfaction.

2610 "RN Supply Predicted To Be Adequate by 1985," AORN J 30(2)
       (August 1979): 312-13.

       Summarizes and discusses the predictions of the Division of
       Nursing, U.S. Public Health Service, SECOND REPORT TO THE
       CONGRESS, MARCH 15, 1979. (0)

2611 Roemer, M.I. and R.J. Roemer. HEALTH CARE SYSTEMS AND COM-
       PARATIVE MANPOWER POLICIES. New York: Marcel Dekker, Inc.,
       1981.

       Examines health care systems and manpower policies of Aus-
       tralia, Canada, Belgium, Norway, and Poland. Compares poli-
       cies in United States to these five.

2612   Rose, M.A. "Factors Affecting Nurse Supply and Demand: An
       Exloration," J NURS ADM 12(2) (February 1982): 31-34.

       Addresses the nursing shortage from an economic standpoint
       by exploring supply and demand factors that influence the
       availability of nurses. (15)

2613   Sekscenski, E. THE HEALTH SERVICES INDUSTRY IN THE UNITED
       STATES: TRENDS IN EMPLOYMENT FROM 1970 TO 1983 WITH PROJEC-
       TIONS TO 1995. Washington, D.C.: Department for Profes-
       sional Employees, AFL-CIO, Pub. No. 84-2, August, 1984.

       Overview of the health service industry. Analyzes trends
       as they relate to the job market for health workers. A union
       publication. (50)

2614   Sigardson, K.M. "Why Nurses Leave Nursing: A Survey of Former
       Nurses," NURS ADM Q 7(1) (Fall 1982): 20-24.

       Reports the results of a survey which examined nurses´ per-
       ceptions about their jobs. The most frequently cited reasons
       for leaving nursing were long hours and understaffing, fol-
       lowed by treatment received from physicians and low pay and
       inadequate benefits. (9)

2615   Smith, R.A. (Ed.). MANPOWER AND PRIMARY HEALTH CARE. Hono-
       lulu: University Press of Hawaii, 1984.

       Work is written for those who plan and implement health
       programs in developing countries. The authors, aware of the
       growing necessity for using health personnel other than doc-
       tors to provide primary health care services, focus on the
       essential issues involved in program development. They detail
       the key elements of a program that trains and deploys com-
       munity health works and intermediate level personnel who pro-
       vide a critical link between central resources and com-
       munities.

2616   Sovie, M.D. "The Economics of Magnetism," NURS ECON 2(2)
       (March/April 1984): 85-92.

       Summarizes the major findings of a study about the ability
       of hospitals to attract and retain nurses. Notes that a hos-
       pital´s magnetism has economic implications that extend beyond
       employment of nurses. Discusses how components of magnetism
       offer economic advantages that may help the institution
       achieve its patient care objectives. (7)

2617   Steck, A.L. "The Nursing Shortage: An Optimistic View," NURS
       OUTLOOK 29(5) (May 1981): 302-4.

       Discusses why nurses leave their jobs and notes that the
       shortage of nurses is an effective demonstration of positive

their jobs create staffing shortages and employers are conse-
quently forced to examine and remedy the causes of nurse dissatisfaction. (9)

2618   "The Nurse Shortage: A National Dilemma," REVIEW OF THE
       FEDERALIZATION OF AMERICAN HOSPITALS 13(2) (April/May 1980):
       12-21.

       Discusses how recruitment and retention have become priority
       goals in the attempts of hospitals to increase their nursing
       staffs. (0)

2619   Deleted.

2620   Wandelt, M., P. Pierce and R. Weddowson.   "Why Nurses Leave
       Nursing and What Can Be Done About It," AM J NURS 81 (1981):
       72-77.

       Reports the results of a study about the nursing shortage
       which was done at the University of Texas.   Discusses such
       issues as staffing, autonomy, professionalism, quality of
       care, and the changes of hospital conditions that would at-
       tract inactive nurses back to the workforce. (0)

2621   Weiss, R.E., G. Sobieck, J.E. Sauer, Jr.   "Nursing Shortage:
       A Solution--A Comprehensive Program of Practical, Cost-Ef-
       fective Remedies," HOSPITAL FORUM 23(6) (September/October
       1980): 19-26.

       Discusses the confusion surrounding the national nursing
       shortage and the fact that the national programs to support
       increased nursing education and retention of nurses in hos-
       pitals have not been successful.   Examines the advantages and
       disadvantages of nurse registries. (0)

2622   White, C.H.   "Nursing Shortage, Turnover and Some Proposed
       Solutions," HOSPITAL FORUM 22(4) (June 1979): 10-13.

       Discusses the shortage of nurses and suggests instead of
       working only towards increasing the supply of nurses, em-
       ployers should examine the job factors that cause such high
       turnover rates among nurses.   Suggests that employers em-
       phasize careers rather than episodic jobs.   Proposes long and
       short-range solutions to the problem of job dissatisfaction.
       (0)

2623   White, D.C.   "The Nurse 'Shortage': The Case of Rhode Is-
       land," NE J HUMAN SERVICES 2(4) (Fall 1982): 40-47.

       Observes that employers of nurses and the federal government
       have divergent opinions regarding the appropriateness of the
       available supply of registered nurses in the United States.
       Utilizes the nurse supply situation in Rhode Island to illus-
       trate on a small scale insights that are difficult to discern
       at the national level. (22)

2624 Yett, D.E. et al. A FORECASTING AND POLICY SIMULATION MODEL
      OF THE HEALTH CARE SECTOR. Lexington, MA.: Lexington Books,
      1979.

      Forecasts, through the use of a model, the supply of nurses
      and the rates of wage adjustments that are likely to occur in
      response to the discrepancies between supply and demand in the
      nursing profession.

2625 Young, K.J. "Professional Commitment of Women in Nursing,"
      WEST J NURS RES 6(1) (Winter 1984): 11-26.

      Discusses the attrition of nurses from the educational pro-
      cess and the occupational world. Explores ways of recruiting
      and retaining nurses who are committed to full-time profes-
      sional careers in nursing. Concludes that women's perceived
      roles regarding marriage and family in our society contribute
      to the problem of nurse attrition. (0)

      See   2109, 2121, 2138.

Private Practice, Independent Practice for Nurses

2626 Agree, B.C. "Beginning an Independent Nursing Practice,"
      AM J NURS 74 (April 1974): 636-42. Reprinted in EXPANDING
      HORIZONS FOR NURSES. Edited by B. Bullough and V. Bullough.
      New York: Springer Publishing Co., 1977, pp. 67-78.

      Looks at eight group and five individual nursing practices
      set up in the 70's and their early successes and failures. (0)

2627 Durham, J.D. and S.B. Hardin. "Promoting Private Practice in a
      Competitive Market," NURS ECON 1(1) (July/August 1983):
      24-28.

      In a competitive health services market, promotion of pri-
      vate practice is an essential activity. Promotion is one
      dimension of marketing, and marketing is a philosophy as well
      as a process. Based on the findings of their Delphi survey
      the authors argue that nurses in private practice have not
      mastered the process of marketing or strategies for practice
      promotion. (25)

2628 Gibson, K.W., J.S. Catterson and P. Skalka. ON OUR OWN.
      New York: Avon Books, 1982.

      Two nurses (Gibson and Catterson) chronicle their efforts to
      set up an independent nursing practice in Chicago which cul-
      minated in a successful lawsuit under the Equal Employment
      Opportunities Act against their former employer who had
      fired them.

2629 Hutchens, C.M. "Looking Ahead: Women and Nursing," IMPRINT
      27(2) (April 1980): 74-75, 79-81.

Provides an overview of the history of nurses and nursing in the United States. Discusses the ongoing controversy over private practice nursing and physician opposition to such practice. (23)

2630   Jacox, A.K. and C.M. Norris. ORGANIZING FOR INDEPENDENT NURS-
       ING PRACTICE. New York: Appleton-Century-Crofts, 1977.

       A compilation of pioneering experiences decribed by nurse
       practitioners. It offers some advice, raises questions, and
       deals with issues such as qualifications, payment, support
       and research.

2631   Kohnke, M. INDEPENDENT NURSING PRACTICE. Garden Grove, CA.:
       Trainex Press, 1974.

       Provides a detailed discussion of the philosophy and mech-
       anics of independent nursing practice. Clearly defines the
       perimeters of professional nursing and differentiatco nurs-
       ing practice from medical practice. Deals with accountability
       to consumers and with consumer advocacy. (34)

2632   Koltz, C.J. PRIVATE PRACTICE IN NURSING: DEVELOPMENT AND
       MANAGEMENT. Germantown, MD.: Aspen Systems Corp., 1979.

       Emphasizes that nurses offer the public a huge resource of
       professional expertise for prevention and treatment of dis-
       ease. Questions why nurses have avoided the fee-for-service
       method that dentists, physicians, physical therapists, and
       other health professionals commonly use. Maintains that
       nurses employed outside of hospitals, in private practice, can
       contribute to upgrading the quality of health care delivery.

2633   Lynch, M.L. ON YOUR OWN: PROFESSIONAL GROWTH THROUGH INDE-
       PENDENT NURSING PRACTICE. Montercy, CA.: Wadsworth Health
       Sciences Division, 1982.

       Provides information on establishing a private nursing
       practice including how a nurse can break from the traditional
       hospital role, if a nurse can earn an adequate living in pri-
       vate practice, and the legal, business, and ethical implica-
       tions of private practice. Resistance (on the part of the
       medical profession and some nurses) to the new roles of nurses
       is discusses as a major barrier to a successful independent
       practice.

2634   Maas, M. and A.K. Jacox. GUIDELINES FOR NURSE AUTONOMY/
       PATIENT WELFARE. New York: Appleton-Century-Crofts, 1977.

       Emphasizes the perspective of nurses as emerging profes-
       sionals. Views the achievement of nurse autonomy and account-
       ability as necessary to nursings' full participation in
       collegial relationships with other health care professionals.
       (37)

2635   Pearson, L.E. "Self-Employment Income: Professional Fees
       and Tax Considerations," NURS ECON 2(1) (January/February
       1984): 52-56.

       Provides information about determining professional fees in
       a competitive marketplace and about self-employment taxes.
       (5)

2636   Riccardi, B.R. and E.C. Dayani. THE NURSE ENTREPRENEUR.
       Reston, VA.: Reston Publishing Co., 1982.

       Provides specific guidelines for management of an autono-
       mous nursing practice. Encourages nurses to assume respon-
       sibility for their professional destiny and to advance in
       business management. Explores how nursing services can be
       made economically affordable and socially acceptable.

       See 897.

Hospital Privileges

2637   American Nurses´ Association. GUIDELINES FOR APPOINTMENT OF
       NURSES FOR INDIVIDUAL PRACTICE PRIVILEGES IN HEALTH CARE
       ORGANIZATIONS. Kansas City, MO.: American Nurses´ Asso-
       ciation, Pub. No. NS-21, 1978.

       Statement by the ANA Commission on Nursing Services out-
       lining the responsibilities of nursing services relative to
       nursing appointments in health care organizations, responsi-
       bilities of the nurse, types of appointments, and nursing
       appointments review committee structure and responsibilities.

2638   Clinton, C., G. Schmittling, T.L. Stern and R.R. Black.
       "Hospital Privileges for Family Physicians: A National
       Study of Office Based Members of the American Academy of
       Family Physicians," J FAMILY PRACTICE 13(3) (1981): 361-71.

       Statistical data on hospital privileges. (13)

2639   Geyman, J.P. "Hospital Privileges of Family Physicians,"
       J FAMILY PRACTICE 13(3) (1981): 325-26.

       Editorial discussing problems of family physicians in ob-
       taining hospital privileges. (12)

2640   Grad, J.D. "Allied Health Professionals and Hospital Privi-
       leges: An Introduction to the Issues," LAW MED HEALTH CARE
       10 (September 1982): 165-67.

       Allied health professionals, including podiatrists, nurse
       practitioners, psychologists, physical therapists, and optome-
       trists are seeking hospital privileges. They face a certain
       amount of physician opposition to these efforts and are turn-
       ing to the courts. (18)

2641   Hayden, M.L. and P. Rowell. "Hospital Privileges: Rationale
       and Process," NURSE PRACT (January 1982): 42-44.

       Explains concept of hospital privileges and suggests pro-
       cess which nurse practitioner can use to obtain privileges.
       (5)

2642   Manley, M.V. "Clinical Privileges for Nonhospital-Based
       Nurses," AM J NURS 81(10) (October 1981): 1822-25.

       Nurses who seek access to patients through departments of
       nursing meet confusion, hostility, and game playing. Indi-
       cates some real questions have to be considered by nursing
       staffs and hospitals that are giving hospital privileges to
       nurse practitioners and others not employed by the hospital.
       (5)

2643   Stern, T.L., G. Schmittling, C. Clinton and R.R. Black.
       "Hospital Privileges for Graduates of Family Practice Resi-
       dency Programs," J FAMILY PRACTION 13(7) (1981): 1013-20.

       Statistical data on hospital privileges for family practice
       residency program graduates. (8)

       See 800, 881.

Nursing Centers

2644   Lang, N.M. "Nurse-Managed Centers: Will They Thrive," AM J
       NURS 83(9) (September 1983): 1290-93.

       Nurse-managed centers, where patient care is integrated
       with research and teaching are portrayed as the wave of the
       future. Some sixty-three centers are in operation. (5)

2645   Mezey,M.D. "Securing a Financial Base," AM J NURS 83(9)
       (September 1983): 1297-98.

       Explores strategies for securing a financial base for nurs-
       ing centers. Recent legislative changes are supporting
       nursing centers as a means of reducing health care costs while
       at the same time improving services to underserved groups. (6)

       See: 1255, 1313, 1659, 1747, 1794.

Home Health Care

2646   American Nurses' Association. HEALTH CARE AT HOME: AN ESSEN-
       TIAL COMPONENT OF A NATIONAL HEALTH POLICY. Kansas City,
       MO.: American Nurses' Association, Pub. No. CH-9, 1978.

       Position paper by the ANA Division on Community Health
       Nursing Practice and Commission on Nursing Service deals with
       health care services to be provided and reimbursed, organi-

zation and structure of home care agencies, necessary controls on services provided, personnel involved in providing
these services, financing, areas of study, and new directions.

2647   Hughes, S.L., D.S. Cordray and V.A. Spiker. "Evaluation of a
       Long-Term Home Care Program," MEDICAL CARE 22(5) (May 1984):
       460-75.

       An evaluation of five programs for home bound elderly per-
       sons who need medical and social services. Persons needing
       this type of care randomly assigned to care or no care. Ex-
       perimental group less likely to be admitted to a nursing
       home. Mortality and hospitalization not significantly diff-
       erent. (31)

2648   Knollmueller, R.N. "Funding Home Care in a Climate of Cost
       Containment," PUBLIC HEALTH NURS 1(1) (March 1984): 16-22.

       Recently, proprietary, private, not-for-profit organiza-
       tions have entered the home care arena. Home care reimburse-
       ment methods are a patchwork, causing confusion and cash flow
       problems. Public funds are administered by different levels
       of government, by several agencies within each level, and with
       various eligibility requirements. Private insurance coverage
       is uneven and limited. (17)

2649   Mundinger, M.O. HOME CARE CONTROVERSY: TOO LITTLE, TOO LATE,
       TOO COSTLY. Rockville, MD.: Aspen Systems Corp., 1983.

       Author critiques home care movement. Argues that the medi-
       care legislation fails to meet the needs of the sick elderly
       because it is based on a medical rather than a nursing model.

2650   National League for Nursing. HOME HEALTH CARE: A DISCUSSION
       PAPER. New York: National League for Nursing, Pub. No.
       21-1689, 1977.

       Examines twenty-two significant issues raised at five HEW
       sponsored regional hearings on the expansion of home health
       care services. Also presents a set of recommendations for
       future direction, as well as including a summary of legisla-
       tion and regulations that affect the proposed expansion.
       Extensive bibliography.

2651   Spegel, A. HOME HEALTH CARE: HOME BIRTHING TO HOSPICE CARE.
       Owing Mills, MD.: National Health Publishing Co., 1983.

       A source book that describes the rapidly growing home health
       care field.

Primary Nursing and Team Nursing

2652   Bloom, J.R. and J.A. Alexander. "Team Nursing: Professional
       Coordination or Bureaucratic Control?," J HEALTH AND SOCIAL
       BEHAVIOR 23(1) (March 1982): 84-95.

Nursing teams are conceptualized as coordination mechanisms that respond to task interdependence within the hospital unit. On larger units the nursing team provides a hierarchical control mechanism, whereas teaming in units characterized by greater staff professionalism provides a means of lateral coordination as well as hierarchical control. (42)

2653 Brown, B.J. PERSPECTIVES IN PRIMARY NURSING. Gaithersburg, MD.: Aspen Systems Corp., 1982.

A collection of twenty-eight articles about primary nursing.

2654 Daeffler, ,R.J. "Patients' Perception of Care Under Team and Primary Nursing," J NURS ADM 5(3) (1975): 20-26.

Patients were more satisfied with their care under primary than team nursing. (24)

2655 Hegyvary, S.T. THE CHANGE IN PRIMARY NURSING: A CROSS CULTURAL VIEW OF PROFESSIONAL PRACTICE. St. Louis: C.V. Mosby, 1982.

A comparative view of nursing in seven countries: Australia, Japan, Belgium, The Netherlands, Norway, Canada and United States--all of which have implemented primary nursing.

2656 Mayer, G. and K. Bailey. THE MIDDLE MANAGER IN PRIMARY NURSING. New York: Springer Publishing Co., 1982.

The role and education of the middle manager in patient-centered systems of nursing care delivery. Concrete suggestions for developing curricula that will improve leadership in primary nursing.

2657 Shukla, R.K. and W.E. Turner, III. "Patients Perception of Care Under Primary and Team Nursing," RES NURS HEALTH 7(2) (June 1984): 93-99.

The relationship between the structure of nursing care and patient satisfaction was assessed after equalizing the quantity and quality of nursing care. Patient satisfaction was not significantly different. (25)

Competition, Competitive Models, Nurses as Alternative to Physicians, HMOs

2658 Blackstone, E.A. "Competition Within the Physicians' Services Industry: Osteopaths and Allopaths," AM J LAW MED 8(2) (Summer 1982): 137-50.

Doctors of osteopathy are the only "full line" competitors of medical doctors. Given the current interest in merger of

the two schools of medicine, this article examines the benefits of having an independent osteopathic school. Conclusion
is that society has an interest in discouraging merger of the
two groups. (89)

2659   Enthoven, A.C. HEALTH PLAN: THE ONLY PRACTICAL SOLUTION TO
       THE SOARING COST OF MEDICAL CARE. Reading, MA.: Addison
       Wesley, 1980.

       Argues that less regulation, more competition, and use of
       rational economic incentives can yield better health care at
       a lower cost.

2660   Fagin, C. "Nursing As An Alternative to High Cost Care," AM
       J NURS 82 (January 1982): 56-60.

       Discusses legislative proposals which seek to stimulate
       competition between various prepaid health care payment
       plans. Notes that state laws and interpretations of nurse
       practice acts hinder nurses from competing in the health care
       market. Summarizes the positive and cost-effective aspects
       of care by nurse midwives and nurse practitioners. (27)

2661   _____. "Nursing's Pivotal Role in Achieving Competition
       in Health Care." FROM ACCOMMODATION TO SELF DETERMINATION:
       NURSING'S ROLE IN THE DEVELOPMENT OF HEALTH CARE POLICY.
       Kansas City, MO.: American Nurses' Association, 1982. Re-
       printed in NURSING ISSUES AND NURSING STRATEGIES FOR THE
       EIGHTIES. Edited by B. Bullough, V. Bullough and M.C.
       Soukup. New York: Springer Publishing Co., 1983, pp. 169-
       78.

       Urges maximizing the potential for nurses' contribution to
       health care system by reimbursement for nursing service. (2)

2662   Fox, P.D., W.B. Goldbeck and J.J. Spies. HEALTH CARE COST
       MANAGEMENT: PRIVATE SECTOR INITIATIVES. Ann Arbor, MI.:
       Health Administration Press, 1984.

       Current strategies for managing the costs of health care
       benefits--from the point of view of purchasers and providers--
       are described and illustrated. The early 1980's have experi-
       enced rapid changes in the health care delivery system. Pri-
       vate employers, for whom health care benefits may exceed
       seven percent of pay, are beginning to take forceful actions
       to manage health care costs, including the adoption of pros-
       pective payment systems and of measures to promote enrollment
       in prepaid health plans. In addition, competition among pro-
       vidors of health care is increasing.

2663   Gabel, J.R. and A.C. Monheit. WILL COMPETITION PLANS CHANGE
       INSURER-PROVIDER RELATIONSHIPS? National Center for Health
       Services Research. Springfield, VA.: National Technical
       Information Service, 1983. Reprinted from MILBANK MEMORIAL
       FUND QUARTERLY/HEALTH AND SOCIETY 61(4) (1983).

Paper examines whether competition proposals are likely to
provide sufficient stimuli to change existing payment relationships between insurers and providers and thereby effec-
tuate a fundamental change in health care delivery. The
choice of this issue reflects the belief that inefficiency
in the health care sector is more than the problem of excess
consumer demand or "moral hazard" from over-insurance. It is
believed that unless insurers change their reimbursement
methods so that providers bear some financial risks for their
resource decisions, the health care system is likely to retain
much of its inherent inefficiency.

2664   Gibson, R.   "Nurse-Midwives and Competition: Testing an Assump-
       tion," NURS ECON 2(1) (January/February 1984): 42-46.

       Some health care observers believe that according hospital
       privileges to nonphysician providers, and to nurse-midwives
       in particular, will inevitably increase health care expendi
       tures. This assumption is used to buttress arguments that
       would restrict the practice of many health care professionals.
       The key issue is the extent to which there can be a sub-
       stitution effect in health care labor markets. (19)

2665   Gray, B.H. (Ed.). THE NEW HEALTH CARE FOR A PROFIT: DOCTORS
       AND HOSPITALS IN A COMPETITIVE MOVEMENT. Washington, D.C.:
       National Academy Press, 1983.

       The Institute of Medicine has begun an in-depth examination
       of the for-profit health care institutions. This work is the
       first with others to be published at a later date. Implica-
       tions of this rapidly escalating trend are discussed.

2666   Greenberg, W. (Ed.). COMPETITION IN THE HEALTH CARE SECTOR:
       PAST, PRESENT, AND FUTURE. Germantown, MD.: Aspen Systems
       Corp.,, 1978.

       Includes papers by economists and social scientists about
       the role of competition in the health care sector. Suggests
       that physicians should have to compete with others in the
       marketplace of ideas and the political process.

2667   Griffith, H.   "Nursing Practice: Substitute or Complement
       According to Economic Theory," NURS ECON 2(2) (March/April
       1984): 105-12.

       Notes that according to economic theory, if nurses' and
       physicians' services are considered substitutes, the demand
       and price for nursing services will increase. If, however,
       nursing services are viewed as complements of physician ser-
       vices, the demand and price for nursing services will de-
       crease. (18)

2668   Harrison, D.H. and J.R. Kimberly. "Private and Public Initia-
       tives in Health Maintenance Organizations," J HEALTH POLI-
       TICS, POLICY AND LAW 7 (Spring 1982): 80-95.

Predicts greater impact of health maintenance organizations on the health care industry. Increased investments
by insurance companies and management companies have streng-
thened HMOs. (32)

2669   Illich, I. MEDICAL NEMESIS. New York: Pantheon Books, 1976.

Argues improvements in health due to public health measures,
rather than medical care. Argues that physicians cost too
much, intrude on life too much, and have too much power. Ob-
jects to the "medicalization of life." Author is a priest,
philosopher and historian.

2670   Mermelstein, R. "Cutting Health Care Costs in California,"
       LAW MED HEALTH CARE 11(4) (September 1983): 177-81.

Summarizes conference dealing with the effect of California
legislation passed in 1982 requiring hospitals to compete with
each other for right to treat patients covered by Medi-Cal.
Results had been to cut costs, although some speakers spoke
of less desirable effects. (11)

2671   Record, J.C. (Ed.). STAFFING PRIMARY CARE IN 1990: PHYSICIAN
       REPLACEMENT AND COST SAVINGS. New York: Springer Publishing
       Co., 1981.

Presents reviews of the state of knowledge about delegation,
comparative productivity, and comparative costs. Compares
data from Kaiser-Permanente with data from the NAMCS (National
Ambulatory Medical Care Survey) with respect to the ratio of
routine to nonroutine office visits. Reports the potential
effect of (NHPs) new health practitioners-physician assistants
and nurse practitioners on the number of physicians needed
in primary care.

2672   Salmon, J.W. "Who Benefits from Competition in Health Care?"
       NURS ECON 1(2) (September/October 1983): 129-34.

Negative view of the efforts by the Reagan administration
to inject competition into the health care delivery system.
Notes that while hospital closings may decrease the problem
of overbedding, essential services are being cut out. (33)

2673   Tennant, F.S. et al. "A Study of the Economic Viability of
       Low Cost Fee for Service Clinics Staffed by Nurse Practi-
       tioners," PUBLIC HEALTH REPORTS 95(4) (1980): 321-23.

A feasibility study done in California which demonstrated
that nurse practitioners in two clinics became financially
self sufficient and reduced ambulatory health care costs in
this fee-for-service system. (13)

2674   Whitney, F. "The GMENAC Report: An Opportunity for Nursing."
       NURSING ISSUES AND NURSING STRATEGIES FOR THE EIGHTIES.
       Edited by B. Bullough, V. Bullough and M.C. Soukup. New
       York: Springer Publishing Co., 1983, pp. 138-54.

Whitney sees ways to overcome the negative recommendations
of the GMENAC Report on extended role nursing. (5)

Physician Assistants

2675 Bliss, A.A., A.M. Sadler and B.L. Sadler. THE PHYSICIAN'S
      ASSISTANT-TODAY AND TOMORROW. Cambridge: Ballinger Pub-
      lishing Co., 1975.

      The history of the physician's assistant concept, the issues
      surrounding the movement and the power struggles with both
      nursing and medicine are recounted. The 1975 work is a
      second edition.

2676 Detmar, D.E. and H.B. Perry. "The Utilization of Surgical
      Physician Assistants: Policy Implications for the Future,"
      SURGICAL CLINICS OF NORTH AMERICA 62(4) (August 1982):
      669-75.

      Reviews the history of the surgical physician assistant,
      summarizes the current status of this field, and discusses
      future policy implications. (27)

2677 Engel, G.V. "An Evaluation of the Continued Viability of
      the Occupation of the Physician's Assistant," J MED ED
      56 (August 1981): 659-62.

      Investigation of the continued viability of the physician's
      assistant in terms of worker satisfaction. Findings suggest
      continued viability in that most physician's assistants are
      satisfied with their work. (9)

2678 Perry, H.B. and B. Breitner. PHYSICIAN ASSISTANTS: THEIR
      CONTRIBUTION TO HEALTH CARE. New York: Human Sciences
      Press, 1982.

      Analysis based on a recent survey conducted by the American
      Academy of Physician Assistants and the Association of Phy-
      sician Assistant Programs, examines recruitment, utilization
      and career structure.

Physicians

2679 Betz, M. and L.O'Connell. "Changing Doctor-Patient Relation-
      ships and The Rise in Concern for Accountability," SOCIAL
      PROBLEMS 31(1) (October 1983): 84-95.

      This paper examines a growing distrust of doctors and the
      resultant call for accountability of the medical profession.
      The structure of exchange between doctors and patients has

changed as a result of population mobility, professionalization, bureaucratization, and specialization. The ideology
of the medical profession is contrasted with that of the
patients. The authors predict that third party social controls will deprofessionalize the medical profession. (54)

2680   Budetti, P.B. "The ´Trickle-Down´ Theory--Is That Any Way
       To Make Policy?" AM J PUB HEALTH 74(12) (December 1984):
       1303-4.

       An editorial questioning government policy aimed at increas-
       ing the physician supply to rural and inner city areas. (5)

2681   Freidon, E. PROFESSION OF MEDICINE: A STUDY OF THE SOCIOLOGY
       OF APPLIED KNOWLEDGE. New York: Dodd, Mead & Co., 1970.

       Study of the concept of profession by means of a detailed
       analysis of medicine. The power of medicine stems partly
       from the knowledge and expertise of physicians and partly
       from structural factors. Questions are raised about the
       power of this profession. A classical work crucial to an
       understanding of professions and the health care delivery
       system.

2682   Hicks, L.L. "Social Policy Implications of Physician Shortage
       Areas in Missouri," AM J PUB HEALTH 71(10) (October 1981):
       116-24.

       A model is used to identify counties in Missouri in which
       the supply of physician services is inadequate to serve the
       resident population. In the model, a formula is used to
       assess the gap between the physician services available in a
       county and the visits which would be required to serve the
       residents. The model is applied to 1976 and 1981 data in
       order to analyze the changes which have occurred within the
       state during that time. The results show that in spite of a
       thirty-four percent increase in the number of physicians prac-
       ticing in Missouri between 1976 and 1981, twenty-four of the
       115 counties in the state experienced a decrease in their
       ability to serve their resident populations adequately. (15)

2683   McNutt, D.R. "GMENAC: Its Manpower Forecasting Framework,"
       AM J PUB HEALTH 71(10) (October 1981): 1116-24.

       Argues that the models developed in the Graduate Medical
       Educational National Advisory Committee Report may have signi-
       ficant utility in future human resource planning at both
       national and local levels. (46)

2684   Reinhardt, U.E. "The GMENAC Forecast: An Alternative View,"
       AM J PUB HEALTH 71(10) (October 1981): 1149-57.

       A response to McNutt. The article is both critical and
       complementary to the report and regards it as a catalyst for
       further thought and research and an advance in the state of
       art of health needs forecasting. (23)

2685 SUMMARY REPORT OF THE GRADUATE MEDICAL NATIONAL ADVISOR
      COMMITTEE, VOLS. 1-7. Washington, D.C.: U.S. Government
      Printing Office, HRA Pub. 81-65-657, 1980.

      Comprehensive study of medical education with recommenda-
      tions for medical educators. Key finding for nursing is a
      predicted future oversupply of physicians.

2686 Wilensky, G.R. and L.F. Rossiter. "The Relative Importance
      of Physician-Induced Demand in the Demand for Medical Care,"
      MILBANK MEMBORIAL QUARTERLY/HEALTH AND SOCIETY 61(6) (1983).

      The increase in the number of physicians entering practice
      in the 1980's will mean that expenditures for medical ser-
      vices will continue their rapid rise if physicians are able
      to induce demand for their services. This paper summarizes
      the empirical evidence regarding physician-induced demand.

NURSING SPECIALTIES

Overview

2687 Downs, F. and D. Brooten. NEW CAREERS IN NURSING. New York:
      Arco Publishing, Inc., 1983.

      An overview of nursing aimed at recruitment of candidates
      into the field. Describes the various levels of nursing and
      the alternative approaches to education and the work roles of
      nurses. Appendices list nursing journals and organizations.
      A resource for high school students and career guidance coun-
      selors.

      See 689, 721, 865, 2117, 2267, 2288.

Nursing Administration

2688 American Nurses' Association. ROLES, RESPONSIBILITIES, AND
      QUALIFICATIONS FOR NURSE ADMINISTRATORS. Kansas City, MO.:
      American Nurses' Association, Pub. No. NS-23, 1978.

      The ANA Commission on Nursing Services describes three
      levels of nursing administration, identifying the responsi-
      bilities characteristic of each level and the educational and
      experiential qualifications desirable for nurses functioning
      in these roles.

2689 _____. A GUIDE FOR NURSES CONSIDERING A CAREER MOVE IN
      NURSING ADMINISTRATION. Kansas City, MO.: American Nurses'
      Association, Pub. No. NS-26, 1979.

      Information developed by the ANA Commission on Nursing
      Services to assist nurse administrators in preparing for a
      position search and examining a prospective position. In-
      cludesquestions candidates should ask and those they should
      be prepared to answer. Selected references.

2690 Fine, R.B. "The Supply and Demand of Nursing Administrators,"
      NURS HEALTH CARE 4(1) (January 1983): 10-15.

      Discusses the need for master's degree preparation in nurs-
      ing administration. The problems of decreasing enrollments
      in nursing schools and job dissatisfaction among nurses in-
      dicate the need for well-prepared nursing administrators who
      are capable of planning new organizational structures and
      educational models. (33)

2691 Friss, L. "Organization Commitment and Job Involvement of
      Directors of Nursing Services," NURS ADM Q 7(2) (Winter
      1983): 1-10.

      Discusses the importance of directors of nursing services
      in the financial and professional success of hospitals.
      Reports the results of a research project which measured and
      analyzed organization commitment, job involvement, and back-
      ground characteristics of nursing directors. (17)

2692 Poulin, M.A. "The Nurse Executive Role: A Structural and
      Functional Analysis," J NURS ADM 14(2) (February 1984):
      9-14.

      A study of 12 nurse executives. (2)

Camp Nursing

2693 American Nurses' Association. STANDARDS FOR NURSING SERVICES
      IN CAMP SETTINGS. Kansas City, MO.: American Nurses' Asso-
      ciation, Pub. No. MCH-8, 1978.

      The ANA Commission on Nursing Services and the Washington
      State Nurses' Association define standards for nursing in camp
      settings to protect the welfare of children and to provide
      direction for nurses employed in camp settings.

Cancer Nursing

2694 American Nurses' Association. STANDARDS OF PEDIATRIC ONCOLOGY
      NURSING PRACTICE. Kansas City, MO.: American Nurses' Asso-
      ciation, Pub. No. MCH-9, 1978.

      The ANA Division on Maternal and Child Health Nursing Prac-
      tice and the Association of Pediatric Oncology Nurses define
      standards for pediatric oncology nursing practice to fulfill
      the profession's obligation to provide and improve the area of
      nursing practice that delivers direct service to children with
      cancer and their families.

2695 _____. OUTCOME STANDARDS FOR CANCER NURSING PRACTICE.
      Kansas City, MO.:American Nurses' Association, Pub. No.
      MS-10, 1979.

      Outcome standards developed by the ANA Division on Medical-
      Surgical Nursing Practice and the Oncology Nursing Society
      for cancer nursing practice as related to prevention and
      early detection, information, coping, comfort, nutrition,
      protective mechanisms, mobility, elimination, sexuality, and
      ventilation. Includes selected bibliography.

Cardiovascular Nursing

2696 American Nurses' Association. STANDARDS OF CARDIOVASCULAR
      NURSING PRACTICE. Kansas City, MO.: American Nurses' As-
      sociation, Pub. No. MS-4, 1981.

The ANA Division on Medical-Surgical Nursing Practice and
the American Heart Association Council on Cardiovascular Nursing define standards for cardiovascular nursing practice to
provide means for evaluating the quality of nursing care received by individuals who have known or predicted alteration
in cardiovascular physiologic function.

Community Health/Public Health Nursing

2697   American Nurses´ Association. STANDARDS OF COMMUNITY NURSING
       PRACTICE. Kansas City, MO.: American Nurses´ Association,
       Pub. No. CH-2, 1974.

       The ANA Division on Community Health Nursing Practice de-
       fines standards necessary for community health nursing prac-
       tice to fulfill the profession´s obligation to promote and
       preserve the health of populations.

2698   _____. A CONCEPTUAL MODEL OF COMMUNITY HEALTH NURSING.
       Kansas City, MO.: American Nurses´ Association, Pub. No.
       CH-10, 1980.

       Statement by the ANA Division on Community Health Nursing
       Practice describing assumptions and beliefs about this area of
       nursing practice, the scope of the practice, and the types of
       practitioners in this area.

2699   Barkauskas, V.H. "Effectiveness of Public Health Nurse Home
       Visits to Primarous Mothers and Their Infants," AM J PUBLIC
       HEALTH 73(5) (May 1983): 573-80.

       Study based on comparison of randomly selected mother-infant
       pairs who had received post partum home visits and those who
       had not received them. No significant differences were noted
       between home visited and not home visited mother infant pairs
       for the majority of health outcome variables. Major, dif-
       ferential health assets and liabilities between groups of
       Black and White mother infant pairs were observed. (18)

2700   Buhler-Wilkerson, K. and S. Reverby. "Can A Time Honored
       Model Solve the Dilemma of Public Health Nursing?" AM J
       PUBLIC HEALTH 74(10) (October 1984): 1081-83.

       Editorial in support of Dreher´s conclusion in article in
       same issue about the benefit of public health nurses providing
       both bedside and preventive care. (9)

2701   Dreher, M. "District Nursing: The Cost Benefits of a Popula-
       tion-Based Practice," AM J PUBLIC HEALTH 74(10) (October
       1984): 1107-11.

       Reports serendipitous findings from an ethnohistorical study
       of public health nursing in rural New England which purports
       to demonstrate that a traditional model of population based
       nursing holds great possibilities for dealing with the nation´s

current and future health problems, particularly health maintenance of the elderly and care of the chronically ill. The
model is examined for the extent to which it is accessible,
available, accountable, acceptable, comprehensive, coordinated
and cost effective and the policy implication of the model for
organization and financing of community health are explored.
(6)

2702 Goeppinger, J. "Primary Health Care: An Answer to the Dilem-
      mas of Community Nursing?" PUBLIC HEALTH NURS 1(3) (Septem-
      ber 1984): 129-40.

      Some issues that are salient to contemporary community nurs-
      ing practice, including goals, levels of practice, roles, and
      settings are presented. Different positions on each issue
      are discussed. The opportunities offered for resolution of
      these issues by the construct of primary health care, as de-
      fined by the World Health Organization (Director-General's
      Report, 1975), are emphasized. (34)

2703 Storfjell, J.L. and P.A. Cruise. "A Model of Community-
      Focused Nursing," PUBLIC HEALTH NURS 1(2) (June 1984): 85-96.

      Describes a study aimed at defining the primary underlying
      dimensions of perceived community-focused practice of com-
      munity health nursing. Three specific regions were identified
      and labeled: (1) client-oriented services, (2) aggregate needs
      identification, and (3) aggregate planning and intervention.
      (27)

Critical Care, Intensive Care Nursing

2704 Noble, M.A. THE ICU ENVIRONMENT: DIRECTIONS FOR NURSING.
      Englewood Cliffs, NJ.: Reston Publishing Co. (Prentice-Hall,
      Inc.), 1982.

      Emphasizes the psychological aspects of intensive care and
      the environment itself. Identifies the unique needs of the
      patients, families, and the staff involved in I.C. and makes
      concrete suggestions for modifying the environment.

2705 "The Organization of Human Resources in Critical Care Units,"
      FOCUS ON CRITICAL CARE 10(1) (February 1983): 43-44.

      Reports the requirement of the Joint Commission on Accredi-
      tation of Hospitals for a collaborative approach to management
      of the critical care units. The American Association of
      Critical Care Nurses and the Society of Critical Care Medicine
      have established an on-going interorganization liaison group.
      (2)

Emergency Nursing

2706 American Nurses' Association. STANDARDS OF EMERGENCY NURSING
      PRACTICE. Kansas City, MO.: American Nurses' Association,
      Pub. No. MS-5, 1975.

450   Nursing Specialties

The ANA Division on Medical-Surgical Nursing Practice and
the Emergency Department Nurses' Association define standards
for emergency nursing practice to provide a means for evaluating the quality of nursing care received by individuals of all
ages with perceived physical or emotional alterations that are
undiagnosed and may require prompt intervention.

Functional Nursing Roles--Patient Teaching,
Clinical Teaching, Advocate

2707   American Nurses' Association. THE REGISTERED NURSE CONSULTANT
       TO THE INTERMEDIATE CARE FACILITY. Kansas City, MO.:
       American Nurses' Association, Pub. No. GE-6, 1977.

       Part I is resource material prepared by the ANA Division on
       Gerontological Nursing Practice designed to assist the regis-
       tered nurse in understanding the role of consultant within the
       intermediate care setting and the process of employment in
       this role. Part II is designed to provide the registered nurse
       an opportunity for self-instruction in identified content areas
       to increase effectiveness in the consultant role. With selected
       bibliography.

2708   Caldera, K., R. Colangelo, M. DiBlasi, D. Garman, S. Kowalczyk,
       S. Mason, M. Murphy, A. Olsen, C. Orr and F. Ouellette.
       "Exploration of the Effects of Educational Level on the
       Nurse's Attitude Toward Discharge Planning," J NURS ED 19(8)
       (October 1980): 24-32.

       A survey of registered nurses working as staff nurses sought
       information regarding their perceptions of the percentage of
       hospital patients requiring discharge teaching, percentage of
       role involved in this task, and perceived discrepancy between
       individual and institutional importance of this task. The
       majority of the nurses indicated they felt most hospitalized
       patients require discharge teaching and most identified five
       minutes a day were spent in this task. No differences were
       found in the educational level of the respondents. (43)

2709   Dubrey, R.J. PROMOTING WELLNESS IN NURSING PRACTICE: A STEP-
       BY-STEP APPROACH TO PATIENT EDUCATION. St. Louis: C.V.
       Mosby Co., 1982.

       Helps nurses integrate patient education into their nursing
       practice by describing goals and objectives for fifteen fre-
       quently encountered health problems. Presents teaching plans
       in behaviorally stated objectives. Incorporates application
       of positive thinking, mental imagery, and affirmation.

2710   Hamric, A.B. and J. Spross (Eds.). THE CLINICAL NURSE SPECIAL-
       IST IN THEORY AND PRACTICE. New York: Grune and Stratton,
       1983.

Contributors present the roles, functions, and opportunities
of the clinical nurse specialist in acute care settings. Also
included are evaluation of the role and certain administrative
issues.

2711   Kohnke, M.F.   ADVOCACY: RISK AND REALITY.   St. Louis: C.V.
       Mosby Co., 1982.

Designed to provide students, faculty and practitioners with
concrete, applicable strategies to think, act, analyze, and
survive in the role of patient advocate.

2712   Redman, B.K.   THE PROCESS OF PATIENT EDUCATION, 5th Ed.   St.
       Louis: C.V. Mosby Co., 1984.

This is the fifth edition of a well-known text focused on
the process of patient education. Discusses the development
and management of the patient education function in health care
institutions. Examines the way patient education interacts
with health policy. Includes chapter summaries and study
questions.

Geriatrics/Gerontology

2713   American Nurses' Association.   NURSING AND LONG-TERM CARE:
       TOWARD QUALITY CARE FOR THE AGING.   Kansas City, MO.:
       American Nurses' Association, Pub. No. GE-4, 1975.

Based on a one year research project conducted by the ANA
Division on Gerontological Nursing Practice to determine the
problems of providing "skilled nursing," and the related problems of alternatives to institutional care, supply and training of qualified personnel, and methods of reimbursement for
quality care.

2714   _____.   STANDARDS OF GERONTOLOGICAL NURSING PRACTICE.
       Kansas City, MO.:   American Nurses' Association, Pub. No.
       GE-2, 1976.

The ANA Division on Gerontological Nursing Practice defines
standards for gerontological nursing practice based on the
premise that knowledge and theories of the aging process, when
applied to nursing practice, will improve the care of the
aged.

2715   _____.   A STATEMENT ON THE SCOPE OF GERONTOLOGICAL NURS-
       ING PRACTICE.   Kansas City, MO.: American Nurses' Associa-
       tion, Pub. No. GE-7, 1981.

The ANA Division on Gerontological Nursing Practice provides
a description of gerontological nursing and the types of
nurses in gerontological practice; includes educational preparation needed for various types of gerontological nursing
practice and implications for research in gerontological
nursing.

2716 _____. A CHALLENGE FOR CHANGE: THE ROLE OF GERONTOLO-
          GICAL NURSING. Kansas City, MO.: American Nurses' Associa-
          tion, Pub. No. GE-9, 1982.

          The ANA Division on Gerontological Nursing Practice presents
          a comprehensive analysis of gerontological nursing's contri-
          bution in providing quality health care for older citizens,
          emphasizing that positive action must be initiated now by and
          on behalf of America's older adults.

2717 Eliopoulos, C. "Self Care Model for Gerontological Nursing,"
          GERIATR NURS 5(8) (November/December 1984): 366-69.

          Using Orem's model, author has constructed a self care model
          for use by the gerontological nurse. (2)

2718 Feldbaum, E.G. and Feldbaum, M.B. "Caring for the Elderly:
          Who Dislikes it Least," J HEALTH, POLITICS, POLICY AND LAW 6
          (Spring 1981): 62-72.

          Study of student nurses and registered nurses who work with
          the aged indicate small percentage of either sample want to
          work with aged persons. Recommendations follow. (14)

2719 Gray, P.L. "Gerontological Nurse Specialist: Luxury or Neces-
          sity," AM J NURS 82 (January 1982): 82-85.

          A report on the results of the use of a GNS in a nursing
          home facility for one year. Concluded that quality of life of
          the residents was enhanced by active participation of a
          clinical nurse specialist. (2)

          See 682.

Maternal/Child Nursing

2720 American Nurses' Association. A STATEMENT ON THE SCOPE OF
          MATERNAL AND CHILD HEALTH NURSING PRACTICE. Kansas City,
          MO.: American Nurses' Association, Pub. No. MCH-10, 1980.

          Statement by the ANA Division on Maternal and Child Health
          Nursing Practice describes this area of nursing practice and
          the types of practitioners in it.

2721 _____. A STATEMENT ON THE SCOPE OF HIGH-RISK PERINATAL
          NURSING PRACTICE. Kansas City, MO.: American Nurses' As-
          sociation, Pub. No. MCH-12, 1980.

          The ANA Council of High-Risk Perinatal Nurses defines the
          role, characteristics, essential knowledge, skills, and pro-
          fessional responsibilities of today's high-risk perinatal
          nurse.

          See 1978.

Medical-Surgical Nursing

2722   American Nurses' Association. STANDARDS OF MEDICAL-SURGICAL
       NURSING PRACTICE. Kansas City, MO.: American Nurses' Asso-
       ciation, Pub. No. MS-1, 1974.

       The ANA Division on Medical-Surgical Nursing Practice de-
       fines standards for medical-surgical nursing practice to pro-
       vide a basic model by which the quality of medical-surgical
       nursing practice may be measured.

2723   _____. A STATEMENT ON THE SCOPE OF MEDICAL-SURGICAL NURSING
       PRACTICE. Kansas City, MO.: American Nurses' Association,
       Pub. No. MS-11, 1980.

       Statement by the ANA Division on Medical-Surgical Nursing
       Practice describing this area of nursing practice and the
       types of practitioners in it.

Neurological Nursing

2724   American Nurses' Association. STANDARDS OF NEUROLOGICAL AND
       NEUROSURGICAL NURSING PRACTICE. Kansas City, MO.: American
       Nurses' Association, Pub. No. MS-8, 1977.

       The ANA Division on Medical-Surgical Nursing Practice and
       the Association of Neurosurgical Nurses define standards for
       neurological and neurosurgical nursing practice to provide a
       means of evaluating the quality of nursing care received by
       individuals who have biopsychosocial alterations due to ner-
       vous system dysfunction.

Nurse Anesthetist

2725   "AANA Membership Survey Results--Fiscal Year 1984," AANA J 52
       (February 1984): 33-40.

       Responses from 16,782 certified registered nurse anesthetist
       members of the American Association of Nurse Anesthetists.
       Most were employed by a hospital, a university, or they worked
       a group practice with anesthesiologists. Most salaries were
       between $25,000 and $40,000. (0)

2726   Cavagnaro, Sr. Mary. "A Comparison Study of Stress Factors As
       They Affect CRNAs," AANA J 51 (June 1983): 290-94.

       Stressors, satisfaction and methods of dealing with stress
       among CRNAs and registered nurses working in critical care
       units compared. (6)

2727   Hirsch, R., W. Forrest, F. Orkin and H. Wollman. HEALTH CARE
       DELIVERY IN ANESTHESIA. Philadelphia: George F. Stickley
       Co., 1980.

Proceedings of a symposium on anesthesia held November, 1977
in Washington, D.C. The object was to define the present
status and future needs of research in anesthesia.

2728   Verville, R.E. "Washington Scene: Congress Passes Nurse Anes-
       thetist 'Pass Through' Amendment on June 27," AANA J 52
       (August 1984): 456-60.

       Amendments to DRG prospective payment provisions of Medicare
       allow nurse anesthetist payments. (0)

       See 720, 745, 2322, 2363.

Nurse-Midwifery

2729   Baxter, L. "Nurse Midwifery Practice: Evolution of Stan-
       dards," J NURSE MIDWIFE 29(6) (November/December 1984):
       351-52.

       Editorial reports a lack of consensus on which procedures
       nurse midwives carry out. (3)

2730   Demkowski, A. "Future Prospects of Nurse Midwifery in the
       United States," J NURSE MIDWIFE 27(2) (March/April 1982):
       9-15.

       Evaluates the future prospects of the nurse-midwifery pro-
       fession by considering factors which support growth as well as
       those which limit advances in the profession. Consumer pre-
       ference for nurse-midwives over physicians is discussed in the
       context of cost containment and the possible effects of a
       physician oversupply. Reimbursement policy, legislation af-
       fecting nurse-midwives, and the contribution to public policy
       goals of nurse midwifery are also covered. (26)

2731   Langwell, K.M., S.D. Wilson, R.T. Deane, R.A. Black and K.F.
       Chin. "Geographic Distribution of Certified Nurse-mid-
       wives," J NURSE MIDWIFE 25(6) (November/December 1980):
       3-11.

       Reports the findings of a study which surveyed the distri-
       bution of nurse-midwives in the U.S. (1)

2732   Meglan, M.C. and H.V. Burst. "Nurse-Midwives Make A Dif-
       ference," NURS OUTLOOK 22 (June 1974): 386-89. Reprinted in
       EXPANDING HORIZONS FOR NURSES. Edited by B. Bullough and V.
       Bullough. New York: Springer Publishing Co., 1977, pp.
       49-54.

       A report on the use of nurse midwives in one target Missis-
       sippi county and their effect in reducing infant mortality.
       (6)

2733   "Nurse Midwives Attract Well-Informed Patients," AORN J 35(7)
       (June 1982): 1418-22.

Comments that the nurse midwife's philosophy about pregnancy and childbirth attracts a well-informed, articulate kind of patient who wants to participate in decisions about her care. Nurse midwives have become increasingly popular and there has been friction with their physician colleagues. (0)

2734   Research and Statistics Committee, American College of Nurse-Midwives. NURSE-MIDWIFERY IN THE UNITED STATES: 1982. Washington, D.C.: American College of Nurse-Midwives, 1984.

Report of 1982 survey of certified nurse midwives. Indicates number of nurse midwives in clinical practice has increased dramatically since 1968.

2735   Roush, R.E. "The Development of Midwifery--Male and Female, Yesterday and Today," J NURSE MIDWIFE 24(3) (May/June 1979): 27-37.

Provides an historical perspective to the development of the modern, certified nurse-midwife. Also includes information about the current status of the midwife, and emphasizes the high quality infant and maternal health care provided by midwives. (29)

2736   Sharp, E.S. and L.E. Lewis. "A Decade of Nurse-Midwifery Practice in a Tertiary University-Affiliated Hospital," J NURSE MIDWIFE 29(6) (November/December 1984): 353-65.

A ten year review of nurse-midwifery practice at Grady Memorial Hospital in Atlanta. Two models of care are described: comprehensive and episodic. Changes in practice over the ten year span are also described. (40)

2737   Sullivan, D. and R. Beeman. "Four Years' Experience With Home Birth by Licensed Midwives in Arizona," AM J PUBLIC HEALTH 6 (June 1984): 641-45.

During four years of program, three percent of home birth clients were hospitalized for complications and another 15 percent received postnatal outpatient care, primarily for second degree lacerations. Five percent of newborns required medical care after delivery and half of these were hospitalized. Complications declined over the four year period due to increased experience, close supervision, and continuing education. (6)

2738   Tom, S. "Nurse Midwifery: A Developing Profession," LAW, MED HEALTH CARE 10(6) (December 1982): 262-66, 282.

An overview of the recent nurse midwifery movement in U.S., including discussion of legal status, quality of care, cost effectiveness, and a list of references. (39)

See 731, 779, 792, 887, 897.

2739 American Nurses' Association. STANDARDS OF PERIOPERATIVE
      NURSING PRACTICE. Kansas City, MO.: American Nurses' Asso-
      ciation, Pub. No. MS-2, 1981.

      The ANA Division of Medical-Surgical Nursing Practice and
      the Association of Operating Room Nurses define standards re-
      lated to nursing practice for individuals who are experiencing
      surgical intervention; encompasses preoperative assessment and
      preparation, intraoperative intervention, and postoperative
      evaluation.

2740 Mailhot, C. and J.L. Biner. "The Operating Room: A Complex
      Challenge for the Nurse Administrator," J NURS ADM 14(4)
      (April 1984): 11-16.

      Overview of current operating room processes and issues. (5)

Orthopedic Nursing

2741 American Nurses' Association. STANDARDS OF ORTHOPEDIC NURS-
      ING PRACTICE. Kansas City, MO.: American Nurses' Associa-
      tion, Pub. No. MS-3, 1975.

      The ANA Division on Medical-Surgical Nursing Practice and
      the Orthopedic Nurses' Association define standards for ortho-
      pedic nursing practice to provide a means for evaluating the
      quality of nursing care received by individuals with known or
      predicted neuro-musculo-skeletal alterations.

Pediatric Nursing

2742 American Nurses' Association. NURSING CARE MODELS FOR ADOLES-
      CENT FAMILIES. Kansas City, MO.: American Nurses' Associa-
      tion, Pub. No. MCH-14, 1984.

      Tells what nurses are doing now about prenatal care for
      adolescents, childbirth and parenting education, care of the
      adolescent family following birth, and nursing research re-
      lated to adolescent pregnancy.

2743 Beal, J. ISSUES AND ADVANCED PRACTICE IN PEDIATRIC NURSING.
      Englewood Cliffs, NJ.: Reston Publishing Co. (Prentice-Hall,
      Inc.), 1983.

      A compilation of unique practice situations that describe
      problem solving and/or the mechanics of practice in areas
      specific to pediatric nursing.

2744 Chinn, P.L. and K.B. Leonard (Eds.). CURRENT PRACTICE IN
      PEDIATRIC NURSING. St. Louis: C.V. Mosby Co., 1980.

      Sixteen nurses write on three topics: developmental changes
      that affect the family, physical and physiological problems
      of children affecting their self concept, and on the expanded
      role of nurses.

Psychiatric, Mental Health Nursing

2745 American Nurses´ Association. PROFESSIONAL DEVELOPMENT IN
      PSYCHIATRIC AND MENTAL HEALTH NURSING. Kansas City, MO.:
      American Nurses´ Association, Pub. No. PMH-2, 1975.

      A collection of 13 papers presented at the 1974 and 1975
      conferences sponsored by the Council of Advanced Practitioners
      in Psychiatric and Mental Health Nursing, dealing with
      specialist certification, legislative issues, and practice and
      research.

2746 _____. STATEMENT ON PSYCHIATRIC AND MENTAL HEALTH NURSING
      PRACTICE. Kansas City, MO.: American Nurses´ Association,
      Pub. No. PMH-3, 1976.

      Statement by the ANA Division on Psychiatric and Mental
      Health Nursing Practice defining psychiatric nursing and its
      interrelationships, in keeping with the contemporary scope and
      roles of practice. Includes selected bibliography.

2747 _____. STANDARDS OF PSYCHIATRIC-MENTAL HEALTH NURSING PRAC-
      TICE. Kansas City, MO.: American Nurses´ Association, Pub.
      No. PHM-1, 1982.

      The ANA Division on Psychiatric and Mental Health Nursing
      Practice defines standards for psychiatric and mental health
      nursing practice.

2748 Koldjeski, D. COMMUNITY MENTAL HEALTH NURSING: NEW DIRECTIONS
      IN THEORY AND PRACTICE. New York: John Wiley & Sons, Inc.,
      1984.

      Presents a conceptual framework for community mental health
      nursing and synthesizes concepts and principles from nursing
      and social psychology theories and integrates with the basic
      science concepts. A new model of community mental health
      nursing is created that can be used to organize and guide
      preventions and interventions with population groups having
      different mental health needs.

2749 Lewis, A. and J. Levy. PSYCHIATRIC LIAISON NURSING: THE
      THEORY AND CLINICAL PRACTICE. Englewood Cliffs, NJ.: Reston
      Publishing Co. (Prentice-Hall, Inc.), 1982.

      Develops a theoretical model of psychiatric liaison nursing
      and uses many clinical examples to show its application to
      nursing practice. Discusess the process of role creation and
      implementation, goals of practice, and "diagnosing the total
      consultation." Suitable both for psychiatric liaison nursing
      students and for clinicians presently in practice.

2750 Smoyak, S.A. and S. Rouslin (Eds.). A COLLECTION OF CLASSICS
      IN PSYCHIATRIC NURSING LITERATURE. Thorofare, NJ.: Slack,
      Inc., 1982.

A selection of thirty-seven articles written by the
luminaries in psychiatric nursing. Authors include the two
editors, as well as A.L. Crawford, D.E. Gregg, M. Leininger,
C.M. Norris, H.E. Peplau, and others. Includes early, unpublished papers and articles written before psychiatric nursing
journals were established. Provides a sense of the field's
early history.

2751   Upton, D. with contributors. MENTAL HEALTH CARE AND NATIONAL
       HEALTH INSURANCE: A PHILOSOPHY OF AND AN APPROACH TO MENTAL
       HEALTH CARE FOR THE FUTURE. New York: Plenum Publishing,
       1983.

       An evaluation of the issues, problems, and controversies in-
       volved in insuring mental health care under national health
       insurance as well as under existing insurance programs.

Rehabilitation Nursing

2752   American Nurses' Association. STANDARDS OF REHABILITATION
       NURSING PRACTICE. Kansas City, MO.: American Nurses' Asso-
       ciation, Pub. No. MS-9, 1977.

       The Division on Medical-Surgical Nursing Practice and the
       Association of Rehabilitation Nurses define standards for
       rehabilitation nursing practice to provide a means of
       evaluating the quality of nursing care received by individuals
       who have an illness or a disability that interrupts or alters
       their physiological function.

2753   Rubin, J. and V. LaPorte (Eds.). ALTERNATIVES IN REHABILI-
       TATING THE HANDICAPPED. New York: Human Sciences Press,
       1982.

       The broad range of viewpoints offered in this work form a
       chronicle of the changes that rehabilitation for the handicap-
       ped is undergoing in the 1980s.

Rheumatology Nursing

2754   American Nurses' Association. OUTCOME STANDARDS FOR RHEUMA-
       TOLOGY NURSING PRACTICE. Kansas City, MO.: American Nurses'
       Association, Pub. No. MS-12, 1983.

       Reflects current knowledge in rheumatology nursing practice,
       focuses on patient outcomes, directed toward helping indivi-
       duals and their families cope with changes imposed by disease
       processes.

School Nursing

2755   American Nurses' Association. SCHOOL NURSES WORKING WITH
       HANDICAPPED CHILDREN. Kansas City, MO.: American Nurses'
       Association, Pub. No. NP-60, 1975.

Statement of the ANA Division on Practice, the American
School Health Association, and the National Association of
School Nurses in response to PL 94-142, the Education for All
Handicapped Children Act of 1975.

2756 _____ STANDARDS OF SCHOOL NURSING PRACTICE. Kansas City,
MO.: American Nurses' Association, Pub. No. NP-66, 1983.

Guidelines supporting the purpose of school nursing, which
is "to enhance the educational process by the modification or
removal of health-related barriers to learning and by promotion of an optimal level of wellness," includes rationale and
structure-process-outcome criteria.

See 724.

Urologic Nursing

2757 American Nurses' Association. STANDARDS OF UROLOGIC NURSING
PRACTICE. Kansas City, MO.: American Nurses' Association,
Pub. No. MS-7, 1977.

The ANA Division on Medical-Surgical Nursing Practice and
the American Urological Association, Allied, define standards
for urologic nursing practice to provide a means of evaluating
the quality of nursing care received by individuals with known
or predicted genitourinary system alterations.

Specialization—Nurse Practitioners

2758 Abdellah, F.G. "The Nurse Practitioner 17 Years Later:
Present and Emerging Issues," INQUIRY 19(2) (Summer 1982):
105-16.

Provides an overview of the present and future issues confronting the nurse practitioner. Nearly two decades after es-
tablishment of the first nurse practitioner program, the nurse
practitioner is a strong figure contributing greatly to the
health care team. Four complex issues are identified as affecting the expansion of the role of the nurse practitioner.
(37)

2759 American Academy of Nursing. PRIMARY CARE BY NURSES: SPHERE
OF RESPONSIBILITY AND ACCOUNTABILITY. Kansas City, MO.:
American Nurses' Association, Pub. No. G-127, 1977.

Papers presented at the 1976 Scientific Session of the
American Academy of Nursing deal with primary care, the role
of nurses in primary care, and the need for education at the
baccalaureate level for primary care nurses.

2760 American Academy of Nursing. PRIMARY CARE IN A PLURALISTIC
SOCIETY: IMPEDIMENTS TO HEALTH CARE DELIVERY. Kansas City,
MO.: American Nurses' Association, Pub. No. G-133, 1978.

A monograph containing papers dealing with the impact of
legal, political, economic, and control factor issues in
primary care nursing. Proceedings of the 1977 Scientific Session of the American Academy of Nursing.

2761 American Nurses´ Association. THE PRIMARY HEALTH CARE NURSE
      PRACTITIONER. Kansas City, MO.: American Nurses´ Associa-
      tion, Pub. No. NP-61, 1980.

      Statement by the ANA Council of Primary Health Care Nurse
      Practitioners describing concepts, educational preparation,
      and practice characteristics of primary health care nurse
      practitioners.

2762 American Nurses´ Association and National Association of
      Pediatric Nurse Associates and Practitioners. NURSE PRAC-
      TITIONERS: A REVIEW OF THE LITERATURE 1965-1982. Kansas
      City, MO.: American Nurses´ Association, 1983.

      A second edition of a comprehensive review of the nurse
      practitioner literature by the Council of Primary Health Care
      Nurse Practitioners of the American Nurses ´ Association and
      The National Association of Pediatric Nurse Associates and
      Practitioners. Citations are grouped into four major cate-
      gories: demography, attitudes and acceptance, impact studies,
      and the psychosocial aspects of the nurse practitioner role.

2763 Billingsley, M.C. et al. "The Extinction of the Nurse Prac-
      titioner: Threat or Reality?" NURSE PRACT 7(9) (October
      1982): 22-23, 26-27, 30.

      Addresses the most serious obstacles facing nurse practi-
      tioners. Among these are: role identity and clinical practice,
      multiple entry levels, multiple titles, consumer awareness,
      energy depletion, legal constraints, reimbursement, physician
      oversupply, and territorial constraints. (12)

2764 Bliss, A.A. and E.D. Cohen (Eds.). THE NEW HEALTH PROFES-
      SIONALS. Germantown, MD.: Aspen Systems Corp., 1977.

      Comprehensive overview of the history, role, legal situ-
      ation, and the issues surrounding nurse practitioners and
      physician´s assistants. Fifty-nine contributors in addition
      to the two editors.

      See 786, 796.

2765 Brown, B.S. "MN for NPs?" PED NURS 6(3) (May/June 1980): 7.

      Editorial discusses pros and cons of master´s degree for
      preparation of nurse practitioners. (2)

2766 Browning, M.H. and D.P. Lewis. THE EXPANDED ROLE OF THE
      NURSE. New York: The American Journal of Nursing Co., 1973.

Reprints of early articles about nurse practitioners, nurses in other expanded roles.

2767   Bullough, B., H. Sultz, O.M.Henry and R. Fiedler. "Trends in Pediatric Nurse Practitioner Education and Employment," PED NURS 10(3) (May/June 1984): 193-96.

Summary of trends related to pediatric nurse practitioners from the three longitudinal studies of nurse practitioners done at the State University of New York-Buffalo. (9)

2768   Bullough, B. "Barriers to the Nurse Practitioner Movement: Problems of Women in a Woman's Field," INT J HEALTH SCIENCE 5 (1975): 2. Reprinted in EXPANDING HORIZONS FOR NURSES. Edited by B. Bullough and V. Bullough. New York: Springer Publishing Co., 1977, pp. 307-18.

The problem of a woman in a woman's field or how coping mechanisms adopted to cope in the male world sometimes work against nurses. (30)

2769   Burns, C.E. and M.K. Thompson. "Developing A Nursing Diagnosis Classification System for PNPs," PED NURS 10(6) (November/December 1984): 411-14.

A nursing diagnosis system incorporating ambulatory pediatric nursing problems and medical diagnoses can aid pediatric nurse practitioners in assessment and intervention as well as delineate their scope of practice. (10)

2770   Butler, C. "The 1983 NAPNAP Membership Survey," PED NURS 10(3) (May/June 1984): 187-90.

In 1983, memberships surveys were mailed to 2,636 NAPNAP members. Approximately fifty-one percent of the members responded. The results describing educational, employment, and salary characteristics of NAPNAP members are presented in this article. (7)

2771   Calkin, J.D. "A Model for Advanced Nursing Practice," J NURS ADM 14(1) (January 1984): 24-30.

A model and a definition of advanced nursing practice and conditions influencing employment of advanced nurse practitioners is presented. (8)

2772   Chen, S.C., V.H. Barkauskas, V.M. Ohlson and E.H. Chen. "Health Problems Encountered by Nurse Practitioners and Physicians," NURS RES 31(3) (May/June 1982): 163-69.

Proportional samples from a total of 39,243 patient visits from sixteen ambulatory care clinics over an eighteen week period indicated that distribution of health problems differed between nurse practitioners and physicians in each clinic. (15)

2773   Committee to Study Extended Roles for Nurses. EXTENDING THE
       SCOPE OF NURSING PRACTICE: SUMMARY AND RECOMMENDATIONS.
       Washington, D.C.: U.S. Government Printing Office, November
       1971, pp. 4-12. Reprinted in EXPANDING HORIZONS FOR NURSES.
       Edited by B. Bullough and V. Bullough. New York: Springer
       Publishing Co., 1977, pp. 12-23.

       An abstract of the 1971 government report which recommended
       that nurses assume more of the tasks associated with the
       primary care of the patient. (0)

2774   Cruikshank, B.M. and T.J. Clow. "Current Status of PNP Educa-
       tion," PED NURS 5(1) (January/February 1980): 9-13.

       Reports data from 1978 survey of pediatric nurse practi-
       tioner educational program. Although common guidelines and
       goals exist, length of programs vary. (12)

2775   Dickenson-Hazard, N. "PNP/A Education of the ´80s," PED NURS
       9(5) (September/October 1983): 335-38, 381.

       The educational preparation of pediatric nurse practi-
       tioners/associates (PNPs/As) has changed since its inception
       in the 1960s. But how has this education changed? And is
       PNP/A education in the 1980s reflected in the certification
       process of the ´80s?

2776   Diers, D. and S. Molde. "Nurses In Primary Care: The New
       Gatekeepers," AM J NURS 83(5) (May 1983): 742-45.

       Primary care given by nurses is different than that given by
       physicians. (11)

2777   Edmunds, M. "Do Nurse Practitioners Still Practice Nursing?"
       NURSE PRACT 9(5) (May 1984): 47, 51.

       Author argues that eight major nursing behaviors constitute
       the nursing component of the nurse practitioner role. (11)

2778   Enggist, R.E. and M.E. Hatcher. "Factors Influencing Consumer
       Receptivity to the Nurse Practitioner," J MEDICAL SYSTEMS
       7(6) (December 1983): 495-512.

       The significance of socio demographic, cognitive attitudinal
       and clinical/medical factors are examined as they influence
       acceptance of the nurse practitioner. (36)

2779   Hallman, E.C. and D. Westlund. "Canadian Nurse Practitioners
       Battle Underutilization," NURSE PRACT 8(6) (June 1983): 45-
       46, 48.

       Initially, nurse practitioners in both Canada and the United
       States were trained to meet physician shortages. This shor-
       tage no longer exists. The issue of optimally utilizing well-
       prepared nurse practitioners is complex and involves physi-
       cian resistance, lack of government initiative and nurses´

attitudes. Isolated examples do exist where nurse practitioners are accepted, cost-effective, competent and well-
utilized. However, many nurse practitioners find it difficult
to practice independently in most urban centers. (27)

2780   Harper, D.C. and M.C. Billingsley. "Organizing for Power,"
       NURSE PRACT (July/August 1983): 24, 26, 28, 30, 33.

       Urges a strong national organization for nurse practitioners.
       Suggests alternatives: restructuring the American Nurses' As-
       sociation Council of Primary Health Care Nurse Practitioners,
       establishing an autonomous organization, an organization af-
       filiated with a medical group, or a network of existing local
       practitioner groups. Advantages and disadvantages of each
       discussed. (10)

2781   Hawkins, J.B.W. and J.A. Thibodeau. THE NURSE PRACTITIONER:
       CURRENT PRACTICE ISSUES. New York: The Tiresias Press,
       Inc., 1983.

       An overview of current issues facing nurse practitioners,
       including sex role stereotyping, power, change, quality as-
       surance, research, the economics of the expanded role, and
       the law as it relates to nurse practitioners. The historical
       background of each issue is reviewed to put current problems
       in context. References and/or bibliography at the end of
       each chapter.

2782   Hayden, M.L., L.R. Davies and E.R. Clore. "Facilitators and
       Inhibitors of the Emergency Nurse Practitioner Role," NURS
       RES 31(5) (September/October 1982): 294-99.

       Sixty-eight respondents provided data about motivating fac-
       tors influencing the decision to seek ENP education and sub-
       sequent job acceptance; current employment status, role con-
       cept, performance and autonomy; and barriers to practice.
       (14)

2783   Hogan, K.A. and R.A. Hogan. "Assessment of the Consumer's
       Potential Response to the Nurse Practitioner Model," J NURS
       ED 21(9) (November 1983): 4-12.

       A survey of employees at Illinois State University revealed
       that respondents would permit nurse practitioners to perform
       traditional nursing roles but these subjects were less accep-
       tant of expanded role activities. Individuals who had
       received nurse practitioner treatment reported a 90 percent
       rate of satisfaction with the services rendered. (14)

2784   Kotthoff, M.E. "In Nursing in the United States: The Primary
       Health Care Nurse Practitioner," INT NURS REV 28(1) (1981):
       24-28.

       Describes health care delivery system in U.S. as it related
       to the development of the primary health care nurse practi-
       tioner. Describes the role of the nurse practitioner. (10)

2785 Kussman, R. "Legal Responsibilities of 'Independent' Pediat-
      ric Nurse Practitioner: Letter to Editor," NE J MED (August
      19, 1978): 316.

      A physician's letter to the editor concerning the liability
      of pediatric nurse practitioners. (0)

2786 Lurie, E.E. "Nurse Practitioners: Issues in Professional
      Socialization," J HEALTH SOCIAL BEHAVIOR 22(1) (March 1981):
      31-48.

      Examines the professional socialization of nurse practi-
      tioners using three theoretical models, none of which fully
      explained the process. The subjects progressed through a two
      step process: formal socialization during the educational
      process and a resocialization on the job. (52)

2787 Munroe, D., J. Pohl, H.H. Gardner and R.E. Bell. "Prescribing
      Patterns of Nurse Practitioners," AM J NURS 82(10) (October
      1982): 1538-47.

      Report of study of the prescribing patterns of six nurse
      practitioners/clinical specialists in one Detroit hospital.
      Prescriptions were consistent with written protocols and
      seemed appropriate. (9)

2788 Nelms, B.C. and R.G. Mullins. "Evolution of Holistic Practice
      in Nurse Practitioners," PED NURS 6(5) (September/October
      1980): 27-31.

      Reports research of changing orientation of nurse practi-
      tioner students during the educational process with an early
      emphasis on the biological aspects of care and a later
      emphasis on the psychosocial aspects. (11)

2789 Noonan, B. "Eight Years in a Medical Nurse Clinic," AM J
      NURS 72 (June 1972): 1128-30. Reprinted in EXPANDING HORI-
      ZONS FOR NURSES. Edited by B. Bullough and V. Bullough.
      New York: Springer Publishing Co., 1977, pp. 34-38.

      Reports the establishment of a Medical Nurse Clinic at Mas-
      sachusetts General Hospital in 1962. Of historical interest.
      Noonan one of the first nurse practitioners. (0)

2790 O'Shea, J.S. and E.W. Collins (Eds.). EFFECTIVENESS OF PEDI-
      ATRIC PRIMARY CARE. Lexington, MA.: The Collamore Press,
      1984.

      A critical assessment of the effectiveness of pediatric
      primary care. The first part examines the issue with regard
      to providers; pediatricians-in-training and fully trained
      pediatricians, family practitioners, pediatric nurse practi-
      tioners, and child health associates. The second part is
      concerned with effectiveness in relation to location: the
      hospital, neighborhood health centers, health maintenance
      organizations, private fee-for-service facilities, and the

telephone. The twenty contributors to the book examine the
issues, assess current methods of treatment and referral, and
point to areas where pediatric primary care could be improved.

2791 Poole, A.L. and S.R. Poole. "The Nurse Practitioner Role in
    Adolescent Health Care," NURSE PRACT 8(9) (October 1983):
    43-44, 46-47, 54.

    This study describes the 12,414 health care problems of
    3,657 adolescent patients visiting twelve family practices
    over a one-year period. Age-sex distribution, visiting pat-
    terns and all categories of morbidity are described for
    patients between thirteen and twenty years of age. Signifi-
    cant sex differences and differences among early, middle and
    late adolescents are also described. This paper proposes
    the need for a competency-based curriculum for NP students and
    offers a list of topics to form the core of such a curriculum.
    (13)

2792 Powers, M.J., A. Jalowiec and P.A. Reichelt. "Nurse Practi-
    tioners and Physician Care Compared for Nonurgent Emergency
    Room Patients," NURSE PRACT 9(2) (February 1984): 39-42, 44,
    45, 48, 52.

    A study of sixty-two emergency room patients who were cared
    for by either a nurse practitioner or a physician. Compliance
    was similar in the two groups but satisfaction with care was
    higher in the nurse practitioner group. (18)

2793 Ramsay, J.A., J.K. McKenzie and D.G. Fish. "Physicians and
    Nurse Practitioners: Do They Provide Equivalent Health
    Care?" AM J PUBLIC HEALTH 72(1) (January 1982): 55-57.

    Data from forty patients attending a hypertension clinic
    staffed by physicians were compared to data from forty
    patients attending a hypertension clinic staffed by nurses
    over a period of fifteen months. Nurses appeared to have more
    success in handling obesity and to achieve better control of
    hypertension. (8)

2794 "Readers Support National Nurse Practitioner Organization,"
    NURSE PRACT (June 1983): 39.

    A survey of nurse practitioner opinion about a potential
    national nurse practitioner organization. (1)

2795 Record, J.C., M. McCally, S.O. Schweitzer, R.M. Blomquest and
    B.D. Berger. "New Health Professions After a Decade and a
    Half: Delegation, Productivity and Costs in Primary Care,"
    J HEALTH POLITICS, POLICY AND LAW 5(3) (Fall 1980): 470-97.

    Summarizes the development of nurse practitioners and
    physician's assistants from the mid-1960's to the present.
    Concludes that nurse practitioners and physician's assistants
    work at high levels of productivity and cost-effectiveness.
    (66)

2796   Rhein, R. "Nurses: Colleagues or Competitors," MEDICAL WORLD
       NEWS 20(14) (July 1979): 65-77.

       Looks at nurse practitioners practicing throughout the U.S.
       from a legal standpoint and as they relate to physicians. (0)

2797   Robyn, D. and J. Hadley. "National Health Insurance and the
       New Health Occupations: Nurse Practitioners and Physicians'
       Assistants," J HEALTH POLITICS, POLICY AND LAW 5 (Fall
       1980): 447-69.

       A discussion of the impact of nurse practitioners and phy-
       sician's assistants on national health insurance and other
       legislation. (43)

2798   Rogers, M. "Nursing: To Be or Not Be," NURS OUTLOOK 20
       (January 1972): 42-46. Reprinted in EXPANDING HORIZONS FOR
       NURSES. Edited by B. Bullough and V. Bullough. New York:
       Springer Publishing Co., 1977, pp. 24-32.

       Urges nursing to present a united front in expanding nursing
       horizons. Nurses are urged to take leadership in evolving
       planning and implementing creative community health services,
       and to avoid the temptation to become nurse practitioners. (6)

2799   Roos, P.D. and M. Crooker. "Variables Affecting Nurse Practi-
       tioner Salaries," NURSE PRACT 8(5) (May 1983): 36, 38, 41-
       42, 44.

       The salaries of 249 graduates of a nurse practitioner pro-
       gram were subjected to a regression analysis. It was found
       that the most important factor affecting salaries is the type
       of practice setting, although educational and geographic vari-
       ables and the length of time the graduate has been an NP also
       have some impact. (9)

2800   Sackett, D.L., W.O. Spitzer, M. Gent. R.S. Roberts et al.
       "The Burlington Randomized Trial of the Nurse Practitioner:
       Health Outcomes of Patients," ANNALS OF INTERNAL MEDICINE
       80 (February 1974): 137-42. Reprinted in EXPANDING HORIZONS
       FOR NURSES. Edited by B. Bullough and V. Bullough. New
       York: Springer Publishing Co., 1977, pp. 55-66.

       Report on a randomized trial comparison of patients treated
       by nurse practitioners vs. more conventional family physicians
       in Burlington, Ontario, Canada. Results argue for effective-
       ness and safety in nurse practitioners as provider of primary
       clinical services. (12)

2801   Scheffler, R.M., S.G. Yoder, N. Weisfeld and G. Ruby. "Phy-
       sicians and New Health Practitioners: Issues for the
       1980's," INQUIRY 16(3) (Fall 1979): 195-229.

       Discusses the federal government's role in developing nurse
       practitioners and physician's assistants and examines the
       major issues of the past and present related to these two

types of health care providers. Concludes that the possibility of an oversupply of physicians exists, and that such
an oversupply would have serious implications for the future
role of nurse practitioners and physician's assistants. (214)

2802 Schorr, T.M. "Editorial: Is That Name Necessary?" AM J NURS 74
      (February 1974): 235. Reprinted in EXPANDING HORIZONS FOR
      NURSES. Edited by B. Bullough and V. Bullough. New York:
      Springer Publishing Co., 1977, pp. 33-34.

      A discussion of the term "nurse practitioner". (0)

2803 Silver, H., L.C. Ford and L.R. Day. "The Pediatric Nurse
      Practitioner Program," J AMER MED ASSOC 204 (1968): 298-302.
      Reprinted in EXPANDING HORIZONS FOR NURSES. Edited by B.
      Bullough and V. Bullough. New York: Springer Publishing
      Co., 1977, pp. 39-48.

      A description of the pediatric nurse practitioner program
      developed at the University of Colorado through a joint ef-
      fort of the Department of Pediatrics of the School of Medicine
      and the School of Nursing. (7)

2804 Smith, D.W. and S.L. Shamansky. "Determining the Market for
      Family Nurse Practitioner Services: The Seattle Experience,"
      NURS RES 32(5) (September/October 1983): 301-305.

      A sample of Seattle residents found that 27.3 percent of the
      respondents intended to use nurse practitioners; evidence
      suggests potential users are primarily women who are rela-
      tively more affluent, better educated, and younger than
      general population. (17)

2805 Spitzer, W.D. "The Nurse Practitioner: Slow Death of a Good
      Idea," NE J MED 310(16) (April 9, 1984): 1049-51.

      An editorial which looks at where the nurse practitioner
      movement in North America is at the present time.

2806 Streff, M.B. and C.E. Streff. "The Counselling Dimension of
      the Nurse Practitioner," PED NURS 8(1) (Janury/February
      1982): 9-13.

      Counselling is an integral part of the pediatric nurse prac-
      titioner's practice. The process for counselling a child,
      adolescent, or parent has several distinct phases; these
      phases may be implemented in a single session or in several
      contacts in the practice setting, depending on the specific
      protocol in that setting. This article presents the counsel-
      ling process and a clinical application. (3)

2807 Sullivan, J.A. "Research on Nurse Practitioners: Process
      Behind the Outcome?" AM J PUBLIC HEALTH 72(1) (January
      1982): 8-9.

An editorial arguing that nurse practitioners show an un-
canny ability to not only provide primary care equivalent to
that of physicians but to offer something special that increases adherence. (9)

2808   Deleted.

2809   Deleted.

2810   Deleted.

2811   Sultz, H.A., M. Zielezny and L. Kinyon. LONGITUDINAL STUDY
       OF NURSE PRACTITIONERS, PHASE I. Bethesda, MD.: U.S. Depar-
       tment of Health, Education and Welfare, DHEW Pub. No. (HRA)
       76-43, March, 1976.

       A study sponsored by the Division of Nursing. Phase I des-
       cribes the nurse practitioner educational programs in opera-
       tion in 1973 and the characteristics of the students enrolled
       in those programs.

2812   Sultz, H.A., M. Zielezny, J.M. Gentry and L. Kinyon. LONGI-
       TUDINAL STUDY OF NURSE PRACTITIONERS, PHASE II. Hyatts-
       ville, MD.: U.S. Department of Health, Education and Welfare.
       DHEW Pub. No. 78-92, September, 1978.

       The second phase of the study follows the cohort of nurse
       practitioner students identified in the 1973 sample after
       graduation to determine their subsequent employment and their
       impact on the health care delivered in the settings they moved
       into.

2813   _____. LONGITUDINAL STUDY OF NURSE PRACTITIONERS, PHASE III.
       Washington, D.C.: U.S. Government Printing Office, HRA Pub.
       81-65-657, 1980.

       Describes a second cohort of nurse practitioner programs and
       students, and follows the students as they work as nurse prac-
       titioners. The study sample focuses on new programs initiated
       after 1973 that were in existence January, 1977.

2814   "The Nurse Practitioner Survey Results," NURSE PRACT 8(2)
       (February 1983): 41-42.

       Reports survey of sample of readers done in 1981 and 1982.
       Demographic data for two years compared. Nurse practitioners
       in all but four states indicated their practice includes pre-
       scribing medications. (0)

2815   Watkins, L.O. and E.H. Wagner. "Nurse Practitioner and Phy-
       sician Adherence to Standing Orders: Criteria for Consulta-
       tion or Referral," AM J PUBLIC HEALTH 72(1) (January 1982):
       22-29.

Examines whether nurse practitioners adhered to consultation referral criteria in standing orders for hypertension, and whether MDs adhered to the task delegation intent expressed in standing orders. Found that they did not always do so but this did not affect acceptable blood pressure control. (13)

2816 Weston, J.L. "Distribution of Nurse Practitioners and Physician Assistants: Implications of Legal Constraints and Reimbursement," PUBLIC HEALTH REPORTS 95(3) (May/June 1980): 253-58.

Studied variables related to distribution of nurse practitioners and physician's assistants. State laws and regulations which regulate employment more important than third party reimbursement. (5)

2817 Witter Du Gas, B. "Nursing's Expanded Role in Canada: Implications of the Joint CMA/CNA Statement of Policy," NURS CLIN NORTH AM 9 (September 1974): 523-33.

History of nurse practitioner movement in Canada. (9)

2818 Wriston, S. "Nurse Practitioner Reimbursement," J HEALTH POLITICS, POLICY AND LAW 6 (Fall 1981): 444-62.

Problems related to nurse practitioner reimbursement under the Rural Health Clinic Services Act of 1977 are addressed. (141)

See: 804, 897, 910, 1434, 1515, 1516, 2320, 2365, 2367.

CLINICAL ISSUES

Abortion

2819   Francke, L.B.   THE AMBIVALENCE OF ABORTION.   New York: Random
       House, 1978.

       A personal and popular account of the guilt and ambivalence
       accompanying an abortion.   Also includes coverage of the right
       to life and pro-choice groups.

2820   Harper, M.W., B.R. Marcom and V.D. Wall.   "Abortion: Do At-
       titudes of Nursing Personnel Affect the Patient's Perception
       of Care," NURS RES 21 (August 1972): 327-31.   Reprinted in
       EXPANDING HORIZONS FOR NURSES.   Edited by B. Bullough and
       V. Bullough. New York: Springer Publishing Co., 1977, pp.
       102-110.

       Found that in many cases care givers attitude toward abor-
       tion has an affect on their care, although this can be over-
       come by their own awareness of their attitudes. (13)

2821   Lader, L. ABORTION.   Indianapolis: Bobbs Merrill Co., 1966.

       Historical and legal background for more recent changes in
       abortion laws and norms.

2822   _____.   ABORTION II: MAKING THE REVOLUTION.   Boston: Beacon
       Press, 1973.

       Describes rapid change in abortion law which occurred in the
       late 1960'a and 1970's.   Analyzes causes of revolution.

2823   Raisler, J.   "Abortion 1980: Battleground for Reproductive
       Rights," J NURSE MIDWIF 25(2) (March/April 1980): 28-32.

       Presents a history of abortion practices and an update on
       abortion legislation.   Both Pro-Choice and Right to Life move-
       ments are analyzed and discussed, and nurse midwives are urged
       to take a strong stand in favor of abortion rights. (17)

2824   Steinhoff, P.G. and M. Diamond. ABORTION POLITICS: THE HAWAII
       EXPERIENCE.   Honolulu: The University of Hawaii Press, 1977.

       Analysis of the controversy and political processes involved
       in the repeal of Hawaii's criminal abortion law.

Aging, Geriatrics

2825   Administration on Aging, Social and Rehabilitation Service,
       U.S. Department of Health, Education and Welfare. WORKS ON
       AGING: A BIBLIOGRAPHY OF SELECTED ANNOTATED REFERENCES,
       COMPILED FOR THE ADMINISTRATION ON AGING. Washington, D.C.:
       U.S. Department of Health, Education and Welfare, 1970.

       This bibliography was prepared to assist practitioners,
       teachers, students, and lay persons working in the field of
       aging.

2826   Barnes, G.M., E.L. Abel et al. ALCOHOL AND THE ELDERLY: A
       COMPREHENSIVE BIBLIOGRAPHY. Westport, CT.: Greenwood Press,
       1980.

       Contents alphabetical by author.

2827   Berardo, F.M. (Ed.). MIDDLE AND LATE TRANSITIONS. Beverly
       Hills, CA.: Sage Publications, Inc., 1982.

       Represents a reorientation in the ways that social scien-
       tists view human development--away from focus on infancy and
       childhood, toward the study of the total life span. Emphasiz-
       ing role transitions and continual development as found in
       common changes during adulthood. Among the topics discussed
       are the historical, economic, and demographic changes which
       have combined to move our population toward the middle of the
       age structure.

2828   Block, M.R., J.L. Davidson and J.D. Grambs. WOMEN OVER FORTY:
       VISIONS AND REALITIES. New York: Springer Publishing Co.,
       1981.

       Provides information concerning erroneous stereotypes of
       women in the aging years in health, sexuality, work, and re-
       tirement.

2829   Herzog, A.R., W.L. Rodgers and J. Woodworth. SUBJECTIVE WELL-
       BEING AMONG DIFFERENT AGE GROUPS. Ann Arbor, MI.: Institute
       for Social Research, 1982.

       Final report of a study sponsored by the National Institute
       of Mental Health on the lifespan patterns of subjective well-
       being. The research also examines the structure of well-being
       and the effects of demographic factors on well-being across
       different age groups; the effects of roles and resources on
       perceived well-being; and the relationship between the activi-
       ties of retired men and women and their feelings of well-being.

2830   Hickey, T. and R.L. Douglass. "Mistreatment of the Elderly
       in the Domestic Setting: An Exploratory Study," AM J PUBLIC
       HEALTH 71(5) (May 1981): 500-507.

Data from an interview study of 228 persons who provide service to the elderly suggests that the incidence of both in-
tentional abuse and unintentional mistreatment is high. (7)

2831   Hicks, B., H. Raisz, J. Segal and N. Doherty. "The Triage
        Experiment in Coordinated Care for the Elderly," AM J PUBLIC
        HEALTH 9 (September 1981): 991-1003.

        Triage teams made up of a nurse clinician and a social
        worker performed assessment, service coordination and monitor-
        ing functions on 307 clients over a two year period and these
        were compared with 195 elderly non triage clients. Triage
        clients had slightly better mental functioning outcomes than
        comparison clients; results of physical and social functioning
        outcomes were inclusive. Utilizations and costs were somewhat
        higher for triage clients but the proportional differernce
        in utilization was greater than the proportional differences
        in cost.(7)

2832   Little, V.C. OPEN CARE FOR THE AGING: COMPARATIVE INTERNA-
        TIONAL APPROACHES. New York: Springer Publishing Co., 1982.

        Using an original conceptual framework and drawing on first-
        hand experiences in Western Samoa, Hong Kong, Japan and Sweden,
        the author presents data on existing services, comparing dif-
        ferent stages in the development of open, community-based care
        systems.

2833   McNelley, R.L. and J.N. Colen. AGING IN MINORITY GROUPS.
        Beverly Hills, CA.: Sage Publications, Inc., 1983.

        Essays explore the demographic distribution of elderly
        people in specific groups--Blacks, Hispanics, American Indians,
        and Asian Americans--and discuss major concerns, including
        housing, income maintenance, mental health, and social service
        delivery. The authors, who belong to the minority groups they
        write about, examine the positive as well as the more diffi-
        cult aspects of aging in minority groups.

2834   Sargent, S.S. NONTRADITIONAL THERAPY AND COUNSELING WITH THE
        AGING. New York: Springer Publishing Co., 1980.

        Programs such as assertiveness training, widows' groups,
        peer counselling, and community workshops. Humanistic and
        behavioral approaches, as well as pastoral psychology are in-
        cluded.

2835   Smyer, M.A. and M. Gatz. MENTAL HEALTH AND AGING: PROGRAMS
        AND EVALUATIONS. Beverly Hills, CA.: Sage Publications,
        Inc., 1983.

        Designed to familiarize policymakers and practitioners with
        a broad range of mental health interventions. Case studies of
        different programs demonstrate how and why each program works.

2836   Thomae, H. and G.L. Maddox. NEW PERSPECTIVES ON OLD AGE: A
       MESSAGE TO DECISION MAKERS, INTERNATIONAL ASSOCIATION OF
       GERONTOLOGY. New York: Springer Publishing Co., 1982.

       This report includes recommendations by I.A.G. for the World
       Congress on Aging of the United Nations in Vienna, Summer
       1982, as well as the research and experience of various coun-
       tries regarding policy issues on care of the elderly.

2837   Yurick, A.G., B.E. Spier, S.S. Robb and N.J. Ebert. THE ACED
       PERSON AND THE NURSING PROCESS, 2nd Ed. Norwalk, CT.:
       Appleton-Century-Crofts, 1984.

       Emphasizes the promotion of health among the elderly and
       support of their functional abilities. Cognitive functioning
       and sensory losses, including changes in vision and hearing,
       problems in elimination and nutrition, and activity patterns
       and abilities are discussed in detail.

       See 682, 2214.

Alternative Models, Holistic Health Care

2838   Blattner, B. HOLISTIC NURSING. Englewood Cliffs, NJ.: Pren-
       tice-Hall, 1981.

       This volume encourages critical appraisal as a responsi-
       bility of both nurse and client. Helps students sort out dif-
       ferent health beliefs and practices. Uses theories, methodo-
       logies, and teaching tools that are consistent with both hol-
       istic health and orthodox medical principles.

2839   Borelli, M.D. and P. Heidt (Eds.). THERAPEUTIC TOUCH. New
       York: Springer Publishing Co., 1981.

       Clinicians and patients share their experiences of thera-
       peutic touch.

2840   Flynn, P.A.R. (Ed.). HEALING CONTINUUM: THE JOURNEYS IN THE
       PHILOSOPHY OF HOLISTIC HEALTH. Englewood Cliffs, NJ.: Pren-
       tice-Hall (Brady), 1981.

       An edited volume with a variety of approaches to health care
       but primary focus is on alternative therapies.

2841   _____. HOLISTIC HEALTH: ART AND SCIENCE OF CARE. Engle-
       wood Cliffs, NJ.: Prentice-Hall (Brady), 1980.

       Designed to integrate ideas from the scientific and non-
       traditional communities, this volume presents and explains the
       concepts and practice of humanistic nursing and alternative
       therapies as an effective means of treating the "whole" person,
       not just the disease or symptom.

2842   Salmon, J.W. (Ed.). ALTERNATIVE MEDICINES: POPULAR AND POLICY
       PERSPECTIVES. New York: Methuen, Inc., 1984.

Offers answers to two essential questions: how do alternative medicines challenge the tenets of conventional scientific
medicine; and could a synthesis of these alternative medicines
and scientific medicine lead to a reformulation of conceptions
of healing?

Biofeedback

2843   Burns, P.A., M.A. Marecki, S.S. Dittmar, and B. Bullough.
       "Kegel's Exercises With Biofeedback Therapy for Treatment
       of Stress Incontinence," NURSE PRACT 10(2) (February 1985):
       28, 33-34, 46.

       Describes an intervention program using biofeedback, and
       measured Kegel's exercises on a small number of women with
       symptoms of stress incontinence. The lessening of symptoms
       became a major factor in continued compliance with the exer-
       cise program.

2844   Fischer-Williams, M. A TEXTBOOK OF BIOLOGICAL FEEDBACK.
       New York: Human Sciences Press, 1981.

       Analysis of the neuro-anatomical and physiological basis of
       biofeedback. Its application to neurological disorders, in-
       cluding pain, stress, seizures, paralysis and insomnia, and
       malfunctions of the cardiovascular, respiratory, endocrine,
       and other physiological systems is discussed in detail.

2845   Wentworth-Rohr, I. SYMPTOM REDUCTION THROUGH CLINICAL BIO-
       FEEDBACK. New York: Human Sciences Press, Inc., 1984.

       Biofeedback as a treatment modality for the reduction of
       selected symptoms is described and discussed.

Compliance

2846   Caplan, R.D., R. Van Harrison, R.V. Wellons and J.R.P. French,
       Jr. SOCIAL SUPPORT AND PATIENT ADHERENCE: EXPERIMENTAL AND
       SURVEY FINDINGS. Ann Arbor, MI.: Institute for Social Re-
       search, 1980.

       An in-depth look at social support and how it affects ad-
       herence to medical regimens, using both experimental and sur-
       vey techniques.

2847   Connelly, C.E. "Economic and Ethical Issues in Patient Com-
       pliance," NURS ECON 2(5) (September/October 1984): 342-47,
       364.

       Patient noncompliance with recommendations for health promo-
       tion and the prevention and treatment of illness significantly
       increases demands for and costs of health care services.
       Despite the economic and health problems resulting from non-
       adherence, nurses are concerned about the ethical implications
       of promoting compliance. (16)

2848   Falvo, D.R. EFFECTIVE PATIENT EDUCATION: A GUIDE TO INCREASED
       COMPLIANCE. Gaithersburg, MD.: Aspen Systems Corp., 1984.

       Issues addressed include: establishing rapport for a thera-
       peutic relationship, assessing individual patient needs, iden-
       tifying psychosocial variables in patient education, building
       communication skills and legal ethical considerations in
       patient education.

2849   Marston, M.V. "Compliance with Medical Regimes: A Review of
       the Literature," NURS RES 19 (1970): 312-23.

       A three part paper which provides an up-to-date summary of
       studies of compliance behavior. Section I is a review of
       methods used to study compliance; Section II is a review of
       demographic, illness and social-psychological variables re-
       lating to compliance; and Section III contains suggestions for
       further research. (86)

2850   Spadaro, D.C. "Factors Involved with Patient Compliance," PED
       NURS 6(4) (July/August 1980): 27-29.

       Definitions of compliance factors involved in compliance
       reviewed. Suggestions for improving compliance given. (15)

2851   Starfield, B., C. Wray, K. Hess, R. Gross, P.S. Birk and B.C.
       D'Lugoff. "The Influence of Patient-Practitioner Agreement
       on Outcome of Care," AM J PUBLIC HEALTH 71(2) (February
       1981): 127-31.

       The findings of this study confirm those of a previous study
       in suggesting that practitioner-patient agreement about prob-
       lems is associated with greater expectations for improvement
       and with better outcome as perceived by patients. In addition,
       they indicate that practitioners also report better outcome
       under the same circumstances. (20)

2852   Yoos, L. "Factors Influencing Maternal Compliance to Anti-
       biotic Regimens," PED NURS 10(2) (March/April 1984): 141-47.

       Noncompliance is one of the major problems faced by health
       care providers today. This study examined a number of strate-
       gies designed to increase maternal compliance to antibiotic
       regimens. Interventions under investigation included educa-
       tion, a reciprocal patient-provider interaction, and decreas-
       ing cost barriers of treatment. (24)

Death, Dying, Bereavement, Hospice Care

2853   American Nurses' Association. NURSING PRACTICE IN THE CARE OF
       THE DYING. Kansas City, MO.: American Nurses' Association,
       Pub. No. NP-65, 1982.

Describes what nursing can do directly and indirectly for the dying client and his significant others. It also explores the legal considerations involved when the nurse interacts with a dying client and his family, in the light of recent cases concerning what is sometimes called the "right to die with dignity."

2854 Buckingham, R.W. and D. Lupu. "A Comparative Study of Hospice Services in the United States," AM J PUBLIC HEALTH 5 (May 1982): 455-63.

Compares two types of hospice and finds those that are best funded are the institutionally based hospices providing both inpatient and home care, greater variety of medical/nursing services, less variety of social-psychological services, using fewer types of volunteers and paid staff. (18)

2855 Cohen, K.P. HOSPICE: PRESCRIPTION FOR TERMINAL CARE. Gaithersburg, MD.: Aspen Systems Corp., 1979.

Provides a picture of how, why and where the hospice movement started, where it is today, the issues that rage around it, and what the future may bring. It looks analytically at fundamentals such as our attitudes toward death and how they influence the kind of life-saving and life-extending techniques we now select.

2856 Corr, C.A. and D.M. Corr (Eds.). HOSPICE CARE: PRINCIPLES AND PRACTICES. New York: Springer Publishing Co., 1983.

The hospice movement is reviewed, models of hospices are presented, and the management of care is discussed. Contributors emphasize client decision making and multidisciplinary care.

2857 DuBois, P.M. THE HOSPICE WAY OF DEATH. New York: Health Sciences Press, Inc., 1980.

Examines new approaches to the understanding and treatment of the terminally ill and the subsequent development of hospices in the U.S. and Europe. Hospices are interdisciplinary programs providing specialized and intensive health and mental health services for the dying and their families.

2858 Epstein, C. NURSING THE DYING PATIENT. Englewood Cliffs, NJ.: Reston Publishing Co. (Prentice-Hall, Inc.), 1975.

Covers heightening self-awareness, the stages of dying, trajectories of dying, death at different ages, the conspiracy of silence, the process of observation, and helping the professional.

2859 Gonda, T.A. and J.E. Ruark. DYING DIGNIFIED: THE HEALTH PROFESSIONALS GUIDE TO CARE. Menlo Park, CA.: Addison-Wesley Publishing Co., 1984.

Comprehensive work on the care of the terminally ill and
their families. Presents the complex situations and feelings
that occur daily among those involved with dying and grieving
patients. Specific, practical techniques for encouraging
open communication and involvement are presented. Psychosocial, cultural, and demographic factors are discussed as
well as special issues such as suicide and children's reactions to death.

2860   Holden, C. "Hospices: For The Dying, Relief From Pain and
       Fear," SCIENCE 193(3) (July 1976): 7.

       Surveys state of hospice movement in U.S. as of 1976. (0)

2861   Kohut, J.M. and S. Kohut, Jr. HOSPICE: CARING FOR THE TER-
       MINALLY ILL. Springfield, IL.: Charles C. Thomas Publisher,
       1984.

       Overview of the hospice concept, with practical information
       on how to set up a hospice, how to train volunteers, how to
       care for the dying patient, and how to handle the stress of
       hospice work.

2862   Martinson, I.M., M. Palta and N.V. Reed. "Death and Dying:
       Selected Attitudes of Minnesota's Registered Nurses," NURS
       RES 27(4) (1978): 226-29.

       Attitudes towards death and dying were studied using a sam-
       ple of 1061 Minnesota nurses. Subjects supported home care
       for dying patients and indicated they would be willing to care
       for both dying adults and children at home, but indicated they
       needed more preparation for the task. (13)

2863   Osterweis, M., F. Solomon and M. Green (Eds.). BEREAVEMENT:
       REACTIONS, CONSEQUENCES, AND CARE. Washington, D.C.:
       National Academy Press, 1984.

       A book prepared by the Committee on The Health Consequences
       of the Stress of Bereavement of the Institute of Medicine.
       Offers guidelines for care givers and family members to help
       the bereaved.

2864   Schraff, S. HOSPICE: THE NURSING PERSPECTIVE. New York:
       National League for Nursing, Pub. No. 20-1967, 1984.

       Provides information on how to finance and start a hospice
       program, supervise professional staff, work with the new Medi-
       care regulations, recruit and retain volunteers and understand
       the hospice philosophy. Includes six case examples.

2865   Thomas, N. and A.S. Cordell. "The Dying Infant: Aiding
       Parents in the Detachment Process," PED NURS 9(5) (Septem-
       ber/October 1983): 355-57.

Meaningful contacts between parents and their infants are important steps in the early grief process. In this article a young mother describes how she cared for her infant son during his illness and death. Nursing intervention used at The Children's Medical Center in Dayton that aid parents undergoing the detachment process and coping with grief are presented; and the importance of a follow-up program is discussed. (8)

2866   Werner-Beland, J. et al. GRIEF RESPONSES TO LONG-TERM ILLNESS AND DISABILITY. Englewood Cliffs, NJ.: Reston Publishing Co. (Prentice-Hall, Inc.), 1980.

Addresses the problem faced by individuals, families, and health professionals who have contact with people with long-term illness or disabilities.

2867   Yeaworth, R.C., F.T. Kapp and C. Winget. "Attitudes of Nursing Students Towards the Dying Patient," NURS RES 23(19) (1974): 21-24.

A questionnaire measuring the attitudes of freshman and senior nursing students about death and dying. Statistically significant data shows seniors more accepting, flexible and open to communication. (6)

Infants, Children

2868   American Nurses' Association. A CALL TO ACTION ON BEHALF OF CHILDREN. Kansas City, MO.: American Nurses' Association, Pub. No. MCH-11, 1980.

Resolutions and statements of concern on topics related to the health and well-being of children, compiled by the ANA Division on Maternal and Child Health Nursing Practice.

2869   Barnes, G.M. ALCOHOL AND YOUTH: A COMPREHENSIVE BIBLIOGRAPHY. Westport, CT.: Greenwood Press, 1982.

Covers the various aspects of alcohol use by youth with emphasis on teenage drinkers. There are approximately 5,000 references to the worldwide literature, both popular and scholarly, primarily from the past forty years (1942-1982), with a few citations from earlier years.

2870   Brown, R.T. and M.E. Wynne. "Sustained Attention in Boys with Attention Deficit Disorder and the Effect of Methylphenidate," PED NURS 10(1) (January/February 1984): 35-39.

This research compared the performance of a group of boys with Attention Deficit Disorder (ADD) to the performance of a group of normal control boys on a screening instrument (Children's Checking Task) measuring sustained attention. The effects of methylphenidate on this measure of sustained attention were also investigated for the boys with ADD. Boys with

ADD demonstrated marked deterioration on the sustained attention task when compared to normal controls. However, methylphenidate therapy for ADD patients significantly improved
their attention performance to a level near that of normal
controls. (21)

2871 Clore, E.R. and Y.S.G. Newberry. "Nurse Practitioner Guidance
      for the Adoptive Family from Birth to Adolescence, Part
      1-5," PED NURS 7(6) (November/December 1981): 16-25.

      A five part article explores the dynamics of the adoptive
      process from the relinquishing mother through the adopted
      child's development as an adolescent. (8)

2872 Gibbons, M.B. "Circumcision: The Controversy Continues,"
      PED NURS 10(2) (March/April 1984): 103-9.

      Although circumcision is the most frequently performed sur-
      gical procedure in this country, the necessity of this proce-
      dure has been widely questioned. By providing the latest in-
      formation regarding circumcision and alternative options,
      nurses can assist parents to make informed decisions. (20)

2873 Griffin, C.C., B.M. Popkin and D.S. Spicer. "Infant Formula
      Promotion and Infant-Feeding Practices, Bicol Region,
      Philippines," AM J PUBLIC HEALTH 74(9) (September 1984):
      992-97.

      A 1978 and 1981 survey in the Bicol region of the Philip-
      pines found that multinationals tended not to affect mother's
      breast feeding practices and behavior directly, but increased
      the probability of them introducing breast milk substitutes
      within the first six months and thus in practicing a program
      of mixed feeding. (6)

2874 Klaus, M.H. and A. Fanaroff. CARE OF THE HIGH-RISK NEONATE,
      2nd Ed. Philadelphia: W.B. Saunders Co., 1979.

      A perinatology text which presents major principles neces-
      sary to care for the sick neonate. Each chapter includes
      questions and case problems.

2875 McClellan, M.A. "On Their Own: Latchkey Children," PED NURS
      10(3) (May/June 1984): 198-202.

      An increasing number of children are left alone to fend for
      themselves after school. Unstructured and unsupervised ac-
      tivity may lead to injury, delinquency, or isolation. Pedia-
      tric and school nurses must take the initiative in investiga-
      ting, developing, and implementing after-school child care
      programs responsive to the needs and problems of these chil-
      dren.

2876 "New Reductions in Infant Mortality: The Challenge of Low
      Birthweight," AM J PUBLIC HEALTH 71(4) (April 1981): 365-66.

Problems related to determining variables involved in the reduction of infant mortality discussed. (7)

2877   Riordan, J. A PRACTICAL GUIDE TO BREASTFEEDING. St. Louis: C.V. Mosby Co., 1983.

Historical and cross cultural sketch of breastfeeding patterns. Suggestions for solving problems related to breastfeeding furnished.

2878   Rothenberg, P.B. and P.E. Varga. "The Relationship Between Age of Mother and Child Health and Development," AM J PUBLIC HEALTH 71(8) (August 1981): 810-17.

Invesigates the relationship between age of mother and children´s health and development at birth and at approximately three years of age using sample composed of Black and Hispanic women and their firstborn children. There were no differences between children of teenage and older mothers in terms of prematurity or birthweight, but the children of younger mothers had higher Apgar scores than those of older mothers. Age of mother was not significantly related to hospitalizations, the need to see a physician regularly, or abnormal weight. The children of teenage mothers scored better than those of older mothers on the total Denver Developmental Screening Test. These findings thus suggest that when relevant background characteristics are controlled, children of teenage mothers are as healthy and develop as well as children of older mothers. (27)

2879   Sosnowitz, B.G. "Managing Parents on Neonatal Intensive Care Units," SOCIAL PROBLEMS 31(4) (April 1984): 390-402.

This paper looks at how staff on neonatal intensive care units manage the parents of sick infants. The information given to parents is manipulated in order to obtain parental behaviors needed by the staff to do their work. The parental role desired by the staff facilitates quick application of medical treatment to the infants with parental consent. Author concludes that parents take responsibility for decisions they do not fully understand and, like clients in all professional relationships, rely on the advice of the experts. (26)

2880   Triplett, J.L. and S.W. Arbeson. "Working With Children of Alcoholics," PED NURS 9(5) (September/October 1983): 317-20.

As unemployment rates climb and family stress increases, more children are likely to experience inconsistent parenting or violence associated with parental alcoholism. Through expanded health histories and astute observations, children at risk can be identified and specific help provided. (8)

2881   Wagner, T.J. and M. Hindi-Alexander. "Hazards of Baby Powder," PED NURS 10(2) (March/April 1984): 124-25.

Aspiration of baby powder, containing talc, has led to nine reported infant deaths, and numerous treatments for cases of severe inhalation. Treatment with steroids may be of some benefit. However, preventive action by parents is essential. (16)

2882 Winchell, C.A. THE HYPERKINETIC CHILD: AN ANNOTATED BIBLIO-GRAPHY 1974-1979. Westport, CT.: Greenwood Press, 1981.

Bibliographies cover the description of the syndrome, etiology, diagnosis, management, and physiological and psychological research, as well as sources on animal models, follow-up studies, sociological aspects, ethical and legal issues, and research and methodology.

2883 Winkelstein, M.L. "Overfeeding in Infancy: The Early Introduction of Solid Foods," PED NURS 10(3) (May/June 1984): 205-8, 236.

Maternal attitudes and knowledge of nutritional requirements can have demonstrable effects on feeding practices. In this study of low-income, inner city mothers, mothers' attitudes about overfeeding were not significantly related to the early introduction of solids. However, mothers who introduced solids early were significantly less knowledgeable about nutrition. (21)

2884 Zimmerman, M.A. "Breast-feeding the Adopted Newborn," PED NURS 7(1) (January/February 1981): 9-12.

Breast-feeding an adopted newborn is possible. This article explains why, gives the steps of preparation and describes the technique. (4)

Men

2885 Swanson, J. and K. Forrest. MEN'S REPRODUCTIVE HEALTH, VOL. 3. New York: Springer Publishing Co., 1984.

Brings together information from the fields of psychology, sociology, urology, nursing, gerontology, public health, and family planning. Covers virtually all aspects of the male role in American society as it relates to reproduction and sexuality.

2886 Tamir, L.M. MEN IN THEIR FORTIES. New York: Springer Publishing Co., 1982.

An empirical study of men facing the experiences and crises of mid-life.

See 1978.

Mental Illness

2887   Arnhoff, F.N. "Social Consequences of Policy Toward Mental
       Illness," SCIENCE 188 (June 1975): 1277-1281. Reprinted in
       EXPANDING HORIZONS FOR NURSES. Edited by B. Bullough and V.
       Bullough. New York: Springer Publishing Co., 1977, pp.
       127-41.

       Argues that from the point of view of individual patient,
       community or home treatment is not necessarily superior either
       in short term or long term effects but when relatives are
       concerned the burden was for many intolerable. Thus some
       questions have to be raised about deinstitutionalization. (50)

2888   Brown, P. THE TRANSFER OF CARE: PSYCHIATRIC DEINSTITUTIONALI-
       ZATION AND ITS AFTERMATH. Boston, MA.: Routledge & Kegan
       Paul, 1985.

       Despite some benefits to mental health care, many serious
       flaws have become apparent in the deinstutionalization of men-
       tal patients and the development of community mental health
       programs. This book analyzes recent mental health practices
       in this country.

2889   Child, A.A., C.M. Murphy and M.C. Rhyne. "Depression in
       Children: Reasons and Risks," PED NURS 6(4) (July/August
       1980): 9-13.

       Literature review examines theories of causality, risk fac-
       tors, and symptoms of depression in children. (18)

2890   Murray, J. and P.R. Abramson. BIAS IN PSYCHOTHERAPY. New
       York: Praeger Publishers, 1983.

       Analyzes the extent to which cultural expectations, stereo-
       types, and prejudices influence the psychotherapeutic process.
       Murray and Abramson are authors of about half the chapters
       with contributors focusing on specialized topics, including
       bias based on sex, race, and sexual identity.

2891   Nelms, B.C. and M.A. Brady. "Assessment and Intervention:
       The Depressed School-age Child," PED NURS 6(4) (July/August
       1980): 15-19.

       To identify, treat or refer depressed or at risk children
       the nurse must have knowledge of normal developmental charac-
       teristics and behaviors and/or factors associated with child-
       hood depression. This article presents a systematic approach
       for assessment and an overview of treatment approaches for the
       depressed and school-age child. (13)

2892   Rosenhan, D.L. "On Being Sane in Insane Places," SCIENCE 179
       (January 19, 1973): 250-58. Reprinted in EXPANDING HORIZONS
       FOR NURSES. Edited by B. Bullough and V. Bullough. New
       York: Springer Publishing Co., 1977, pp. 111-26.

The experience of eight pseudo patients in a mental hospital setting. Dramatizes problems related to institutionalization. (21)

See 830.

Sexuality

2893 Bullough V. and B. Bullough. "Sexuality and the Nurse," IMPRINT (February 1974): 17-19, 30-33. Reprinted in EX-PANDING HORIZONS FOR NURSES. Edited by B. Bullough and V. Bullough. New York: Springer Publishing Co., 1977, pp. 82-90.

Discusses various issues in sexuality which the nurse might be called upon to deal with. (0)

2894 Hicks, C. "Taking the Lid Off...Sexuality and the Nurse," NURS TIMES 76(39) (1980): 1681-82.

Sexuality was the subject of the annual ANS Conference. Sex counselor Anne Dickson emphasized the need for nurses to be aware of their own myths and attitudes. She also highlighted important counseling skills for nurses to utilize with their patients. (0)

2895 Hogan, R.M. HUMAN SEXUALITY: A NURSING PERSPECTIVE. New York: Appleton-Century-Crofts, 1980.

Variety of sexual issues presented from a nursing perspective, including life cycle changes in sexual expression, alternative life styles, sexual assault, abortion and pregnancy, nursing role in illness and disability discussed.

2896 Lief, H.I. and T. Payne. "Sexuality Knowledge and Attitudes," AM J NURS 75(11) (1975): 2026-29.

The importance of education in sexualty relating to quality nursing care is studied by looking at sexuality in terms of knowledge and attitude. Results show nursing students to be more knowledgeable and liberal than graduate nurses.(21)

2897 Tabeek, E.S. and M.G. Conroy. "Teaching Sexual Awareness to the Significantly Disabled School-Age Child," PED NURS 7(5) (September/October 1981): 21-25.

This article explores some aspects of a program in sexuality awareness initiated at a hospital school for physically disabled children. The objectives of this program did not include specific sexual capacity and fulfillment, but rather dealt with the least sensitive areas and provided a baseline of factual information to permit students, faculty and health professionals commonalities for communication and discussion. This increased awareness was the impetus for the development of several other programs at the hospital school. (7)

2898   Woods, N.F. HUMAN SEXUALITY IN HEALTH AND ILLNESS. St.
       Louis: C.V. Mosby Co., 1983.

       Provides the health care professional with information on
       the trends and research in the field of sexuality. Discus-
       sions emphasize psychosocial aspects.

Social, Psychological Aspects of Care, Stress
Management, Crisis Intervention

2899   Caplan, R.D., A. Abbey, D.J. Abramis, F.M. Andres, T.L. Con-
       way and J.R.P. French, Jr. TRANQUILIZER USE AND WELL-BEING:
       A LONGITUDINAL STUDY OF SOCIAL AND PSYCHOLOGICAL EFFECTS.
       Ann Arbor, MI.: Institute for Social Research, 1984.

       Presents the results of a comprehensive study of the social
       and psychological effects of diazepam. Through a longitudinal
       survey of 675 respondents, the researchers examined the effects
       of the tranquilizer's use on quality of life, anxiety, per-
       ceived performance, stress, social support, perceived control,
       coping and defense.

2900   Cornwall, J. HARD EARNED LIVES. New York: Methuen, Inc.,
       1985.

       This work explores the relationship between people's ideas
       and theories about their health and the social and economic
       factors governing their lives.

2901   Dracup, K. "Psychosocial Aspects of Coronary Heart Disease:
       Implications for Nursing Research," WEST J NURS RES 4(3)
       (Summer 1982): 257-71.

       A survey of past major studies on psychological and social
       factors relating to coronary disease and the gaps and problems
       remaining. Commentary by M. Jacobs, S. Cunningham, V. Car-
       rieri and response (pp. 272-76). (56)

2902   Eisenberg, M., F. Sutkin and M. Jansen. CHRONIC ILLNESS AND
       DISABILITY THROUGH THE LIFE SPAN: EFFECTS ON SELF AND FAMILY.
       New York: Springer Publishing Co., 1984.

       Examines the impact of chronic and disabling conditions on
       the individual within the family context.

2903   Garland, L. and C.T. Bush. COPING BEHAVIORS AND NURSING.
       Englewood Cliffs, NJ.: Reston Publishing Co. (Prentice-Hall,
       Inc.), 1982.

       A comprehensive treatment of frequently encountered coping
       behaviors. Offers a conceptual approach to identifying and
       responding to both adaptive and maladaptive coping mechanisms.
       Covers both psychological and physiological stressors and
       responses.

2904 Getty, C. and W. Humphreys. UNDERSTANDING THE FAMILY: STRESS
      AND CHANGE IN AMERICAN FAMILY LIFE. New York: Appleton-
      Century-Crofts, 1981.

      Explores the complex needs and problems of modern families.
      Organized around four topics: family role relationships,
      ethnicity, traumatic disruptions of family life, and working
      with families. Edited with twenty-seven contributors.

2905 Gow, K.M. HOW NURSES' EMOTIONS AFFECT PATIENT CARE: SELF-
      STUDIES BY NURSES. New York: Springer Publishing Co., 1982.

      In this unique text, nurses describe and analyze helpful and
      unhelpful encounters with patients.

2906 Hilbert, R.A. "The Cultural Dimensions of Chronic Pain:
      Flawed Reality Contruction and The Problem of Meaning,"
      SOCIAL PROBLEMS 31(4) (April 1984): 365-78.

      Chronic pain sufferers tend to feel frustrated and socially
      isolated. They encounter further difficulties in social set-
      tings where problems regarding the management of pain remain
      unsolved. The problems of chronic pain sufferers suggest a
      form of suffering which transcends physical pain. (51)

2907 Hoff, L.A. PEOPLE IN CRISIS: UNDERSTANDING AND HELPING, 2nd
      Ed. Menlo Park, CA.: Addison-Wesley Publishing Co., 1984.

      Examines what crisis is, how to recognize it, and what to do
      about it. A multidisciplinary coverage of the crisis situa-
      tions common to today's society: violence, man-made disasters,
      and life transitions.

2908 Kneisl, C.R. and H.S. Wilson. HANDBOOK OF PSYCHOSOCIAL NURSING
      CARE. Menlo Park, CA.: Addison-Wesley Publishing Co., 1984.

      Pocket-sized volume is alphabetically arranged to offer the
      practicing nurse quick access to essential information on
      psychosocial assessment and intervention strategies.

2909 Lazarus, R.S. and S. Folkman. STRESS, APPRAISAL, AND COPING.
      New York: Springer Publishing Co., 1984.

      Builds on the concepts of cognitive appraisal and coping to
      present theory of the psychology of stress. As an integrative
      analysis, it encompasses the many dimensions of stress-related
      problems, including those related to health care.

2910 Lear, M.W. HEARTSOUNDS. New York: Simon and Schuster, 1980.

      The author, a journalist, tells of her physician husband's
      struggles to live after a massive heart attack. He lives
      through by-pass surgery, several serious complications, and a

series of hospitalizations as his condition worsens. The work
has a ring of truth. Most of the nurses are described in
positive but realistic terms. The work provides important
insights about the health care delivery system from the point
of view of the patient and his loved ones.

2911   Manfredi, C. and M. Pickett. "The Take Time Series´: A Prog-
       ram on Coping With Stress," NURS FORUM 20(3) (1981): 322-28.

       Describes three programs designed to assist individuals in
       low socioeconomic groups cope with stress. Programs used
       relaxation, involvement, and audio perception as focal topics
       for coping with stress. (5)

2912   Mumford, E., H. Schlesinger and G.V. Glass. "The Effects of
       Psychological Intervention on Recovery from Surgery and
       Heart Attacks: An Analysis of the Literature," AM J PUBLIC
       HEALTH 72(2) (February 1982): 141-51.

       A general survey of medical, nursing, and other literature
       dealing with psychological intervention and which demonstrates
       the importance of such intervention. (65)

2913   Ryan, J. "The Neglected Crisis," AM J NURS 84(10) (October
       1984): 1257-58.

       Spiritual support can be important to some patients in
       crisis situations. (7)

Suicide

2914   Battin, M.P. and R. Maris (Eds.). SUICIDE AND ETHICS. New
       York: Health Sciences Press, Inc., 1983.

       Issues related to suicide and suicide prevention are dis-
       cussed from a variety of points of view, including philoso-
       phers and a psychiatrist.

2915   Linzer, N. (Ed.). SUICIDE: THE WILL TO LIVE VS. THE WILL TO
       DIE. New York: Human Sciences Press, Inc., 1984.

       Examination of the rise of suicide among all age groups in
       society. Addressing the "before" and "after" of suicide, it
       discusses detection, prevention, and intervention both with
       potential suicides and bereaved survivors. Perspectives are
       offered by psychiatrists, psychologists, social workers, and
       nurses.

2916   Shneidman, E.S. SUICIDE THOUGHTS AND REFLECTIONS, 1960-1980.
       New York: Human Sciences Press, Inc., 1981.

       This collection of the author´s work on suicide prevention
       over a twenty year period. Gathered from a variety of sources,
       the selections cover definitional, taxonomic, psychodynamic,
       cognitive-logical, and psychotherapeutic aspects of suicidal
       phenomena.

Victims of Rape, Violence, Abuse, Neglect

2917   Alexander, C.S. "The Responsible Victim: Nurses´ Perceptions
       of Victims of Rape," J HEALTH & SOCIAL BEHAVIOR 21(1)
       (March 1980): 22-31.

       Considers how judgments made by hospital nurses (N=312)
       regarding victim responsibility are influenced by the type of
       crime (i.e., rape or beating), the victim´s marital status,
       her dress, her relationship with the assailant, evidence of
       her resistance, the extent of her injuries, and psychological
       attributes and sociodemography characteristics of the nurse.
       Findings suggest that the assignment of blame differs sig-
       nificantly for those victims described as "respectable."
       Psychological attributes of the nurse emerged as the strongest
       predictors of victim blaming. (49)

2918   Campbell, J.C. and J.C. Humphreys. NURSING CARE OF VICTIMS OF
       FAMILY VIOLENCE. Englewood Cliffs, NJ.: Reston Publishing
       Co. (Prentice-Hall, Inc.), 1984.

       Uses a nursing process format. It addresses the nursing
       care of victims of family violence, including victims of child
       abuse, wife abuse, incest, and abuse of the elderly.

2919   Campbell, J. "Misogyny and Homicide of Women," ADV NURS
       SCIENCE 3(2) (January 1981): 67-85.

       Observes that misogyny is a basic part of the violence
       against women and nature in American society. Encourages
       nurses to create and support wife-abuse shelters and to dili-
       gently identify and report violence against women. (81)

2920   Foley, T.S. and M.A. Davies. RAPE: NURSING CARE OF VICTIMS.
       St. Louis: C.V. Mosby Co., 1983.

       The nurse´s role in caring for victims of rape and child
       abuse is presented. A series of exercises is presented to
       help nurses deal with their own reactions to the situations so
       they can better help their clients.

2921   Halpern, S., D.J. Hicks and T.L. Crenshaw. RAPE: HELPING THE
       VICTIM. Oradell, NJ.: Medical Economics Co., 1978.

       Short, easy to understand manual on the processes that can
       be used to assist the rape victim.

2922   Kalisch, B.J. CHILD ABUSE AND NEGLECT: AN ANNOTATED BIBLIO-
       GRAPHY. Westport, CT.: Greenwood Press, 1978.

       This bibliography is an attempt to control the vast litera-
       ture on the battered child that has appeared particularly
       since 1960. There is a detailed table of contents as well as
       author and key word indexes.

2923   McCown, D.E. "Father/Daughter Incest: A Family Problem,"
       PED NURS 7(4) (July/August 1981): 25-28.

       Describes problem, outlines interventions. (11)

2924   Pagelow, M.D. WOMAN-BATTERING: VICTIMS AND THEIR EXPERIENCES.
       Beverly Hills, CA.: Sage Publications, 1981.

       Reports experiences and perceptions of a sample of women
       victims and she integrates this data into a larger theoretical
       framework, challenging current myths about woman-battering.

2925   Scully, D. and J. Marolla. "Convicted Rapists' Vocabulary of
       Motive: Excuses and Justifications," SOCIAL PROBLEMS 31(5)
       (June 1984): 530-44.

       Analyzes the excuses and justifications which a sample of
       convicted incarcerated rapists used to explain themselves and
       their crimes. Justifications attempted to present their own
       behavior as situationally appropriate and, using a number of
       common rape stereotypes, to make their victims appear culpable.

2926   Warner, C.G. (Ed.). RAPE AND SEXUAL ASSAULT: MANAGEMENT AND
       INTERVENTION. Gaithersburg, MD.: Aspen Systems Corp., 1980.

       Tells how to examine the accused, assess the victim's
       ability to cope with the impact of the assault, counsel family
       and friends, help the victim cope with fear, guilt, and much
       more. Concrete suggestions, ideas for treatment and proce-
       dures essential within your area of expertise.

Women's Health, Pregnancy, Childbirth, Menarche,
Menopause

2927   Abel, E.L. NARCOTICS AND REPRODUCTION: A BIBLIOGRAPHY. West-
       port, CT.: Greenwood Press, 1983.

       Lists materials dealing with the effects of the use of
       heroin, morphine, methadone, and related narcotic drugs on
       reproduction. Materials dealing with sexual behavior, sexual
       function, and sexual physiology have been included; however,
       the majority of the citations focus on the effects of nar-
       cotics on the fetus.
       Introduction traces the history of narcotic drugs, the in-
       cidence of their use among pregnant women, and the possible
       side effects of that use.

2928   _____. SMOKING AND REPRODUCTION: A COMPREHENSIVE BIBLIO-
       GRAPHY. Westport, CT.: Greenwood Press, 1982.

       Following the introduction which discusses briefly how
       tobacco smoking has acquired its popularity and what various
       effects nicotine has on sexual behavior, the bibliography is
       divided into alphabetical sections by authors names.

Clinical Issues   489

2929   Brown, B.S. "Tampons, Teen-Agers and Toxic Shock," PED NURS
       7(3) (May/June 1981): 7.

       Advises practitioners to teach patients to wear tampons only
       intermittently and to be aware of symptoms of toxic shock. (4)

2930   Bullough, V.L. "Age at Menarche: A Misunderstanding," SCIENCE
       213(17) (July 1981): 365-66.

       Through a misinterpretation of historical data the age of
       menarche in the nineteenth century is erroneously taken to
       have been seventeen years. This error has resulted in unwar-
       ranted beliefs about change in female sexual maturation in the
       U.S. in the twentieth century. (21)

2931   Collier, P. "Health Behaviors of Women," NURS CLIN NORTH AM
       17(1) (March 1982): 121-26.

       Reviews both historical and current perspectives on women's
       health and illness behaviors. Notes that health care pro-
       viders should be facilitators of positive health in women and
       discusses the nursing role in assessing women's health and in
       preventive care. (18)

2932   Committee on Assessing Alternative Birth Settings, Institute
       of Medicine and National Research Council. RESEARCH ISSUES
       IN THE ASSESSMENT OF BIRTH SETTINGS. Washington, D.C.:
       National Academy Press, 1982.

       A literature review and overview of what is now known about
       current childbirth settings, including out of hospital set-
       tings. Sponsored by the Institute of Medicine and the Board
       of Maternal Child and Family Research of the National Research
       Council this study is aimed at providing baseline data to
       plan for a funded research project.

2933   Devereux, M.E. "Equal Employment Opportunity Under Title VII
       and The Exclusion of Fertile Women From the Toxic Work-
       place," LAW MED HEALTH CARE 12(4) (September 1984): 164-72.

       Discusses difficulty of applying Title VII of the 1964 civil
       rights law to the unborn fetus, particularly since there is
       difficulty reconciling this goal with protection of the
       woman's right to work. (77)

2934   Estok, P.J. "Balancing the Power: Improving Health Care for
       Women," MATERN CHILD NURS J 6(2) (March/April 1981): 91-96.

       Discusses how nurses can help women change the power balance
       of the physician/client relationship in order to improve
       health care for women. (16)

2935   Fox, G.L. (Ed.). THE CHILDBEARING DECISION: FERTILITY ATTI-
       TUDES AND BEHAVIOR. Beverly Hills, CA.: Sage Publications,
       Inc., 1982.

Essays explore fertility decision making from diverse disciplinary perspectives. The authors assess contemporary
findings--decisions and factors such as socialization, sex
roles, work, personal values, and marital status.

2936 Gold, E.B. (Ed.). THE CHANGING RISK OF DISEASE IN WOMEN: AN
      EPIDEMIOLOGIC APPROACH. Lexington, MA.: The Collamore Press,
      1984.

      The epidemiologic aspects of disease risk in women related
      to the changing social and professional roles of women. The
      differing risk for women for certain cancers, cardiovascular
      disease, diabetes, psychiatric disorders, as well as menstrual
      and fertility disorders are covered. The book brings together
      the work of investigators from a variety of disciplines, in-
      cluding epidemiology, clinical medicine, and the basic
      sciences.

2937 Golub, S. MENARCHE. Lexington, MA.: Lexington Books, D.C.
      Heath and Co., 1983.

      Review of current research related to menarche.

2938 Mackey, M. (Ed.). WOMEN'S HEALTH RESEARCH: AN EXCHANGE OF
      IDEAS. Chicago: University of Illinois, College of Nursing,
      1980.

      Provides a directory of groups interested in women's health.
      Addresses such areas as women as research subjects and women
      as health care consumers.

2939 Marieskind. H. WOMEN IN THE HEALTH SYSTEM: PATIENTS, PRO-
      VIDERS, AND PROGRAMS. St. Louis: C.V. Mosby Co., 1980.

      Presents facts and statistics on women's health and discus-
      ses women's involvement, both as providers and consumers,
      within the health care system.

2940 McCrea, F.B. "The Politics of Menopause: The 'Discovery' of a
      Deficiency Disease," SOCIAL PROBLEMS 31(1) (October 1983):
      111-23.

      Menopause, defined as a deficiency disease by physicians in
      the 1960s, when synthetic estrogen became widely available.
      Estrogen therapy, promoted by physicians and the pharmaceu-
      tical industry, was linked to cancer and other health problems
      in the mid-1970s. Feminists argued that menopause was a nor-
      mal aging process. This paper looks at how these opposing
      definitions of menopause evolved and examines the efforts of
      women to fight off the stigma of the disease label.

2941 McKay, S. and C.R. Phillips. FAMILY-CENTERED MATERNITY CARE:
      IMPLEMENTATION STRATEGIES. Gaithersburg, MD.: Aspen Systems
      Corp., 1983.

A sourcebook on family center facilities across the U.S. and
Canada and how to staff, supply, and organize your own family-
centered maternity-child program. Forms, procedures, protocols, guidelines, and goals from hospitals and birthing centers.

2942   Moore, E.C. "Women and Health, United States, 1980," PUBLIC
       HEALTH REPORTS 95(5) (1980): Supplement, 1-84.

       Documents the progress that has been made in the health
       status of American women. Focuses on women's roles as con-
       sumers and providers of health care. (127)

2943   Morris, N.M. "The Biological Advantages and Social Disadvan-
       tages of Teenage Pregnancy," AM J PUBLIC HEALTH 71(8)
       (August 1981): 796.

       Editorial. (3)

2944   Norris, R.V. with C. Sullivan. PMS: PREMENSTRUAL SYNDROME.
       New York: Rawson, 1983.

       This book is a comprehensive treatment of premenstrual syn-
       drome (PMS) as a physical disorder rather than the psycho-
       somatic one. The authors write sympathetically and from a
       feminist point of view about cases treated by professionals
       at PMS program centers and elsewhere. The syndrome is de-
       fined, and some of the problems that accompany it are des-
       cribed.

2945   Peeples, M.D. and C.A. Miller. "Monitoring and Assessment in
       Maternal and Child Health: Recommendations for Action at the
       State Level," J HEALTH POLICY AND LAW 8(2) (Summer 1983):
       251-76.

       Recent administration-sponsored changes in federal health
       policy and funding may harbor adverse effects for the health
       of mothers and children, and for the capabilities of state-
       level programs to serve them appropriately. Careful monitor-
       ing is required to assess the nature, extent, and impact of
       those changes. This paper examines several monitoring efforts
       in maternal and child health and recommends additional action
       at the state level to meet urgent information requirements.
       (29)

2946   Rickel, A.U., M. Gerrard and I. Iscoe. SOCIAL AND PSYCHO-
       LOGICAL PROBLEMS OF WOMEN: PREVENTION AND CRISIS INTERVEN-
       TION. New York: Hemisphere Publishing Corp., 1984.

       Combines research, theory, and clinical experience to
       analyze the psychology of women in the multi-faceted profes-
       sional and personal aspects of their lives. Intervention
       techniques are presented in the book designed to prevent and
       handle prevailing crises and future problems.

2947   Rubin, R. MATERNAL IDENTITY AND THE MATERNAL EXPERIENCE.
       New York: Springer Publishing Co., 1984.

       Focus is on the complex process of the woman's changing
       sense of self identity during the maternal experience from
       pregnancy to bonding.

2948   Sagov, S.E., R.I. Feinbloom, P. Spindel and A. Brodsky. HOME
       BIRTH: A PRACTITIONER'S GUIDE TO BIRTH OUTSIDE THE HOSPITAL.
       Gaithersburg, MD.: Aspen Systems Corp., 1983.

       Argues home birth is a safe alternative for properly
       screened and prepared women. Covers management, logistical,
       economic, political, and clinical issues. Presents profes-
       sional standards of maternity care and shows how midwife-phy-
       sician teams can provide quality and continuity of care with
       hospital backup.

2949   Sandelowski, M. PAIN, PLEASURE, AND AMERICAN CHILDBIRTH:
       FROM THE TWILIGHT SLEEP TO THE READ METHOD, 1914-1960.
       Westport, CT.: Greenwood Press, 1984.

       American childbirth practices were largely governed by the
       desire to minimize pain and suffering until the advent of the
       Read method. The method of natural childbirth developed by
       Dr. Grantly Dick-Read promised not only a painless birth, but
       also a pleasurable birth experience. According to Sandelow-
       ski, the shift from childbirth pain to pleasure did not result
       in any real change in American childbirth views and practices.
       She maintains that childbirth continued to be considered an
       abnormal condition subject to professional surveillance and
       intervention.

2950   Stillion, J. DEATH AND THE SEXES: AN EXAMINATION OF DIFFEREN-
       TIAL LONGEVITY, ATTITUDES, BEHAVIORS, AND COPING SKILLS.
       New York: Hemisphere Publishing Corp., 1984.

       Examines research regarding the sex differential in death
       and reviews possible causes from biological, psychosocial, and
       environmental perspectives. Also discusses sex-role sociali-
       zation as it may relate to murder, suicide, early male death
       rates, death attitudes and death anxiety of males and females,
       bereavement, and sex differences in widowhood. Death educa-
       tion practices are examined.

2951   Wyshak, G. "Evidence for a Secular Trend in Age of Menarche,"
       NEW ENGLAND J MED 306(17) (1982): 1033. Reprinted in OB/GYN
       18(3) (1984): 239.

       Argues for a declining age of menarche. (20)

2952   Zelnik, M., J.F. Kantner and K. Ford. SEX AND PREGNANCY IN
       ADOLESCENCE. Beverly Hills, CA.: Sage Publications, Inc.,
       1981.

The authors analyze the results of their two national surveys, focusing on the sexual behavior of young women between
the ages of fifteen and nineteen and the choices that preceded
teenage pregnancies and childbirth. Patterns in sexual activity, contraceptive use and nonuse, pregnancy, abortion, and
unwed motherhood are discussed.

See 654.

Other Issues

2953 Ahana, D. and M.M. Kunishi. CANCER CARE PROTOCOLS FOR HOS-
      PITAL AND HOME CARE USE. New York: Springer Publishing C,
      1981.

      Basic interventions for nurses with an emphasis on the con-
      tinuity and coordination of care between hospital and home.

2954 Baker, J. A.I.D.S.: EVERYTHING YOU MUST KNOW ABOUT ACQUIRED
      IMMUNE DEFICIENCY SYNDROME: THE KILLER EPIDEMIC OF THE 80'S.
      Saratoga, CA.: R & E Publishers, 1983.

      Since AIDS (Acquired Immune Deficiency Syndrome) was diag-
      nosed in 1981, there has been an outpouring of literature on
      it. This book summarizes what was known about AIDS as of the
      Fall of 1983.

2955 Davis, J.H. and A.M. Juhasz. "The Human/Companion Animal
      Bond: How Nurses Can Use This Therapeutic Resource," NURS
      HEALTH CARE 5(9) (November 1984): 497-501.

      Review of literature. (40)

2956 Fagerhaugh, S.Y. and A. Strauss. POLITICS OF PAIN MANAGEMENT:
      STAFF-PATIENT INTERACTION. Menlo Park, CA.: Addison-Wesley
      Publishing Co., 1977.

      Thesis of the book is that interactions between staff and
      patient and even between staff members are important variables
      in the management of pain. Persons with chronic pain are the
      least well cared for, but people with any type of illness who
      are labelled "problem patients" are neglected. Case studies
      used to illustrate. Research base is primarily field research.

2957 Gross, S. and S. Garb (Eds.). CANCER TREATMENT AND RESEARCH
      IN HUMANISTIC PERSPECTIVE: ETHICAL AND SOCIAL ISSUES. New
      York: Springer Publishing Co., 1984.

      A forum of authoritative views on the pressing humanistic
      concerns that accompany the onset and treatment of cancer.
      Topics include the ethics of drug experimentation, ineffective
      therapies, pain management, the staff-patient relationship,
      and the personal needs and struggles of cancer-care profes-
      sionals, patients, and families.

2958   Kiester, E., Jr. "A Little Fever Is Good For You," SCIENCE
       5(9) (November 1984): 168-73.

       Describes early research with iguanas that identified the
       importance of fever in combatting infection. Subsequent re-
       search identified endogenous pyrogen, released from white
       blood cells which raises temperature and withdraws iron from
       the bloodstream with an infection. This line of research is
       leading to less use of antipyretics with ordinary illnesses.
       (O)

2959   Locker, D. DISABILITY AND DISADVANTAGE: THE CONSEQUENCES OF
       CHRONIC ILLNESS. New York: Methuen, Inc., 1983.

       Based on structured interviews with rheumatoid arthritis
       sufferers, the author's discussion pursues two themes: that
       chronic illness and coping with its limitations severely erode
       the sufferers' personal, material, and social resources, and
       that the resources and problem-solving strategies adopted by
       disabled persons intervene between impairment, disability, and
       disadvantage.

2960   _____. SYMPTOMS AND ILLNESS: THE COGNITIVE ORGANIZATION
       OF DISORDER. New York: Methuen, Inc., 1981.

       This volume argues that meaning is central to social life
       and that illness must be understood as a social phenomenon
       composed of the meanings that people create. Using the re-
       sults of studies, Locker demonstrates that there is no neces-
       sary relationship between events in the biological realm and
       the social meanings imputed to them. He shows how our common
       understanding of health and disease structures our experience
       of the world.

2961   McGill, K.A. "Knowledges and Attitudes of Staff Nurses Con-
       cerning Alcoholism." Dissertation Abstracts International,
       39/19-B. Ann Arbor University Microfilms, 1978, No. 79-
       09008, 4814.

       Relates selected demographic factors to the knowledge and
       attitudes of staff nurses concerning alcohol. Results showed
       attitudes and knowledge are significantly influenced by
       racial/ethnic origin, religion, total years in nursing, educa-
       tion, and information.

2962   Prottas, J.M. "Obtaining Replacements: The Organizational
       Framework of Organ Procurement," J HEALTH POLITICS, POLICY
       AND LAW 8(2) (Summer 1983): 235-50.

       In the last ten years there has grown up in the U.S. the
       most extensive organ procurement system in the world. This
       system, consisting of approximately 120 organ procurement
       agencies, retrieved 4435 cadaveric kidneys for transplant pur-
       poses in 1981. The nation's organ procurement agencies vary
       greatly in terms of size, organizational structure, and effec-
       tiveness. On average, those agencies not formally part of a

transplant hospital appear to be the most effective. This can be accounted for by their superior operational flexibility and their pursuit of a "marketing" strategy. Success in organ procurement requires that medical professionals in nontransplant hospitals, and the potential donors' families, be motivated to assist in the organ procurement process. (27)

Abbott, A. 2016
Abdellah, F.G. 2758
Abel, E.L. 2927, 2928
Abraham, I.L. 1898
Abrahams, N. 272
Abrams, N. 24
Abruzzese, R.S. 1393
Abu-Saad, H. 1143, 1144, 1145, 1146
Accord, L. G. 2037
Ackerman, A.M. 1300, 1301
Adams, D.E. 1302
Aday, L.A. 2381
Administration on Aging. 2825
Agate, J. 578
Agree, B.C. 2626
Ahana, D. 2953
Ahmed, M.C. 2382
Aiken, L. 1, 2383, 2384, 2559, 2560, 2561
Aikens, C.A. 25
Ainsworth, T.H. 2504
Alessi, D.J. 2093
Alexander, C.S. 2917
Alexander, J.W. 2226
Alhadeff, G. 1265
Alichnie, M.C. 1147
Allbritten, D. 1181, 2505
Allen, D.V. 548
Allen, M. 26
Allen, M.E.M. 1084
Allen, P. 27
Alley, L. 2562
Almore, M.G. 1658
Alutto, J.A. 2038
Alvarez, R. 2438
Alward, R.R. 1354
American Academy of Nursing. 924, 2121, 2227, 2368, 2385, 2386, 2387, 2388, 2389, 2519, 2759, 2760
American Association of Occupational Health Nurses. 28
American Medical Association. 2390, 2487

American Nurses' Association. 2, 3, 4, 5, 29, 30, 31, 32, 33, 34, 35, 36, 366, 621, 766, 767, 768, 769, 770, 771, 772, 869, 884, 885, 886, 1067, 1068, 1388, 1488, 1863, 1864, 1899, 1900, 1901, 1902, 1903, 2039, 2040, 2041, 2094, 2197, 2198, 2306, 2307, 2317, 2340, 2369, 2370, 2371, 2372, 2373, 2374, 2391, 2439, 2506, 2507, 2508, 2509, 2510, 2511, 2512, 2563, 2564, 2637, 2646, 2688, 2689, 2693, 2694, 2695, 2696, 2697, 2698, 2705, 2706, 2707, 2713, 2714, 2715, 2716, 2720, 2721, 2722, 2723, 2724, 2739, 2741, 2742, 2745, 2746, 2747, 2752, 2754, 2755, 2756, 2757, 2761, 2762, 2853, 2868
American Nurses' Foundation. 2392
Ames, S.A. 1303
Anderson, A. 1085
Anderson, B. 2042
Anderson, E. 1238
Anderson, N.E. 1304, 1866
Andrews, S. 1591
Angel, G. 2140
Annas, G.J. 37, 274, 275, 276, 277, 443, 654, 817, 818, 819, 840, 841, 842, 863, 2268, 2554
Appelbaum, P.S. 820
Apperson, M. 821
Applegate, M.I. 38
Aquino, N.S. 1086
Archer, S.E. 1239
Arlton, D.M. 1659
Armiger, B. 622
Armstrong, M.L. 1592
Arney, W.R. 1394
Arnhoff, F.N. 2887
Arnold, J. 1660
Arnold, N. 2566
Aroian, J. 1395
Aroskar, M.A. 39, 40, 41, 42, 43, 278, 444, 507, 1531, 2228

Artinian, B.M.   1532, 1904
Ashley, J.A.   2141, 2142
Ashworth, P.   508
Atkinson, L.D.   1905
Atwood, A.H.   1661
Atwood, J.R.   1906
Auld, M.   2269
Auster, D.   1087
Awtrey, J.   1089
Aydelotte, M.K.   925
Bach, C.A.   1183
Bachman, R.   2488
Backer, B.A.   445
Bahr, R.T.   2440
Bailar, J.C.   1907
Baj, P.A.   981
Baker, A.   1089
Baker, C.M.   959, 982, 1305
Baker, J.   2954
Baker, N.   887, 888
Baker, R.   2229
Bakke, K.   406
Baldwin, B.A.   1662
Baldwin, S.   1355
Balint, J.   1266
Ballard, S.   1908
Balogh, E.   1090
Balzar, J.   2567
Bandman, E.L.   44, 45, 446
Banks, J.   1306
Baram, M.S.   822
Barkauskas, V.H.   926, 2699
Barnes, E.G.   879
Barnes, G.M.   2826, 2869
Barnes, S.Y.   1091
Baron, C.H.   549
Barrett, J.E.   1307
Bartsch, J.   46
Bartscher, P.W.   1663
Batchelor, E.   550
Batey, M.V.   870
Bath, R.   2489
Battin, M.P.   2914
Bauman, K.   1664, 1665
Baumgart, A.J.   2143
Baxter, L.   2729
Bayles, M.D.   551
Beal, J.   2743
Beale, A.V.   1148
Beare, P.G.   1593, 1594
Beason, C.   2043
Beauchamp, T.   47, 48, 447
Becktell, P.   1666, 16667
Begun, J.W.   773
Behm, R.J.   1807

Bejsovec, J.L.   279
Beletz, E.E.   2044, 2045
Bell, D.F.   1808, 1809
Bell, E.A.   1668
Bell, N.K.   280
Bell, S.   552
Belle, D.   2441
Belock, S.   1396
Benda, E.   1092, 1669, 2270
Benedikter, H.   1909
Benjamin, M.   49
Benner, P.   1397, 2122
Benner, R.V.   1810
Benoliel, J.Q.   1595
Berardo, F.M.   2827
Berendt, H.   1670
Berg, D.L.   448
Bergman, R.   50
Bergstrom, N.   1910
Berk, M.L.   2442
Berkowitz, M.W.   591
Bernstein, A.H.   449, 880
Besch, L.B.   281
Betz, C.L.   1671
Betz, M.   2679
Beyers, M.   2096
Bigbee, J.L.   871, 872
Bihldroff, J.P.   282
Bille, D.A.   1596
Billings, D.M.   1672
Billingsley, M.C.   2763
Binder, J.   2393
Binger, J.L.   1149, 1398, 1911
Bingham, S.   2144
Bissell, L.   367, 2341
Blackford, N.   2271
Blackstone, E.A.   2658
Blainey, C.G.   1093
Blake, B.L.K.   368
Blaker, G.   2097
Blanchard, S.L.   960
Blatchley, M.E.   1653
Blattner, B.   2838
Blazeck, A.M.   1240
Bliss, A.A.   2675, 2764
Bloch, B.   1597
Block, D.   623
Block, M.R.   2828
Bloom, J.R.   2046, 2047, 2652
Blumenreich, G.A.   720
Bock, J.   2230
Boehret, A.C.   1004
Bomberger, A.S.   1399
Bonday, K.N.   1811
Borelli, M.D.   2839

Borgman, M.F.   1356, 1533
Borovies, D.L.   1400
Bowler, J.E.   2145
Bowman, M.   2272
Bowman, R.A.   2199
Bowyer, E.A.   721
Boyar-Naito, V.   1401
Boyd, K.M.   283
Boyer, C.M.   1402, 1403
Boyer, J.M.   2048
Boyle, J.F.   553
Bradley, J.C.   1912
Bradshaw, C.E.   1673
Branch, M.F.   2308, 2443
Brandon, A.N.   1598
Brannigan, C.N.   1184
Brett, J.L.   2098
Breyer, F.J.   1812
Bridges, M.J.   1674
Bridgewater, S.C.   983
Brink, P.J.   2444
Broadhurst, J.   51
Brock, A.M.   1308
Brody, H.   52
Brogan, J.M.   53
Bronner, M.   1094
Brook, R.H.   2394
Brooten, D.   2017
Brossart, J.   2490
Brower, H.T.   1522, 1523
Brower, T.   2356
Brown, B.J.   927, 928, 1005, 2653
Brown, B.S.   889, 2318, 2352,
   2357, 2765, 2929
Brown, E.   1006
Brown, E.L.   929
Brown, H.   2445, 2446
Brown, J.   2447
Brown, J.S.   1913
Brown, M.S.   2358, 2359
Brown, N.   554
Brown, P.   2888
Brown, R.T.   2870
Brown, S.J.   1534
Brown, S.T.   1185
Brown, V.   2309
Browne, W.P.   2395
Browning, M.H.   2766
Brownlee, A.T.   2448
Bruer, J.T.   1914
Brusich, J.   1535
Brykczynski, K.   1404
Buckeye State Nurses Association.
   1868
Buckingham, R.W.   2854

Buckley, J.   1150
Budetti, P.B.   2680
Bueche, M.N.   1186
Buhler-Wilkerson, K.   2700
Buldt, B.W.   2146
Bullough, B.   6, 7, 8, 54, 655,
   656, 657, 658, 774, 775, 776,
   777, 843, 873, 874, 890, 914,
   1060, 1389, 1390, 1869, 2018,
   2147, 2450, 2767, 2768
Bullough, V.L.   9, 931, 932,
   2148, 2149, 2449, 2491, 2893,
   2930
Bureau of Health Professions.
   2310
Burgess, G.   1536
Burke, S.   2200
Burns, C.E.   2769
Burns, P.   2843
Buschmann, M.B.T.   1599
Bush, T.A.   1405
Busl, L.D.   1187
Butler, C.   2770
Butters, S.   1406
Cabiniss, S.H.   55
Cadmus, N.E.   56
Cahall, J.B.   1600
Caldera, K.   2708
Calkin, J.D.   1309, 2771
Camooso, C.   1310, 1814
Campazzi, B.C.   722
Campbell, C.   2231
Campbell, J.   2918
Campbell, J.C.   2919
Campbell, J.M.   891
Campos-Outcalt, D.   844
Canadian Nurses Association 57, 58
Cantor, M.M.   1268
Caplan, R.D.   2846, 2899
Capron, A.M.   407
Capuzzi, C.   2201, 2375
Carmack, B.J.   1095
Carnegie, M.E.   284
Carozza, V.   1409
Carpenito, L.J.   1915
Carper, B.A.   59
Carrington, B.W.   2049, 2311
Carrol, A.M.   60
Carter, J.H.   2513
Carter, L.B.   961
Castiglia, P.T.   2123
Castillo, M.H.   2312
Castle, J.   1269
Castledine, G.   450
Castles, M.R.   61, 1601

Caterinicchio, R.P.   2520
Catholic Hospital Association.
  62
Caulkins, S.   2492
Cavagnaro, Sr. M.   2726
Cawley, M.A.   451
Cazalas, M.W.   659
Cearns, E.   2273
Chambers, C.M.   1071
Chamings, P.A.   1675
Chapman, C.M.   285
Chapman, J.J.   1676
Chase, B.M.   1537
Chaska, N.L.   10, 933, 962, 2019
Chavigny, K.H.   509, 723, 1677
Chayet, N.L.   660
Checkoway, B.   2202
Chee, M.   452
Chen, M.K.   2396
Chen, S.C.   2772
Chenevert, M.   2150
Chicadoz, G.H.   1241
Child, A.A.   2889
Chinn, P.L.   408, 1916, 1917,
  2744
Chiriboga, D.A.   1918
Choi, S.C.   1096
Christensen, D.B.   875
Christensen, G.J.   1061
Christensen, R.A.   453
Christian, P.L.   1678
Christman, L.   63, 934, 1062,
  1188, 1242
Christopher, R.   2151
Christy, T.E.   1243, 1870
Ciocci, G.   2568
Cizmek, C.   1538
Claerbaut, D.   1097, 1151
Clark, C.C.   1679, 2536
Clark, M.D.   1680
Clark, P.E.   1919
Clark, T.   1815
Clarke, L.M.   1681
Clarkson, J.A.   1189
Claus, K.E.   2537
Clayton, G.M.   1603
Cleland, V.S.   2152
Clemen, S.   1311
Clements, I.W.   1410
Clinton, C.   2638
Clore, E.R.   2871
Cogliano, J.F.   579
Cohen, A.G.   2050
Cohen, B.J.   1190
Cohen, K.P.   2855

Cohn, K.   2051
Cohn, S.   510
Cohn, S.D.   724, 728, 778, 779,
  845, 892
Cohrssen, J.J.   823
Colangelo, M.   2052
College of Nurses of Ontario.   65
Collier, P.   2931
Collins, M.B.   1411
Collins, P.B.   1191
Collins, V.J.   454
Colls, J.P.   1604
Collison, C.R.   1244
Committee for a Study of the
  Health Care of Racial/Ethnic
  Minorities and Handicapped Per-
  sons.   2451
Committee for the Study of Nurs-
  ing Education.   935
Committee on Assessing Alterna-
  tive Birth Settings.   2932
Committee on the Grading of Nurs-
  ing Schools.   936
Committee to Study Extended Roles
  for Nurses.   2773
Connant, L.H.   624
Connelly, C.E.   369, 2847
Conners, V.L.   1682
Connors, D.D.   2153
Conway, M.E.   984, 2397
Conway-Rutowski, B.   937
Coombe, E.I.   1683
Cooper, C.G.   864
Cooper, S.S.   1414, 1415, 1416
Corcoran, S.   625
Corea, G.   2538
Corless, I.B.   2319
Corning, P.A.   2398
Cornwall, J.   2900
Corr, C.A.   2856
Cotanch, P.H.   1063
Cote, A.A.   286
Coudret, N.A.   1192
Cousins, N.   2539
Cowan, C.E.   2155
Coward, H.   66
Cowart, M.E.   67, 1358, 1684
Cowen, D.L.   876
Cox, C.L.   580
Craig, J.L.   1685
Crancer, J.   1686
Cranford, R.E.   68
Craven, M.E.   69
Crawford, M.E.   1193
Creason, N.   1012, 1194

Creighton, H. 70, 71, 370, 371,
  511, 626, 661, 662, 663, 664,
  725, 846, 916, 1195
Crisham, P. 72, 73
Cronenwett, L.R. 1920
Cronin-Stubbs, D. 1312
Crooks, E. 2054
Crowder, E. 74
Cruikshank, B.M. 2320, 2774
Culang, T.G. 1313
Culliton, B.J. 555
Cummings, D. 1605
Cunning, B.R. 1687
Curran, C.L. 963, 1152, 1417,
  1418, 1816
Curran, C.R. 1196
Curran, W.J. 75, 665, 726
Curtin, L. 6, 76, 77, 78, 79,
  80, 81, 287, 372, 373, 536,
  556, 2521, 2569, 2570
Cushing, M. 374, 409, 410, 455,
  512, 666, 667, 727, 728, 729,
  730, 825
Dachelet, C.Z. 1817
Daeffler, R.J. 2654
Dagenais, F. 1921
Dalme, F.C. 1098
Daly, M. 2156
Damen, J. 1314
Damrosch, S.P. 1922
Daniel, I.Q. 375
Darby, C. 82
Dardick, L. 2493
Davenport, N.J. 1197
Davidhizar, R. 1688
Davidson, M.E. 1689
Davis, A.J. 83, 84, 85, 86, 87,
  88, 89, 90, 91, 288, 289, 376,
  411, 412, 513, 514, 537, 557,
  581, 627, 628, 629, 630, 631,
  632, 633, 634, 635
Davis, C.K. 2399, 2522
Davis, F. 2020
Davis, J.H. 1540, 2955
Davis, K. 2400
Davis, P.S. 456
Davis, W.E. 1153
Davitz, J. 1923, 2124
Dawson, J.D. 92
Dayani, E.C. 2203
Dean, N.R. 1818
Dean, P.R. 1819
Deane, R.T. 2571
Dear, M.R. 1315
DeGraw, D.K. 2055

DelBueno, D.J. 1541, 2100
Demetrulias, D. 1820
Demkowski, A. 2730
Dempsey, P.A. 1924
Dennis, C.M. 1198
Denny, E.O. 1316
Densford, K.J. 94
Derby, V.L. 1013
Derdiarian, A.K. 1542, 1925
Derwinski, B. 1317
deSantis, G. 2021
Detherage, K.S. 1014
Detmar, D.E. 2676
Devereux, M.E. 2933
Devlin, K. 1606
Dexter, P. 1607
Dexter, P.A. 964
Dick, D.J. 1690
Dickens, M.R. 1245
Dickenson-Hazard, N. 2775
Dickman, R.L. 290
Diers, D. 2022, 2101, 2776
Dieterle, J.A. 1359
Dilday, R.C. 95
Diminno, M. 1500
DiRienzo, J.N. 1691
Dittmar, C.C. 2102, 2103
Dobbie, B.J. 1360
Dobson, S. 2452
Dock, S. 377
Dodd, M.J. 1821
Dodge, G.H. 917
Dodge, J.S. 291
Dolan, A.K. 2056
Donabedian, D. 1318, 1608
Donaldson, M.L. 1692
Donaldson, S.K. 1609
Donegan, J.B. 2157
Donnelly, G.F. 12, 96, 2204
Donohue, M.P. 292
Donovan, C.T. 515
Donovan, L. 2104, 2573
Donovan, M. 1419
Donovan, P. 780
Doona, M.E. 97, 98
Doudera, A.E. 413, 457, 538
Douglas, D. J. 965
Douglas, J.M. 2057
Downs, F. 1489, 2687
Downs, F.S. 636, 637, 1693,
  1926
Doyle, E. 781
Dracup, K. 2901
Drake, D.C. 414
Drane, J.F. 516

Dreher, M. 1610, 2701
Drice, A.D. 1154
Driscoll, V.M. 2401
Duane, N.F. 1694
Dubin, L.F. 1611
Dubois, P.M. 2857
Dubrey, R.J. 2709
Duespohl, T.A. 13
Dunbley, P.H. 1073
Duncan, G.J. 2453
Dunham, A. 2454
Dunlop, D. 1612
Dunn, A.M. 2205
Dunn, L.J. 638
Durand, B. 99
Durbak, I. 2574
Durham, J.D. 1361, 2627
Durrant, L. 1099
Dustan, L.C. 1155
Duxbury, M.L. 2125
Easterling, J.F. 2058
Eccard, W.L. 668
Edelstein, R.R. 1420, 2206
Edelwich, J. 558
Edgell, B. 100
Edgil, A.E. 101
Edmunds, L. 1421
Edmunds, M. 2321, 2777
Edmunds, M.W. 2105
Edmundson, M.A. 1501
Ehrenreich, B. 2158, 2159,
  2160, 2161
Eichelberger, K.M. 1927
Eichhorn, E. 1422
Eisenberg, M. 2902
Eisenbud, M. 2555
Elder, R.G. 559
Eliopoulos, C. 2717
Elkind, A.K. 2342, 2343
Ellis, J.R. 14
Ellis, S. 2274
Ellis, T.S. 415
Elsea, S.J. 517
Emanuel, W.J. 2059
Emerson, W. 2060, 2061
Engel, G.L. 1928
Engel, G.V. 2677
Enggist, R.E. 2778
English, J. 1613
Ennen, A.L. 782
Ensor, B.E. 378
Enthoven, A.C. 2659
Epstein, C. 2858
Epstein, S.S. 2556
Erde, E.L. 379

Erickson, H. 1362, 1929
Eschbach, D. 966
Estok, P.J. 2934
Ethics Committee, American Aca-
  demy of Neurology. 458
Evaneshko, V. 1930
Evans, A.D. 1695
Evans, D. 2232
Everson, S.J. 1319
Ezell, A.S. 967, 985
Fabayo, A.O. 1289
Fagerhaugh, S.Y. 2956
Fagin, C. 986, 1614, 1931,
  2575, 2660, 2661
Falkson, J.L. 2402
Falvo, D.R. 2848
Faron, A. 1696
Farrell, J.J. 1697
Farrell, M. 1019
Fasano, N. 938, 1246
Fawcett, J. 1932
Fay, P. 293
Feeley, E. 1320
Fegan, W.A. 560
Feldbaum, E.G. 2718
Feldman, E. 847
Feldstein, P.J. 2062, 2576, 2577
Feliu, A.G. 380
Fenner, K.M. 104
Fenwick, R.D. 2494
Ferguson, C.K. 1156
Ferguson, V. 294, 295
Fernandes, R.C. 2233
Ferrell, B. 1100
Fiesta, J. 669
Fine, R.B. 2690
Fineberg, K.S. 731
Finley, B. 1101, 1698
Finneran, M.D. 987
Fischer-Williams, M. 2844
Fishbein, E.G. 1102
Fishel, A.H. 968, 1103
Fitzpatrick, J.L. 1933
Fitzpatrick, M.L. 1502, 2023,
  2162
Flaherty, M.J. 105, 106, 381
Flanagan, L. 2063
Fleming, J. 1615
Fleming, J.W. 1199
Fletcher, J. 459
Flynn, B.C. 1503
Flynn, J.P. 1699
Flynn, P. 1200
Flynn, P.A.R. 2840, 2841
Foley, T.S. 2920

Folta, J. 15, 2455
Fondiller, S.H. 1875
Fong, M.L. 1157
Fontes, H.M. 1934
Foote, R.H. 1104
Ford, J.G. 107
Forrest, L. 2313
Forsyth, D. 1700
Fortune, M. 969
Foster, H.S. 881
Fouts, J. 1321
Fowler, G. 1822
Fox, D.J. 1935, 1936
Fox, G.L. 2935
Fox, P.D. 2662
Fox, R.N. 1937
Fralic, M.F. 2578
Francis, M.B. 1701
Francke, L.B. 2819
Frazer, J. 1616
Freeman, L.H. 1423
Freidson, E. 2681
Frey, E.F. 108
Fried, C. 826
Friedan, B. 2163
Friedman, F.B. 2322
Friedman, W.H. 1702
Friss, L. 2106, 2691
Fritz, E.L. 1363
Frohock, F.M. 561
Fromer, M.J. 109, 110, 296,
    460, 562, 563, 592
Fry, S.T. 518, 593, 639, 2376
Fuller, E.O. 1938
Fulton, K. 382, 2344
Furrow, B.R. 519, 827, 848
Fuszard, B. 2126
Gabel, J.R. 2663
Gadow, S. 111, 112, 113, 297,
    461, 520, 582, 583, 1939
Gaevert, H.S. 1201
Galarowicz, L. 1484
Gallant, D.M. 640
Galliford, S. 1364
Galloway, B. 2495
Galton, M. 114
Ganos, D. 115
Garant, C.A. 2207
Garesche, E.F. 116
Gargaro, W.J. 298, 299, 300,
    301, 462
Garland, L. 2903
Garrity, M. 1202
Garrow, D. 416
Gartner, A. 2540

Garvey, J. 1365, 1366, 1367
Gaut, D.A. 1940
Gay, J.T. 1203
Gaylin, W. 828
Gendrop, S.C. 463
Gennaro, S. 1823
George, J. 1941
George, J.E. 670
Georgopoulos, B.S. 2405
Gerber, R. 1424
Gerds, G. 117
Getty, C. 2904
Geyman, J.P. 2639
Gibbons, M.B. 2872
Gibson, K.W. 2628
Gibson, R. 2664
Gideon, J. 2064
Gikuuri, J.P. 302
Gilbert, C. 594
Ginzberg, E. 1023, 2127
Girard, N.L. 1703
Gladwin,, M.E. 118
Glantz, L.H. 564, 849
Glaser, W.A. 2403
Goad, S. 2404
Goddard, H. 1425
Goeppinger, J. 2702
Goertzen, I. 119
Gold, E.B. 2936
Goldmark Report. 939
Goldstein, J.O. 1270
Goldwater, M. 894, 2208
Golub, S. 464, 2937
Gonda, T.A. 2859
Gonzalez-Swafford, M.J. 2456
Goodall, P.A. 120
Goodrich, A.W. 121
Goodwin, J.O. 1543
Goodwin, L.D. 1942
Gordon, I.T. 1617
Gordy, H.E. 1704
Gorenberg, B. 1943
Gorney-Fadiman, M.J. 1490
Gorovitz, S. 122
Gortner, S.R. 1944, 1945
Gould, E.O. 1824
Gounley, M.E. 123
Gow, K.M. 2905
Grace, H. 970, 1491, 1492,
    1493, 1876
Grad, J.D. 2640
Graham, B. 1322
Graham, L.E. 1426
Grand, N.K. 384
Grassi-Russo, N. 1105

Gray, B.H.   2665
Gray, P.L.   2719
Greenberg, W.   2666
Greenlaw, J.   303, 304, 305, 385,
   386, 387, 465, 521, 671, 672,
   732, 733, 734, 735, 736, 2275,
   2276, 2277
Greenleaf, N.P.   2164, 2579
Greenstein, L.R.   466
Gress, L.D.   1427
Griffin, C.C.   2873
Griffith, H.   895, 2667
Griffith, J.W.   988, 1705, 1706
Grissum, M.   2165
Grobe, S.J.   783
Grodin, M.A.   417
Groff, B.   2278
Gross, L.C.   1368
Gross, S.   2957
Gross, S.J.   784
Grosser, L.R.   2234
Grosskopf, D.   1707
Grosso, C.   2457
Gruzalski, B.   124
Guenther, J.   467
Guerin, D.H.   1618
Gulino, C.K.   125, 126
Gumley, C.J.   2279
Gunn, I.P.   2323
Gunter, L.M.   584
Gustafson, D.D.   1825
Gustafson, J.M.   418
Guy, J.   2065
Hacker, L.J.   127
Hackler, E.T.   737
Hackley, B.K.   896
Hadley, R.D.   128
Haggerty, L.   1708
Haggerty, V.C.   785
Hair, B.B.   1709
Halberstam, M.J.   306
Hale, S.L.   1369
Hall, B.A.   989, 1710
Hall, K.V.   1544
Hall, V.C.   786, 787
Halleran, C.   2209
Hallman, E.C.   2779
Halpern, S.   2921
Hamilton, P.A.   2541
Hamric, A.B.   2710
Hannon, J.   1504
Hansen, H.R.   788
Harbin, R.E.   468
Harper, D.C.   2780
Harper, M.W.   2820

Harris, C.H.   419
Harrison, D.H.   2668
Harron, F.   129, 130, 131
Hartigan, E.G.   595
Hartin, J.M.   1711
Hartley, C.L.   940
Harwood, A.   2458
Hassell, J.   1826
Hassett, M.   1712
Haug, M.   2543
Haughey, B.P.   1946
Haukenes, E.   1323
Haussman, R.   1947
Hautman, M.A.   1827
Havighurst, C.   882
Hawken, P.L.   990
Hawkins, J.W.   1324, 1545, 1877,
   2781
Hay, H.S.   132
Hayden, M.L.   2641, 2782
Hayes, E.J.   133
Hayes, E.R.   1158
Haymes, H.   1428
Hayter, J.   1546, 1948
Hazzard, M.E.   1619
Healey, J.M.   307
Hegyvary, S.T.   2655
Heide, W.S.   2166
Hein, E.C.   1620
Heit, P.   1621
Heitler, G.   673
Heller, B.R.   1204
Helmuth, M.R.   1205
Hemelt, M.D.   674, 675
Hendershot, G.E.   565
Henderson, G.   2459
Henderson, V.   134, 1949
Herr, S.S.   829, 830
Herrington, J.V.   1547
Herron, Sr. C.   1429
Hershey, N.   676, 738, 739, 740,
   789, 790, 897
Herzog, A.R.   2829
Heymann, P.B.   420
Hickey, T.   2830
Hicks, B.   2831
Hicks, C.   2460, 2894
Hicks, L.L.   2682
Hicks, M.   2107
Higgins, P.G.   1370
Higgs, Z.R.   991
Hilbert, G.K.   1290
Hilbert, R.A.   2906
Hill, L.   1622
Hill, L.L.   2542

Hillder, M.D.   135
Hillier, S.   2345, 2346
Hillsmith, K.E.   1371
Himmelberger, A.H.   1325
Hinkley, C.   2235
Hinshaw, A.S.   1430, 1548
Hipps, O.S.   1430, 1548
Hirsch, R.   2727
Hitchens, E.W.   1828
Hodgson, C.   2461
Hoeffer, B.   136
Hoekelman, R.A.   2324
Hoff, L.A.   2907
Hoffman, S.   1372
Hogan, K.A.   2783
Hogan, R.M.   2895
Hogue, E.   741, 831
Holden, C.   2860
Holder, A.R.   308, 677, 742
Holgate, P.   678
Holloran, S.D.   1431
Hollshwander, C.H.   992, 1247
Holm, K.   1248, 1713, 1952
Holmstrom, L.L.   1953
Holt, F.X.   2280
Holtzclaw, B.J.   1159
Holzemer, W.L.   1206, 1494
Horacek, L.A.   1714
Horan, D.J.   421, 469
Horn, B.   2462
Horsley, J.E.   388, 470, 471
Hott, J.R.   2236
House, C.S.   596
Howell, F.   1271
Hoyt, J.D.   850
Huber, J.   2167
Huber, M.L.   941
Huckabay, L.M.   1715, 1829, 1830
Huckstadt, A.A.   1716
Hughes, B.S.   791
Hughes, L.   2237
Hughes, S.L.   2647
Hull, R.T.   140, 141, 142, 143,
   144, 145, 389, 2168
Humphrey, C.   2024
Humphrey, P.   1717
Hunt, J.   2238
Hutchens, C.M.   2629
Hutcheson, J.D.   1160
Huttmann, B.   309, 472, 473
Hyde, E.   792
Hymovich, D.P.   1954
Hynes, K.M.   146
Ibbotson, P.   2066
Illich, I.   2669

Imbus, S.H.   310
Infante, M.   1718, 1955
Irish, A.C.   2496
Iversen, S.M.   1719
Jackson, N.E.   1720
Jacobi, E.M.   1721
Jacobs, A.M.   1831
Jacobson, B.   2347
Jacobson, S.F.   641
Jacox, A.   942, 2067, 2406, 2430
Jaffe, S.   390, 2348
Jaffee, M.   1549
Jameton, A.   147, 148
Janzen, S.   1722
Jarratt, V.R.   971
Jeffers, J.M.   1326
Jefferson, L.V.   391, 2349
Jeglin-Mendez, A.M.   1723
Jennings, C.P.   898
Jenny, J.   311
Jernigan, D.K.   1724
Johnson, D.E.   1956
Johnson, J.   972, 2108
Johnson, M.H.   1623
Johnson, P.   474, 475
Johnson, R.   1725
Johnson, S.H.   679
Johnson, W.L.   2580, 2581, 2582,
   2583
Johnston, T.   1726, 2281
Joiner, C.   2128
Jonas, S.   2407
Jones, A.   680
Jones, B.   2068
Jones, D.A.   1624
Jones, E.E.   2463
Jones, E.M.   2282
Jones, E.W.   597, 1550
Jones, F.M.   1432
Jones, J.H.   642
Jones, K.R.   2524
Jonsen, A.   422
Jordan, C.H.   2210
Judd, J.M.   1625
Kahn, A.M.   1106
Kalisch, B.   2211, 2239, 2240,
   2241, 2325, 2584, 2922
Kalisch, P.   16, 2242, 2243,
   2244, 2245, 2246, 2247, 2248,
   2249, 2250, 2251, 2585
Kammer, C.H.   1727
Kander, M.L.   681
Kane, R.L.   2464
Kantner, J.E.   2283
Kanungo, R.N.   2129

Kapp, M.B.   682, 832, 851
Kaserman, I.   149
Kasley, V.   476
Kasper, A.S.   2169
Kastenbaum, B.K.   313
Katz, B.F.   392, 2069
Kauffman, M.   1728
Kayser-Jones, J.   1108, 1109
Keane, M.   477
Keane, N.P.   150
Keating, S.   794
Keenan, T.   2326
Kehrer, B.H.   744
Keller, M.L.   1505
Kelley, D.N.   151, 152
Kelley, K.   314
Kelley, L.K.   1207
Kellmer, D.M.   598
Kelly, C.   17
Kelly, L.Y.   2360
Kelly, M.A.   1957
Kennedy, C.W.   2252
Kennedy, M.M.   2212
Kennedy, S.L.   2284
Kerr, A.H.   683
Kerr, J.A.C.   1958
Ketefian, S.   153, 154, 599
Kieffer, M.J.   745
Kielinen, C.E.   1208
Kiester, E., Jr.   2958
Kilchenstein, L.   1551
Kilmon, C.   1506
Kim, H.S.   1328, 1960, 1961
Kim, J.J.   1962
Kim, M.J.   1959
King, E.C.   1832, 1833
King, I.M.   1963
King, V.G.   1552
Kinkela, G.G.   795
Kinsey, D.C.   1209
Kintgen-Andrews, J.   1553
Kirchhoff, K.T.   1834
Kishi, K.I.   1729, 1964
Kissam. P.C.   796
Kjervik, D.K.   539, 1329
Klaus, M.H.   2874
Klein, C.A.   684, 746, 747
Klein, C.A.   747
Kleinberg, D.A.   1433
Kleinberger, H.   423
Kluge, E.W.   155, 2070
Klutas, E.M.   522
Kneisl, C.R.   2908
Knollmueller, R.N.   2648
Knopke, H.J.   1161

Knowles, R.D.   2544
Knowlton, C.N.   1554
Koehler, M.L.   1835
Kohnke, M.   315, 316, 317, 2631,
   2711
Kohut, J.M.   2861
Koldjeski, D.   2748
Koltz, C.J.   2632
Korup, V.   1626
Kosik, S.H.   318
Kostro-Marolda, K.   319
Kotchek, L.   1555
Kotthoff, M.E.   2784
Kowalski, K.   1434
Kraegel, J.M.   2408
Kramer, M.   1272, 1556, 1730,
   1731, 2586
Kratz, C.   643
Kraus, A.S.   478
Krause, E.A.   2071
Krawczyk, R.   600, 1557, 1732
Krueger, J.C.   320, 1965
Kruger, D.H.   2072
Kruse, L.C.   1733, 1836
Kubler-Ross, E.   479, 480
Kucera, W.R.   797, 833
Kuhn, J.K.   1249, 1734
Kupchak, Sr. B.   2213
Kuramoto, A.   1524
Kushner, K.P.   156
Kussman, R.   2785
LaBar, C.   899
Laben, J.K.   685
Lacefield, W.E.   1210
Lachman, V.D.   2353
Lader, L.   2821, 2822
LaForet, E.G.   601
LaMancusa, M.   1735
Lamerton, R.   481, 540
LaMonica, E.L.   1435, 1627
Lanara, V.A.   157
Lancaster, J.   1966
Landfield, J.S.   158
Lane, G.H.   1628
Lang, N.M.   2644
Lang, R.H.   2409
Langford, T.L.   1250
Langham, P.   602
Langwell, K.M.   2731
Larocco, S.   1436
Laroche, E.   2285
Larsen, J.   2170
Larson, E.   1967
Lash, A.A.   1033
LaViolette, S.   2073

Law, S. 748
Lawrence, J.A. 523
Lawrence, J.C. 2497
Lawton, A.H. 585
Lazarus, R.S. 2909
Lazinski, H. 1034
Lear, M.W. 2910
Lebacqz, K. 321, 1968
Leddy, S. 1330
Lee, A. 2253, 2254, 2327, 2587
Lee, L.A. 1837
Lee, P.R. 2410
Leftwich, R.E. 1211
Lehrer, S.S. 1736
Leininger, M. 943, 1035, 1969,
   1970, 2465, 2466
LeMaitre, G.D. 2130
Lemin, B. 2286
Lenhart, R.D. 1212
Lenburg, C.B. 1525, 1526, 1527
Lenow, J.L. 566
Lentsche, P.M. 586
Lenz, E.R. 1213
Leonard, A. 1110, 1629
Leone, L.P. 1111
Leslie, F.M. 1971
Lesnik, M.J. 686
Lestz, P. 524
Levenstein, A. 159, 2074
Levine, A.D. 2557
Levine, E. 2588
Levine, I. 2287
Levine, L.B. 1558
Levine, M. 160
Levine, M.E. 525
Levinson, R.M. 1737
Lewin, E. 2171
Lewis, A. 2749
Lewis, E.N. 2589
Lewis, E.P. 18, 322, 323
Lewis, M.C. 2288
Lewis, P. 2289
Lewis, S.M. 1630
Lidz, C.W. 834
Lieb, R. 2214
Lief, H.I. 2896
Lillard, J. 1112
Limandri, B.J. 993
Limbert, P.M. 162
Lindeman, C.A. 1972
Lindsey, A.M. 1973, 1974
Link, C.R. 2467, 2590, 2591,
   2592, 2593
Linzer, N. 2915
Little, M. 1113

Little, V.C. 2832
Locker, D. 2959, 2960
Lockett, B.A. 2215
Logan, W. 2594
Lombardi, T. 749
Loomis, M.E. 1975
Lopez, K.A. 1738
Lorber, J. 424, 2172
Lord, A.S. 1739
Lorenz, F.J. 2075
Loss, L. 2468
Loustav, A. 1838
Lovell, M.C. 2173, 2174, 2328
Lowe, A.G. 2361
Ludemann, R. 1976
Luft, H.S. 2469
Luginbill, C. 1214
Lukasik, C. 2362
Lum, J.L. 2595
Lumpp, F. 163, 164
Lumpp, S. 165
Lurie, E.E. 2786
Luther, D.C. 1373
Lutjens, L.R. 2411
Lynaugh, J. 1631, 1878
Lynch, M.L. 2633
Lynk, W.J. 687
Lysaught, J.P. 19, 1879
Maas, M. 2634
MacAvoy, S. 1839
Machan, T.R. 688
MacIntyre, A. 324
Mackey, M. 2938
MacPhail, J. 1251
MacPherson, K.I. 2175
Macrae, N. 2412
Magilvy, K. 1632
Mahler, H. 2363
Mahon, K. 166, 603
Mahoney, J. 167
Mailhot, C. 2740
Malarkey, L. 1114
Malinski, V.M. 1977
Mallick, M.J. 1633
Mallison, M.B. 798
Maloney, E.M. 526
Malter, S. 567
Mancini, J. 1115
Mancini, M. 325, 689, 690
Manfredi, C. 2911
Manley, M.V. 2642
Manson, J.N. 326, 865
Manuel, R.C. 2470
Mappes, E.J.K. 168
Mappes, T.A. 169

Maraldo, P. 2597
Marchewka, A.E. 327
Marcinek, M.A. 482
Marieskind, H. 256, 2939
Marks, L.N. 2292
Marmor, et al. 835
Marriner, A. 1215, 1840
Marston, M.V. 2849
Marten, M.L. 1634
Martens, K.H. 1740
Martin, E.J. 994
Martin, R.M. 170
Martin, S. 2255
Martinez, R.A. 2471
Martinson, I.M. 2862
Mason, D.J. 1741
Masson, V. 944
Matejski, M.P. 171, 1507, 1559
Matheson, H.L.V. 568
Mathias, J. 2364
Mauger, B.L. 945
Mauksch, I.G. 946, 1116, 1216,
  1252, 2025
Maurer, T. 2498
Maury-Hess, S. 1292
May, J.J. 2525
May, K.A. 327, 328
May, K.M. 1495
Mayer, G. 1635, 2656
McAllister, J. 172
McBride, H. 1374
McCaffrey, C. 1439
McCaffrey, D.P. 691
McCarthy, D.G. 483
McCarthy, N.C. 1742
McCarthy, P.A. 1253
McCarty, P. 901
McClellan, M.A. 2875
McCloskey, J.C. 1273
McClure, M.L. 393, 1880
McConnell, E. 2131
McConnell, T.C. 173
McCormick, K.A. 1636
McCormick, R.A. 174
McCown, D.E. 1978, 2923
McCrann, D.D. 330
McCrea, F.B. 2940
McCullought, L. 175
McDaniels, O.B. 1560
McEvoy, M.D. 1561
McFadden, C.J. 176
McFarland, D.E. 2216
McGill, C. 1440
McGill, K.A. 2961
McGoram, S. 1743

McGrath, B.J. 1375
McGriff, E.P. 1881
McGrory, A. 2257, 2258
McGuire, M.A. 2329
McIsaac, I. 177
McKay, R.C. 644
McKay, S. 2941
McKay, S.R. 1117, 1744
McKenna, M. 2472
McKenzie, C.M. 1745
McKibbin, R.C. 2109, 2110
McKinlay, J.B. 178, 692
McKinley, J. 2413
McLane, A.M. 1508
McMorrow, M.E. 1118
McNally, J.M. 1162
McNeil, J. 947
McNelley, R.L. 2833
McNutt, D.R. 2683
McQuaid, E.A. 1074
McQueen, J. 1217
McShea, M.M. 179
McTernan, E.J. 2598
McVey, W.E. 180
Meaux, C.A. 2314, 2315
Mechanic, D. 2414, 2415, 2330
Meglan, M.C. 2732
Meisenhelder, J.B. 1274, 1441
Mejia, A. 2599
Melcolm, N. 1841
Meleca, C.B. 1442
Melnyk, K.A.M. 1979
Melosh, B. 2176
Memmer, M.K. 1746
Mendelson, M.M.A. 2416
Mermelstein, R. 2670
Merritt, S.L. 1331
Metress, J.F. 2473
Metzger, B.L. 1980
Meyer, P.B. 645
Mezey, M. 1747
Mezey, M.D. 973, 2645
Middleton, C. 181
Milio, N. 1981, 2417, 2418
Millar, S. 2076
Miller, B.K. 331
Miller, R.D. 693
Miller, Sr. P. 995
Miller, S.R. 1982
Miller, T. 1748
Milliken, B. 2293
Mills, B.B. 1254
Milunsky, A. 852
Mindel, C.H. 2474

Minehan, P.L.   1443
Mitchell, C.A.   1749
Mitchell, J.J.   604, 1750
Mitchell, K.   646
Mittleman, R.   527
Molloy, J.T.   2026
Monheit, A.C.   799
Moniz, D.M.   800, 877
Monninger, E.   1842
Montag, M.   1293, 1294, 1295
Mooney, M.M.   182, 1983
Mooneyhan, E.L.   1376
Moore, B.M.   1163
Moore, D.S.   1119
Moore, E.   2217
Moore, E.C.   2942
Moore, J.   2294
Moore, J.B.   1036
Moraczewski, A.S.   569
Morgan, J.N.   2475
Moritz, D.A.   1562
Morris, A.L.   948
Morris, L.   1751
Morris, N.M.   2943
Morris, P.B.   1120
Morrish, M.   1444
Morrison, B.L.   1121
Morton, A.   2295
Moscovice, I.   2600
Moser, D.   425
Moses, E.   2601
Moskowitz, S.   866, 867, 2111
Moyer, R.L.   1752
Muff, J.   2177, 2259, 2260
Muldary, T.W.   2331
Mulligan, J.E.   2178
Mullins, A.C.   2514
Mumford, E.   2912
Mundinger, M.O.   2218, 2649
Munhall, P.   605, 1637, 1984
Munro, B.H.   1275
Munroe, D.   2787
Munzig, N.C.   426
Murchison, I.   694
Murdaugh, C.   1638
Murdock, J.E.   1639
Murphy, C.   183
Murphy, C.P.   184, 185, 186, 187
Murphy, J.F.   996, 1496
Murphy, M.A.   188
Murphy, M.L.   1445
Murphy, N.   1509, 1640
Murphy, P.   394, 2332
Murphy, S.A.   1510, 1843
Murray, J.   2890

Murray, L.M.   1276, 1753
Murray, R.   1446
Mutzebaugh, C.A.   1754
Muyskens, J.L.   189, 190, 2077
Muzio, L.G.   1377
Myers, L.B.   1655
Nahm, H.E.   949
Natapoff, J.N.   1641
National Advisory Council on
   Vocational Education.   1884
National Association for Prac-
   tical Nurse Education and
   Service.   191
National Commission for the
   Study of Nursing and Nursing
   Education.   1885
National Commission on Nursing.
   20
National Health Publishing.   695
National Institute of Health.
   1985
National League for Nursing.
   21, 192, 332, 333, 2219,
   2545, 2650
Nations, W.C.   334
Nayer, D.D.   974, 1378
Nelms, B.C.   2788, 2891
Nelson, J.K.N.   1512
Nelson, L.F.   1844
Nelson, M.J.   193
Neubauer, D.W.   335
Neuman, B.   1379, 1986
Newman, M.A.   1987
Newton, L.   2261
Newton, L.H.   2027
Newton, M.   395
Nichols, A.W.   194, 803
Niedringhalls, L.   1164
Nieswiadomy, R.M.   1218
Nightingale, F.   2179
Noble, M.A.   1642, 2704
Noonan, B.   2789
Norberg, A.   541
Norman, E.M.   1447
Norman, K.A.   1755
Norris, C.G.   1165
Norris, R.V.   2944
Northrop, C.   647, 912
Notter, L.   1988
Notter, L.E.   1528
Nousianen, T.   2078
Novicky, D.   2603
Numerof, R.E.   2079
Nurses Network.   2180
Nuttall, P.   2296

Oberle, J. 570
Oberst, M.T. 336, 337, 648
O'Brien, L. 196
O'Connor, A. 1220
O'Connor, A.B. 1448, 1449, 1450
O'Donnell, M. 2499, 2500
O'Donnell, M.P. 2420
O'Flynn, A.I. 1989
O'Grady, D.J. 1643
O'Heath, K.A. 2262
Oiler, C. 1990
O'Kane, P.K. 1221
Olivieri, P. 1845
Olson, E.M. 1332
Olson, J. 484
Olson, M. 1451
O'Neil, E.A. 696, 751, 805
O'Neil, P.A. 197
O'Reilly, D.P. 2181
Orem, D.E. 1991
Orgel, G.S. 338
O'Rourke, K.A. 2081
Orque, M.S. 2476
O'Shea, H.S. 1222
O'Shea, J.S. 2790
Osler, W. 198
Ossler, C.C. 1255
Osterveis, M. 2863
Ostheimer, N.C. 199
Ostmoe, P.M. 1122, 1333
Ostrand, L. 1223
O'Sullivan, A.L. 697
Outtz, J.H. 1166
Overstreet, L.P. 1846
Packard, K.L. 1123
Packer, J. 1563
Paduano, M.A. 1167, 1756, 1757
Page, G.G. 1758
Page, S. 1224
Pagelow, M.D. 2924
Palmer, M.E. 1452
Pankratz, L. 339
Pappert, M.S. 340
Parasuraman, S. 2132
Pardue, S.F. 1334, 1513
Paris, J.J. 427, 428, 486
Parlocha, P. 1124
Parson, L. 542
Parsons, E. 200
Parsons, M.A. 1225
Parsons, S. 201
Partridge, K.B. 2028
Partridge, R. 998, 1888
Patey, E.H. 487
Patterson, P. 429

Patterson, R.J. 1759
Patton, M.Q. 1992
Paul, W. 2501
Pavalon, E.I. 202
Payton, R.J. 203, 341, 606, 607
Pearson, A. 2263
Pearson, L.E. 2115, 2635
Pena, J.J. 2515
Penberty-Valentine, M. 2421
Pence, T. 204
Pender, N.J. 2546
Penticuff, J.H. 528
Peoples, M.D. 2945
Peplau, H.E. 342, 543
Perry, C.M. 205
Perry, H.B. 2678
Perry, S. 913
Perry, S.E. 752, 1226, 1760
Personett, J.D. 2606
Peters, J.D. 698
Peterson, C.J. 952, 953
Peterson, M.L. 905
Petrowski, D.D. 1761
Phaneuf, M.C. 2516
Phillips, J.R. 1227
Pickard, M.R. 1453
Pinch, W.J. 1564
Pisani, J. 1889
Plasterer, H.H. 1762
Player, J.M. 2116
Pletsch, P.K. 1763
Plomann, M.P. 2527
Podjasek, J.H. 1497
Podnieks, E. 587
Podratz, R.O. 918, 1228
Pogoncheff, E. 2502
Pohlman, K. 1890
Pollock, C. 919, 920
Ponak, A.M. 2082
Poole, A.L. 2791
Popoff, D. 488
Porter, K. 207
Porter-O'Grady, T. 2422
Portes, K.K. 1847
Porth, C. 1229
Pothier, P. 430
Poulin, M.A. 208, 2029, 2692
Powell, P.J. 2117
Powers, M.J. 2792
Prato, S.A. 209
Prescott, P.A. 2607, 2608
President's Commission. 343
Price, J.L. 2609
Price, R. 344
Prottas, J.M. 2962

Prussin, J.A.   2423
Ptaszynski, E.M.   1764
Puetz, B.   1454, 2030
Pugh, E.L.   2182
Pulcini, J.   906
Purtilo, R.B.   211
Putt, A.M.   1993
Pyne, R.H.   212
Quaife, F.M.   213
Quick, J.D.   2424
Quinn, N.   345
Quiring, J.   1335, 1565
Rabb, J.D.   215
Rabkin, M.T.   489
Raisler, J.   2823
Raker, L.   1278
Ramphal, M.   1336
Ramsay, J.A.   2793
Ramsey, P.   490
Randolph, B.M.   2183
Rawnsley, M.M.   954, 1566
Rea, K.   431
Reakes, J.C.   1765
Rebone, J.W.   432
Record, J.C.   2671, 2795
Redman, B.K.   999, 1567, 2712
Reed, F.C.   1380
Reed, J.C.   1568
Reed, S.B.   1381
Regan, J.H.   1766
Regan, W.A.   398, 753
Rehr, H.   216
Reich, W.   217
Reilly, D.   218, 219, 608, 609
Reinhardt, U.W.   2684
Reppucci, N.D.   699
Research and Statistics Committee
    American College of Nurse-
    Midwives.   2734
Rhein, R.   2796
Rhinehart, N.W.   1486
Rhode, M.A.   1569
Rhodes, A.M.   700
Riccardi, B.R.   2636
Richard, E.   1570
Richardson, L.   2477, 2478
Rickel, A.U.   2946
Riddell, D.   975
Riehl, J.P.   1994
Rimer, B.   2354
Rinaldi, L.   1455
Rinke, L.T.   1051, 1337
Riordan, J.   2877
Ritter, H.A.   2333
Roach, M.S.   221

Roach, W.H.   754
Robb, I.H.   222
Robb, S.   346
Robb, S.S.   347
Robbins, D.   492, 529
Roberts, C.S.   433
Roberts, M.   2220
Roberts, S.L.   2184
Robertson, J.   853
Robertson, J.A.   434, 854
Robyn, D.   2118, 2797
Rocereto, L.R.   701
Rockwell, V.T.   1456
Roell, S.M.   1457
Roemer, M.I.   2425, 2611
Roemer, R.   702, 806, 2426
Rogers, M.   2797
Rogers, M.E.   1996
Romalis, S.   2547
Romanell, P.   223
Ronald, J.S.   1338
Roos, P.D.   2799
Rorabaugh, M.L.   2365
Rose, M.   2133
Rose, M.A.   2612
Rosen, E.   224
Rosenhan, D.L.   2892
Rosenkoetter, M.   1339
Rosko, M.D.   2528
Rosoff, A.J.   836
Roth, C.   2334
Roth, M.D.   399
Rothenberg, L.S.   435
Rothenberg, P.B.   2878
Rothman, 2083
Rothweiler, T.M.   1571
Rothwell, S.   2084
Rotkovitch, R.   2085
Rottenberg, S.   807
Rottkamp, B.C.   1280
Roush, R.E.   2735
Rowland, R.   2185
Rowley, P.T.   571
Roy, A.L.   1848
Roy, C.   1572, 1997, 1998
Royal College of Nursing of the
    United Kingdom.   649
Rozovsky, F.A.   837
Rozovsky, L.E.   348
Rubenfeld, M.G.   703, 1052
Rubenstein, H.S.   755
Rubin, J.   2753
Rubin, R.   2947
Rudov, M.H.   2479
Rudy, C.A.   921

Ruffen, J.E. 2480
Ruffing, M.A. 1340
Rule, J.B. 226
Russel, F. 227
Russell, O.R. 493
Russell, R. 494
Rutkowski, A.D. 2086, 2428
Ryan, J. 2913
Ryan-Merritt, M. 1767
Ryden, M.B. 610
Rynerson, B.C. 1768, 1769
Sackett, D.L. 2800
Sadoff, R.L. 704
Safier, G. 955, 2031
Sagov, S.E. 2948
Sain, T.R. 2087
Salman, S.L. 756, 757, 758
Salmon, J.W. 2672, 2842
Salvage, J. 2264, 2316
Salzer, J.L. 2366
Sandelowski, M. 2186, 2949
Sanders, S.H. 1644
Sandroff, R. 349, 400, 495,
  572, 2187
Sanford, S. 2529
Santora, D. 1573
Sargent, S.S. 2834
Sargis, N.M. 1126
Sasmor, J.L. 1282, 2429
Sateren, J.L. 1574
Saucier, C.P. 2548
Saylor, A.A. 1230
Scanlon, K.M. 759
Schalenberg, C. 1770
Scheffer, B. 1771
Scheffler, R.M. 2801
Schilling, M.J. 612
Schleutermann, J.A. 1772
Schlotfeldt, R. 1498
Schmalenberg, C.E. 976
Schmidt, M.S. 1080
Schnall, D.J. 23
Schoen, D. 1168, 1283, 1893
Schoenrock, N.B. 613
Schoffstall, C. 1382
Schoolcraft, V. 1849
Schor, I. 1459
Schorr, T.M. 228, 229, 573,
  2802
Schowalter, J.E. 436
Schraff, S. 2864
Schrock, R.A. 230, 544
Schroeder, D.M. 1460
Schroy, I.J. 1773
Schulkin, J. 545

Schweitzer, B. 705, 706, 707,
  808, 809, 907
Schwirian, P.M. 1169
Scott, D.W. 650
Scott, H. 2188
Scott, R. 231
Sculco, C.D. 1575
Scully, D. 2925
Scully, D.H. 2549
Seidl, A.H. 1774
Seigel, H. 1341, 1461, 2032
Seither, F.F. 1170
Sekscenski, E. 2613
Sexton, D.L. 1999, 2430
Sexton, R. 401
Shaffer, F.A. 2530, 2531
Shaffer, M.K. 1462, 1656, 1850
Shamansky, S.L. 1775, 2378,
  2550
Sharp, E.S. 2736
Sharpe, D. 2297, 2298
Shaw, M.W. 855
Shelley, S.I. 2000
Shelly, J.A. 232
Shelp, E.E. 233, 234
Shelton, B.J. 1342
Shepard, I.M. 868
Shepard, M.W. 496
Sherer, B.K. 1463
Sheridean, J.E. 2517
Sherman, J.E. 1258, 1514
Sherwood, J. 2221
Shine, M.S. 1343
Shneidman, E.S. 2916
Shockley, J. 1464
Short, T.L. 2532
Shufer, S. 437
Shukla, R.K. 2657
Shumaker, D. 1776
Siantz, M.L. 235, 546
Sidel, R. 2431
Sidley, N.T. 708
Siegel, H. 1515
Sigardson, K.M. 2614
Sigman, P. 236
Silva, M.C. 237, 238, 239, 350
Silver, H. 2803
Sime, A.M. 1127, 1171
Simmons, P.D. 240
Simmons, R.S. 2189
Simms, L.M. 1529
Simpson, R. 547
Sklar, C. 351, 352, 574, 760
Slaninka, S.C. 1383
Slavinsky, A. 1128, 1391

Smallegan, M.J. 1777
Smania, M.A. 1851
Smeltzer, C. 1645
Smith, B.J. 353
Smith, C. 354
Smith, C.E. 1465, 1576, 1778
Smith, C.M. 1466
Smith, D.B. 709
Smith, D.W. 2804
Smith, E.D. 614
Smith, G.R. 1259, 1260, 1577
Smith, I.K. 1769
Smith, L. 497
Smith, M.C. 1852
Smith, R.A. 2615
Smith, S. 241
Smith, S.J. 242
Smith, W.D. 2481
Smitherman, C. 2001
Smoyak, S.A. 2190, 2750
Smullen, B.B. 1129
Smurl, J.F. 243
Smyer, M.A. 2835
Smythe, E.E.M. 2551
Snavely, B.K. 2299
Snowden, L.R. 2482
Snyder, D.J. 1284
Sobol, E.G. 1173
Solomons, H.C. 1231
Sommerfeld, D.P. 1780
Sorcinelli, M.D. 1232
Sorenson, G. 1261
Sorrel, L. 2088
Sosnowitz, B.G. 2879
Soukup, M.C. 1285, 1781
Soules, H.M. 1286
Southby, J.R. 651
Southwick, A.F. 710
Sovie, M. 956, 1467, 1468,
  2134, 2616
Spadaro, D.C. 2850
Sparks, S.M. 1646, 1782, 1783
Spector, E. 2483
Spegel, A. 2651
Spevlin, G. 498
Spicker, S. 244
Spilotro, S. 1262
Spink, L.M. 1000
Spitzer, W.D. 2805
Spratlen, L.P. 1784
Spross, J. 530
Spruck, M. 1344, 1785
Stacklum, M.M. 1130
Stafford, M.J. 245
Stamper, J. 1853

Stanley, A.T. 246, 355, 615,
  616
Stanley, L. 402
Stanton, M.P. 1854
Starck, P.L. 1578
Starfield, B. 2851
Starr, P. 2432
Staunton, M. 247
St. Denis, H.A. 611
Stecchi, J.M. 1855
Steck, A.L. 2617
Steel, J.E. 2335, 2379
Steele, S.M. 248
Steiger, N. 2552
Stein, K.Z. 1579
Stein, L.I. 2336
Stein, R.F. 1131, 1856
Steiner, M.J. 1786
Steinfels, M.O. 617
Steinhoff, P.G. 2824
Stern, T.L. 2643
Sternberg, M.J. 249, 618
Stetler, C.B. 2002
Steurer, K. 531
Stevens, B.J. 2003, 2222
Stevens, K.R. 2223
Stewart, I. 957
Stewart, I.M. 619
Stewart, P.H. 1787
Stillion, J. 2950
Stinson, R. 438
Stoia, J.P. 1788
Stoller, E.P. 1132
Stoner, M.H. 1516
Storch, J.L. 356
Storfjell, J.L. 2703
Storlie, F.J. 499
Storms, D.M. 2265
Story, B.W. 1174
Strauser, C.J. 1789
Strauss, M.B. 1647
Strauss, S.S. 1133
Streff, M.B. 2806
Strickland, O.L. 575
Strong, C. 439
Stuart, C.T. 922
Stuart-Siddall, S. 1648, 1790
Stuebbe, B. 1134
Styles, M.M. 1392, 2033
Suess, L.R. 1345
Sullivan, D. 2737
Sullivan, G.C. 1517
Sullivan, J.A. 2807
Sultz, H.A. 1518, 1519, 1520,
  2811, 2812, 2813

Swansburg, R.C.   2266
Swanson, E.A.   1057, 1791
Swanson, J.   2885
Sward, K.M.   250, 251
Sweeney, J.   1896
Sweeney, M.A.   1470, 1649,
  1857, 2004
Sweeney, S.S.   1233
Swenar, C.   1471
Swendsen, L.A.   1346
Sweezy, S.R.   652
Tabeek, E.   2897
Tagg, P.   2300
Tagliacozzo, R.   2350
Talbott, S.W.   2191
Tamir, L.M.   2886
Tappen, R.M.   1234
Tarnow, K.G.   1792
Tarpey, K.S.   1793
Tate, B.L.   252
Taub, S.   253, 856
Taubenheim, A.M.   1794
Taylor, S.W.   1795
Telesco, M.   2089
Tennant, F.S.   2673
Thaker, H.H.   2119
The Committee on the Legal and
  Ethical Aspects of Health Care
  for Children.   440
The Task Force on Supportive
  Care.   858
Thoford, S.M.   711
Thomae, H.   2836
Thomas, B.   1347, 1530, 1580
Thomas, C.   811
Thomas, M.J.   812
Thomas, N.   2865
Thomas, S.P.   1581
Thompson, H.O.   532
Thompson, H.S.   533
Thompson, J.B.   254, 255
Thompson, L.   2135
Thompson, M.A.   1582
Thompson, M.J.   883
Thomstad, B.   2337
Tien, J.   1136
Tilden, V.P.   653, 1657, 1796
Tiollotson, D.M.   1384
Titus, A.C.   761
Tollett, S.M.   1348
Tom, S.   2738
Tooley, M.   576
Toth, R.S.   813
Trandel-Korenchuk, D.   712, 713,
  764, 814, 2192

Trandel-Korenchuk, K.M.   357,
  2301
Triplett, J.L.   2880
Tripp, S.   908
Tripp-Reimer, T.   2484
Trocchio, J.   714
Trussel, P.B.   2005
Tuma, J.L.   358
Tumminia, P.A.   1137
Turnbull, E.   1235, 1583
Turner, J.T.   2034
Tyrer, L.B.   577
Tyler, L.W.   1650
Ulin, P.R.   1521, 1651, 2367
Ulione, M.S.   1797
Uphold, C.R.   1138
Upton, D.   2751
U.S. Department of Health and
  Human Services, Public Health
  Service.   2433
Uustal, D.B.   256, 257, 258
Vacek, P.   1287
Valentine, N.M.   1798
VanBree, N.S.   1349
Vance, C.N.   2193
Vanderzee, H.   2533
VanDoren, J.A.   1487
VanMeter, M.   1385
Van Ort, S.R.   1236
Varveri, P.S.   1476
Vaughn, J.C.   1297
Veatch, R.   259, 260
Veninga, R.L.   2434
Ventura, M.R.   2136
Ventura, W.P.   1175
Verville, R.E.   715, 2728
Vestal, C.   2802
Viers-Henderson, V.   2485
Viles, S.M.   765
Vinson, K.S.   1176
Vitagliano, A.   1477
Vito, K.O.   620, 1584
Vogt, J.F.   2137
Vogt, R.B.   1799
Voight, J.W.   1350, 1585
Wagner, D.   2224
Wagner, D.L.   977
Wagner, T.J.   2881
Wahlquist, G.I.   1263
Waitzkin, H.   2435
Wakefield-Fisher, M.   1264
Wald, F.S.   1652
Wales, S.K.   1586
Walker, D.   978
Walker, L.   1587

Walker, L.O.   2006
Walkington, J.F.   1588
Wallace, S.E.   500
Walljasper, D.   1478
Walsh, M.   359
Walshe-Brennan, K.S.   360
Walters, C.R.   1800
Walton, D.N.   501
Waltz, C.F.   1139, 1858
Wandelt, M.   2007, 2138, 2518, 2620
Warner, C.G.   2926
Warner, K.E.   2436
Warner, S.L.   261
Wasch, S.   1479
Watchorn, C.   815
Waters, J.   859
Watkins, L.O.   2815
Watson, A.B.   361
Watson, C.   2303
Watson, J.   1140, 1351, 2194
Waugh, D.   262
Way, H.   263
Weber, L.J.   264, 502
Weingard, M.   2120
Weinstein, E.L.   1177, 1178
Weir, R.F.   441, 503
Weisensee, M.G.   1801
Weiss, K.   2553
Weiss, R.E.   2621
Weiss, S.J.   2338
Weisstub, D.N.   717
Welborn, P.   1802
Welch, L.B.   1589, 1803
Wells, D.   2091
Wells, H.   265
Wells, R.   266
Wentworth-Rohr, I.   2845
Werley, J.   2008
Werner, J.   979
Werner-Beland, J.   2866
Wessell, M.L.   1804
West, M.   958
Westfall, D.   860
Weston, J.L.   910, 2816
Westwick, C.R.   1859
Wetle, T.   588
Wexler, D.B.   718
Whelan, E.   1298
Whitaker, J.G.   923
White, C.   980
White, C.H.   2622
White, C.M.   2380
White, D.C.   2632
White, T.A.   2503

White, W.D.   838
Whiteworth, R.A.   504
Whitman, H.   534
Whitman, M.   2035
Whitney, F.   2674
Wierczorek, R.R.   2225
Wilensky, G.R.   2486, 2686
Wiley, K.   2009
Wiley, L.   719
Wilkes, E.   362
Will, G.F.   505
Williams, A.   2355
Williams, D.C.   2622
Williams, F.C.   268
Williams, M.A.   1141
Williams, M.L.   1860
Williams, R.A.   2339
Williams, R.M.   1386
Williamson, J.A.   1299
Willian, M.K.   2534
Wilson, H.S.   1179, 2010, 2011
Wilson, J.S.   1481
Winchell, C.A.   2882
Winger, C.   506
Winkelstein, M.L.   2883
Winkler, L.   269
Winslow, G.R.   270, 2036
Wise, P.   1482
Wisniewski, S.C.   2195
Witt, P.   405
Witter Du Gas, B.   2817
Wolanin, M.O.   589
Wolf, G.A.   2139
Wolff, M.A.   816
Wolfle, L.M.   1861
Wood, J.H.   1897
Wood, V.   1237
Woods, N.F.   2898
Wooldridge, P.J.   2012
Woolley, A.S.   1142, 2267
Wray, D.A.   2304
Wright, W.   2013
Wriston, S.   911, 2818
Wu, R.   1387, 1590
Wutchous, S.M.   1805
Wyshak, G.   2951
Wysocki, A.B.   2014
Yardley, B.   2305
Yarling, R.R.   363, 364, 590, 861
Yeaw, E.M.J.   1806
Yeaworth, R.C.   535, 2867
Yett, D.E.   2624
Yoos, L.   2852
Young, D.A.   2535
Young, K.J.   2625

Younger, J.B.   2437
Youngner, S.J.   365
Yura, H.   2015
Yurick, A.G.   2837
Zachary, R.   442
Zaslow, J.   862
Zebelman, E.   1483
Zelnik, M.   2952
Zettiniq, P.   1352
Ziegenfuss, J.T.   839
Ziel, S.   2196
Zimmerman, A.   2092
Zimmerman, M.A.   2884
Zuzich, A.   271